Bone Fracture: Advances in Orthopedics

Bone Fracture: Advances in Orthopedics

Editor: Brandon Gomez

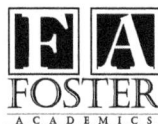

FA
FOSTER
ACADEMICS

www.fosteracademics.com

www.fosteracademics.com

FA FOSTER
ACADEMICS

Cataloging-in-Publication Data

Bone fracture : advances in orthopedics / edited by Brandon Gomez.
   p. cm.
Includes bibliographical references and index.
ISBN 978-1-63242-761-8
1. Fractures. 2. Orthopedics. 3. Bones--Diseases. I. Gomez, Brandon.
RD101 .B66 2019
617.15--dc23

Foster Academics,
118-35 Queens Blvd., Suite 400,
Forest Hills, NY 11375, USA

ISBN 978-1-63242-761-8 (Hardback)

Contents

Preface

The purpose of the book is to provide a glimpse into the dynamics and to present opinions and studies of some of the scientists engaged in the development of new ideas in the field from very different standpoints. This book will prove useful to students and researchers owing to its high content quality.

Medical conditions in which there are partial or complete breaks in the continuity of the bones are known as bone fractures. They are usually caused by force impact, trauma injury, and some medical conditions, such as osteoporosis, osteopenia, osteogenesis imperfect, etc. As there is an absence of nociceptors in the bone tissue, so there are no specific symptoms associated with bone fractures. However, bone fractures can be extremely painful in some cases. Tests like, radiographic imaging, computed tomography (CT) scan and magnetic resonance imaging (MRI) are some of the most common tests to diagnose bone fractures. The book aims to shed light on some of the unexplored aspects of bone fracture and the recent researches in the field of orthopedics. From theories to research, case studies related to all contemporary topics of relevance of this area of study have been included in this book. It aims to serve as a resource guide for students, doctors and experts alike and contribute to the growth of the discipline.

At the end, I would like to appreciate all the efforts made by the authors in completing their chapters professionally. I express my deepest gratitude to all of them for contributing to this book by sharing their valuable works. A special thanks to my family and friends for their constant support in this journey.

Editor

Higher Fish Intake Is Associated with a Lower Risk of Hip Fractures in Chinese Men and Women: A Matched Case-Control Study

Fan Fan[1,◑], Wen-Qiong Xue[1,6◑], Bao-Hua Wu[1,2], Ming-Guang He[3], Hai-Li Xie[1], Wei-Fu Ouyang[1,4], Su-lan Tu[1,5], Yu-Ming Chen[1]*

1 Guangdong Provincial Key Laboratory of Food, Nutrition and Health, School of Public Health, Sun Yat-sen University, Guangzhou, People's Republic of China, 2 Guangzhou Orthopaedics Trauma Hospital, Guangzhou, People's Republic of China, 3 Zhongshan Ophthalmic Center, Sun Yat-sen University, Guangzhou, People's Republic of China, 4 Guangdong General Hospital, Guangzhou, Guangdong, People's Republic of China, 5 Orthopaedics Hospital of Baishi District, Jiangmen, Guangdong, People's Republic of China, 6 Sun Yat-sen University Cancer Center, Guangzhou, People's Republic of China

Abstract

Objectives: Fish is rich in nutrients that are favorable to bone health, but limited data are available regarding the relationship between fish intake and hip fractures. Our study examined the association between habitual fish intake and risk of hip fractures.

Methods: A case-control study was performed between June 2009 and June 2012 in Guangdong Province, China. Five hundred and eighty-one hip fracture incident cases, aged 55 to 80 years (mean: 71 years), were enrolled from four hospitals. 1:1 matched controls by gender and age ($\pm$3 years) were also recruited from communities and hospitals. Face-to-face interviews were used to obtain habitual dietary intake and information on various covariates.

Results: Univariate conditional logistic regression analyses showed significantly dose-dependent inverse correlations between the risk of hip fractures and the intake of fresh-water fish, sea fish, mollusca, shellfish, and total fish in all of the subjects (p-trend: <0.001–0.016). After adjusting for covariates, the associations were slightly attenuated but remained significant for all (p-trend: <0.001–0.017) except for fresh-water fish (p = 0.553). The ORs (95%CI) of hip fractures for the highest (vs. lowest) quartile were 0.80 (0.48–1.31) for fresh-water fish, 0.31 (0.18–0.52) for sea fish, 0.55 (0.34–0.88) for mollusca and shellfish, and 0.47 (0.28–0.79) for total fish, respectively. Stratified and interaction analyses showed that the association was more significant in males than in females (*p*-interaction = 0.052).

Conclusion: Higher intake of seafood is independently associated with lower risk of hip fractures in elderly Chinese. Increasing consumption of sea fish may benefit the prevention of hip fractures in this population.

Editor: Nick Harvey, University of Southampton, United Kingdom

Funding: The study was jointly supported by the National Natural Science Foundation of China (No. 30872100, 81072299) and the 5010 Program for Clinical Researches of Sun Yat-sen University (No. 2007032). The funders had no role in study design, data collection and analysis, decision to publish, or preparation of the manuscript.

Competing Interests: The authors have declared that no competing interests exist.

* E-mail: chenyum@mail.sysu.edu.cn

◑ These authors contributed equally to this work.

Introduction

Hip fractures are considered to be the most severe complication of osteoporosis, and have attracted increased attention because of poor prognosis such as leading to chronic pain, increasing the risk of mortality (20–24% patients die in the first year following injury) [1] and disability (40% of survivors lose the ability to walk) [1] and enhancing medical burdens (USD17.14 billion in China in 2011) [2]. The number of incident cases is expected to increase from 1.66 million in 1990 to 4.50–6.26 million per year in 2050 [3]. Given the serious individual and economic consequences of hip fractures, prevention strategies are essential.

Nutritional factors play a key role in the maintenance of optimal bone health [4]. Fish is a major food group worldwide, with a mean intake of 90~200 g/d (raw weight) consumed in Chinese coastal areas according to the 2002 National Nutritional Survey [5]. Fish is a major source of high-bioavailability protein, n-3 polyunsaturated fatty acids (PUFA), fat-soluble vitamins (such as A and D), and minerals (e.g., calcium, zinc, selenium, and iodine). Many of these nutrients may have beneficial effects on bone health [4]. Some studies have examined the association between fish consumption and bone health, but have generated inconsistent results. Many studies have shown that higher fish or seafood consumption may produce greater bone mineral density (BMD) [6–9]. Others have explored the effects of fish consumption on fractures, but the inconsistent results are thought to be the result of various study designs and populations or weak effects [9–12]. The majority of these studies, however, were performed in Western populations; thus, limited data have rendered findings on the effects of fish consumption on the risk of bone fractures inconclusive in Asian populations. This study examines the association of habitual intake of total fish and different types of fish with the risk of hip fractures in middle-aged and elderly Chinese in Guangdong Province, a coastal region of China.

Materials and Methods

Study population

This 1:1 matched case-control study was performed between June 2009 and June 2012 in Guangdong Province, China. Eligible cases were required to be hip fracture incident patients within 2 weeks of diagnosis (according to the medical records), confirmed by X-ray image, aged between 55 and 80 years, and living in Guangdong Province for more than 10 years. We attempted to contact all of the eligible patients hospitalized at the following hospitals: Guangzhou Orthopaedics Trauma Hospital, Guangdong General Hospital, First Affiliated Hospital of Sun Yat-sen University, and the Orthopaedics Hospital of Baishi District in Jiangmen city, Guangdong Province. Subjects with the following conditions were excluded: (i) pathological or high-energy fractures (for example, automobile accidents or a fall from above chair height); (ii) substantial changes in dietary habits within the previous 5 years; (iii) chronic disease that might affect dietary habits such as diabetes, stroke, coronary disease, cancer, cognitive disorder, liver cirrhosis, renal failure, thyroid disorder, or chronic diarrhea; (iv) current use of exogenous estrogens exceeding 3 months, corticosteroids, thiazine, or other medications known to affect endocrine balance; and (v) poor vision that might affect routine activities. Each case was matched by one control with the same gender and age (±3 years). Apparently healthy community residents in the same cities and inpatients who had been hospitalized within 1 week with one of the following diseases were accepted as control subjects: influenza, pneumonia, benign ophthalmic or otorhinolaryngologic tumor, and acute surgical disease or cataract in one eye. With the exception of a history of any fracture, the same selection criteria were applied to the control subjects that were applied to the case-patients. Written informed consent was obtained from all participants before the interviews and the ethics committee of the School of Public Health of Sun Yat-sen University approved the study.

Data collection

Face-to-face interviews were conducted by experienced interviewers with relevant knowledge. We used a structured questionnaire to collect the following information: 1) sociodemographic characteristics (e.g., education, occupation, marital status); 2) lifestyle habits (e.g., smoking, alcohol drinking, tea consumption, physical activity); 3) habitual dietary consumption in the previous 12 months before diagnosis (case-patients) or interview (control subjects); 4) history of chronic diseases and medications; and 5) history of menstruation and child-bearing for female participants. Subjects were also asked whether they had taken calcium or multivitamin supplements daily for at least six consecutive months in the past ten years, and how long they had use the supplements. Each interviewer completed an equal proportion of interviews between case and control groups.

We used a 79-item food-frequency questionnaire (FFQ), validated by a local source population (the correlation coefficient between the FFQ and six 3-day dietary records within 6 months was 0.30 for fish [13]), to assess dietary consumption. The mean intake of food per day, week, month, or year in the year prior to

the diagnosis or interview was reported. For seasonal foods, participants were asked to report how many months of the year they consumed each item. Photographs of food portion sizes were provided to help participants estimate the amount of food intake. Fish intake was evaluated by using the following items: (1) freshwater fish (e.g., grass carp, black carp, bullhead, crucian carp, mandarin fish, etc.); (2) sea fish (e.g., pomfret, grouper, golden thread fish, hairtail, etc.); (3) mollusca (e.g., squid, cuttlefish, oyster, scallop); (4) shrimp and crab. Based on the similarities in nutrient composition, we classified seafood into three groups: freshwater fish, sea fish, and mollusca and shellfish. Daily intakes of dietary energy and nutrients were calculated according to the 2002 China Food Composition Table [14].

Statistical analysis

All data were imputed doubly by two investigators independently using Epidata 3.1. To achieve an approximately normal distribution for the statistical analysis, logarithmic transformation was used in the daily energy intakes, and square root transformation was applied to the other dietary exposures. Dietary intakes were adjusted for daily total energy intake using the residual method. We divided subjects into gender-specific quartiles (Q1–Q4) based on the distribution of dietary intake among the control group, and then applied the gender-specific cutoffs to the cases.

Conditional logistic regressions were conducted, with the bottom quartile group defined as the reference group. Tests were considered statistically significant at $p<0.05$ (two-tailed), and odds ratios (ORs) with their corresponding 95% confidence intervals (CIs) were yielded in both univariate and multivariate analyses. The ordinal values for the dietary intake categories were included as continuous variables in linear trend tests. Demographic characteristics and other potential osteoporosis risk factors were evaluated by paired t-tests (continuous variables) or paired χ^2 tests (categorical variables), which, with $p\leq0.05$, would be induced into the multivariate models as confounders by the forward stepwise method. The intakes of other food groups (cereals, soybeans, fresh vegetables, fruits, dairy products, nuts, and livestock and poultry meat) and total energy were also included in the multivariate adjustments.

Stratified analyses were conducted according to gender and the sources of control. Women's menstrual histories (years since menopause and oral contraceptive and estrogen use) were adjusted for in the multivariate analysis. Multiplicative interactions were estimated by the likelihood ratio test.

Results

Table 1 shows the process of participant selection. 581 cases with 581 matched controls were analyzed. Of the 581 cases, 396 had femoral neck fractures while the other 185 had intertrochanteric fractures. Of the 581 controls, 398 were recruited from communities and 183 were recruited from hospitals.

The cases and controls had similar gender distributions due to the paired design. The controls were more likely than the case patients to have a higher BMI, education level, and household income in addition to the following: no family history of fracture, engaging in mental work, drinking tea, being married, increased physical activity, and the consumption of multivitamin and calcium supplements. Female case-patients tended to exhibit less physical activity, more years since menopause, and less use of oral contraceptives or estrogen than their matched controls (Table 2).

The mean intakes of main food groups are shown in Table 3. In the control group, the mean values for the energy-adjusted consumption of freshwater fish from quartile 1 to quartile 4 were

Table 1. Process of participant selection.

	Cases	Matched controls	
		Community	Hospital
Screened	1137	708	307
Excluded (in total)	556	310	124
Diseases affecting dietary habits	246	154	52
Diseases affecting routine activities	133	96	22
Pathological or high-energy fractures.	44	0	0
Unable to communicate.	23	8	10
Refused to participate	94	0	20
Unreasonable energy intakes*	16	5	7
History of any fracture	0	47	13
Included in the analyses	581	398	183

*Reasonable range: 800–4000 kcal/d for males and 500–3500 kcal/d for females.

2.69, 10.90, 17.86, and 39.10 (g/d) in males and 3.00, 10.49, 20.76, and 55.81 (g/d) in females, while the mean values for sea fish in the same quartiles were 0.54, 3.05, 6.47, and 35.07 (g/d) in males and 0.12, 1.40, 6.10, and 26.93 (g/d) in females.

Univariate conditional logistic regression analyses showed significantly dose-dependent inverse associations between the intake of total fish and all fish subtypes and the risk of hip fracture in all of the subjects (p-trend: <0.001–0.016). After adjusting for age, BMI, socioeconomic factors, physical activity, passive smoking, tea drinking, and dietary factors, significant associations remained for total fish and other fish subtypes, with the exception of freshwater fish. Compared to the lowest quartile, the ORs (95%CI) of hip fractures for the highest quartile were 0.80 (0.48–1.31) for fresh-water fish, 0.31 (0.18–0.52) for sea fish, 0.55 (0.34–0.88) for mollusca and shellfish, and 0.47 (0.28–0.79) for total fish in the multivariate model, respectively (Table 4).

Stratified and interaction analyses demonstrated that the effect of sea fish intake was much more significant in males than in females (OR for Q4 vs. Q1: 0.10 vs. 0.36, p interaction: 0.052). The associations of total fish and its subtypes with hip fracture did not differ in subgroups stratified by control sources (Table 5).

Discussion

This matched case-control study, with 581 cases and 581 controls, revealed that the intake of fish and shellfish had a statistically significant protective effect on the risk of hip fracture. The favorable effect of sea fish was much stronger than that of freshwater fish. Fish are a major source of animal food in the traditional diet among the coastal regions of mainland China. Our finding suggests that an increase in fish consumption, especially sea fish, may benefit the prevention of hip fractures in this population.

Most but not all previous studies have supported the hypothesis that a greater intake of fish is favorable for the prevention of osteoporosis. A large population-based study in China by Zalloua et al. [6] found that increasing seafood consumption (>250 vs. <250 g/week) was significantly associated with greater BMD at the total body and hip in women (p<0.01). Farina et al. [7] found that high intakes (≥3 vs. <3, servings/wk) of fish were associated with the maintenance of femur neck BMD in both men and women in their 4-year Framingham Osteoporosis Study. Similar results were observed in cross-sectional studies in Hong Kong

postmenopausal women [8] and in 1,305 participants aged ≥65 years from a U.S. cardiovascular health study [9]. However, fracture studies have produced inconsistent results. In the Nurses' Health Study involving 72,337 post-menopausal women, a dose-response relationship was noted between a higher intake of dark fish (sea fish) and lower risk of hip fracture (p-trend = 0.03) [10]. A similar result was observed in a case-control study of hip fractures (294 cases and 498 controls) in Japan [11], but not in a cohort study with a 12-year follow up in 4,573 people in Japan [12] or in the Cardiovascular Health Study with 5,045 participants and an 11-year follow up [9] possibly due to limited study size. Generally consistent with the majority of previous studies, our findings showed that greater intakes of sea fish and shellfish had a protective effect against the risk of hip fracture.

The positive effects of fish can be partially attributed to rich nutrients that support bone health. Fish and shellfish are good sources of high-bioavailability protein, which many studies have found may positively affect bone health by improving calcium absorption, increasing insulin-like growth factor I, and improving lean body mass [15]. Other researchers have proposed that excess protein may have an adverse effect on bone by increasing acid load [16,17]. The potential renal acid load (PRAL) values (mEq/ 100 g) in sea fish (8.29) and freshwater fish (8.25) were slightly lower than those in pork (9.9) and beef (10.0) [14,18]. The beneficial effects of seafood may be due to the high-bioavailability protein it contains and a relatively lower acid-load generated by the displacement of meat protein. Another important nutrient that may play a role in this association is calcium. Calcium has been considered the key nutrient for bone health. A meta-analysis of eighteen studies reported a positive association between dietary calcium and risk of hip fracture (OR = 0.96, 95% CI: 0.93–0.99) [19]. The level of calcium in fish was much higher than in other meat [14]. Thus, the positive effect of seafood might be partially explained by its high calcium content.

We found that the favorable effect of sea fish on hip fracture was more substantial than that of freshwater fish, as was observed in a population-based cross-sectional study on fish and BMD in Hong Kong [8]. The beneficial effect was reported in sea fish but not in fresh-water fish on BMD in Chinese women in the cross-sectional study [6] and on the incidence of hip fracture in the Nurses Health Study cohort [10]. Why sea fish have a more favorable effect on bone health than freshwater fish remains uncertain. The differential effect between sea fish and freshwater fish is unlikely to be explained by high-quality protein and calcium, because their presence in the two types of fish was similar. Vitamin D and n-3 polyunsaturated fatty acid might partially explain the difference between sea fish and freshwater fish. Sea fish are richer in vitamin D than freshwater fish and vitamin D has long been thought to enhance the effects of calcium on bone health [20]. The human body most commonly obtains vitamin D from the diet or skin exposure to sunlight. However, the endogenous production of vitamin D tends to decrease with age and elderly people become more dependent on dietary sources to maintain adequate vitamin D status [21]. Second, sea fish are richer sources than freshwater fish of the long-chain n-3 fatty acids eicosapentaenoic acid and docosahexaenoic. Many studies have shown the beneficial effects of n-3 fatty acids on bone health in both humans and animals [22–24]. The possible mechanisms for the beneficial effects of dietary n-3 fatty acids on bone are extensive and include increasing calcium absorption [25,26], increasing the synthesis of bone collagen [27], inhibiting bone resorption [25], decreasing urinary calcium excretion [27], and modulating the action of inflammatory cytokines, e.g., interleukin-1, interleukin-6, and tumor necrosis factors [28–30]. Thus, the varied effect of both types of

Table 2. Demographics, lifestyle characteristics, and select hip fracture risk factors of study population in Guangzhou, China.

	Men (148 pairs)			Women (433 pairs)		
	Cases	Controls	p	Cases	Controls	p
Age, y	70.03±6.96	69.49±6.99	*0.016*	71.37±6.62	71.39±6.48	0.898
Body mass index, *kg/m²*	20.93±2.11	23.21±2.36	*<0.001*	21.40±3.90	22.93±3.07	*<0.001*
Marital status, *N(%)*			*0.006*			*<0.001*
Married	116(78.4)	130(88.4)		230(53.6)	296(69.0)	
Unmarried/Divorced/Widowed	32(21.6)	17(11.6)		199(46.4)	133(31.0)	
Education level, *N(%)*			*0.001*			*<0.001*
Primary school or below	80(54.1)	48(32.7)		277(64.9)	209(48.9)	
Secondary school	23(29.6)	36(29.4)		42(9.8)	81(19)	
High school or above	45(30.4)	63(42.9)		108(25.3)	137(32.1)	
Occupation[a], *N(%)*			*0.022*			*0.002*
Full mental work	31(20.9)	36(24.3)		64(14.8)	80(186)	
Main mental work	28(18.9)	48(32.4)		64(14.8)	99(23.0)	
Main physical labor	33(22.3)	25(16.9)		72(16.7)	60(13.9)	
Full physical labor	49(33.1)	36(24.3)		208(48.3)	153(35.5)	
Other	7(4.7)	3(2.0)		23(5.3)	39(9.0)	
Household income, *Yuan/month/person, N(%)*			*0.004*			*<0.001*
≤500	7(4.8)	2(1.4)		35(8.1)	10(2.3)	
501~2000	65(44.2)	40(27.0)		197(45.8)	147(34.2)	
2000~3000	54(36.7)	79(53.4)		147(34.2)	195(45.3)	
>3000	21(14.3)	27(18.2)		51(11.9)	78(18.1)	
Social status, *N(%)*			*0.008*			*0.001*
Bad	44(29.7)	23(15.5)		103(23.9)	61(14.1)	
General	54(36.5)	67(45.3)		206(47.8)	234(54.0)	
Good	50(33.8)	58(39.2)		122(28.3)	138(31.9)	
Family history of fractures, *N(%)*			0.087			0.137
Father	9(6.1)	5(3.4)		17(3.9)	12(2.8)	
Mother	13(8.8)	5(3.4)		53(12.3)	36(8.3)	
Orientation of house[b], *N(%)*			*0.043*			0.211
Exposure to the sun	122(82.4)	129(90.2)		337(78.9)	321(75.2)	
Smoking status[c], *N(%)*	69(46.6)	54(36.5)	0.077	17(3.9)	7(1.6)	0.064
Passive smoking[d], *N(%)*	45(30.4)	20(13.5)	*<0.001*	95(22.0)	76(17.6)	0.081
Alcohol drinker[e], *N(%)*	28(18.9)	18(12.2)	0.143	10(2.3)	16(3.7)	0.327
Tea drinker[f], *N(%)*	60(40.5)	86(58.1)	*0.003*	139(32.2)	169(39.1)	*0.042*
Calcium supplement user, *N(%)*	18(12.2)	39(26.4)	*0.001*	134(30.9)	171(39.5)	*0.006*
Multivitamin user, *N(%)*	11(7.4)	39(26.4)	*<0.001*	36(8.3)	103(23.8)	*<0.001*
Physical activity[g], *MET• h/d*	69.01±47.91	71.28±43.59	0.624	76.35±45.30	88.36±64.37	*0.001*
Years since menopause, y				22.48±7.56	21.19±8.96	*0.001*
Oral contraceptive user, *N(%)*				25(6.0)	76(18.3)	*<0.001*
Estrogen user, *N(%)*				7(1.7)	42(10.1)	*<0.001*

Continuous variables were described by means ±standard deviation.
[a]Occupation: "mental work" refers to those works which need less physical activity, such as administrators, managers, clerks, professionals or other white collars.
[b]House orientations: 'head' referred to the orientation of the living room. Housing with east, south, southeast, southwest, northeast, and northwest orientations designated a head in the sun and other orientations designated a head in the shade.
[c]Smoking was defined as having smoked ≥1 cigarette daily for at least six consecutive months.
[d]Passive smoking was defined as being exposed to other's tobacco smoking for ≥5 minutes daily in the previous five years.
[e]Alcohol drinkers were defined as having had wine ≥1 time(s) daily for at least six consecutive months.
[f]Tea drinkers were defined as drinking at least one cup of tea per week in the previous six months.
[g]Physical activities included daily occupational, leisure-time, and household-chores, evaluated by metabolic equivalent (MET) hours per day.

Table 3. Intake of main food groups for study population in Guangzhou, China[a].

	Men (148 pairs)		p	Women (433 pairs)		p
	Cases	Controls		Cases	Controls	
Dietary energy, kcal/d	1388±345	1402±385	0.668	1274±381	1323±360	**0.044**
Cereals	699±121	689±148	0.513	656±134	630±136	*0.001*
Soy protein	3.11±3.99	4.67±4.71	*0.001*	2.36±3.06	3.44±3.73	*<0.001*
Vegetables	232±106	289±130	*<0.001*	241±120	288±130	*<0.001*
Fruits	39.8±30.6	66.6±56.8	*<0.001*	52.7±42.9	67.3±57.7	*<0.001*
Milk and dairy products	46.7±71.6	77.1±101.9	*0.002*	71.6±113.4	95.4±94.7	*<0.001*
Nuts	9.28±10.52	12.42±13.71	*0.023*	6.75±11.03	11.66±16.65	*<0.001*
Meat	87.7±51.9	63.2±31.5	*<0.001*	80.2±52.7	64.0±39.6	*<0.001*
Poultry	22.6±16.5	17.8±12.3	*0.004*	19.0±15.0	19.6±16.8	0.629
Total fish	26.2±22.9	34.5±26.5	*0.002*	26.4±22.3	34.6±33.3	*<0.001*
Freshwater fish	16.4±15.3	17.6±17.2	0.490	17.0±16.1	22.5±32.0	*0.001*
Sea fish	4.94±11.64	11.28±17.92	*<0.001*	5.72±12.00	8.62±13.75	*0.001*
Mollusca and shellfish	4.57±7.97	5.57±8.93	0.200	3.39±6.98	3.71±5.94	0.463

Continuous variables were described by means ±SD and evaluated by t-test.
[a]Mean intakes of food groups were adjusted for daily energy intake using the residual method. The mean of daily energy intake was 1355 kcal (male) or 1278 kcal (female).

Table 4. Odds ratio (95% CIs) of hip fractures for quartiles of seafood intake in Guangzhou, China.

	Quartiles of dietary energy-adjusted intake				P for trend
	1 (referent)	2	3	4 (highest)	
Freshwater fish					
Intake (M/F), g/d	2.69/3.00	10.90/10.49	17.86/20.76	39.10/55.81	
N (cases/control)	180/145	130/146	155/145	116/145	
OR I (95%CI)	1.00	0.70(0.51–0.98)	0.82(0.59–1.15)	0.60(0.42–0.86)	*0.016*
OR II (95%CI)	1.00	0.98(0.63–1.54)	1.19(0.74–1.90)	0.80(0.48–1.31)	0.553
Sea fish					
Intake (M/F), g/d	0.54/0.12	3.05/1.40	6.47/6.10	35.07/26.93	
N (cases/control)	224/145	159/146	119/145	79/145	
OR I (95%CI)	1.00	0.69(0.51–0.95)	0.49(0.35–0.69)	0.31(0.22–0.46)	*<0.001*
OR II (95%CI)	1.00	0.64(0.41–1.00)	0.46(0.29–0.72)	0.31(0.18–0.52)	*<0.001*
Mollusca and shellfish					
Intake (M/F), g/d	0.27/0.08	1.83/0.73	4.15/2.88	16.04/11.15	
N (cases/control)	211/145	145/145	112/146	113/145	
OR I (95%CI)	1.00	0.70(0.51–0.95)	0.49(0.35–0.70)	0.50(0.35–0.71)	*<0.001*
OR II (95%CI)	1.00	0.62(0.41–0.96)	0.49(0.30–0.78)	0.55(0.34–0.88)	*0.004*
Total fish					
Intake (M/F), g/d	9.75/7.88	22.85/20.95	35.25/36.33	70.15/73.42	
N (cases/control)	196/145	152/145	145/146	88/145	
OR I (95%CI)	1.00	0.75(0.54–1.03)	0.66(0.47–0.93)	0.40(0.28–0.85)	*<0.001*
OR II (95%CI)	1.00	0.89(0.57–1.38)	1.04(0.64–1.67)	0.47(0.28–0.79)	*0.017*

Intake (M/F): Mean intake of seafood in male/female controls.
OR I, OR II: from conditional logistic model. OR I: without further adjustment; OR II: adjusted for BMI, education, marital status, occupation, household income, social status, house orientation, family history of fractures, passive smoking, tea drinking, calcium supplement user, multivitamin user, physical activity, daily energy intake, and energy-adjusted intakes of other food groups (including cereals, soybeans, vegetables, fruits, fresh meats, fresh poultry, nuts, milk and dairy products) by stepwise forward method. 95%CI: 95% confidence interval.

Table 5. Odds ratio (95% CIs) of hip fractures for quartiles of seafood stratified by gender, source of controls, and fracture sites in Guangzhou, China.

Variable	Pair N	Quartiles of dietary energy-adjusted intake				p-trend	p-interaction
		1 (referent)	2	3	4 (highest)		
Freshwater fish							
Gender							0.189
Male	148	1.00	1.09(0.19–6.38)	1.82(0.29–11.38)	2.30(0.41–12.82)	0.270	
Female	433	1.00	0.82(0.47–1.43)	1.08(0.60–1.95)	0.52(0.28–0.97)	0.212	
Source of controls							0.143
Community	398	1.00	1.07(0.56–2.03)	1.76(0.90–3.45)	1.21(0.60–2.46)	0.510	
Hospital	183	1.00	1.35(0.64–2.87)	1.01(0.47–2.19)	0.60(0.26–1.38)	0.215	
Sea fish							
Gender							0.052
Male	148	1.00	0.24(0.06–1.02)	0.03(0.01–0.19)	0.10(0.02–0.47)	0.015	
Female	433	1.00	0.86(0.51–1.48)	0.72(0.40–1.29)	0.36(0.18–0.69)	0.003	
Source of controls							0.768
Community	398	1.00	0.47(0.25–0.90)	0.34(0.17–0.68)	0.29(0.14–0.58)	<0.001	
Hospital	183	1.00	0.75(0.35–1.60)	0.30(0.13–0.68)	0.18(0.06–0.54)	<0.001	
Mollusca and shellfish							
Gender							0.540
Male	148	1.00	0.51(0.09–2.74)	0.89(0.17–4.61)	0.08(0.01–1.37)	0.252	
Female	433	1.00	1.00(0.59–1.69)	0.47(0.26–0.87)	0.59(0.32–1.06)	0.016	
Source of controls							0.403
Community	398	1.00	0.37(0.20–0.69)	0.39(0.20–0.77)	0.59(0.31–1.12)	0.039	
Hospital	183	1.00	0.54(0.25–1.17)	0.34(0.15–0.79)	0.25(0.09–0.68)	0.002	
Total fish							
Gender							0.864
Male	148	1.00	1.24(0.29–5.41)	2.10(0.41–10.73)	0.41(0.07–2.43)	0.665	
Female	433	1.00	1.06(0.61–1.86)	1.18(0.65–2.12)	0.42(0.22–0.78)	0.037	
Source of controls							0.389
Community	398	1.00	0.86(0.50–1.66)	1.19(0.58–2.44)	0.57(0.28–1.15)	0.200	
Hospital	183	1.00	0.95(0.47–1.91)	1.36(0.63–2.91)	0.25(0.09–0.70)	0.075	

Odds ratios (95% CI): from multivariate conditional logistic regression models. Covariates adjusted for: see ORII in Table 3. For women, years since menopause, oral contraceptive user, estrogen user were further adjusted for by the stepwise forward method.

fish on bone health might be partially explained by the different content of vitamin D and n-3 fatty acids in the population.

We explored whether the beneficial effects of sea fish varied with gender, control sources, or fracture sites. The association between the intake of sea fish and the risk of hip fracture was more substantial in males than in females (OR, comparing extreme quartiles: 0.10 vs. 0.36, p-interaction: 0.052). This difference might stem from a large between-individual variation in the sea fish intakes of males and females (mean difference of intake between Q4 and Q1 in males vs. females, g/d: 34.53 vs. 26.81).

Our study has the following limitations. First, the time sequence between the exposure and outcome may be uncertain in the case-control study. However, it is unlikely to have an inverse time sequence because (i) only new cases were selected, (ii) we excluded both cases and controls with chronic diseases that might change dietary habits or nutritional factors, and (iii) adults generally maintain a long-term stable dietary habit [31,32]. Second, hospital-based case-control studies are prone to selection biases. We controlled the selection bias by using multiple cases sourced

from four different hospitals and controls from various hospitals and the community. The stratified analysis showed similar associations between hospital- and community-based controls. Third, while it is difficult for elderly participants to accurately recall habitual dietary intake, a differentially biased report of the fish intake between cases and controls is unlikely because the beneficial effects of fish consumption on bone health is not publically confirmed or well-known. We also controlled the interviewer bias through standardized training and by having the interviewers conduct an equal proportion of case and control interviews. Finally, apart from age and gender, other socioeconomic factors and food intakes were not balanced between the cases and controls. Thus, we used a multivariate model to control the possible confounders.

Conclusions

Our findings show that a higher intake of seafood is significantly and independently associated with a lower risk of hip fracture in the elderly. Therefore, increasing sea fish consumption may benefit the prevention of hip fracture in the elderly.

Acknowledgments

We are grateful for the help of the doctors and nurses in the above-mentioned hospitals in facilitating both the recruitment of participants and the interviews.

References

1. Leibson CL, Tosteson AN, Gabriel SE, Ransom JE, Melton LJ (2002) Mortality, disability, and nursing home use for persons with and without hip fracture: a population-based study. J Am Geriatr Soc 50: 1644–1650.
2. Mithal A Dhingra V, Lau E(2009) The Asian Audit: Epidemiology, Costs and Burden of Osteoporosis in Asia 2009. IFO.
3. Pongchaiyakul C, Songpattanasilp T, Taechakraichana N (2008) Osteoporosis: overview in disease, epidemiology, treatment and health economy. J Med Assoc Thai 91: 581–594.
4. New SA, Bonjour JP, New SA, Bonjour JP (2003) Nutritional Aspects of Bone Health. Cambridge CB4 0WF, UK: The Royal Society of Chemistry.
5. Jin SG, editor(2008) 2002 national nutrition and health survey in Chinese residents: Part X Beijing: People's Medical Publishing House. 62–66 p.
6. Zalloua PA, Hsu YH, Terwedow H, Zang T, Wu D, et al. (2007) Impact of seafood and fruit consumption on bone mineral density. Maturitas 56: 1–11.
7. Farina EK, Kiel DP, Roubenoff R, Schaefer EJ, Cupples LA, et al. (2011) Protective effects of fish intake and interactive effects of long-chain polyunsaturated fatty acid intakes on hip bone mineral density in older adults: the Framingham Osteoporosis Study. Am J Clin Nutr 93: 1142–1151.
8. Chen YM, Ho SC, Lam SS (2010) Higher sea fish intake is associated with greater bone mass and lower osteoporosis risk in postmenopausal Chinese women. Osteoporos Int 21: 939–946.
9. Virtanen JK, Mozaffarian D, Cauley JA, Mukamal KJ, Robbins J, et al. (2010) Fish consumption, bone mineral density, and risk of hip fracture among older adults: the cardiovascular health study. J Bone Miner Res 25: 1972–1979.
10. Feskanich D, Willett WC, Colditz GA (2003) Calcium, vitamin D, milk consumption, and hip fractures: a prospective study among postmenopausal women. Am J Clin Nutr 77: 504–511.
11. Suzuki T, Yoshida H, Hashimoto T, Yoshimura N, Fujiwara S, et al. (1997) Case-control study of risk factors for hip fractures in the Japanese elderly by a Mediterranean Osteoporosis Study (MEDOS) questionnaire. Bone 21: 461–467.
12. Fujiwara S, Kasagi F, Yamada M, Kodama K (1997) Risk factors for hip fracture in a Japanese cohort. J Bone Miner Res 12: 998–1004.
13. Zhang CX, Ho SC (2009) Validity and reproducibility of a food frequency Questionnaire among Chinese women in Guangdong province. Asia Pac J Clin Nutr 18: 240–250.
14. Yang YX, Wang GY, Pan XC (2002) China Food Composition Table. Beijing: Peking University Medical Press.
15. Kerstetter JE, Kenny AM, Insogna KL (2011) Dietary protein and skeletal health: a review of recent human research. Curr Opin Lipidol 22: 16–20.
16. Dargent-Molina P, Sabia S, Touvier M, Kesse E, Breart G, et al. (2008) Proteins, dietary acid load, and calcium and risk of postmenopausal fractures in the E3N French women prospective study. J Bone Miner Res 23: 1915–1922.
17. Sellmeyer DE, Stone KL, Sebastian A, Cummings SR (2001) A high ratio of dietary animal to vegetable protein increases the rate of bone loss and the risk of fracture in postmenopausal women. Study of Osteoporotic Fractures Research Group. Am J Clin Nutr 73: 118–122.
18. Remer T, Manz F (1995) Potential renal acid load of foods and its influence on urine pH. J Am Diet Assoc 95: 791–797.
19. Cumming RG, Nevitt MC (1997) Calcium for prevention of osteoporotic fractures in postmenopausal women. J Bone Miner Res 12: 1321–1329.
20. Tang BM, Eslick GD, Nowson C, Smith C, Bensoussan A (2007) Use of calcium or calcium in combination with vitamin D supplementation to prevent fractures and bone loss in people aged 50 years and older: a meta-analysis. Lancet 370: 657–666.
21. Prentice A (2004) Diet, nutrition and the prevention of osteoporosis. Public Health Nutr 7: 227–243.
22. Maggio M, Artoni A, Lauretani F, Borghi L, Nouvenne A, et al. (2009) The impact of omega-3 fatty acids on osteoporosis. Curr Pharm Des 15: 4157–4164.
23. Salari P, Rezaie A, Larijani B, Abdollahi M (2008) A systematic review of the impact of n-3 fatty acids in bone health and osteoporosis. Med Sci Monit 14: RA37–44.
24. Claassen N, Coetzer H, Steinmann CM, Kruger MC (1995) The effect of different n-6/n-3 essential fatty acid ratios on calcium balance and bone in rats. Prostaglandins Leukot Essent Fatty Acids 53: 13–19.
25. Claassen N, Potgieter HC, Seppa M, Vermaak WJ, Coetzer H, et al. (1995) Supplemented gamma-linolenic acid and eicosapentaenoic acid influence bone status in young male rats: effects on free urinary collagen crosslinks, total urinary hydroxyproline, and bone calcium content. Bone 16: 385S–392S.
26. Haag M, Magada ON, Claassen N, Bohmer LH, Kruger MC (2003) Omega-3 fatty acids modulate ATPases involved in duodenal Ca absorption. Prostaglandins Leukot Essent Fatty Acids 68: 423–429.
27. Kruger MC, Horrobin DF (1997) Calcium metabolism, osteoporosis and essential fatty acids: a review. Prog Lipid Res 36: 131–151.
28. Sun D, Krishnan A, Zaman K, Lawrence R, Bhattacharya A, et al. (2003) Dietary n-3 fatty acids decrease osteoclastogenesis and loss of bone mass in ovariectomized mice. J Bone Miner Res 18: 1206–1216.
29. Caughey GE, Mantzioris E, Gibson RA, Cleland LG, James MJ (1996) The effect on human tumor necrosis factor alpha and interleukin 1 beta production of diets enriched in n-3 fatty acids from vegetable oil or fish oil. Am J Clin Nutr 63: 116–122.
30. Ferrucci L, Cherubini A, Bandinelli S, Bartali B, Corsi A, et al. (2006) Relationship of plasma polyunsaturated fatty acids to circulating inflammatory markers. J Clin Endocrinol Metab 91: 439–446.
31. Macdonald HM, New SA, Reid DM (2005) Longitudinal changes in dietary intake in Scottish women around the menopause: changes in dietary pattern result in minor changes in nutrient intake. Public Health Nutr 8: 409–416.
32. Macdonald HM, New SA, Golden MH, Campbell MK, Reid DM (2004) Nutritional associations with bone loss during the menopausal transition: evidence of a beneficial effect of calcium, alcohol, and fruit and vegetable nutrients and of a detrimental effect of fatty acids. Am J Clin Nutr 79: 155–165.

Author Contributions

Obtained the fundings: YMC. Conceived and designed the experiments: YMC. Performed the experiments: FF WQX BHW HLX WFO SLT. Analyzed the data: YMC FF. Contributed reagents/materials/analysis tools: MGH. Wrote the paper: YMC FF.

2

Impaired Angiogenesis during Fracture Healing in GPCR Kinase 2 Interacting Protein-1 (GIT1) Knock Out Mice

Guoyong Yin[1,3⑨], Tzong-Jen Sheu[2⑨], Prashanthi Menon[1], Jinjiang Pang[1], Hsin-Chiu Ho[2], Shanshan Shi[2], Chao Xie[2], Elaine Smolock[1], Chen Yan[1], Michael J. Zuscik[2], Bradford C. Berk[1]*

1 Aab Cardiovascular Research Institute and the Department of Medicine, University of Rochester Medical Center, Rochester, New York, United States of America, 2 Center for Musculoskeletal Research and the Department of Orthopaedics and Rehabilitation, University of Rochester Medical Center, Rochester, New York, United States of America, 3 Orthopaedic Department, The First Affiliated Hospital of Nanjing Medical University, Jiangsu, China

Abstract

G protein coupled receptor kinase 2 (GRK2) interacting protein-1 (GIT1), is a scaffold protein that plays an important role in angiogenesis and osteoclast activity. We have previously demonstrated that GIT1 knockout (GIT1 KO) mice have impaired angiogenesis and dysregulated osteoclast podosome formation leading to a reduction in the bone resorbing ability of these cells. Since both angiogenesis and osteoclast-mediated bone remodeling are involved in the fracture healing process, we hypothesized that GIT1 participates in the normal progression of repair following bone injury. In the present study, comparison of fracture healing in wild type (WT) and GIT1 KO mice revealed altered healing in mice with loss of GIT1 function. Alcian blue staining of fracture callus indicated a persistence of cartilagenous matrix in day 21 callus samples from GIT1 KO mice which was temporally correlated with increased type 2 collagen immunostaining. GIT1 KO mice also showed a decrease in chondrocyte proliferation and apoptosis at days 7 and 14, as determined by PCNA and TUNEL staining. Vascular microcomputed tomography analysis of callus samples at days 7, 14 and 21 revealed decreased blood vessel volume, number, and connection density in GIT1 KO mice compared to WT controls. Correlating with this, VEGF-A, phospho-VEGFR2 and PECAM1 (CD31) were decreased in GIT1 KO mice, indicating reduced angiogenesis with loss of GIT1. Finally, calluses from GIT1 KO mice displayed a reduced number of tartrate resistant acid phosphatase-positive osteoclasts at days 14 and 21. Collectively, these results indicate that GIT1 is an important signaling participant in fracture healing, with gene ablation leading to reduced callus vascularity and reduced osteoclast number in the healing callus.

Editor: Luc Malaval, INSERM U1059/LBTO, Université Jean Monnet, France

Funding: This work was supported by NIH/NHLBI R01 HL063462 (to BCB), National Natural Science Foundation of China Grant #81271988 (to GY), NIH/NIAMS P50 AR054041-5471 (to MJZ) and NIH/NIAMS P30 AR061307. The funders had no role in study design, data collection and analysis, decision to publish, or preparation of the manuscript.

Competing Interests: The authors have declared that no competing interests exist.

* E-mail: brad_berk@urmc.rochester.edu

⑨ These authors contributed equally to this work.

Introduction

Fracture healing is a complex process involving an early inflammatory phase, recruitment, expansion and differentiation of mesenchymal cells, and production of cartilage and bone matrix in a temporally regulated manner [1–3]. After fracture, the repair process begins with hematoma formation and an inflammatory response [2]. In this early inflammatory phase, lack of blood vessels causes a regional hypoxic environment leading to the formation of a cartilagenous template that initiates a process of differentiation that recapitulates endochondral ossification [4]. Included are the proliferation and differentiation of mesenchymal progenitor cells into chondrocytes [1,5] which facilitate deposition of extracellular matrix components at the fracture site resulting in the formation of the transient soft callus [4]. In an initial remodeling phase, the avascular cartilagenous callus is converted into a vascularized and mineralized tissue that is remodeled by osteoclasts during an initial cartilage resorption phase [6], and then later in a bone remodeling phase that sculpts the healed skeletal element into the anatomically appropriate shape [7–9]. The importance of vascular invasion during endochondral bone

formation has been established, with defects in bone vasculature having been reported in osteoporosis and rickets [10]. Thus, not surprisingly, during skeletal repair, neoangiogenesis driven by vascular endothelial growth factor (VEGF) is required to support nutrient and oxygen transport, with tissue oxygenation being required for osteogenic differentiation [11–16]. Further suggesting the need for this angiogenic cascade of events in the repair process, pharmacologic inhibition of angiogenesis has been shown to impair fracture healing by reducing/delaying callus mineralization [17].

G protein coupled receptor kinase 2 (GRK2) interacting protein 1 (GIT1) was originally identified by its binding to GRK2 and its effects on adrenergic receptor endocytosis [18]. GIT1 has five functional domains, including a zinc finger domain responsible for ARF-GAP activity, three ankyrin repeats, a Spa2 homology domain (SHD), a synaptic localization domain (SLD), and a conserved carboxyl-terminal region that interacts with paxillin (PBS) [19]. Through these domains, GIT1 interacts with diverse proteins including ARF6, MEK, phospholipase C-γ (PLCγ), p21-activated kinase (PAK)-interacting exchange factor (PIX) and paxillin [20,21]. GIT1 has diverse biological functions, which we have shown to include a critical role in pulmonary vascular development by regulating VEGF induced PLCγ and ERK1/2 activation [22]. GIT1 is also upregulated in atherosclerotic plaques and regulates endothelial cell and vascular smooth muscle cell migration [23]. Recently, we identified an important role of GIT1 in bone physiology based on its regulation of osteoclast sealing zone formation, a critical step required for the function of this cell [24]. Based on the observations that GIT1 plays an important role in angiogenesis and osteoclast function, both of which are critical for bone repair, we hypothesized that GIT1 is an important molecular player in the bone healing process.

In the present study, we established that loss of GIT1 alters the fracture healing process. Homozygous GIT1 knockout (GIT1 KO) mice display a persistence of cartilagenous callus evidenced by preservation of Alcian Blue staining and type 2 collagen content. Chondrocyte differentiation was impacted by loss of GIT1, with PCNA and TUNEL staining revealing decreased proliferation and apoptosis of chondrocytes. We used microcomputed tomography (microCT) to investigate overall callus volume and vascular parameters and discovered that GIT1 KO mice have reduced vessel volume and vessel number, which correlated with decreased expression of VEGF-A and VEGFR2. We also examined osteoclst numbers in the callus, and document a reduced number of TRAP-stained cells during the remodeling phases of healing in mice with loss of GIT1 function. Overall, findings documented in this report establish that GIT1 is important for the normal progression of the bone healing program via effects on callus vascularization and osteoclast number, improtant determinants for callus mineralization and remodeling respectively.

Materials and Methods

Ethics Statement

To ensure the humane treatment of mice in this study, all experiments involving mice were performed with the approval and supervision of the University Committee on Animal Resources, the AALAC-, OLAW- and USDA-approved IACUC at the University of Rochester Medical Center.

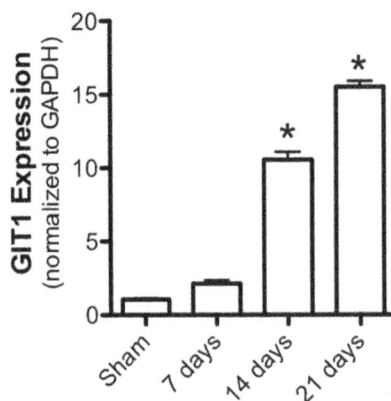

Figure 1. GIT1 mRNA is expressed during fracture healing. WT mice were administered femur fractures and fractured femora were harvested for isolation of mRNA from the callus at 7, 14, and 21 days post-injury. qPCR was performed to examine the profile of GIT1 expression. Bars represent mean GIT1 expression level relative to GAPDH +/− SEM (N = 4, *p<0.05).

Animals

Homozygous GIT1 knockout (GIT1 KO) mice were generated on the C57/BL6 background as described in Pang et al [22]. Chimeric mice generated were backcrossed for more than 7 generations. GIT1 KO mice at age of 10–12 weeks were used for femoral fracture with WT littermates used as controls. It is important to note that because of the high rate of perinatal lethality in GIT1 KO mice due to a pulmonary defect [22] and because of sensitivity to anesthesia, we were limited to an experimental strategy that included only 3 KO mice at each of 3 harvest time points post-fracture: 7, 14 and 21 days.

Mouse Femur Fracture Model

Femur fractures in mice were performed as described in Xie et al [25]. Briefly, mice were anesthetized using a mixture of ketamine and xylazine delivered via intraperitoneal injection. The skin and the underlying tissues over the left knee were incised. A 25-gauge needle was inserted through the patellar tendon and into the medullary canal of the femur. A mid-diaphyseal fracture was created via three-point bending using an Einhorn device [1]. After fracture, 0.5 mg/kg buprenorphine (Abbott labs, North Chicago, Illinois) was administered subcutaneously to each mouse daily for 3 days to control pain. Radiographs were obtained on 7, 14, and 21 days under anesthesia using a Faxitron X-ray system (Faxitron X-ray, Wheeling, Illinois).

Quantitative Real Time PCR (qPCR)

Fracture calluses from WT mice (n = 4) per time point (7, 14, 21 days) were carefully excised from the lower limb. The soft tissue surrounding the calluses was removed and the samples were flash-frozen in liquid N_2. Frozen samples were placed in a Tissuelyser (Qiagen, Venlo, Netherlands) along with 1 mL of TRIzol (Invitrogen, Carlsbad, CA). Homogenization was performed using a frequency of 30 Hz for a time of 3 minutes. The samples were checked for adequate disruption and the mRNA was purified according to the TRIzol System protocol. The concentration of stock mRNA was determined in triplicate using a Nanodrop photospectrometer. The mRNA was diluted in RNase-free water and aliquoted into working dilutions of 0.5 μg/μL. A cDNA library was synthesized using 0.5 μg of callus mRNA by a commercially available reverse transcription kit (Invitrogen, Carlsbad, CA). qPCR analyses were performed using murine-specific primers for *GIT1* and *GAPDH*. The qPCR reactions were performed using SyberGreen (ABgene, Rochester, NY) in a RotorGene real time PCR machine (Corbett Research, Carlsbad, CA). GIT1 expression was normalized using GAPDH expression as an internal control.

Microcomputed Tomography Imaging

Microcomputed tomography imaging (microCT) was performed to assess mineralized callus volume and vascularity as we have previously described [25–28]. Vascular networks at the cortical bone junction and around the fractures were examined using microCT analysis combined with perfusion of a lead chromate based contrast agent [29]. Briefly, Microfil MV-122 (Flow Tech, Inc., Carver, Massachusetts) contrast media, a radiopaque silicone rubber compound containing lead chromate, was perfused via the heart along with 4% paraformaldehyde following an initial vascular flush with heparinized saline. After perfusion, the fractured femur was removed and scanned using a microCT imaging system (VivaCT 40; Scanco Medical AG, Basserdorf, Switzerland) at resolution of 10.5 μm to image bone and vasculature. The samples were subsequently decalcified for 21 days using a 10% EDTA solution. After complete decalcification, the samples were scanned again to image only vascularization within the callus. By registering the 2-D slices before and after decalcification, contour lines were drawn to define a VOI that only included the vasculature in or immediately adjacent to the fracture callus itself. The reconstructed scan images were globally thresholded based on intensity values to render 3-D images of the vasculature in new bone callus, excluding the vessels in the surrounding tissues. Three-dimensional morphometric analysis, based on direct distance transform methods, was subsequently performed on the 3-D images using algorithms that are commonly used to model trabecular bone morphology. This facilitated quantification and analysis of vascular network morphology including vessel volume, number, spacing, and connection density. It should be noted that all measurements of the vascular network were constrained by the limit of resolution of the scanner (10 μm) and the permeability of the networks to the viscous Microfil. Careful heparinization and consistent application of perfusion conditions were established to ensure comparability between mice.

Histology and Histomorphometry

Fractured femora harvested for microCT analysis were processed for histology as previously described [30]. Briefly, femora were disarticulated at the knee and hip, denuded of soft tissue, and fixed at RT in 10% NBF for 72 hours. After three washes in phosphate buffered saline (PBS), fixed femora were decalcified in 10% EDTA for 7 to 14 days. Tissues were then processed using a Tissue-Tek VIP 6 tissue processor (Sakura Finetek USA, Inc., Torrance, CA, USA) and embedded in paraffin. Serial 3 μm thick sagittal sections were obtained from a 60 μm region spanning the center of the fracture callus. Three sections, each separated by approximately 25 to 50 μm, were stained with Alcian Blue Hematoxylin/Orange G and histomorphometric analysis was performed using a point counting method as described previously [31]. Briefly, blinded sections were analyzed using a standardized eyepiece grid under the 10× objective to determine the percent of total callus area composed of cartilage and woven bone. Cartilage was defined as tissue with positive Alcian Blue stain. Woven bone was counted whenever a trabecular structure was observed, regardless of staining. Cortical bone and internal (i.e. intramedullary) callus were not included in these analyses. At each intersection of a horizontal and vertical grid line, the identity of the underlying tissue was determined, with the outcomes for every intersection documented and counted. Based on the number of counted intersections on each slide, the relative area of each tissue type as a percentage of the callus area (i.e. grid intersections that fell within the callus domain) was calculated.

Immunohistochemistry

Previously published methods were employed for immunohistochemical analysis of PCNA and VEGFR2 expression [32] and type 2 collagen expression [33]. Briefly, for either antigen, sections were incubated at 60°C for 30 minutes, followed by deparaffinization in xylene and hydration in gradient ethanol. Sections were permeabilized in PBS containing 0.2% Triton X-100 (Sigma, St. Louis, MO) for 10 min, washed in PBS, blocked with 3% H_2O_2 in methanol for 30 minutes, and 3% goat serum in PBS for 30 minutes. Sections were then incubated with primary antibodies overnight at 4°C. The next day, sections were washed with PBS and incubated with biotinylated secondary antibodies (Vector Laboratories, Burlingame, CA) in blocking buffer for 30 minutes. After washing with PBS, ABC reagent (Vector Laboratories) was added for 30 minutes and sections were washed again before

detection with AEC reagent (Vector Laboratories). Negative controls were performed on adjacent sections by omitting primary antibodies. All sections were analyzed using an Olympus VS120 Whole Slide Imager and quantification was performed using the automated Visiopharm Integrator System (Visiopharm, Hoersholm, Denmark) and its associated software.

Immunofluorescence

Slides from WT and GIT1 KO femure fractures were deparaffinized in xylene, rehydrated in graded ethanol, and rinsed in distilled, deionized H_2O as described above. For PECAM1 (CD31) detection, slides were boiled for 15 minutes in citrate buffer (Zymed Laboratories, San Francisco, CA), cooled for 20 minutes, and washed in PBS for 5 minutes. Slides were then blocked with normal goat serum containing 5% BSA in PBS for 30–60 minutes and incubated overnight with primary antibodies diluted 1:100 in blocking buffer. After two rinses with PBS, the sections were incubated in the dark for 1 hour at 37°C with rabbit secondary antibody diluted 1:500 in normal rabbit serum. Slides were rinsed in PBS before the addition of Topro3 nuclear stain (Invitrogen, Grand Island, NY) and then mounted with Prolong Gold mounting media (Invitrogen). Confocal images were captured using Zeiss LSM 510 Axioskop 2 microscope (Zeiss Microimaging, Thornwood, NY) and analyzed with Zen 2007 software (Zeiss, San Diego, CA).

Osteoclast Quantification

Three sections per callus were stained for tartrate-resistant acid phosphatase (TRAP) using a previously described method [34]. Briefly, after deparaffinization and rehydration with distilled water, sections were incubated at 37°C for 25 minutes in a solution of anhydrous sodium acetate (Sigma), L-(+) tartaric acid (Sigma), glacial acetic acid, fast red violet LB salt (Sigma), naphthol AS-MX phosphate (Sigma), ethylene glycol monoethyl ether (Sigma), and distilled water. Sections were rinsed in distilled water, counterstained with hematoxylin for 10 seconds and then placed in ammonia water for 5 seconds. Quantification was completed using the 10× objective and Osteomeasure software (Osteo-Metrics, Inc., Decatur, GA) to contour bone perimeter within the callus and identify osteoclast number as a percentage of covered bone surface perimeter and as a number of cells per mm of bone surface. Osteoclasts were defined as multi-nucleated, TRAP-positive cells seated on a bone surface.

Statistical Analysis

All values are expressed as mean +/− SEM. Statistical differences between groups were detected using either ANOVA (when >2 experimental groups were compared) or two-tailed unpaired Student's t tests (when only 2 experimental groups were compared). A p-value less than 0.05 (p<0.05) was considered significant.

Results

GIT1 is Expressed during Fracture Healing

To establish that GIT1 is expressed and regulated during the fracture healing process, qPCR was performed on mRNA isolated from the healing callus of WT mice at days 7, 14 and 21 post-fracture. Consistent with previously published work identifying GIT1 function in vascular tissue and osteoclasts, GIT1 is upregulated significantly by day 14 and remains highly-expressed at day 21 (Fig. 1). These timepoints correspond to callus revascularization, cartilage remodeling and woven bone remodeling in the temporal progression of healing. These results set the

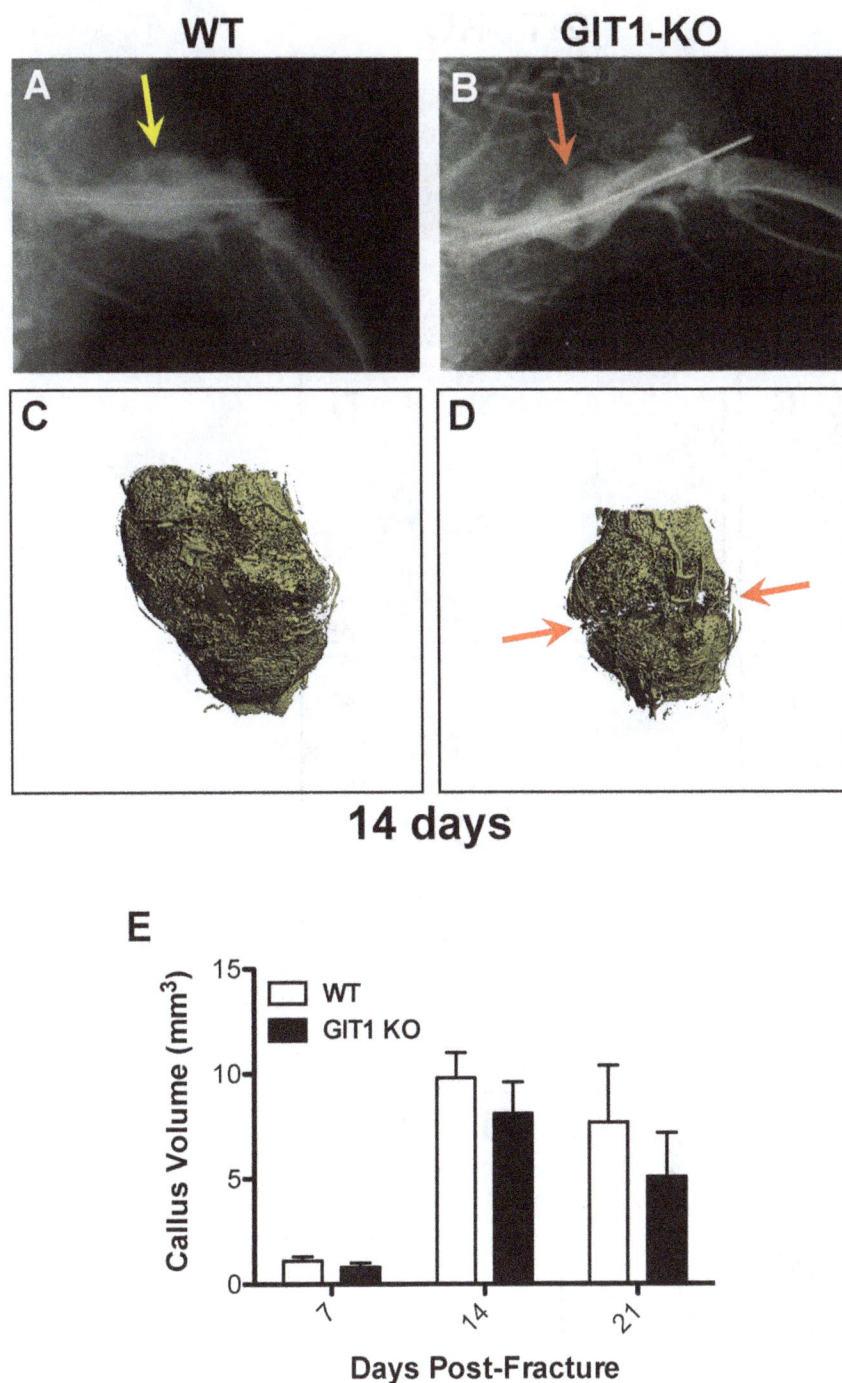

Figure 2. Disjunction persists at 14 days post-fracture in GIT1 KO mice. Femur fractures were induced in 10-week-old WT and GIT1 KO mice. Fractured femora were harvested for analysis at 7, 14, and 21 days post-injury. Radiographs obtained at the 14 day time point consistently revealed radiolucency in GIT1 KO calluses (B, red arrow) compared with calluses from WT mice (A, yellow arrow). This was supported by microCT analysis, which revealed lack of bridging mineral in GIT1 KOs (D, red arrows) compared to a connected shell of mineral in WT controls (C). Further quantification of callus geometry via microCT indicated that there were no differences in mineralized callus volume between WT and GIT1 KO mice (E). Bars represent mean callus volume (mm^3) +/− SEM (N = 3, *p<0.05).

stage for study of bone healing in mice in the context of GIT1 loss-of-function.

Fracture Healing is Impaired in GIT1 KO Mice

To begin investigating the role of GIT1 in the fracture healing process, we induced femoral fractures in WT and GIT1 KO mice

and assessed the healing process by radiographical evaluation and microCT analysis of mineralized callus volume. At day 14, loss of radiolucency at the fracture site in WT mice suggested the normal pacing of repair (Fig. 2A), while the healing process was delayed in GIT1 KO mice (Fig. 2B, red arrow). Representative microCT reconstructions confirm persistence of disjunction in GIT1 KO

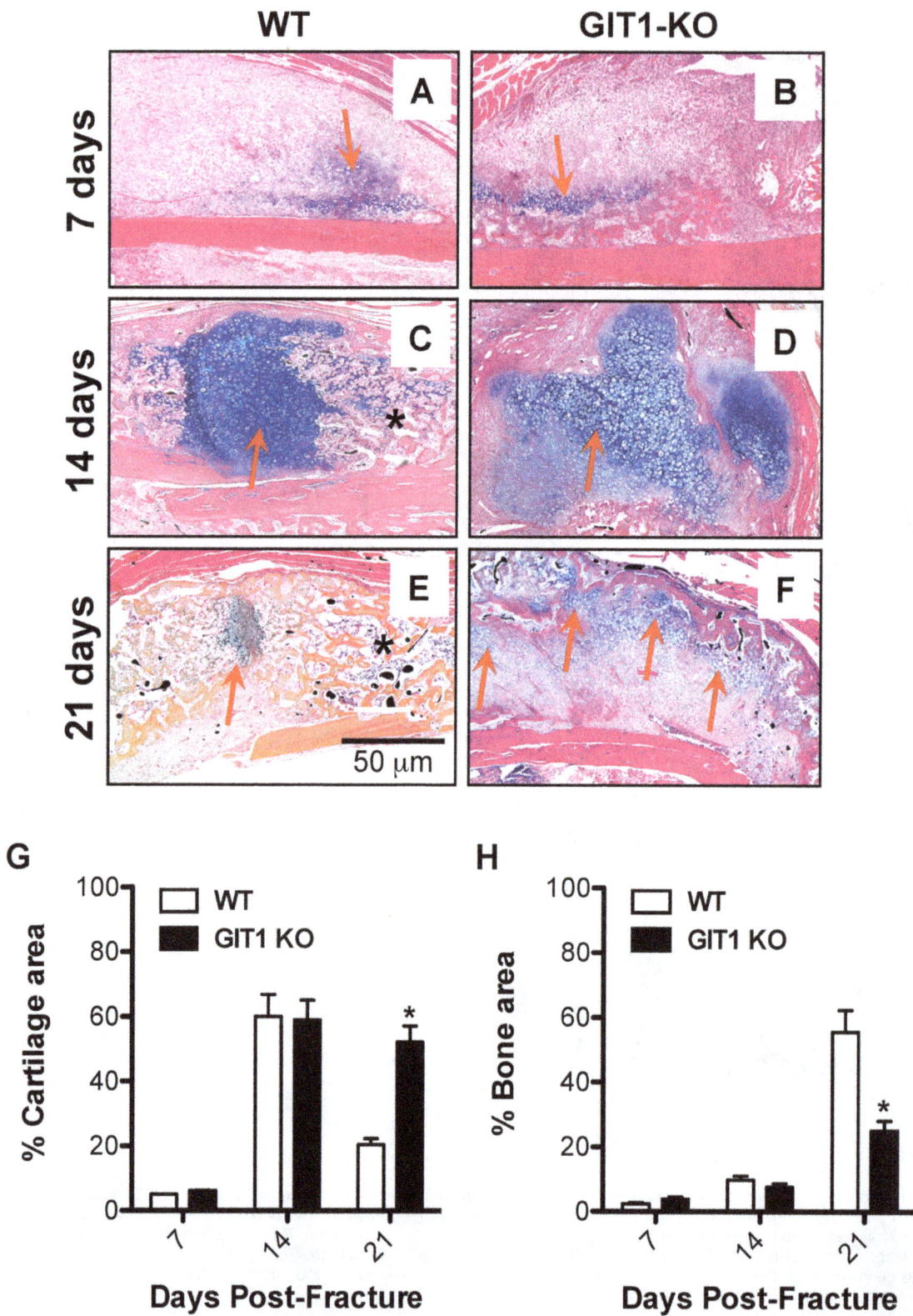

Figure 3. Cartilage persists and woven bone callus is delayed in GIT1 KO mice. Histological analysis of fracture callus cartilage content was performed via Alcian Blue Hematoxylin/Orange G staining. Representative stains of calluses from WT and GIT1 KO mice at 1, 2 and 3 weeks post-fracture are displayed (A–F). Red arrows denote Alcian Blue-stained cartilagenous matrix and asterisks denote mineralized woven bone. Histomorphometry was performed on triplicate sections from multiple mice, with % Cartilage Area (G) and % Bone Area (H) quantified. Bars represent % Area (cartilage or bone) +/− SEM (*p<0.05, N=3).

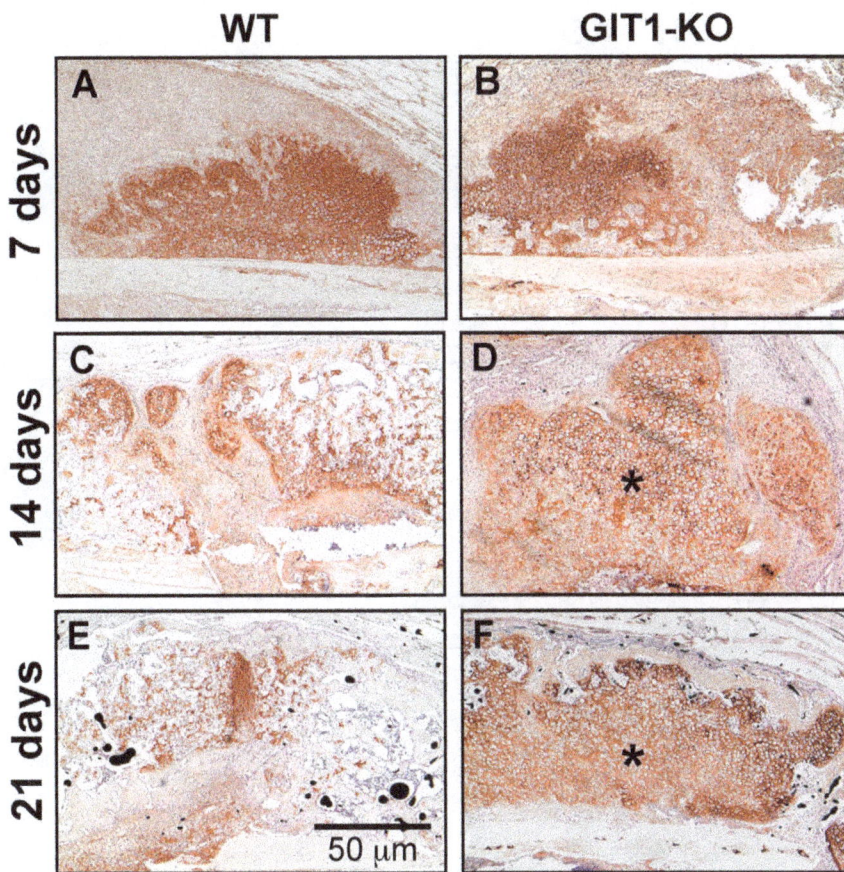

Figure 4. Type 2 collagen-containing matrix persists in GIT1 KO mice. Tissue sections cut from WT and GIT1 KO mice were analyzed for COL2A1 content using an immunohistochemistry approach. Representative stains at 7, 14 and 21 days post-fracture are depicted, with asterisks denoting areas within the callus at 2 and 3 weeks post-fracture in GIT1 KO mice (D and F respectively) that have more robust/persistent staining.

mice (Fig. 2D, red arrows indicating disjunction) compared to WT mice (Fig. 2C) at 14 days post-fracture, although quantification of mineralized callus volume in cohorts of animals failed to achieve significance at any timepoint, only revealing a trend toward a decrease (Fig. 2E).

Chondrocyte Maturation is Delayed in Fracture Callus of GIT1 KO Mice

Alcian Blue was used to stain extracellular matrix surrounding chondrocytes within the fracture callus, with representative sections depicted (Fig. 3A–F). At days 7 and 14 post-fracture, cartilage matrix content in WT mice (Fig. 3A and 3C) was similar to that in GIT1 KO mice (Fig. 3B and 3D). However, unlike in WT mice (Fig. 3E), cartilaginous callus in GIT1 KO mice was still present at day 21 (red arrows, Fig. 3F). Histomorphometric quantification of callus cartilage and bone content confirmed that at 21 days post-fracture, GIT1 KO mice had persistent cartilage (Fig. 3G) that was at the expense of woven bone (Fig. 3H).

To further examine the cartilage phenotype, we performed COL2A1 immunohistochemistry in WT and GIT1 KO mice at 7, 14 and 21 days post-fracture. Representative stained sections are displayed in Fig. 4, with GIT1 KO mice trending toward persistence of COL2A1 at 14 and 21 days (Fig. 4D and 4F) compared to matched sections from WT mice (Fig. 4C and 4E). These results suggest that cartilage persists in the fracture callus of GIT1 KO mice at the expense of woven bone formation.

Chondrocyte Proliferation and Apoptosis is Reduced in Fracture Callus of GIT1 KO Mice

To explore the possible association between persistent cartilagenous callus and changes in chondrocyte proliferation and apoptosis, we performed PCNA immunostaining and TUNEL immunofluorescence respectively. At days 7 and 14, PCNA-positive cells were more abundant in the cartilaginous soft callus of WT mice (Fig. 5A and 5C) relative to calluses from GIT1 KO mice (Fig. 5B and 5D). Histomorphometry confirmed this, establishing that GIT1 KO chondrocytes were less proliferative at 7 and 14 days post fracture (Fig. 5E). Regarding apoptosis, representative TUNEL-stained sections reveal that the percentage of TUNEL-positive cells (relative to DAPI) was reduced in GIT1 KO chondrocytes at both day 14 and 21 post-fracture (Fig. 6A–H). Again, this was confirmed quantitatively (Fig. 6I), indicating that GIT1 KO chondrocytes are less apoptotic during the time period of healing that normally involves remodeling of the cartilagenous callus (i.e. conversion to bone) and associated programmed death of chondrocytes. While GIT1 appears to have a role in modulating proliferation and death of chondrocytes, it is not clear how these combined phenotypes (reduced mitosis and death in the GIT1 KO group) account for the net persistence of the cartilagenous callus and the delay in its conversion to woven bone.

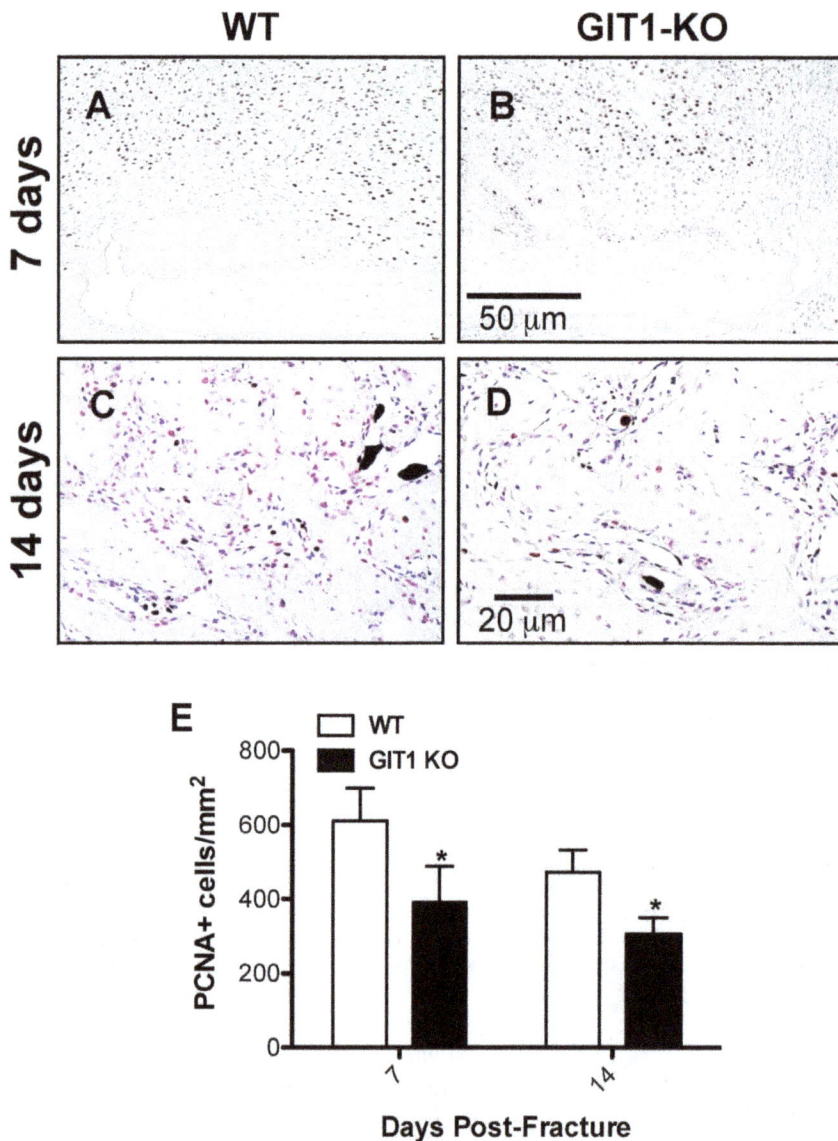

Figure 5. Chondrocyte proliferation is reduced in GIT1 KO mice. Representative PCNA staining is shown at 7 and 14 days post-fracture in WT mice (A and C) and at 7 (B) and 14 days (D) post-fracture in GIT1 KO mice (B and D respectively). Histomorphometry was performed on triplicate sections from multiple mice to quantify the number of PCNA-positive cells per unit callus area (E). The data is presented as mean of the number of PCNA positive cells/mm^2+/− SEM (*p<0.05, N=3).

Blood Vessel Volume and Number are Decreased in Fracture Callus of GIT1 KO Mice

Based on our previously published results demonstrating a pulmonary vascular deficit in GIT1 KO mice, we hypothesized that delayed bone repair in these animals could be due to impaired angiogenesis in the fracture callus. Therefore, we performed quantitative vascular microCT analyses to evaluate neovascularization at day 7, 14, and 21 post-fracture in WT and GIT1 KO mice. Representative reconstructions indicated reduced callus vascularity in KO mice compared to the WT cohort, with GIT1 KO mice displaying a marked reduction in vessel volume, number, and connectivity (Fig. 7A–F). These apparent changes were supported by quantifation of various vascular parameters, substantiating that compared to the WT cohort, GIT KO mice had reduced vessel volume (Fig. 7G), reduced vessel number (Fig. 7H), increased spacing between vessels (Fig. 7I) and reduced

connection density (Fig. 7J). It should be noted that the quantification of reduced vessel connectivity (i.e. connection density) is influenced by the efficiency of vessel perfusion with contrast agent, and there may not be adequate filling in vascular beds with smaller vessel diameters, reducing the accuracy of the connectivity algorithm and conclusions that are drawn from it.

Neovascularization is Impaired in the Fracture Callus of GIT1 KO Mice

To further evaluate angiogenesis, we analyzed vessel number using an antibody against PECAM1 (CD31), an endothelial cell marker. A strong signal was observed in vessels of the callus from WT mice at days 7 and 14 (Fig. 8A and 8C). In contrast, the number of PECAM1$^+$ vessels was dramatically reduced in GIT1 KO mice (Fig. 8B and 8D). Quantification of the number of blood vessels revealed a 60% reduction in GIT1 KO mice (Fig. 8E) at

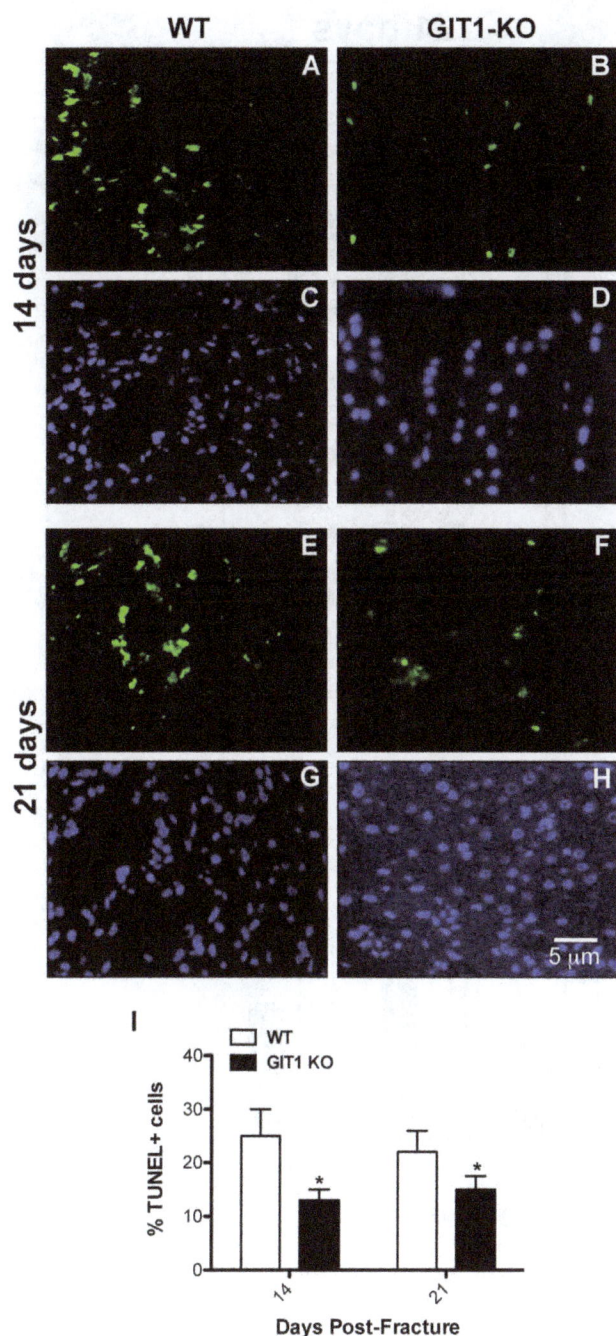

Figure 6. Chondrocyte TUNEL staining is reduced in GIT1 KO mice. Chondrocyte apoptosis was assessed in WT and GIT1 KO mice at 14 and 21 days post-fracture. Representative TUNEL immunofluorescence and DAPI staining at both time points is presented in WT mice (A/C and E/G respectively) and in GIT1 KO mice (B/D and F/H respectively). Quantitative histomorphometric analyses of the number of TUNEL-positive cells per unit area in triplicate sections from three WT and GIT1 KO mice at 14 and 21 days post-fracture are presented (I). Bars represent the percent of TUNEL positive cells/mm^2+/− SEM (*p<0.05, N = 3).

both 7 and 14 days post-fracture. In order to examine why vessel parameters (from the vascular microCT findings, Fig. 7) and vessel density (PECAM1) were lower in GIT1 KO mice, we first analyzed the amount of phospho-VEGFR2 expressed in the callus.

Compared to WT mice, the phospho-VEGFR2 positivity was reduced in GIT1 KO mice at 14 and 21 days post-fracture (Fig. 9A–D). Quantification in multiple mice from each cohort supported this, revealing a 50% reduction in GIT1 KO mice at days 14 and 21 (Fig. 9E). Since the active form of VEGF receptor was significantly decreased at 14 and 21 days, we next examined VEGF expression levels. Representative immunohistochemistry at 14 days post-fracture depicts reduced VEGF expression in GIT1 KO callus compared to WT controls (Fig. 9F–G). Taken together, these findings indicate that GIT1 is critical for VEGF induced microvessel sprouting in fracture callus, and GIT1 deficiency impairs neoangiogenesis in response to injury.

Osteoclast Number is Reduced in GIT1 KO Fracture Callus

As mentioned, alterations in callus chondrocyte proliferation and apoptosis cannot explain the healing phenotype seen in GIT1 KO mice. Since we have previously established that osteoclast differentiation and activity is impaired in GIT1 KO mice [24], we therefore focused on assessing osteoclast numbers. To assess osteoclast number, histology-based quantification of the number of TRAP-positive cells was performed in callus samples from both WT and GIT1 KO mice at days 7, 14 and 21 post-fracture. Although there was no difference in the number of the TRAP positive cells and the amount of cartilaginous callus (Alcian blue) between WT (Fig. 10A and 10C) and GIT1 KO mice (Fig. 10B and 10D) mice at day 7, differences were observed at days 14 and 21. The increased percentage of cartilaginous callus in GIT1 KO mice compared to WT mice at day 21 (Fig. 3) was concordant with what appeared to be a marginally decreased TRAP positivity in the GIT1 KO cohort at day 14 (Fig. 10C, 10D, 10G and 10H), and a significant decrease in TRAP staining at day 21 (Fig. 10E, 10F, 10G and 10H). This net reduction in osteoclast number in GIT1 KO mice could account for the larger amount/persistence of cartilage callus in these animals that we have observed via Alcian Blue staining (seen in both Fig. 10 and Fig. 3).

Discussion

Delayed and/or failed fracture repair are major public health issues that impact populations in the United States and throughout the world. Musculoskeletal deficits that result from delayed healing post-injury and post-surgery limits the performance of normal daily activities, compromises the function of various organ systems, and has a debilitating impact on psychological health and social function [35–41]. Given the scope of this public health crisis, it is the goal of researchers in the field to further understand the molecular basis for normal and pathologic healing with the aim of developing novel therapeutic strategies.

Endochondral-based healing, which predominates in the repair of long bones, requires the correct temporospatial coordination of a series of molecular and cellular events [42]. From a tissue architecture perspective, these events are organized into four overlapping phases – (1) inflammation, (2) soft (cartilaginous) callus formation, (3) resorption of cartilage and hard (woven bone) callus formation, and (4) woven bone remodeling. Mesenchymal stem cells (MSCs) and chondro−/osteo-progenitor populations that primarily reside in the periosteum are essential throughout fracture repair [43,44]. The transition from soft to hard callus requires angiogenesis, because increased tissue oxygen concentration is necessary for osteoprogenitors to mineralize the matrix. Additionally, functional osteoclasts are needed to remove the cartilage matrix during woven bone formation and to remodel the woven bone callus to ultimately recapitulate the normal structure of the injured element.

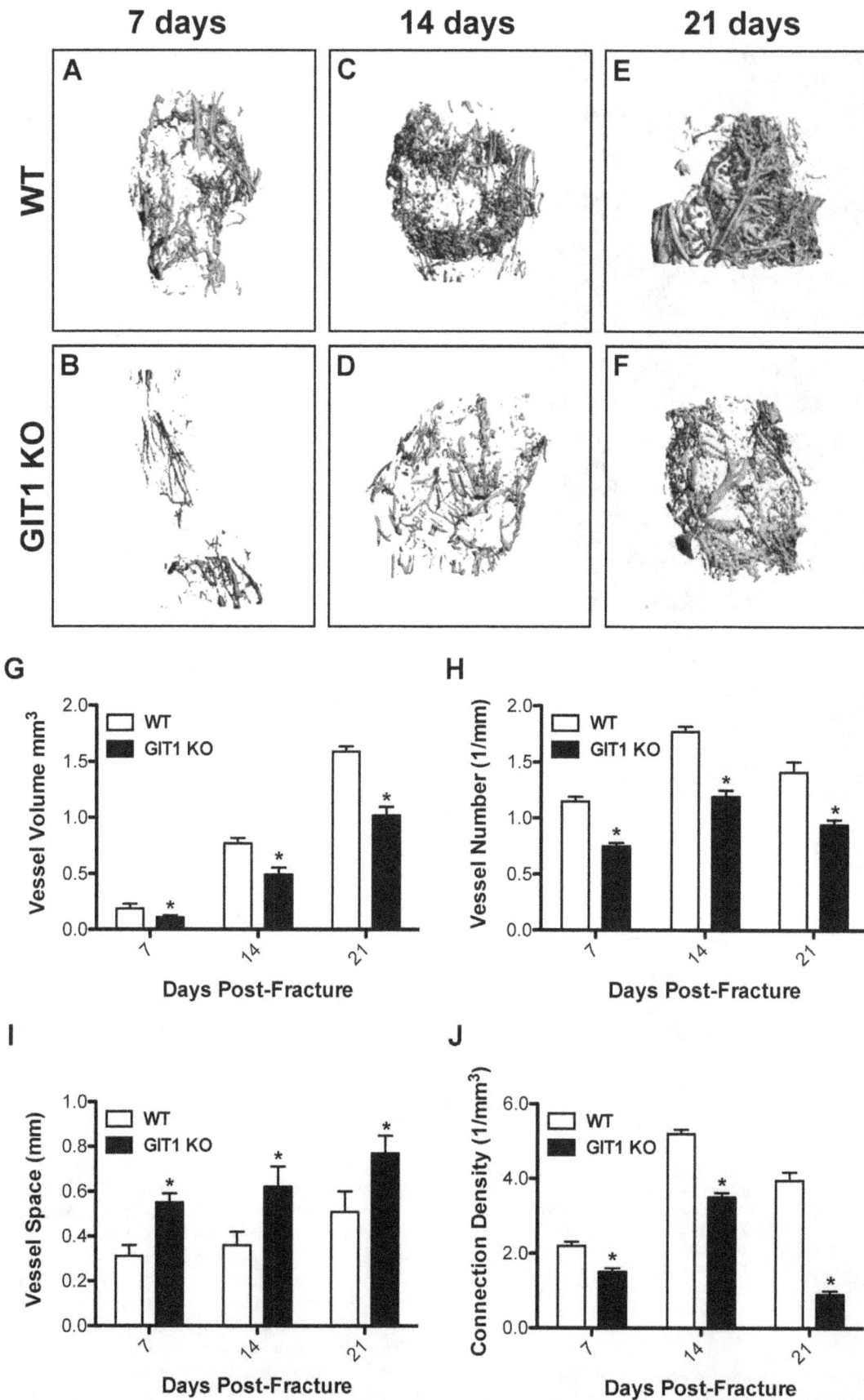

Figure 7. Fracture callus vascularity is reduced in GIT1 KO mice. To visualize and quantify callus vascularity, WT and GIT1 KO mice were perfused with lead chromate microfilm perfusion reagent. Harvested femora were decalcified and representative vascular microCT reconstructions

from each experimental group at 7, 14 and 21 days post-fracture are presented. Reduced vascularity in GIT1 KO mice (A, C, E) compared to WT control mice (B, D, F) was evident at all time points. Quantification of callus vascular parameters, including Vessel Volume (G), Vessel Number (H), Vessel Spacing (I) and Connection Density (J) supported these findings, with GIT1 KO mice possessing reduced callus vessel volume, vessel number and connection density and increased space between vessels compared to callus from WT mice. Bars represent mean for each value +/− SEM (N = 3, *p< 0.05).

Our group has recently documented a critical role for GIT1 in pulmonary vascular development [22] and in the formation of functional osteoclasts via regulation of sealing zone formation [24].

Given these unique roles for GIT1, both critical for normal tissue morphogenesis in fracture repair, we became interested in the function of this protein during the bone healing process. Based on

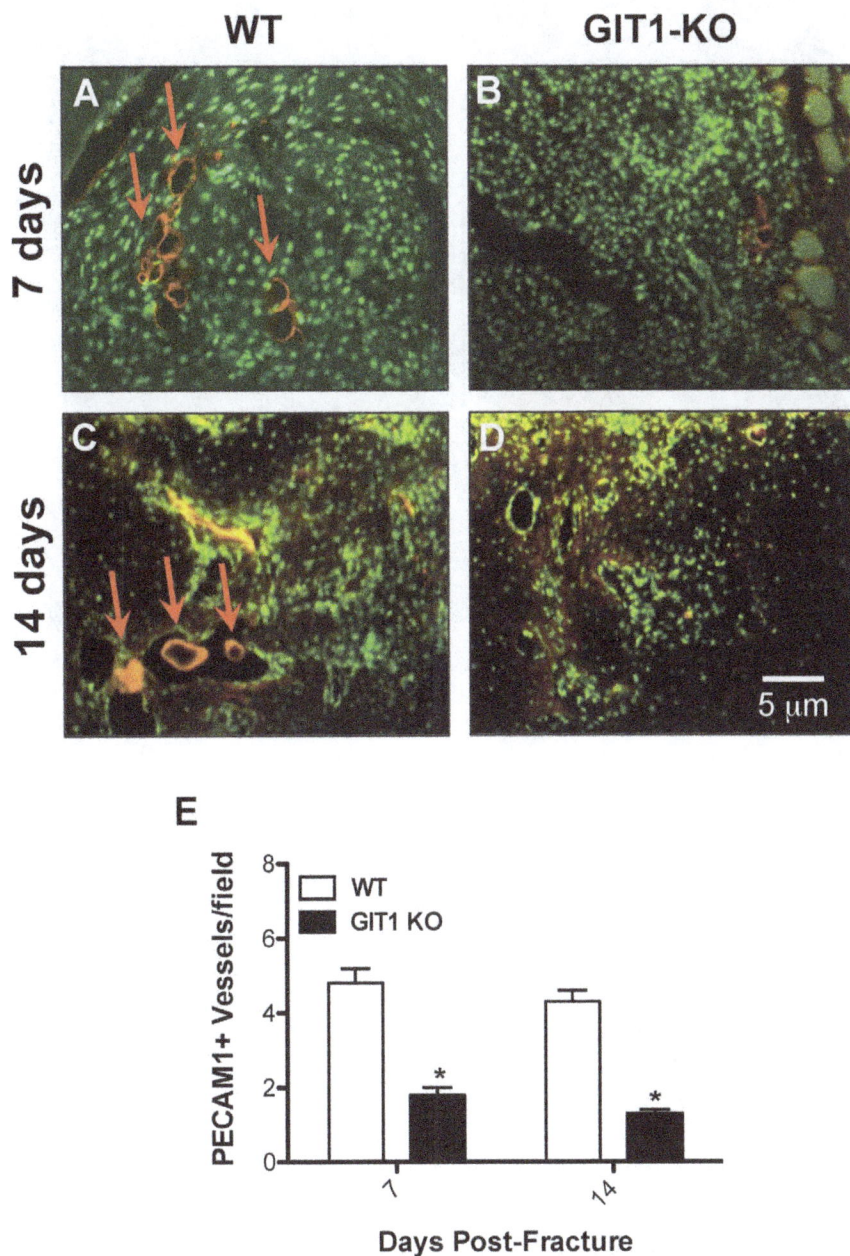

Figure 8. PECAM1+ blood vessel number is reduced in GIT1 KO mice. Representative PECAM1 immunofluorescence is presented at 7 and 14 days post-fracture in WT mice (A and C) and GIT1−/− mice (B and D). Histomorphometry was performed to quantify the average number of positively-stained blood vessels present in each field of view on each section analyzed. Three sections (from 3 levels within each callus, 25–50 μm apart) were viewed using the 10× objective, with counts being collected from 3 fields of view in each section. All counts from each callus (9 fields total) were averaged. Vessel counting using this approach confirmed the immunofluorescence in panels A–D, with WT calluses possessing between 2 and 3-fold more PECAM1+ vessels than GIT1 KO calluses at both time points (E). Bars represent mean number of PECAM1+ vessels/field +/− SEM (*p<0.01, N = 3).

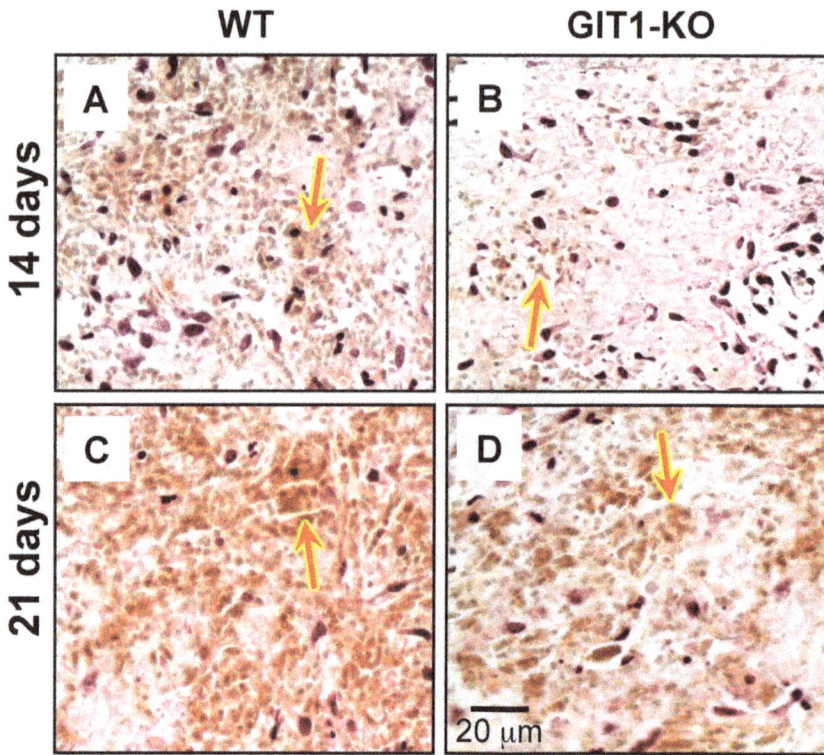

pVEGF Receptor

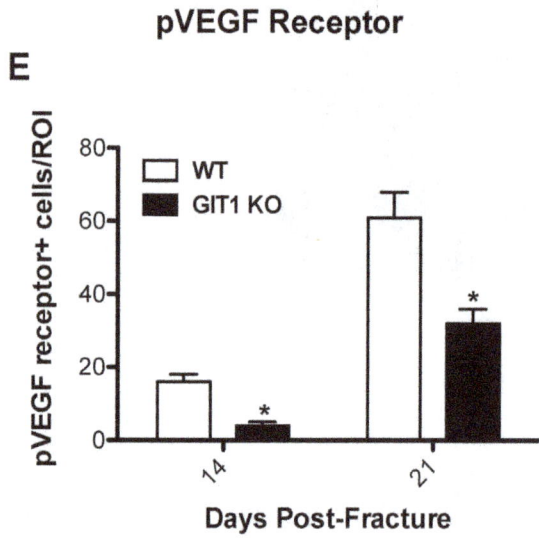

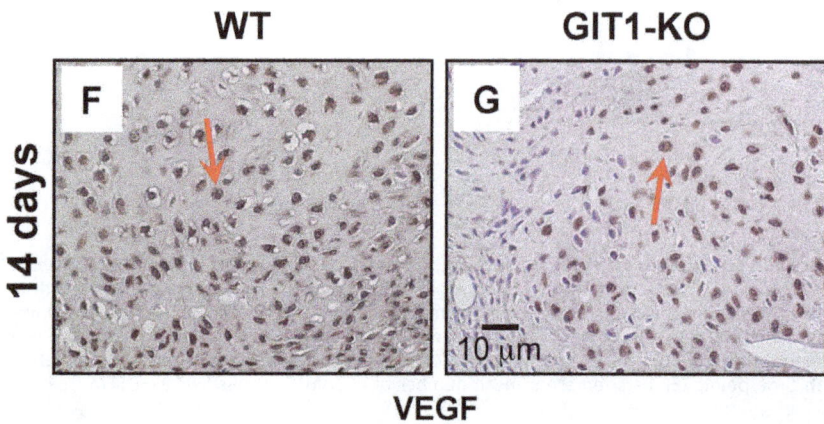

VEGF

Figure 9. VEGF signaling is reduced in GIT1 KO mice. Phospho-VEGF receptor immunostaining was performed on fracture calluses from WT and GIT1 KO mice at 2 and 3 weeks post-fracture. Panels A-D depict representative staining profiles, with Phospho-VEGF receptor-positive cells staining red as indicated by red arrows. Histomorphometry was performed to quantify the number of Phospho-VEGF receptor-positive cells per unit callus area (E). Data is presented as the mean number of positive cells per unit area (i.e. region of interest) +/− SEM (*p<0.01, N = 3). Additionally, immunohistochemistry was performed of assess VEGF levels in fracture calluses from WT (F) and GIT1 KO mice (G). Representative histological sections of calluses at 2 weeks post-fracture are presented, depicting reduced expression in KO mice. VEGF positive cells are stained reddish-brown as indicated by red arrows.

our previous work, we hypothesized that loss of GIT1 function will lead to delayed healing in a mouse model of femur fracture due to i) impaired neovascularization of the callus and ii) inhibited cartilage and woven bone remodeling due to reduced osteoclast number and/or function. Supporting this hypothesis, our results indicate that GIT1 deficiency leads to a fracture healing defect that is driven by two primary effects: altered neovascularization of the callus in early-mid stage healing, and reduced osteoclast number during primary and secondary callus remodeling.

Regarding blood vessels in the callus, successful bone repair requires the revascularization of injured tissues to provide oxygen, facilitate metabolic waste management, and deliver a population of circulating precursor cells that may contribute to healing either directly or in a paracrine manner. Angiogenesis during the repair process is thought to be modulated by VEGFs and their cognate receptors VEGFR1 and VEGFR2. It has been demonstrated that delivery of VEGF during mouse femur fracture healing enhances vascular ingrowth into the callus and accelerates repair by promoting bony bridging [45]. This has been confirmed in allograft bone healing, where VEGF gene therapy accelerates the healing process [26]. Conversely, inhibition of new blood vessel formation by injecting TNP-470, an endostatin-like anti-angiogenesis agent [46], prevented fracture healing in a rodent fracture model [17]. Here, we show for the first time that GIT1 may be an important regulator of angiogenesis during fracture repair, thus having a direct impact of the progression of the healing process. Previously we demonstrated that GIT1 is required for activation of PLC-γ and ERK1/2 in endothelial cells and osteoblasts, leading to the regulation of VEGF expression in osteoblasts through the GIT1-ERK1/2 signaling axis [47]. In the present study, we demonstrate that loss of GIT1 results in reduced VEGF expression and phospho-VEGFR2 (active form) in the fracture callus. We also found that GIT1 deficiency significantly decreased small vessel connectivity density and PECAM1 expression in the fracture callus. Correlated with this, vascular microCT analyses revealed reduced overall vessel volume, number and connection density coupled with increased spacing between vessels. These results suggest that the impaired fracture healing process in GIT1 KO mice is at least in part related to impaired VEGF-induced angiogenesis, implicating GIT1 as central regulator of angiogenesis in the context of bone healing.

In addition to the resulting vascular defect described above, the loss of GIT1 function likely also contributes to impaired fracture healing due to altered primary and secondary remodeling because of a defect in osteoclast formation and/or function. We have previously published that GIT1 is required for appropriate osteoclast function via its role in regulating cytoskeletal-related ruffled border and sealing zone formation [24]. Following the formation of the cartilagenous callus, an initial phase of osteoclast-driven remodeling removes the cartilage template, which is then replaced by mineralized woven bone matrix. This occurs in response to macrophage colony-stimulating factor (M-CSF), RANK ligand (RANKL) and osteoprotegerin (OPG) [6]. This initial woven bone matrix is subsequently replaced by organized lamellar bone through a second remodeling process that is the final step in achieving an anatomically correct skeletal element. This

second remodeling process is also governed by osteoclasts, which become dominant in this final stage due to the induction of IL-1 and TNF-α and the subsequent expansion of the functional osteoclast population [7,8] via RANKL in the remodeling callus [9]. In this report, histomorphometric analysis revealed persistent cartilaginous callus that could be the result of delayed cartilage matrix removal due to reduced osteoclast number (and possibly activity) in GIT1 deficient mice that was seen at day 14 and 21 (i.e. during primary and secondary callus remodeling). This phenotype could be related to both the reduced number of osteoclasts observed in the callus area as well as reduced formation of resorbing zones (ruffled border), a known phenotype following loss of GIT1 [24]. Overall, these findings suggest that osteoclast-dependent callus remodeling is likely at least partially impaired in GIT1 KO mice. The molecular basis of this effect may involve several mechanisms including altered RANKL and OPG expression, or cytoskeletal defects that alter osteoclast function, a subject requiring further study.

In addition to these central defects in fracture healing seen in GIT1 KO mice, we also observed an alteration in normal chondrogenic differentiation and cartilage persistence. While expression of Sox9, the master inducer of chondrogenesis, was not altered (data not shown), there was reduced chondrocyte proliferation and apoptosis (Fig. 7 and 8). This was in conjunction with enhanced Alcian Blue staining and cartilage persistence coupled with delayed woven bone formation (Fig. 5) and type 2 collagen immunoreactivity (Fig. 6). Since it is not known if there is a direct role for GIT1 in normal chondrocyte physiology, we postulate that these defects could be indirect and downstream of impaired neovascularization of the callus and/or reduced osteoclast formation and function. Further effort is required to determine any potential direct effects of GIT1 deficiency on chondrocyte differentiation.

In conclusion, data is presented in this report that supports a previously unappreciated role for GIT1 as a regulator of bone fracture healing. GIT1 deficiency leads to decreased revascularization of the fracture callus, decreased chondrocyte proliferation and apoptosis, and reduced osteoclast number. Since the fragility of the GIT1 KO model severely limited the completion of a full evaluation of healing including a higher N for histologic and microCT analyses, mRNA profiling of the callus to further establish molecular mechanism, and performance of biomechanical testing, further study into the role of GIT1 in fracture repair is required. The development of a floxed GIT1 KO model allowing temporal and tissue-specific gene ablation would facilitate the next step in the study of mechanism that would alleviate the high rate of mortality leading to the low number of mice available to populate the experimental groups included in this study. Despite this shortcoming, the results presented clearly define GIT1 as a contributor to bone repair. We speculate that agents targeting activation of GIT1 could be exploited to i) improve callus vascularization in the early phases of healing, and ii) accelerate osteoclast-driven remodeling steps, in particular the resorption of cartilagenous callus that is required to clear the path for deposition of woven bone and stabilization of the fracture site.

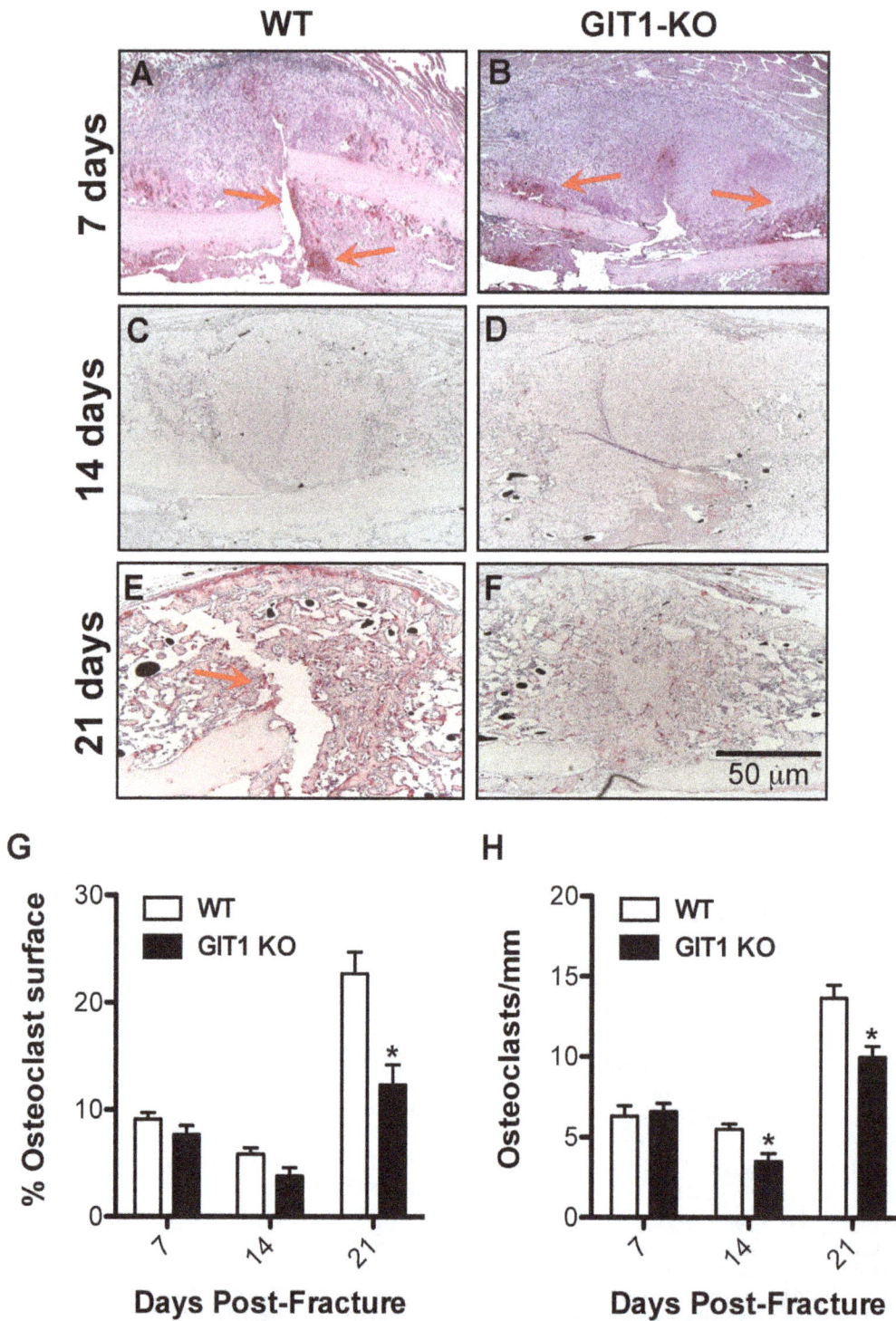

Figure 10. Osteoclast number is reduced in GIT1 KO mice. The presence of osteoclasts in the fracture callus of WT and GIT1 KO mice was assessed at 7 (A and B respectively), 14 (C and D respectively) and 21 days (E and F respectively) post-fracture via TRAP staining. Histomorphometry to quantify percentage of osteoclast surface (G) and osteoclast number per unit bone surface (H) was also performed on triplicate sections from multiple mice, with bars representing the mean for each parameter +/− SEM (*p<0.05, N=3).

Acknowledgments

We thank Dr. Tianfang Li and Dr. Yufeng Dong for helpful suggestions and thoughtful discussion of data, and we thank Michael Thullen for assistance with all microCT analysis of mineralized and vascular tissues.

Author Contributions

Conceived and designed the experiments: GY TJS MJZ BCB. Performed the experiments: GY TJS. Analyzed the data: GY TJS PM JP HH SS CX ES CY MJZ BCB. Contributed reagents/materials/analysis tools: GY TJS ES MJZ BCB. Wrote the paper: GY TJS.

References

1. Einhorn TA (1998) The cell and molecular biology of fracture healing. ClinOrthop: S7–21.

2. Gerstenfeld LC, Cullinane DM, Barnes GL, Graves DT, Einhorn TA (2003) Fracture healing as a post-natal developmental process: molecular, spatial, and temporal aspects of its regulation. JCell Biochem 88: 873–884.

3. Marsell R, Einhorn TA (2011) The biology of fracture healing. Injury 42: 551–555.

4. Thompson Z, Miclau T, Hu D, Helms JA (2002) A model for intramembranous ossification during fracture healing. Journal of Orthopaedic Research 20: 1091–1098.

5. Li G, White G, Connolly C, Marsh D (2002) Cell proliferation and apoptosis during fracture healing. J Bone Miner Res 17: 791–799.

6. Kon T, Cho TJ, Aizawa T, Yamazaki M, Nooh N, et al. (2001) Expression of osteoprotegerin, receptor activator of NF-kappaB ligand (osteoprotegerin ligand) and related proinflammatory cytokines during fracture healing. Journal of Bone and Mineral Research 16: 1004–1014.

7. Mountziaris PM, Mikos AG (2008) Modulation of the inflammatory response for enhanced bone tissue regeneration. Tissue Eng Part B Rev 14: 179–186.

8. Ai-Aql ZS, Alagl AS, Graves DT, Gerstenfeld LC, Einhorn TA (2008) Molecular mechanisms controlling bone formation during fracture healing and distraction osteogenesis. J Dent Res 87: 107–118.

9. Gerstenfeld LC, Sacks DJ, Pelis M, Mason ZD, Graves DT, et al. (2009) Comparison of effects of the bisphosphonate alendronate versus the RANKL inhibitor denosumab on murine fracture healing. J Bone Miner Res 24: 196–208.

10. Maes C, Kobayashi T, Selig MK, Torrekens S, Roth SI, et al. (2010) Osteoblast precursors, but not mature osteoblasts, move into developing and fractured bones along with invading blood vessels. Dev Cell 19: 329–344.

11. Pufe T, Wildemann B, Petersen W, Mentlein R, Raschke M, et al. (2002) Quantitative measurement of the splice variants 120 and 164 of the angiogenic peptide vascular endothelial growth factor in the time flow of fracture healing: a study in the rat. Cell Tissue Res 309: 387–392.

12. Eckardt H, Bundgaard KG, Christensen KS, Lind M, Hansen ES, et al. (2003) Effects of locally applied vascular endothelial growth factor (VEGF) and VEGF-inhibitor to the rabbit tibia during distraction osteogenesis. J Orthop Res 21: 335–340.

13. Ferguson C, Alpern E, Miclau T, Helms JA (1999) Does adult fracture repair recapitulate embryonic skeletal formation? Mechanisms of Development 87: 57–66.

14. Glowacki J (1998) Angiogenesis in fracture repair. Clin Orthop Relat Res: S82–89.

15. Gerber HP, Vu TH, Ryan AM, Kowalski J, Werb Z, et al. (1999) VEGF couples hypertrophic cartilage remodeling, ossification and angiogenesis during endochondral bone formation. NatMed 5: 623–628.

16. Athanasopoulos AN, Schneider D, Keiper T, Alt V, Pendurthi UR, et al. (2007) Vascular endothelial growth factor (VEGF)-induced up-regulation of CCN1 in osteoblasts mediates proangiogenic activities in endothelial cells and promotes fracture healing. Journal of Biological Chemistry 282: 26746–26753.

17. Hausman MR, Schaffler MB, Majeska RJ (2001) Prevention of fracture healing in rats by an inhibitor of angiogenesis. Bone 29: 560–564.

18. Premont RT, Claing A, Vitale N, Freeman JL, Pitcher JA, et al. (1998) beta2-Adrenergic receptor regulation by GIT1, a G protein-coupled receptor kinase-associated ADP ribosylation factor GTPase-activating protein. Proc Natl Acad Sci U S A 95: 14082–14087.

19. Natarajan K, Yin G, Berk BC (2004) Scaffolds direct Src-specific signaling in response to angiotensin II: new roles for Cas and GIT1. Mol Pharmacol 65: 822–825.

20. Haendeler J, Yin G, Hojo Y, Saito Y, Melaragno M, et al. (2003) GIT1 mediates Src-dependent activation of phospholipase Cgamma by angiotensin II and epidermal growth factor. J Biol Chem 278: 49936–49944.

21. Yin G, Haendeler J, Yan C, Berk BC (2004) GIT1 functions as a scaffold for MEK1-extracellular signal-regulated kinase 1 and 2 activation by angiotensin II and epidermal growth factor. Mol Cell Biol 24: 875–885.

22. Pang J, Hoefen R, Pryhuber GS, Wang J, Yin G, et al. (2009) G-protein-coupled receptor kinase interacting protein-1 is required for pulmonary vascular development. Circulation 119: 1524–1532.

23. Wang J, Taba Y, Pang J, Yin G, Yan C, et al. (2009) GIT1 mediates VEGF-induced podosome formation in endothelial cells: critical role for PLCgamma. Arterioscler Thromb Vasc Biol 29: 202–208.

24. Menon P, Yin G, Smolock EM, Zuscik MJ, Yan C, et al. (2010) GPCR kinase 2 interacting protein 1 (GIT1) regulates osteoclast function and bone mass. J Cell Physiol 225: 777–785.

25. Xie C, Liang B, Xue M, Lin AS, Loiselle A, et al. (2009) Rescue of impaired fracture healing in COX-2−/− mice via activation of prostaglandin E2 receptor subtype 4. AmJPathol 175: 772–785.

26. Ito H, Koefoed M, Tiyapatanaputi P, Gromov K, Goater JJ, et al. (2005) Remodeling of cortical bone allografts mediated by adherent rAAV-RANKL and VEGF gene therapy. NatMed 11: 291–297.

27. Zhang X, Xie C, Lin AS, Ito H, Awad H, et al. (2005) Periosteal progenitor cell fate in segmental cortical bone graft transplantations: implications for functional tissue engineering. Journal of Bone and Mineral Research 20: 2124–2137.

28. Dhillon RS, Xie C, Tyler W, Calvi LM, Awad HA, et al. (2013) PTH-enhanced structural allograft healing is associated with decreased angiopoietin-2-mediated arteriogenesis, mast cell accumulation, and fibrosis. J Bone Miner Res 28: 586–597.

29. Duvall CL, Taylor WR, Weiss D, Guldberg RE (2004) Quantitative microcomputed tomography analysis of collateral vessel development after ischemic injury. Am J Physiol Heart Circ Physiol 287: H302–310.

30. Zhang X, Schwarz EM, Young DA, Puzas JE, Rosier RN, et al. (2002) Cyclooxygenase-2 regulates mesenchymal cell differentiation into the osteoblast lineage and is critically involved in bone repair. JClinInvest 109: 1405–1415.

31. Naik AA, Xie C, Zuscik MJ, Kingsley P, Schwarz EM, et al. (2009) Reduced COX-2 expression in aged mice is associated with impaired fracture healing. Journal of Bone and Mineral Research 24: 251–264.

32. Konishi H, Wu J, Cooke JP (2010) Chronic exposure to nicotine impairs cholinergic angiogenesis. Vasc Med 15: 47–54.

33. Arasapam G, Scherer M, Cool JC, Foster BK, Xian CJ (2006) Roles of COX-2 and iNOS in the bony repair of the injured growth plate cartilage. J Cell Biochem 99: 450–461.

34. Boyce BF, Xing L (2008) Functions of RANKL/RANK/OPG in bone modeling and remodeling. Arch Biochem Biophys 473: 139–146.

35. Alarcon T, Gonzalez-Montalvo JI, Gotor P, Madero R, Otero A (2011) Activities of daily living after hip fracture: profile and rate of recovery during 2 years of follow-up. Osteoporos Int 22: 1609–1613.

36. Brenneman SK, Barrett-Connor E, Sajjan S, Markson LE, Siris ES (2006) Impact of recent fracture on health-related quality of life in postmenopausal women. J Bone Miner Res 21: 809–816.

37. Ding R, McCarthy ML, Houseknecht E, Ziegfeld S, Knight VM, et al. (2006) The health-related quality of life of children with an extremity fracture: a one-year follow-up study. J Pediatr Orthop 26: 157–163.

38. Giannoudis PV, Harwood PJ, Kontakis G, Allami M, Macdonald D, et al. (2009) Long-term quality of life in trauma patients following the full spectrum of tibial injury (fasciotomy, closed fracture, grade IIIB/IIIC open fracture and amputation). Injury 40: 213–219.

39. Lonnroos E, Kautiainen H, Sund R, Karppi P, Hartikainen S, et al. (2009) Utilization of inpatient care before and after hip fracture: a population-based study. Osteoporos Int 20: 879–886.

40. Olerud P, Ahrengart L, Soderqvist A, Saving J, Tidermark J (2010) Quality of life and functional outcome after a 2-part proximal humeral fracture: a prospective cohort study on 50 patients treated with a locking plate. J Shoulder Elbow Surg 19: 814–822.

41. Silverman SL, Shen W, Minshall ME, Xie S, Moses KH (2007) Prevalence of depressive symptoms in postmenopausal women with low bone mineral density and/or prevalent vertebral fracture: results from the Multiple Outcomes of Raloxifene Evaluation (MORE) study. J Rheumatol 34: 140–144.

42. Schindeler A, McDonald MM, Bokko P, Little DG (2008) Bone remodeling during fracture repair: The cellular picture. Semin Cell Dev Biol 19: 459–466.

43. Zhang X, Naik A, Xie C, Reynolds D, Palmer J, et al. (2005) Periosteal stem cells are essential for bone revitalization and repair. JMusculoskeletNeuronalInteract 5: 360–362.

44. Zuscik MJ, O'Keefe RJ (2009) Skeletal Healing. In: Rosen CJ, editor. Primer on the Metabolic Bone Diseases and Disorders of Mineral Metabolism: American Society of Bone and Mineral Research. 61–65.

45. Street J, Bao M, deGuzman L, Bunting S, Peale FV Jr, et al. (2002) Vascular endothelial growth factor stimulates bone repair by promoting angiogenesis and bone turnover. ProcNatlAcadSciUSA 99: 9656–9661.

46. Moulton KS, Heller E, Konerding MA, Flynn E, Palinski W, et al. (1999) Angiogenesis inhibitors endostatin or TNP-470 reduce intimal neovascularization and plaque growth in apolipoprotein E-deficient mice. Circulation 99: 1726–1732.

47. Rui Z, Li X, Fan J, Ren Y, Yuan Y, et al. (2012) GIT1Y321 phosphorylation is required for ERK1/2- and PDGF-dependent VEGF secretion from osteoblasts to promote angiogenesis and bone healing. Int J Mol Med 30: 819–825.

3

Coffee Consumption and Risk of Fracture in the Cohort of Swedish Men (COSM)

Helena Hallström[1,3], **Alicja Wolk**[2], **Anders Glynn**[3], **Karl Michaëlsson**[1], **Liisa Byberg**[1]*

1 Department of Surgical Sciences, Section of Orthopaedics, Uppsala University, Uppsala, Sweden, **2** Institute of Environmental Medicine, Division of Nutritional Epidemiology, Karolinska Institutet, Stockholm, Sweden, **3** Risk and Benefit Assessment Department, National Food Agency, Uppsala, Sweden

Abstract

Background: Recent research in a large cohort of women showed that coffee consumption is not associated with increased risk of fracture. Whether this is the case also among men is less clear.

Methods: In the Cohort of Swedish Men (COSM) study, 42,978 men aged 45–79 years old at baseline in 1997 answered a self-administered food frequency questionnaire covering coffee consumption and a medical and lifestyle questionnaire covering potential confounders. Our main outcomes first fracture at any site and first hip fracture were collected from the National Patient Registry in Sweden. The association between coffee consumption and fracture risk was investigated using Cox's proportional hazards regression.

Results: During a mean follow-up of 11.2 years, 5,066 men had a first fracture at any site and of these, 1,186 (23%) were hip fractures. There was no association between increasing coffee consumption (per 200 ml) and rate of any fracture (hazard ratio [HR] 1.00; 95% confidence interval [CI] 0.99–1.02) or hip fracture (HR 1.02; 95% CI 0.99–1.06) after adjustment for potential confounders. For men consuming ≥4 cups of coffee/day compared to those consuming <1 cup of coffee/day, HR for any type of fracture was 0.91 (95% CI 0.80–1.02) and for hip fracture: 0.89 (95% CI 0.70–1.14).

Conclusions: High coffee consumption was not associated with an increased risk of fractures in this large cohort of Swedish men.

Editor: Bamidele O. Tayo, Loyola University Medical Center, United States of America

Funding: This work was funded by the Swedish Research Council. The funder had no role in study design, data collection and analysis, decision to publish, or preparation of the manuscript.

Competing Interests: The authors have declared that no competing interests exist.

* E-mail: liisa.byberg@surgsci.uu.se

Introduction

Osteoporotic fractures - the ultimate manifestation of osteoporosis - are affecting a growing number of elderly individuals globally [1]. Both men and women are affected by osteoporosis, but despite a lower risk of osteoporotic fractures in men, the morbidity and mortality seem to be greater in men having experienced such fractures [2].

A number of dietary factors have been discussed in the aetiology of osteoporosis, including consumption of caffeine-containing beverages [3–6], especially coffee, which has a relatively high concentration of caffeine [7]. Some studies have demonstrated an association between caffeine intake and calcium homeostasis in humans [8,9] and negative effects on osteoblast function in vitro [10–12]. Epidemiological studies investigating the relation between coffee, tea consumption and caffeine intake and the risk of fractures are fairly abundant in women but scarce in men. Results from the three previous cohort studies in men have shown no association [13,14], and a decreased risk of fracture [15], also summarized in a recent meta-analysis [16].

The incidence of fractures is high in Sweden, also among men [17]. In an international comparison intake of coffee (and thus intake of caffeine) is similarly high in Sweden [18]. Thus, studying the relation between coffee consumption and the risk of fractures in Sweden may be optimal [19]. We recently published results from the so far largest epidemiological study concerning coffee consumption and fracture risk in women. We found that whereas a high coffee consumption is associated with slightly lower bone mineral density (BMD), this is not manifested in an increased risk of fracture [20]. We have also previously demonstrated an association between high coffee consumption and a decrease in bone mineral density (BMD) in older men [21]. Importantly, however, fractures in elderly are not only the consequence of osteoporosis but factors related to the risk of falling are also of importance [22,23].

The primary aim of this investigation was to study the association between coffee intake and the risk of incident fractures in a large prospective population-based cohort of Swedish men 45–79 years old at the beginning of the study. A secondary aim was to evaluate whether risk of fracture in relation to coffee consumption was affected by calcium intake.

Methods

Study Population

The Cohort of Swedish Men (COSM) was created in the autumn of 1997 [24]. All male residents (n = 100,303, aged 45–79 years) of Örebro and Västmanland Counties in central Sweden were invited to participate in the study. Along with the invitation, they received written information about the study and a self-administered questionnaire that included almost 350 items on diet and other lifestyle factors (e.g., socio-demographic data, waist and hip circumference, total physical activity, self-perceived health status, smoking status, alcohol consumption and use of dietary supplements).

Of the invited 100,303 men, 48,850 (49%) returned the questionnaire. The COSM is regarded as representative of Swedish men in this age range in terms of distribution of age, educational level and prevalence of overweight. From the baseline population, participants with incorrect or incomplete national registration numbers (n = 205) and those who reported an implausible energy intake (±3 SD of mean log-transformed energy, n = 567) were excluded. In addition, the following categories were excluded: men diagnosed with cancer other than non-melanoma skin cancer (n = 2,592) before baseline at 1 January 1998 or men who had passed away before 1 January 1998, as based on computerised linkage of the cohort to the National Cancer Register and the Population Register. Finally, we excluded an additional 2,361 men from the analyses in that these individuals had not stated their consumption of coffee even though non-use was a response possibility. Thus, the final sample for inclusion in the study was 42,978 men (Figure 1).

Written informed consent was obtained from the study participants and the study was approved by the Regional Ethical Review Board at Karolinska Institutet, Stockholm, Sweden.

Dietary Assessment

Using a 96-item food frequency questionnaire (FFQ), dietary intake data were assessed at baseline (1997). Average frequency of consumption of coffee (number of cups consumed per day or week) during the previous year was recorded by the participants. Eight possible categories were used to report consumption frequency: never/seldom, 1–3 times per month, 1–2 times per week, 3–4 times per week, 5–6 times per week, once a day, 2 times a day and ≥3 times per day.

To calculate intake of nutrients the frequency of consumption of each food item was multiplied by the nutrient content of appropriate age-specific portion sizes obtained from the Swedish Food Agency Database [25]. Adjustment of nutrient intake using the residual method [26] was performed for total energy intake (2,200 kcal, which was the mean in men in the validation study of the FFQ [27], see below). The cup size was standardized to 200 ml (200 g) of coffee beverage. The FFQ-based information on coffee has been validated against data from fourteen 24-hour recall interviews over 1 year in a group of 248 men (Spearman's correlation coefficient = 0.71) [28].

Ascertainment of Fractures

Ascertainment was made of all first incident cases of any fracture (International Classification of Disease [ICD-10] codes S02, S12, S22, S32, S42, S52, S62, S72, S82, S92) and first incident cases of hip fracture (ICD-10 codes S720, S721, S722) registered in the National Patient Register [29] and regional hospital diagnosis registers between 1 January 1998 and 31 December 2010. Complete matching is enabled by use of the

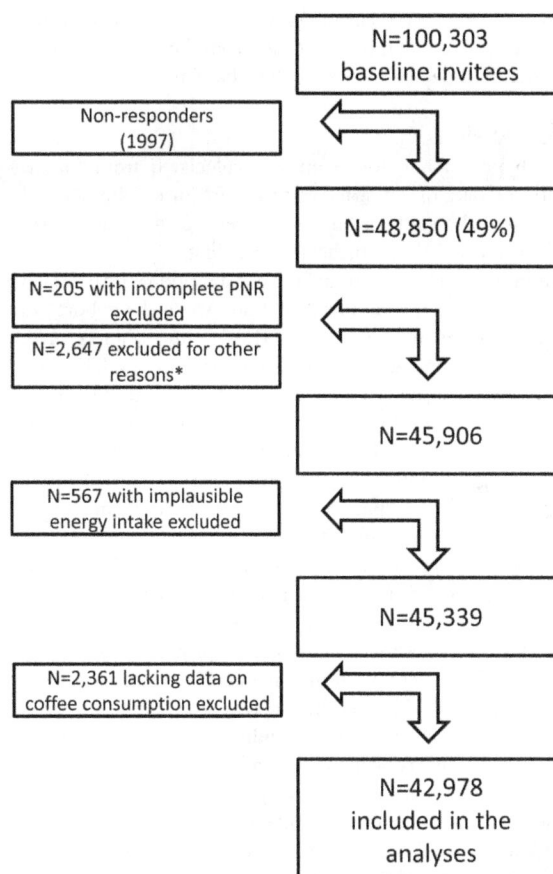

Figure 1. A flow chart describing the Cohort of Swedish Men (COSM). *Reasons for exclusions were: erroneous personal identification number, questionnaires not dated, erroneous dates of moving out of the study area or death, and a cancer diagnosis (except for non-melanoma skin cancer and only before the baseline questionnaire). Implausible energy intake was defined as ±3SD from the mean value of the log-transformed reported energy intake. Finally, individuals with lacking data on coffee consumption were excluded in the analyses. PNR: personal identification number.

unique personal registration number provided to all Swedish citizens.

Lifestyle and Comorbidity

Information about lifestyle variables, such as height (at age 20 years), weight, education, civil status, employment, alcohol consumption, smoking habits, cortisone use and physical activity, was obtained from the questionnaire.

According to five predefined categories, the participants recorded occupational physical activity, home/housework, walking/cycling duration per day and exercise duration per week during the past year before they were enrolled in the study [30]. To calculate total physical activity the reported time spent at each activity per day was multiplied by its typical energy expenditure requirements expressed in metabolic equivalents (MET). MET, expressed as kcal/kg/h, is the metabolic equivalent of sitting quietly for 1 hour [30]. The total sum of MET hours was used to create a MET (24-hour) score per day [30]. This variable was used in the statistical analyses. Validation of this method has been carried out and the Spearman correlation coefficient between the questionnaire and the activity records was 0.6 for the total activity score [30,31]. Smoking habits were reported as smoking status (never, past, current). We calculated Charlson's weighted comorbidity index [32,33] based on diagnoses from the National Patient Register that had been registered before baseline.

Statistical Analysis

For each participant, follow-up was calculated from January 1998 until the date of any fracture or hip fracture, date of death, date of leaving the study regions or the end of the study period (31st of December 2010), whichever came first.

When individual data on coffee consumption were lacking (n = 2,361/45,339, corresponding to about 5% of the cohort), the participants affected were not retained as non-consumers in the analyses. It was found to be more appropriate to exclude them from the analyses because in a previous study [34] only 11% of the missing cases for coffee consumption were actually non-consumers. In the event individual data were lacking for covariates other than coffee consumption, multiple imputations were performed by applying the Markov Chain Monte Carlo multiple method to construct baseline values (all <5%).

To analyse the relation between consumption of coffee and risk of first fracture event (any fracture and hip fracture), crude- and multivariable-adjusted hazard ratios (HR) and 95% confidence intervals (CI) were estimated by Cox's proportional hazards regression. Analyses were performed with coffee consumption as a continuous variable, with each unit corresponding to 200 ml (or one cup) of coffee. To compare our results with previous studies we also categorised coffee consumption into four categories (<1, 1, 2–3 and ≥4 cups daily). We further investigated the influence of very high coffee intake, i.e. ≥8 cups of coffee/day. For each category of coffee intake, age-adjusted failure curves (set at age 60 years corresponding to the mean baseline value) to illustrate fracture incidences were constructed by using the Kaplan-Meier method. Log-log plots for confirmation of the proportionality assumption were produced. The basic model used to estimate HRs included age. A multivariable model additionally included intakes of total energy, calcium, retinol, vitamin D, potassium, phosphorus, protein and alcohol, body mass index, height, physical activity (MET 24-hour score) (all continuous), intake of any vitamins, cortisone use, educational level (≤9, 12, >12 years, other), smoking status (never, former, current), previous fractures (yes or no) and Charlson's comorbidity index (continuous) [32,33]. Because intake of sleeping pills and 5α-reductase inhibitors or α1-receptor antagonists (indication mainly benign prostatic hyperplasia) only marginally affected the relations, these potential covariates were not included in the final multivariate model.

To analyse potential non-linear trends restricted cubic-spline Cox's regression analyses were performed to flexibly model the associations between coffee intake and fracture risk [35]. Four knots placed at percentiles 5, 35, 65 and 95 of coffee consumption were used. The reference level was set to the lowest category of coffee intake (<1 cup of coffee/day). The results of these analyses are presented as smoothed curves with 95% CIs.

Statistical interactions between coffee consumption and calcium intake or age were assessed by creating a product term of the two and assessing whether this contributed to improved model fit by likelihood ratio testing. These interactions were further evaluated by performing stratified analyses using pre-defined cut-offs for calcium intake (below or above 800 mg/day, the recommended intake in Sweden) and for age (<50, 50–70 and ≥70 years).

All statistical analyses were performed using Stata version 11 (Stata Corp LP, Collage Station, TX, USA).

Results

Baseline characteristics of the cohort are shown in Table 1. Forty-three per cent of the participants reported a daily consumption of 2–3 cups per day and 41% consumed 4 cups of coffee or more daily. The remaining 16% consumed 1 cup of coffee or less daily. In contrast, the consumption of tea was low. Among tea drinkers (57% of the participants in the cohort), 77% consumed 1 cup of tea or less per day.

A first fracture at any site was observed in 5,066 participants (11.8% of the cohort) during a median of 11.3 years of follow-up and 483,508 person years. During a median of 11.7 years of follow-up for hip fractures, there were 1,186 incident cases (2.8% of the cohort). For each category of coffee consumption (<1, 1, 2–3 and ≥4 cups per day), the age-adjusted incidence proportions of any fracture and hip fracture during follow-up are depicted in Figure 2. Smoking was more prevalent in the highest consumption category of coffee (≥4 cups daily) in comparison with categories with lower coffee consumption. Energy intake was somewhat higher in the category of participants drinking ≥4 cups of coffee daily than in the reference category.

When coffee exposure served as a continuous variable, no association was noted between increasing coffee consumption and rate of any fracture (HR 1.00; 95% CI 0.99–1.02) or hip fracture (HR 1.02; 95% CI 0.99–1.06) per 200 ml of coffee after multivariate adjustment. Similarly, no associations were found between increasing consumption and rate of any fracture or hip fracture after categorising coffee consumption into the four categories. HR for any fracture for men consuming ≥4 cups vs. <1 cup per day was 0.91 (95% CI 0.80–1.02) after multivariate adjustment. For hip fracture, the corresponding HR was 0.89 (95% CI 0.70–1.14) (Table 2).

Moreover, even a consumption of eight cups of coffee or more per day, in comparison with <1 cup per day, was not associated with an increased risk of any fracture (HR 0.92; 95% CI 0.77–1.02) or hip fracture (HR 0.94; 95% CI 0.64–1.38). The prevalence of high consumption (≥8 cups) was 3.0%.

As shown in Figure 3, no non-linear associations between consumption of coffee and incidence of any fracture or hip fracture could be observed.

We observed no indication of the presence of effect modification by calcium intake on the association between coffee consumption and fracture risk (P = 0.46 for any fracture and P = 0.28 for hip fracture). There was no indication of an interaction between age and coffee consumption (P = 0.11 for any fracture and P = 0.28 for hip fracture). The stratified analyses gave similar results as the full analysis (not shown).

Discussion

No significant association was found between consumption of coffee and incidence of fractures in this large prospective cohort of Swedish men. Furthermore, this result was not modified by either calcium intake or age.

The results from this investigation in men are in line with the results in our recent study of a large cohort of Swedish women. In this study a coffee consumption of ≥4 cups daily was associated with a decrease in BMD, but this decrease did not translate into an increased risk of fractures [20]. We previously observed lower BMD of the proximal femur with higher consumption of coffee in men [21]. Epidemiological research in men regarding coffee consumption and risk of fracture is rather scarce. The male part of the multicentre MEDOS case-control study by Kanis et al, 1999 [36], collected 730 hip fracture cases and 1,132 controls from Southern Europe. In this study no

Table 1. Baseline characteristics of study subjects by coffee consumption.

	Number of cups of coffee per day			
	<1 cup	1 cup	2–3 cups	≥4 cups
N (%)	2,318 (5.4)	4,514 (10.5)	18,366 (42.7)	17,780 (41.4)
Age at entry (yrs)	60.1 (9.6)	61.8 (9.6)	61.3 (9.8)	58.8 (9.4)
BMI at entry (kg/m^2)	25.7 (3.7)	26.0 (3.4)	25.7 (3.3)	25.9 (3.3)
Average intake per day[a]				
Energy (kcal)	2,522 (879)	2,522 (879)	2,577 (775)	2,846 (852)
Calcium (mg)	1,416 (496)	1,423 (454)	1,458 (452)	1,495 (475)
Supplemental Calcium (mg)[b]	315 (485)	281 (380)	261 (332)	267 (394)
Total calcium[c]	1,457 (533)	1,453 (481)	1,485 (469)	1,518 (492)
Vitamin D (µg)	6.44 (3.01)	6.80 (3.60)	6.65 (2.97)	6.62 (2.80)
Retinol (µg)	1,751 (894)	1,804 (1019)	1,754 (872)	1719 (878)
Potassium (mg)	3,827 (703)	3,871 (680)	3,941 (640)	4,086 (669)
Protein (g)	102.0 (16.2)	102.2 (15.4)	102.1 (14.8)	102.7 (15.1)
Phosphorus (mg)	2043 (353)	2048 (333)	2068 (332)	2080 (349)
Alcohol (g)[d]	7.7 (22.3)	9.3 (19.7)	8.9 (20.0)	9.2 (21.4)
Coffee (g)[d]	84 (58)	212 (55)	552 (113)	999 (377)
Tea (g)[d,e]	273 (485)	271 (352)	253 (294)	117 (295)
Leisure time PA level, n (%)				
1 (lowest)	214 (9.8)	500 (11.9)	1,627 (9.4)	1,873 (11.4)
2	404 (18.6)	714 (17)	2,913 (16.9)	2,598 (18)
3	801 (36.7)	1,517 (36)	6,508 (37.7)	5,963 (36.3)
4 (highest)	761 (34.9)	1,481 (35.2)	6,199 (35.9)	5,648 (34.4)
Smoking status, n (%)				
Current	394 (17.3)	795 (17.8)	3,778 (20.8)	5,684 (32.5)
Former	835 (36.6)	1,769 (39.6)	7,214 (39.8)	6,847 (39.1)
Never	1,051 (46.1)	1,901 (42.6)	7,149 (39.4)	4,986 (28.5)
Two or more Charlson's comorbidities, n (%)	133 (5.7)	260 (5.8)	820 (4.5)	598 (3.4)
Educational level, n (%)[f]				
≤9 years	1,423 (61.7)	3,036 (67.5)	12,534 (68.5)	12,790 (72.1)
>9–12 years	1,363 (15.7)	652 (14.5)	2,532 (13.8)	2,377 (13.4)
>12 years	510 (22.1)	792 (17.6)	3,160 (17.3)	2,503 (14.1)
Other	110 (0.4)	21 (0.5)	77 (0.4)	65 (0.4)
Fracture before baseline, n (%)	327 (14.1)	515 (11.4)	2,184 (11.9)	2,176 (12.2)
Proscar use, n (%)	160 (2.6)	152 (3.4)	1,493 (2.7)	1,366 (2.1)
Cortisone use, n (%)	130 (5.6)	192 (4.3)	1,725 (4.0)	1, 732 (4.1)
Marital status, single, n (%)	566 (29.4)	910 (20.2)	3,023 (16.5)	3,013 (17.0)

Data shown are mean (SD) or n (%) where indicated.
[a]Energy-adjusted average nutrient data,
[b]Users of calcium supplements,
[c]All participants – mean values for calcium supplements were used,
[d]Median(SD),
[e]Number reporting consumption of tea: 22,942,
[f]Educational level "other" refers to vocational or other education.

association between past coffee consumption or caffeine intake recalled after the fracture event and the risk of hip fracture was demonstrated. In a study by Kiel *et al* [13], a part of the Framingham cohort was investigated to assess intake of caffeine and risk of hip fracture. In males, caffeine intake corresponding to two cups of coffee or four cups of tea was associated with an increased risk of hip fracture, although this was not statistically significant and based on a limited number of fractures (n = 22).

In a large Norwegian cohort study including over 20,000 men with mean age 47 years, dietary factors in relation to hip fracture incidence were examined [14]. With 11 years of follow-up and 56 incident hip fracture cases, the authors did not observe an association between coffee intake and fracture risk. In a prospective cohort of Swedish middle-aged men (n = 7,495) followed for 30 years and aiming at identifying risk factors for hip fracture, Trimpou *et al* [15] found that coffee consumption

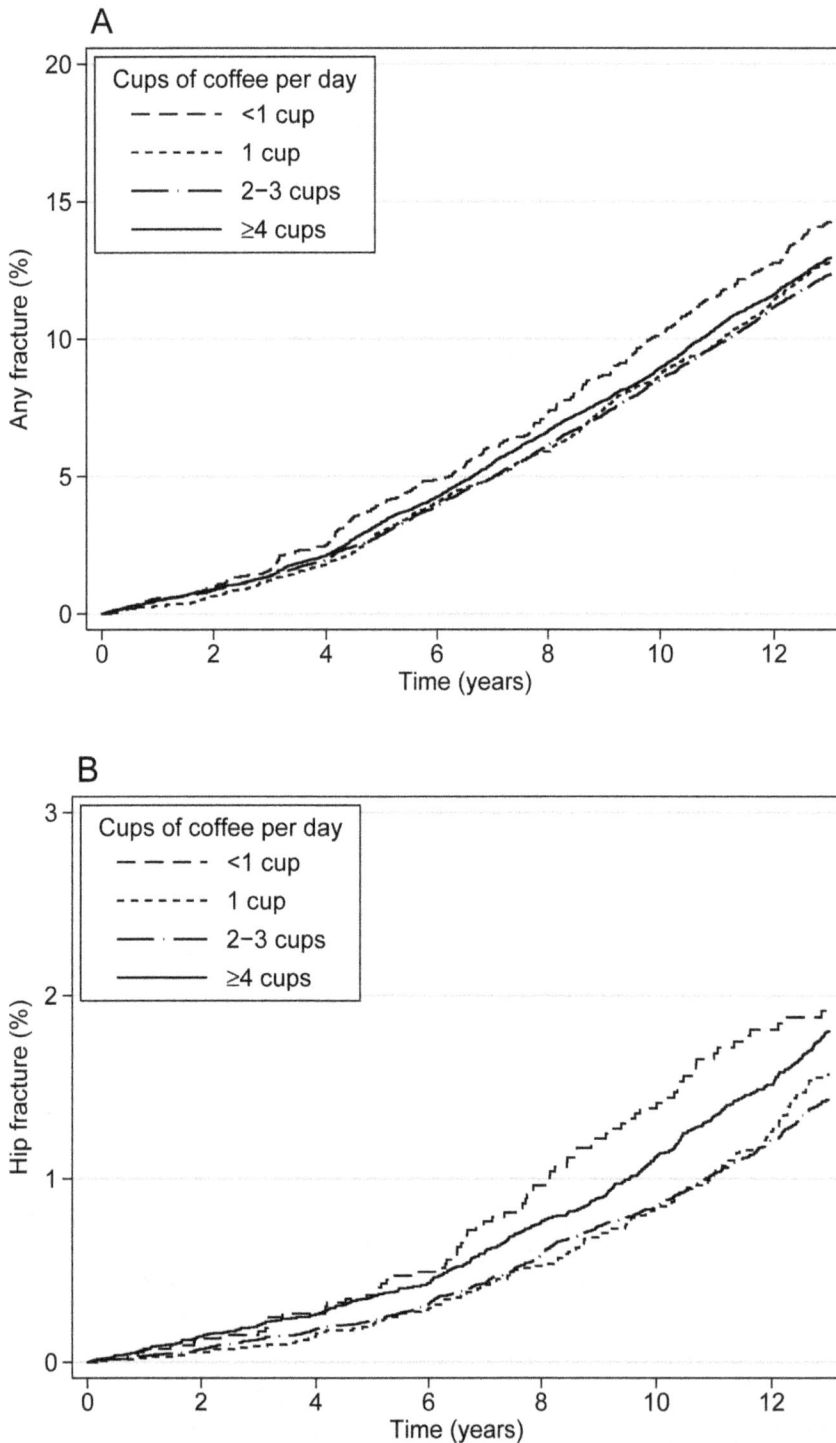

Figure 2. Fracture incidence in the Cohort of Swedish Men (COSM). Incidences of any fracture (Panel A) and hip fracture (Panel B) in relation to follow-up using Kaplan-Meier failure curves adjusted to age 60 for the four consumption categories of coffee (<1, 1, 2–3 and 4 cups or more per day).

was associated with a lower risk of hip fracture (n fractures = 451). There seemed not to be a dose-response effect in the unadjusted analysis and in the multivariate analysis, coffee consumption was dichotomized into any consumption and no consumption. The authors state that this association could be explained by adverse characteristics among those who did not

drink coffee. The three cohort studies with information on estimates in men have been summarized in a recent meta-analysis [16], suggesting a decreased risk of hip fracture with increasing coffee consumption. The analysis is greatly influenced by the Trimpou study [15] with a weight of 76%. To summarise, the few available cohort studies in men have limitations because

Table 2. Coffee consumption and risk of any fracture and hip fracture in the Cohort of Swedish Men (COSM).

	Number of cups of coffee per day				Coffee per 200 ml (Continuous)
	<1 cup	1 cup	2–3 cups	≥4 cups	
Number of fractures	311	548	2,166	2,041	5,066
Person-years at risk	25,770	49,717	205,143	202,877	483,508
Rate/1000 person-years	12.1	11.0	10.6	10.1	10.5
Age-adjusted HR (95% CI)	1.00 (reference)	0.86 (0.75–0.98)	0.83 (0.74–0.94)	0.87 (0.77–0.98)	1.01 (0.99–1.02)
Adjusted HR (95% CI)[a]	1.00 (reference)	0.89 (0.78–1.02)	0.88 (0.78–0.99)	0.91 (0.80–1.02)	1.00 (0.99–1.02)
Number of hip fractures	78	135	526	447	1,186
Person-years at risk	26,959	51,807	213,260	211,106	503,131
Rate/1000 person-years	2.9	2.6	2.5	2.1	2.4
Age-adjusted HR (95% CI)	1.00 (reference)	0.76 (0.57–1.00)	0.73 (0.58–0.93)	0.85 (0.67–1.08)	1.03 0.99–1.06)
Adjusted HR (95% CI)[a]	1.00 (reference)	0.78 (0.59–1.03)	0.79 (0.62–1.00)	0.89 (0.70–1.14)	1.02 (0.99–1.06)

CI: confidence interval, HR: hazard ratio.
[a]Covariates included were: intake of total energy, calcium, retinol, vitamin D, potassium, phosphorus, protein, alcohol, body mass index, height, physical activity (MET 24-hour score) (all continuous), intake of any vitamins, cortisone use, educational level (≤9, 12, >12 years, other), smoking status (never, former, current), previous fractures (yes or no) and Charlson's comorbidity index (continuous).

of few fractures [13,14], that the only exposure considered was caffeine as a pooled estimate, *i.e.* the exposure calculation included not only coffee [13], or that coffee consumption was considered as any vs. no consumption [15]. The present study exceeds by far the total number of hip fractures in previous cohort studies and also had the possibility to study a large number of fractures of any type (we observe 1,186 hip fractures and 5,066 fractures of any type).

Strengths and Limitations

One of the most important strengths of our study is that we had the opportunity to collect data from a large population-based cohort of middle-aged and elderly men during a mean follow-up of 11.3 years. Such a follow-up is sufficiently long to observe an adequate number of fractures. Because all fractures were identified by the use of registers, we believe that the risk of not having detected men with a fracture during follow-up is small. There was considerable variation in consumption of coffee in this cohort with a large number of participants consuming high amounts of coffee, which improves the chances of detecting associations. In this context it should be noted that the consumption of decaffeinated coffee is very low in Sweden (<1%) [37]. Moreover, we did not focus on intake of caffeine, but on consumption of coffee, which might be another advantage in that several studies have indicated that tea could have a positive influence on BMD [38–40] and fracture risk [36], probably because of the fluoride, phytoestrogen or antioxidant content of tea [39]. Finally, it should be possible to generalise our results to all men in Sweden because the participants well represent the source population [41].

We also acknowledge a number of potential limitations. Because this investigation is based on data from one single FFQ, some degree of error in the exposure measurement cannot be excluded. Attenuation of a true association is likely in that the potentially resulting misclassification probably would be non-differential. Fractures associated with high trauma were not excluded because a comparable increased risk of both low- and high-trauma fracture with decreasing bone density in the elderly has been indicated [42]. However, there has been discourse as to whether inclusion of

both high and low impact fractures will result in a lower risk estimate compared with low trauma fractures only [43]. Despite controlling for known major risk factors for fractures, including comorbidity, it is still possible that residual confounding could have influenced the results of this study. For instance, we could not adjust for vitamin D status or sunlight exposure in the current study. However, we have previously shown that the effect of coffee intake on BMD was not stronger among women with low vitamin D status [20]. The importance of the dietary source of protein (*i.e.* animal or vegetable) on the association between coffee consumption and fracture could not be assessed in the present study. There is to date no consensus on the relation between dietary protein and fracture risk [44] but recent systematic reviews and meta-analyses suggest that the postulated dietary acidic load exaggerated by protein intake does not have a causal effect on bone health [45,46]. Carriers of a genetic variant of the vitamin D receptor might be more vulnerable toward the effects of caffeine on bone [47]. In fact, results from our previous study suggest that genetically determined differences in caffeine metabolism might be of importance for how BMD is affected by coffee/caffeine [21]. However, in this study genotyping of the participants was not performed. Furthermore, we did not have the possibility to measure BMD in this cohort. Such a measurement might have been of interest because in an earlier study we obtained evidence of a modest decrease in BMD of the proximal femur among elderly men (aged 72 years) drinking 4 cups of coffee or more per day [21]. In the context of previous research, in which no association between coffee consumption and fracture risk has been observed, the small impact in the relation between BMD and coffee does not seem to influence the risk of fracture among men on the population level. Intervention on causes of fracture other than coffee consumption would probably have a larger impact on fracture incidence.

Conclusion

In conclusion, we did not observe an increased risk of osteoporotic fractures in this large cohort of Swedish middle-aged

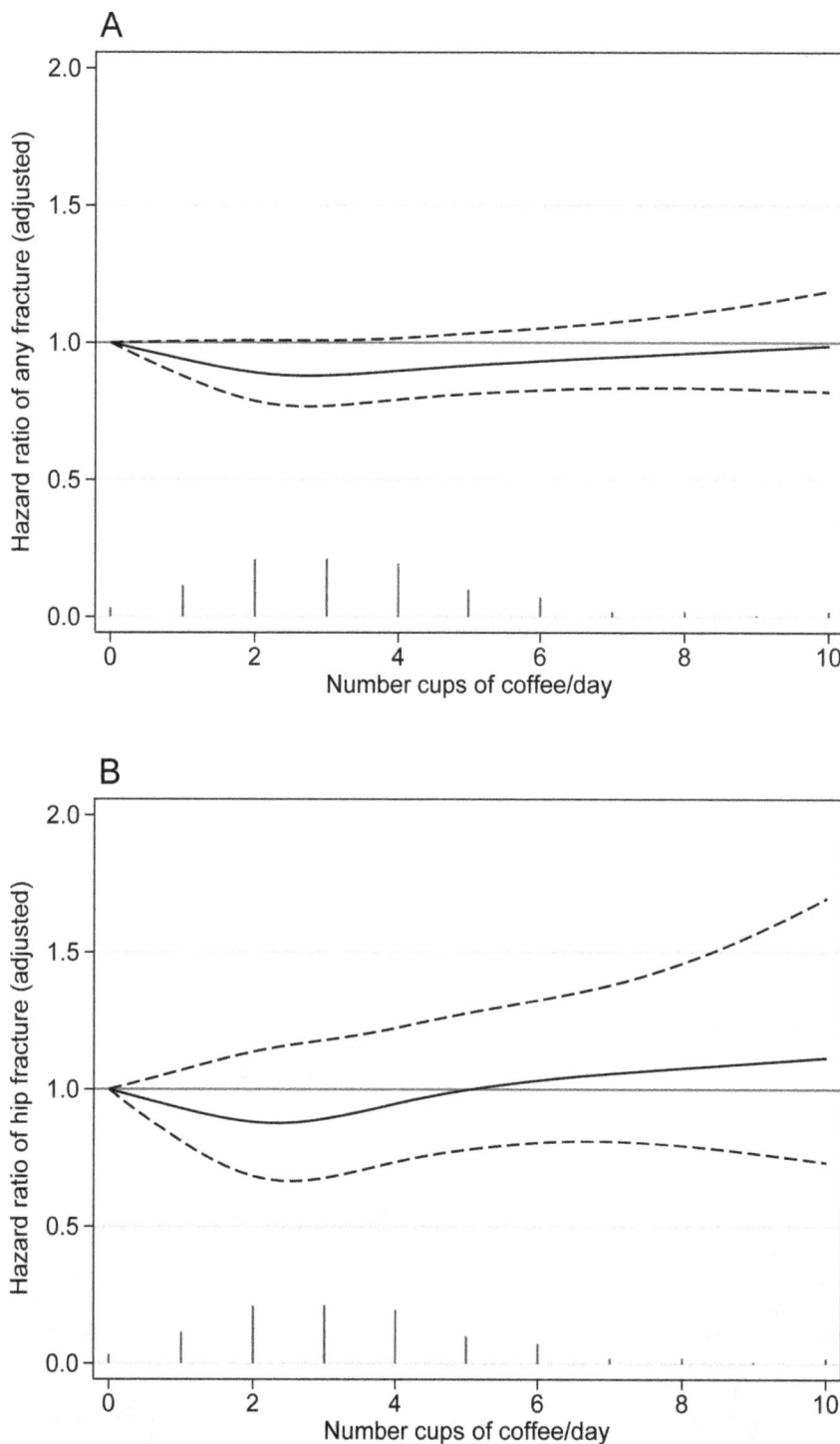

Figure 3. Association between coffee consumption and fracture risk. Multivariate-adjusted hazard ratios (HR) with 95% confidence intervals (CI) (dashed lines) of any fracture (Panel A) and hip fracture (Panel B) by coffee consumption. The vertical bars represent the distribution of coffee intake. The smoothed curves were fitted with a restricted cubic spline model with a consumption of <1 cup of coffee as the reference. Adjustments were made for intake of energy, protein, calcium, retinol, vitamin D, phosphorus, potassium and alcohol, body mass index, height, physical activity (MET-24 h score) (all continuous), intake of any vitamins, cortisone use, educational level (≤9, 12, >12 years, other), smoking status (never, former, current), previous fractures (yes or no) and Charlson's comorbidity index (continuous).

and elderly men. Calcium intake did not influence risk for fracture of any type or hip fracture.

Author Contributions

Conceived and designed the experiments: HH KM. Analyzed the data: HH LB. Wrote the paper: HH LB KM. Recruited participants: AW.

Interpreted the data: HH LB KM AG. Obtained funding: AW KM. Supervised the study: LB. Approved final version: HH KM AW AG LB.

References

1. Johnell O, Kanis JA (2006) An estimate of the worldwide prevalence and disability associated with osteoporotic fractures. Osteoporos Int 17: 1726–1733.
2. Dy CJ, Lamont LE, Ton QV, Lane JM (2011) Sex and Gender Considerations in Male Patients With Osteoporosis. Clin Orthop Relat Res 469: 1906–1912.
3. Lane NE (2006) Epidemiology, etiology, and diagnosis of osteoporosis. Am J Obstet Gynecol 194: S3–11.
4. Michaëlsson K, Lithell H, Vessby B, Melhus H (2003) Serum retinol levels and the risk of fracture. N Engl J Med 348: 287–294.
5. Heaney RP (2002) Effects of caffeine on bone and the calcium economy. Food Chem Toxicol 40: 1263–1270.
6. Kanis JA, Johansson H, Johnell O, Oden A, De Laet C, et al. (2005) Alcohol intake as a risk factor for fracture. Osteoporos Int 16: 737–742.
7. Mandel HG (2002) Update on caffeine consumption, disposition and action. Food Chem Toxicol 40: 1231–1234.
8. Massey LK, Opryszek MS (1990) No effects of adaptation to dietary caffeine on calcium excretion in young women. Nutr Res 10: 741–747.
9. Barger-Lux MJ, Heaney RP (1995) Caffeine and the calcium economy revisited. Osteoporos Int 5: 97–102.
10. Tsuang YH, Sun JS, Chen LT, Sun SC, Chen SC (2006) Direct effects of caffeine on osteoblastic cells metabolism: the possible causal effect of caffeine on the formation of osteoporosis. J Orthop Surg Res 1: 7.
11. Lu PZ, Lai CY, Chan WH (2008) Caffeine Induces Cell Death via Activation of Apoptotic Signal and Inactivation of Survival Signal in Human Osteoblasts. Int J Mol Sci 9: 698–718.
12. Zhou Y, Guan XX, Zhu ZL, Guo J, Huang YC, et al. (2010) Caffeine inhibits the viability and osteogenic differentiation of rat bone marrow-derived mesenchymal stromal cells. Br J Pharmacol 161: 1542–1552.
13. Kiel DP, Felson DT, Hannan MT, Anderson JJ, Wilson PW (1990) Caffeine and the risk of hip fracture: the Framingham Study. Am J Epidemiol 132: 675–684.
14. Meyer HE, Pedersen JI, Loken EB, Tverdal A (1997) Dietary factors and the incidence of hip fracture in middle-aged Norwegians. A prospective study. Am J Epidemiol 145: 117–123.
15. Trimpou P, Landin-Wilhelmsen K, Oden A, Rosengren A, Wilhelmsen L (2010) Male risk factors for hip fracture-a 30-year follow-up study in 7,495 men. Osteoporos Int 21: 409–416.
16. Liu H, Yao K, Zhang W, Zhou J, Wu T, et al. (2012) Coffee consumption and risk of fractures: a meta-analysis. Arch Med Sci 8: 776–783.
17. Kanis JA, Oden A, McCloskey EV, Johansson H, Wahl DA, et al. (2012) A systematic review of hip fracture incidence and probability of fracture worldwide. Osteoporos Int 23: 2239–2256.
18. Fredholm BB, Battig K, Holmen J, Nehlig A, Zvartau EE (1999) Actions of caffeine in the brain with special reference to factors that contribute to its widespread use. Pharmacol Rev 51: 83–133.
19. Andersson HC, Hallström H, Kihlman BA (2004) Intake of caffeine and other methylxanthines during pregnancy and risk for adverse effects in pregnant women and their foetuses. TemaNord 2004: 565. Copenhagen: Nordic Council of Ministers. 387 p. Available: http://www.norden.org/sv/publikationer/publikationer/2004-565/publicationfile. Accessed 2014 April 28.
20. Hallström H, Byberg L, Glynn A, Lemming EW, Wolk A, et al. (2013) Long-term Coffee Consumption in Relation to Fracture Risk and Bone Mineral Density in Women. Am J Epidemiol 178: 898–909.
21. Hallström H, Melhus H, Glynn A, Lind L, Syvänen AC, et al. (2010) Coffee consumption and CYP1A2 genotype in relation to bone mineral density of the proximal femur in elderly men and women: a cohort study. Nutr Metab (Lond) 7: 12.
22. Jarvinen TL, Sievanen H, Khan KM, Heinonen A, Kannus P (2008) Shifting the focus in fracture prevention from osteoporosis to falls. BMJ 336: 124–126.
23. Wagner H, Melhus H, Gedeborg R, Pedersen NL, Michaelsson K (2009) Simply ask them about their balance–future fracture risk in a nationwide cohort study of twins. Am J Epidemiol 169: 143–149.
24. The Cohort of Swedish Men (COSM). Available: http://ki.se/ki/jsp/polopoly.jsp?d=22104&l=en. Accessed 2014 February 3.
25. Bergström L, Hagman U, Ericsson H, Bruce Å (1991) The food composition database KOST: the National Food Administration's information system for nutritive values of food. Vår Föda: 439–447.
26. Willett WC, Howe GR, Kushi LH (1997) Adjustment for total energy intake in epidemiologic studies. Am J Clin Nutr 65: 1220S–1228S; discussion 1229S–1231S.
27. Messerer M, Johansson SE, Wolk A (2004) The validity of questionnaire-based micronutrient intake estimates is increased by including dietary supplement use in Swedish men. J Nutr 134: 1800–1805.
28. Discacciati A, Orsini N, Andersson SO, Andren O, Johansson JE, et al. (2013) Coffee consumption and risk of localized, advanced and fatal prostate cancer: a population-based prospective study. Ann Oncol 24: 1912–1918.
29. Calltorp J, Adami HO, Astrom H, Fryklund L, Rossner S, et al. (1996) Country profile: Sweden. Lancet 347: 587–594.
30. Norman A, Bellocco R, Bergstrom A, Wolk A (2001) Validity and reproducibility of self-reported total physical activity-differences by relative weight. Int J Obes Relat Metab Disord 25: 682–688.
31. Larsson SC, Rutegard J, Bergkvist L, Wolk A (2006) Physical activity, obesity, and risk of colon and rectal cancer in a cohort of Swedish men. Eur J Cancer 42: 2590–2597.
32. Charlson ME, Pompei P, Ales KL, MacKenzie CR (1987) A new method of classifying prognostic comorbidity in longitudinal studies: development and validation. J Chronic Dis 40: 373–383.
33. Quan H, Sundararajan V, Halfon P, Fong A, Burnand B, et al. (2005) Coding algorithms for defining comorbidities in ICD-9-CM and ICD-10 administrative data. Med Care 43: 1130–1139.
34. Hansson LM, Galanti MR (2000) Diet-associated risks of disease and self-reported food consumption: how shall we treat partial nonresponse in a food frequency questionnaire? Nutr Cancer 36: 1–6.
35. Heinzl H, Kaider A (1997) Gaining more flexibility in Cox proportional hazards regression models with cubic spline functions. Comput Methods Programs Biomed 54: 201–208.
36. Kanis J, Johnell O, Gullberg B, Allander E, Elffors L, et al. (1999) Risk factors for hip fracture in men from southern Europe: the MEDOS study. Mediterranean Osteoporosis Study. Osteoporos Int 9: 45–54.
37. European Coffee Federation (2013) European Coffee Report 2012/13. Available: http://www.ecf-coffee.org/images/European_Coffee_Report_2012-13_European_chapter.pdf. Accessed 2014 January 31.
38. Hegarty VM, May HM, Khaw KT (2000) Tea drinking and bone mineral density in older women. Am J Clin Nutr 71: 1003–1007.
39. Wu CH, Yang YC, Yao WJ, Lu FH, Wu JS, et al. (2002) Epidemiological evidence of increased bone mineral density in habitual tea drinkers. Arch Intern Med 162: 1001–1006.
40. Chen Z, Pettinger MB, Ritenbaugh C, LaCroix AZ, Robbins J, et al. (2003) Habitual tea consumption and risk of osteoporosis: a prospective study in the women's health initiative observational cohort. Am J Epidemiol 158: 772–781.
41. Norman A, Bellocco R, Vaida F, Wolk A (2002) Total physical activity in relation to age, body mass, health and other factors in a cohort of Swedish men. Int J Obes Relat Metab Disord 26: 670–675.
42. Mackey DC, Lui LY, Cawthon PM, Bauer DC, Nevitt MC, et al. (2007) High-trauma fractures and low bone mineral density in older women and men. Jama 298: 2381–2388.
43. Sanders KM, Pasco JA, Ugoni AM, Nicholson GC, Seeman E, et al. (1998) The exclusion of high trauma fractures may underestimate the prevalence of bone fragility fractures in the community: the Geelong Osteoporosis Study. J Bone Miner Res 13: 1337–1342.
44. Mangano KM, Sahni S, Kerstetter JE (2014) Dietary protein is beneficial to bone health under conditions of adequate calcium intake: an update on clinical research. Curr Opin Clin Nutr Metab Care 17: 69–74.
45. Fenton TR, Lyon AW, Eliasziw M, Tough SC, Hanley DA (2009) Meta-analysis of the effect of the acid-ash hypothesis of osteoporosis on calcium balance. J Bone Miner Res 24: 1835–1840.
46. Hanley DA, Whiting SJ (2013) Does a high dietary acid content cause bone loss, and can bone loss be prevented with an alkaline diet? J Clin Densitom 16: 420–425.
47. Rapuri PB, Gallagher JC, Nawaz Z (2007) Caffeine decreases vitamin D receptor protein expression and 1,25(OH)2D3 stimulated alkaline phosphatase activity in human osteoblast cells. J Steroid Biochem Mol Biol 103: 368–371.

4

Hip Structural Parameters over 96 Weeks in HIV-Infected Adults Switching Treatment to Tenofovir-Emtricitabine or Abacavir-Lamivudine

Hila Haskelberg[1]*, Nicholas Pocock[2], Janaki Amin[1], Peter Robert Ebeling[3], Sean Emery[1], Andrew Carr[2], on behalf of the STEAL Study Group

1 The Kirby Institute, University of New South Wales, Sydney, Australia, 2 St. Vincent's Hospital, Sydney, Australia, 3 North West Academic Centre, University of Melbourne, Melbourne, Australia

Abstract

Background: Therapy with tenofovir is associated with lower bone mineral density (BMD), higher markers of bone turnover and increased fracture risk in HIV-infected adults. Bone structural parameters generated by hip structural analysis may represent a separate measure of bone strength, but have not been assessed in HIV.

Methods: Dual-energy X-ray absorptiometry (DXA) scans from 254 HIV-infected adults randomised to simplify their existing dual nucleoside analogue reverse transcriptase inhibitor therapy to coformulated tenofovir-emtricitabine or abacavir-lamivudine were analysed using DXA-derived hip structural analysis software. Hip structural parameters included femoral strength index, section modulus, cross-sectional area, and cross-sectional moment of inertia. We used one-way ANOVA to test the relationship between nucleoside analogue type at baseline and structural parameters, multivariable analysis to assess baseline covariates associated with femoral strength index, and t-tests to compare mean change in structural parameters over 96 weeks between randomised groups.

Results: Participants taking tenofovir at baseline had lower section modulus (-107.3 mm^2, p = 0.001), lower cross-sectional area (-15.01 mm^3, p = 0.001), and lower cross-sectional moment of inertia ($-2,036.8$ mm^4, p = 0.007) than those receiving other nucleoside analogues. After adjustment for baseline risk factors, the association remained significant for section modulus (p = 0.008) and cross-sectional area (p = 0.002). Baseline covariates significantly associated with higher femoral strength index were higher spine T-score (p = 0.001), lower body fat mass (p<0.001), lower bone alkaline phosphatase (p = 0.025), and higher osteoprotegerin (p = 0.024). Hip structural parameters did not change significantly over 96 weeks and none was significantly affected by treatment simplification to tenofovir-emtricitabine or abacavir-lamivudine.

Conclusion: In this population, tenofovir use was associated with reduced composite indices of bone strength as measured by hip structural analysis, but none of the structural parameters improved significantly over 96 weeks with tenofovir cessation.

Editor: Yi-Hsiang Hsu, Harvard Medical School, United States of America

Funding: This work was supported by The Kirby Institute (formerly the National Centre in HIV Epidemiology and Clinical Research) funded by the Australian Government Department of Health and Ageing. The Kirby Institute is affiliated with the Faculty of Medicine, University of New South Wales. The funders had no role in study design, data collection and analysis, decision to publish, or preparation of the manuscript.

Competing Interests: The authors have read the journal's policy and have the following conflicts: Sean Emery is a Editorial Board member. Hila Haskelberg and Janaki Amin declare no conflict of interest. Nicolas Pocock received consultancy fees from Merck, Sanofi Aventis and Servier; and has served on an advisory board for Merck. Peter Ebeling's institution has received research funding from Merck; consultancy fees from Gilead Sciences and GlaxoSmithKline/ ViiV Healthcare; and has served on an advisory board for Merck. Sean Emery has received research grant support from Abbvie, Gilead Sciences, Merck Research Laboratories, Pfizer, and ViiV Healthcare. Andrew Carr has received research funding from ViiV Healthcare, and Merck; consultancy fees from Gilead Sciences, ViiV Healthcare, MSD and Roche; lecture and travel sponsorships from Gilead Sciences, MSD, and ViiV Healthcare; and has served on advisory boards for Gilead Sciences, MSD, and ViiV Healthcare.

* E-mail: hhaskelberg@kirby.unsw.edu.au

Introduction

Low bone mineral density (BMD) and higher rates of fractures have been reported in HIV-infected adults compared with general population controls [1,2], and have been particularly associated with tenofovir (TDF) therapy [3]. BMD as measured by dual-energy X-ray absorptiometry (DXA) is the gold standard for clinical assessment of bone fragility. The relationship between decreased BMD and increased risk of fractures is well established [4]. BMD, however, only accounts for about 50% of fracture risk [5] and does not describe other components of bone quality such as geometric configuration, which can be estimated by DXA-derived hip structural analysis (HSA) [6,7]. HSA software

Hip Structural Parameters over 96 Weeks in HIV-Infected Adults Switching Treatment...

31

Table 1. Hip structural parameters included in this analysis [8].

Measure	Derivation	Comments
Femoral strength index	Calculated as strength/stress, where, strength = 185–0.34 (age - 45) and stress is moment*y/CSMI+force/CSA	Indicates the bone's resistance to fracture from forces generated during a fall on the greater trochanter
Hip axis length (HAL, mm)	The distance along the femoral neck axis, extending from the bone edge at the base of the trochanter to the bone edge at the inner pelvic brim	Suggested to be a measure of the degree to which the femur extends beyond the pelvis, increasing risk for impact, though relationship to fractures is unclear
Buckling ratio	Ratio of the outer radius to the cortical thickness	Indicator of cortical stability under compressive loads
Section Modulus (Z, mm^3)	CSMI divided by half the width of the femoral neck	A measure of bending strength
Cross-sectional area (CSA; mm^2)	Represents the area of mineral packed together in the defined cross section of the femoral neck	Proportional to bone's ability to resist axial compressive force
Cross-sectional moment of inertia (CSMI; mm^4)	calculated using the mass distribution derived from the absorption curve	Bone's ability to resist bending forces

generates a femoral strength index, an integral measure that combines BMD, femur geometry, age, height and weight and aims to reflect the bone's ability to withstand forces generated during a fall [8].

A cross-sectional analysis of hip osteoporotic fractures and composite indices of femoral neck strength in healthy women found decreased measures of femoral neck strength in women with fractures [9]. In addition, structural parameters were found to predict hip fracture in postmenopausal women after adjusting for both clinical risk factors and BMD [10–13]. Yet the role of these measures as independent predictors of hip fracture remains controversial, particularly in men [14].

Studies of osteoporosis and fractures in HIV-infected adults have mainly focused on BMD; the effects of HIV and its treatment on other measures of bone quality are unclear. Walker Harris et al. [15] have recently found in a cross-sectional study that HIV/HCV-co-infected men had significantly lower measures of hip strength at the narrow neck and shaft when compared to healthy controls. Lower lean body mass accounted for most of the differences between groups after adjusting for race, age, smoking status, height, and weight [15]. In a longitudinal study of perinatally HIV-infected youth (n = 31; 9–18 y), neither bone geometry nor strength was significantly different compared with healthy controls [16].

In the STEAL study, patients randomized to simplify their existing dual nucleoside reverse transcriptase inhibitor (NRTI) therapy to coformulated tenofovir-emtricitabine (TDF-FTC) had greater BMD decreases and greater bone turnover marker increases over 96 weeks than those who were randomised to abacavir-lamivudine (ABC-3TC) [17]. STEAL provides an opportunity to examine bone structure cross-sectionally and longitudinally, and in particular any effect of TDF. We hypothesised that there would be a significant difference between TDF-FTC and ABC-3TC in measures of bone structure, as assessed by DXA-derived Hip Structural Analysis. The aim of this analysis was to estimate and compare changes in bone structural parameters by randomised arm from baseline to 96 weeks. A secondary objectives was were to determine the relationship between femoral strength index and baseline clinical and biochemical characteristics, and to explore the relationship between markers of bone turnover and changes in the above measures of bone structure

Methods

Study design

STEAL was an open-label, prospective, randomized, non-inferiority study that compared simplification of current NRTIs to fixed-dose combination TDF-FTC or ABC-3TC over 96 weeks in 357 adults with plasma HIV viral load <50 copies/mL [17]. The supporting CONSORT checklist and STEAL protocol are available as supporting information; see Checklist S1, and Protocol S1

Ethics Statement

The study was approved by each site's Human Research and Ethics Committee and registered at Clinicaltrials.gov (NCT00192634). The specific ethics committees that gave approval for the STEAL study are: St Vincent's Hospital Human Research Ethics Committee (HREC), South Eastern Sydney/Illawarra Area Health Service HREC, Harbour HREC of Northern Sydney Central Coast Health, North Coast Area Health Service HREC, Sydney West Area Health Service HREC, Sydney South West Area Health Service HREC, Alfred Hospital EC, Southern Health HREC, Melbourne Health HREC, The Prince Charles Hospital HREC, Cairns & Hinterland Health Service District EC, Gold Coast Health Service District HREC, Royal Brisbane and Women's Hospital HREC, Flinders Clinical Research EC, Royal Adelaide Hospital Research EC, Royal Perth Hospital EC. Each participant signed a written informed consent before enrolment.

DXA and hip structural analysis

DXA measurements of the right hip and lumbar spine BMD were performed for each participant at baseline, week 48, and week 96, using a standardized protocol. The following were recorded: hip and spine BMD, T-scores and Z-scores, total body fat tissue and lean tissue masses. DXA instruments varied between study sites and for this analysis, only data from GE-Lunar scanners were used.

Archived lunar image files of the right femur were analysed by a trained individual blinded to antiretroviral therapy, using the HSA software Lunar Prodigy enCORE 2011 version 13.60.033 (GE Healthcare). The HSA software provides a line of pixels traversing the bone axis which gives a projection of the surface area of bone in the cross section. The results reported in this analysis are from the femoral neck. The HSA software automatically assesses all cross sections in the femoral neck and identifies the plane that is

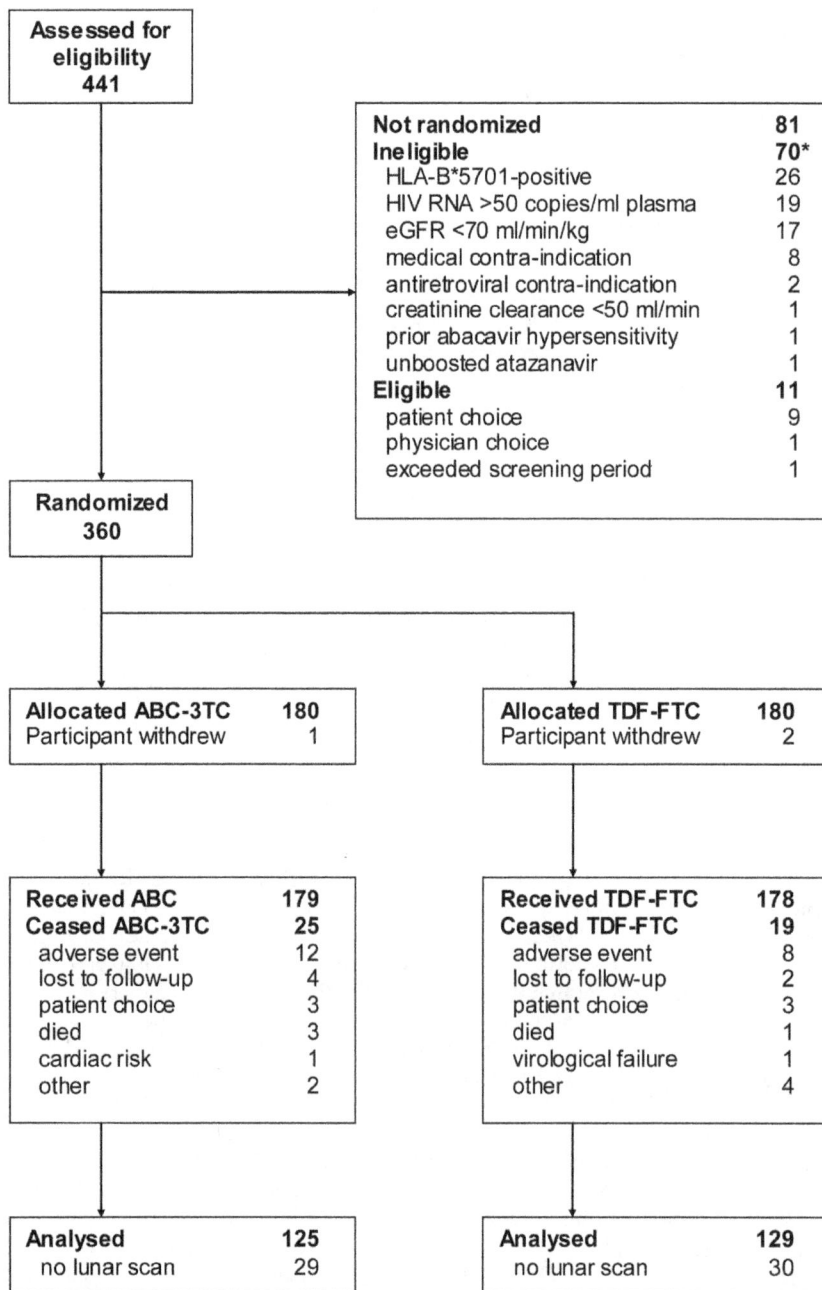

```
┌──────────────┐
│ Assessed for │
│ eligibility  │
│     441      │
└──────────────┘
```

Not randomized	81*
Ineligible	**70***
HLA-B*5701-positive	26
HIV RNA >50 copies/ml plasma	19
eGFR <70 ml/min/kg	17
medical contra-indication	8
antiretroviral contra-indication	2
creatinine clearance <50 ml/min	1
prior abacavir hypersensitivity	1
unboosted atazanavir	1
Eligible	**11**
patient choice	9
physician choice	1
exceeded screening period	1

```
┌──────────────┐
│  Randomized  │
│     360      │
└──────────────┘
```

Allocated ABC-3TC	**180**		**Allocated TDF-FTC**	**180**
Participant withdrew	1		Participant withdrew	2

Received ABC	**179**		**Received TDF-FTC**	**178**
Ceased ABC-3TC	**25**		**Ceased TDF-FTC**	**19**
adverse event	12		adverse event	8
lost to follow-up	4		lost to follow-up	2
patient choice	3		patient choice	3
died	3		died	1
cardiac risk	1		virological failure	1
other	2		other	4

Analysed	**125**		**Analysed**	**129**
no lunar scan	29		no lunar scan	30

Figure 1. Patient disposition.

the weakest, by calculating the mass distribution derived from an X-ray absorption curve [8]. Specifically, the following structural parameters were obtained: hip axis length (HAL, mm), femoral strength index, buckling ratio, section modulus (Z, in mm^3), cross-sectional moment of inertia (CSMI, in mm^4), and cross sectional area (CSA, in mm^2) (Table 1).

Laboratory markers

Plasma and serum samples were collected at baseline and at weeks 12, 24, 48, 72 and 96 (following a 10-hour overnight fast, except at week 12) and stored at $-70°C$. Markers of bone resorption (C-terminal cross-linking telopeptide of type 1 collagen [βCTX]), bone formation (procollagen type 1 N-terminal propep-

tide [P1NP]; bone-specific alkaline phosphatise [BALP]) and regulators of bone turnover (osteoprotegerin [OPG] and receptor activator of nuclear factor kappa ligand [RANKL]) were evaluated. The following were assessed at baseline only: interleukin-6, oestradiol, free testosterone and 25-hydroxy vitamin D. Assays are described elsewhere [18]. BTMs were batch-tested after study completion in one laboratory.

Statistical analyses

All analyses were performed on the per-protocol data so as to evaluate the biological effects of exposure to randomised therapy. "Per-protocol" is defined as available data collected on partici-

Table 2. Baseline characteristics.

Baseline characteristics	NRTI at study entry			Randomization		Main Study (n = 357)
	ABC (n = 53)	TDF (n = 74)	Other (n = 127)	ABC-3TC (n = 125)	TDF-FTC (n = 129)	
Age (years)	48.7±8.4	42.8±8.5	44±8.4	45.8±8.9	44.3±8.4	45.1±8.6
Male (%)	98	99	98	99	98	98
Ethnicity – white (%)	92	88	79	84	85	86
HIV duration (years)	13.4±5.6	8.7±5.7	9.9±5.7	10.0±5.7	10.5±6.1	10.2±6.0
CD4+ count	613±257	609±257	612±248	629±259	595±245	612±282
ART exposure						
NRTI duration (years)	8.0±4.1	4.1±3.1	5.8±2.8	5.8±3.5	5.8±3.5	5.8±3.6
Current protease inhibitor (%)	26	28	19	24	22	23
Anthropometric factors						
Weight (kg)	76.8±11.5	72.9±12.2	77.7±12.8	76.0±12.9	76.2±12.2	76.8±12.6
Fat mass (kg)	16.2±6.8	14.9±7.2	16.5±7.7	15.7±7.3	16.2±7.5	16.8±7.9
Bone mineral density						
Right hip (g/cm²)	1.06±0.14	1.00±0.11	1.04±0.13	1.04+0.13	1.02+0.13	
Lumbar Spine (g/cm²)	1.26±0.14	1.16±0.15	1.21±0.16	1.2±0.16	1.2±0.15	
Bone turnover markers						
βCTx (ng/L)	256±152	314±157	226±134	252±154	265±145	
BALP (µg/L)	16.8±8.4	23.6±11.6	17.9±10.3	19.3±10.1	19.4±11.2	
P1NP (µg/L)	45.7±19.1	67.7±22.8	50.1±21.9	53.1±23.9	55.7±22.6	
OPG (pmol/L)	3.8±1.1	4.0±1.4	3.8±1.1	3.9±1.3	3.8±1.1	
RANKL (pmol/L)	0.2±0.3	0.2±0.2	0.3±0.5	0.2±0.3	0.2±0.4	
Hip structural parameters						
Femoral strength index	1.68±0.43	1.57±0.34	1.60±0.38	1.60±0.37	1.62±0.39	
Hip axis length (mm)	118.1±6.9	116.8±7.1	118.9±8.5	118.2±7.4	118.1±8.2	
Buckling ratio	3.9±1.6	4.4±1.5	4.2±1.8	4.2±1.7	4.2±1.7	
Section modulus (mm³)	873±196	766±147	836±180	832±175	815±182	
Cross-sectional area (mm²)	174±28	159±20	169±26	167±25	167±26	
Cross-sectional moment of inertia (mm⁴)	16235±5032	14198±3387	15705±4222	15473±4127	15283±4368	

Note. Results are expressed as mean ± standard deviation or %.
Abbreviations: **ABC-3TC**, abacavir-lamivudine; **BALP**, bone-specific alkaline phosphatase; **βCTx**, C-terminal cross-linking telopeptide of type 1 collagen; **BMD**, bone mineral density; **NNRTI**, non-nucleoside reverse transcriptase inhibitor; **NRTI**, nucleoside reverse transcriptase inhibitor; **OPG**, osteoprotegerin; **P1NP**, procollagen type 1 N-terminal propeptide; **RANKL**, Receptor Activator of Nuclear Factor Kappa Ligand; **TDF-FTC**, tenofovir-emtricitabine.

pants while on randomised strategy as defined in the STEAL protocol.

The associations between baseline covariates (including demographic, HIV-related factors, antiretroviral therapy, body composition, bone remodelling regulators, sex hormones, and vitamin D), and absolute baseline femoral strength index were analysed using linear regression. Multivariable model was built using backward, stepwise methods. Covariates that achieved a p-value <0.1 in univariate analysis were assessed for inclusion in the model. In an exploratory analysis, one-way ANOVA was used to assess the relationship between type of NRTI at study entry (ABC, TDF, or other) and all structural measures at baseline. To test this relationship further, linear regression models were a-priori adjusted for covariates known to be related to bone status i.e. age, sex, ethnicity, smoking, height, total body fat mass, total body lean mass, and HIV infection duration to account for possible associations with hip structural analysis outcomes. Structural parameters at week 48 and week 96 were compared with baseline using paired t-tests. Randomized groups were compared for

changes in structural measures by t-tests at 48 weeks and 96 weeks. Results are reported as regression coefficients i.e. differences between groups. Statistical significance was defined as a 2-sided α of 0.05. Statistical analyses were performed with STATA (StataCorp. 2011. Stata Statistical Software: Release 12. College Station, TX: StataCorp LP USA).

Results

Patient disposition is outlined in Figure 1. Of 357 participants enrolled in the parent study, 285 had GE-lunar Prodigy scans data available at baseline; 17 discontinued ABC-3TC and 14 discontinued TDF-FTC by week 96. Therefore, the analysed per-protocol population comprised the remaining 254 participants (71% of main study population). Baseline characteristics of the population analysed were similar to those of all study participants [19] and well balanced between arms (Table 2). At study entry, 29% of the participants (n = 74) were taking TDF-containing regimen, 21% (n = 53) were on ABC-containing regimen and 50%

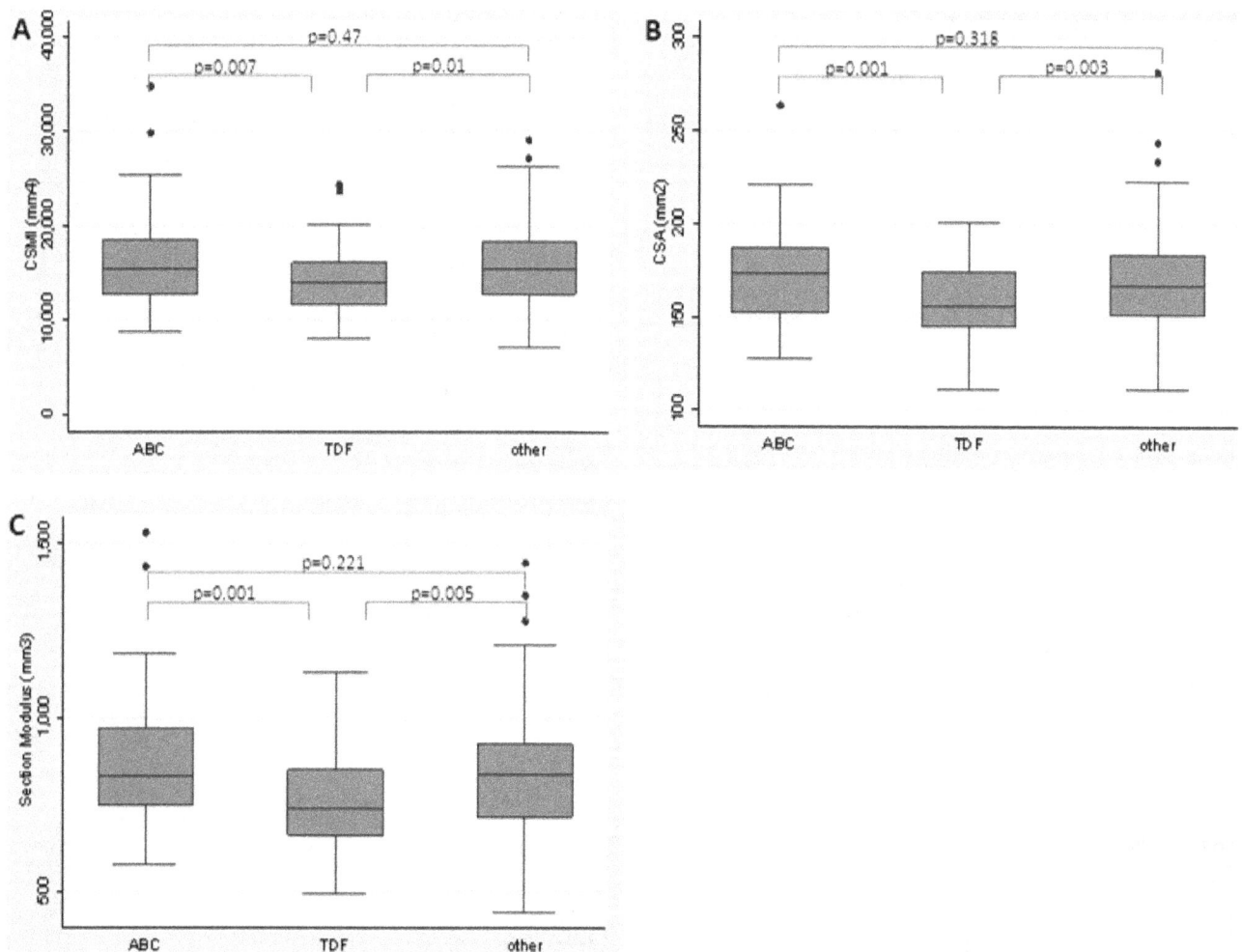

Figure 2. Hip structural parameters at baseline by type of NRTI at study entry (A) CSMI (bone's ability to resist bending), (B) CSA (bone's ability to resist axial compressive force) and (C) section modulus (bending strength). Abbreviations: CSA, cross-sectional area; CSMI, cross-sectional moment of inertia.

(n = 127) were taking other NRTIs (typically two of the following: 3TC, FTC, zidovudine, didanosine, stavudine).

Hip structural parameters at baseline

Baseline CSMI, CSA, and section modulus were all significantly different across the three sub-groups of NRTI types at baseline [CSMI: $F_{(2,208)} = 26.98$, p = 0.013; CSA: $F_{(2,251)} = 6.59$, p = 0.002; section modulus: $F_{(2,251)} = 6.51$, p = 0.002].

Compared to the ABC group, participants that entered the study on TDF had lower baseline CSMI (coefficient: -2036.8 mm^4; 95% CI: -3520.8 to -552.7; p = 0.007), lower CSA (-15.01 mm^2; 95% CI: -23.8 to -6.2; p = 0.001), and lower section modulus (-107.3 mm^3; 95% CI: -169.1 to -45.4; p = 0.001) (Figure 2). After adjustment, the association remained significant for CSA (-13.7 mm^2; 95% CI: -21.3 to -6.2; p = 0.002) and section modulus (-83.1 mm^3; 95% CI: -135.5 to -30.6; p = 0.008), but not for CSMI (-1168.85 mm^4; 95% CI: -2366.9 to 29.2; p = 0.159).

Baseline covariates significantly associated with higher femoral strength index at baseline in multivariable analysis were higher spine T-score (p trend = 0.001), lower body fat mass (p trend < 0.001), lower bone alkaline phosphatase (BALP; p = 0.025), and higher osteoprotegerin (OPG; P = 0.024; Table 3).

Changes in hip structural parameters over 96 weeks

For all structural measures besides HAL, there was no significant difference between baseline and week 48 or between baseline and week 96 for the whole cohort. The absolute increase in HAL from baseline was statistically significant at week 48 though not at week 96 [(diff: 0.25; 95% confidence intervals [CI]: 0.09 to 0.41; p = 0.002); (diff: 0.16; 95% CI: -0.005 to 0.33; p = 0.058, respectively)]. There was no difference between randomised arms in absolute change at week 48 or week 96 (Table 4).

Analysing the effect of randomisation by the NRTI sub-groups, patients that were on ABC at baseline and switched to TDF (n = 24) had significantly greater decreases of CSA (coeff: -6.7 mm^2; 95% CI: -12.3 to -1.0; p = 0.021) and CSMI (coeff: -675.1 mm^4; 95% CI: -1298.4 to -51.7; p = 0.034) at week 48 compared with those who continued on ABC (n = 26). There were no significant differences from baseline to week 96. No significant change was found for 74 patients on TDF at baseline who either stayed on TDF or switched to ABC.

Table 3. Covariates associated with femoral strength index at baseline

Covariate	Univariate analysis					Multivariate model (n = 228)			
	N	Coef. femoral strength index	95% Conf. Interval	P>|z|	overall P value	Coef. femoral strength index	95% Conf. Interval	P>|z|	overall P value
HIV RNA (copies/ml)	254	0	(−0.00 to 0.00)	0.09		0	(−0.00 to 0.00)	0.191	
No PI - NNRTI*	195	0				0			
PI	59	−0.12	(−0.23 to −0.01)	0.027		−0.09	(−0.20 to 0.01)	0.079	
Spine BMD wk0 - quartiles									
0.788–1.061*	54	0				0			
1.062–1.180	60	0.17	(0.03 to 0.31)	0.016		0.15	(0.01 to 0.28)	0.034	
1.181–1.292	71	0.22	(0.09 to 0.35)	0.001		0.27	(0.14 to 0.40)	<0.001	
1.293–1.798	69	0.2	(0.06 to 0.33)	0.004	0.005	0.18	(0.06 to 0.31)	0.005	0.003
Total body lean tissue mass wk0 - quartiles									
32464–51980 g*	67	0				0			
51981–56673 g	57	0	(−0.13 to 0.14)	0.977		0.03	(−0.10 to 0.16)	0.677	
56674–61811 g	62	−0.1	(−0.23 to 0.03)	0.129		−0.05	(−0.18 to 0.08)	0.436	
61812–79671 g	68	−0.09	(−0.21 to 0.04)	0.191	0.09	−0.04	(−0.17 to 0.10)	0.614	0.391
Total body fat tissue mass wk0 - quartiles									
1110–10590 g*	69	0				0			
10591–15428 g	59	−0.17	(−0.29 to −0.04)	0.008		−0.19	(−0.32 to −0.07)	0.002	
15429–20942 g	64	−0.25	(−0.37 to −0.13)	<0.001		−0.31	(−0.43 to −0.19)	<0.001	
20943–46433 g	62	−0.36	(−0.48 to −0.24)	<0.001	<0.001	−0.38	(−0.50 to −0.25)	<0.001	<0.001
Alkaline phosphatase (mmol/l)	253	0	(−0.00 to −0.00)	0.039		0	(−0.00 to 0.00)	0.886	
BALP Wk0	228	0	(−0.01 to 0.00)	0.066		−0.01	(−0.01 to −0.00)	0.03	
OPG Wk0	228	0.04	(0.00 to 0.09)	0.032		0.04	(0.00 to 0.08)	0.038	
RANK-L Wk0	228	0.15	(0.02 to 0.28)	0.021		0.13	(0.01 to 0.25)	0.032	

Table 4. Mean change in hip structural parameters over 96 weeks by randomisation

Hip structural parameters	Abacavir-lamivudine	Tenofovir-emtricitabine	Mean difference (95% confidence interval)	P
Femoral strength index	−0.02	−0.01	0.01 (−0.05 to 0.07)	0.704
Hip axis length (mm)	0.3	0.03	−0.27 (−0.6 to 0.6)	0.109
Buckling ratio	−0.06	−0.3	−0.2 (−0.7 to 0.1)	0.220
Section modulus (mm^3)	2.2	0.2	−2.0 (−16.8 to 12.7)	0.787
Cross-sectional area (mm^2)	1.3	−0.2	−1.5 (−3.8 to 0.6)	0.155
Cross-sectional moment of inertia (mm^4)	−42.4	−3.8	38.6 (−276 to 353)	0.810

Discussion

To our knowledge, this is the first longitudinal study to investigate DXA-derived structural properties of the femoral neck in HIV-infected adults. In this cohort of predominantly young HIV-infected men, participants that were taking TDF at study entry had decreased composite indices of bone strength, as estimated by hip structural analysis, compared to ABC and other NRTIs. Independent baseline factors associated with lower femoral hip strength index at baseline included lower bone formation markers and lower body fat mass. The majority of structural parameters did not improve over 96 weeks of follow-up and nor were they significantly affected by treatment simplification to TDF-FTC or ABC-3TC.

Most studies of HIV-infected adults have shown that they are at greater risk of fractures when compared with healthy population controls [1,2], yet the pathogenesis of HIV-associated bone disease is multifactorial and not fully understood. In the STEAL cohort, four participants experienced fractures, two in each treatment arm [17]. In a number of randomized controlled studies, the initiation or a switch to ART was associated with 6–12 months of bone loss, which then stabilizes [17,19]. In post-menopausal women, treatment with a bisphosphonate resulted in significant improvements in hip geometric parameters after one [20] and two years [21] of treatment. The finding in our cohort that most of the structural indices did not significantly change following ART switch, supports the finding by Tuck et al. that some bone geometrical measures are relatively stable over time in men [14]. Furthermore, our data also corroborate a recent population-based study (n = 1760), which found that a decline in BMD was counteracted by an increase in bone size, resulting in only a small decrease of up to 0.5% in composite indices of hip strength (as measured by DXA-derived hip structural analysis), resulting in a partial preservation of bone strength in men from peak value to age 90 years [22].

In our study, higher OPG was independently associated with higher femoral strength index. The RANKL/RANK/OPG signalling pathway has a critical role in bone remodelling; specifically, OPG inhibits bone resorption [23]. Our results are consistent with the Framingham Offspring Study in HIV-uninfected adults (n = 1165 men), which found that increased OPG was independently positively associated with indices of hip strength in men [24]. Higher OPG levels may reflect a compensatory reaction to accelerated bone resorption and deterioration of cortical bone [25]. This may also explain the observation that there were no significant changes over the 2 years of follow-up in majority of structural parameters in our cohort. We also found that lower body fat mass was an independent predictor of higher femoral strength index, which is consistent with the index's formula – negative correlation between the strength (resistance to fracture forces) relative to load (forces placed on the hip during a fall).

Unlike the previous cross-sectional study of hip geomerty in HIV/HCV co-infected adults [15], we found no association between any of the structural parameters and lower lean mass. However, it is difficult to directly compare the two studies. Firstly, chronic hepatitis C monoinfection has been independently associated with unbalanced bone turnover and reduced bone quality [26]. Secondly, the population studied by Walker-Harris was mostly African-American (86%) while 85% of our cohort was Caucasian and probably less than 10% had HCV co-infection. And finally, the participants in the HIV/HCV cohort were evaluated at three locations at the proximal femur using a Hologic scanner, which employs a different HSA method to assess strength at the femoral neck than the Lunar software used in our study.

Despite being younger with shorter duration of HIV and shorter exposure to ART, participants that were on TDF at study entry had significantly lower CSA (bone's ability to resist bending) and section modulus (bending strength) at baseline than those receiving other NRTIs. Switching from TDF lead to an increase in BMD [27], in our study, however, TDF cessation did not lead to a significant improvement in any structural parameter of the hip over 96 weeks. The Study of Osteoporotic Fractures (n = 7474) found that that a 1 SD decrease in CSA increased the risk of incident hip fracture by 1.80–1.93, depending on which covariates were included in the model [13]. There is a body of literature demonstrating a greater effect of TDF-based regimens on decreasing BMD [17,19,28] and increased fracture risk [3]. As the reduced composite indices of bone strength that were found with TDF, did not improve after treatment switch, it may imply that prevention of loss in bone strength is more important than switching treatment to improve these bone measures. It was recently found by Bedimo at el. [3] that cumulative exposure to TDF was an independent predictor of increased risk of osteoporotic fractures (yearly HR 1.12; 95% CI 1.03–1.21). The possible effects of long-term exposure to TDF on bone structure require further investigation in patients initiating antiretroviral therapy.

Our study has several limitations. There is an inherent limitation in using DXA, which produces two-dimensional images, to assess three-dimensional measures of hip geometry and the calculated strength indices [6]. Furthermore, relative changes in the cortical versus cancellous bone are not detected by DXA. However, the DXA-derived HSA method is currently more available and affordable than the three-dimensional techniques (such as finite element modelling), and allows the evaluation of femoral neck structure in additional to BMD. Our finding regarding the association to TDF was only found in the uncontrolled cross-sectional analysis at baseline. Another limitation is the generalizability of our findings: our cohort comprised mainly Caucasian men and we only analysed data from GE-Lunar scanners, therefore limiting our ability to extend our findings to different populations or to other methods that assess hip strength. Lastly, the short follow-up period and small sample size precluded the investigation of fracture risk. Nevertheless, our study includes a comprehensive set of bone-related data - bone turnover markers, BMD and hip structure, which allows us a greater understanding of the skeletal status of this cohort.

To conclude, HIV-infected adults who were on TDF at study entry, had reduced composite indices of bone strength (as assessed by hip structural analysis), compared with other NRTIs groups. Treatment simplification to TDF-FTC or ABC-3TC had no significant effect on hip structural parameters over 96 weeks of follow-up. This study suggests that hip structural parameters may not improve with TDF cessation in our cohort's age group and their assessment does not add any predictive value to BMD in clinical management of HIV-infected adults. Yet, differences in the length, width, and angle of the femoral neck may increase fracture risk with ageing; further longer prospective studies of bone structure in larger cohorts of individuals with HIV may shed more light on the pathogenesis of bone disease in HIV-infection.

Acknowledgments

The content is solely the responsibility of the authors and the views expressed in this publication do not necessarily represent the position of the Australian Government.

STEAL Study Group (as listed in [17])

STEAL study investigators – Anthony Allworth, Jonathan Anderson, David Baker, Mark Bloch, Mark Boyd, John Chuah, David Cooper, Stephen Davies, Linda Dayan, William Donohue, Nicholas Doong, Dominic Dwyer, John Dyer, Robert Finlayson, Michelle Giles, David Gordon, Mark Kelly, Nicholas Medland, Richard Moore, David Nolan, David Orth, Jeffrey Post, John Quin, Tim Read, Norman Roth, Darren Russell, David Shaw, David Smith, Don Smith, Alan Street, Ban Kiem Tee, Ian Woolley.

We extend our grateful thanks to all the participants and the study co-ordinators.

Author Contributions

Conceived and designed the experiments: HH, NP, AC. Performed the experiments: HH, NP. Analyzed the data: HH. Contributed reagents/materials/analysis tools: NP. Wrote the paper: HH. All authors reviewed all data and analyses, and reviewed the manuscript.

References

1. Hansen A-BE, Gerstoft J, Kronborg G, Larsen CS, Pedersen C, et al. (2012) Incidence of low and high-energy fractures in persons with and without HIV infection: a Danish population-based cohort study. AIDS 26: 285–293 210.1097/QAD.1090b1013e32834ed32838a32837.
2. Triant VA, Brown TT, Lee H, Grinspoon SK (2008) Fracture prevalence among human immunodeficiency virus (HIV)-infected versus non-HIV-infected patients in a large U.S. healthcare system. J Clin Endocrinol Metab 93: 3499–3504.
3. Bedimo R, Maalouf NM, Zhang S, Drechsler H, Tebas P (2012) Osteoporotic fracture risk associated with cumulative exposure to tenofovir and other antiretroviral agents. AIDS 26: 825.
4. Kanis JA (2002) Diagnosis of osteoporosis and assessment of fracture risk. Lancet 359: 1929–1936.
5. Marshall D, Johnell O, Wedel H (1996) Meta-analysis of how well measures of bone mineral density predict occurrence of osteoporotic fractures. BMJ 312: 1254–1259.
6. Beck T (2003) Measuring the structural strength of bones with dual-energy X-ray absorptiometry: principles, technical limitations, and future possibilities. Osteoporosis International 14: 81–88.
7. Lou Bonnick S (2007) Hsa: Beyond bmd with dxa. Bone 41: S9–S12.
8. Yoshikawa T, Turner C, Peacock M, Slemenda C, Weaver C, et al. (1994) Geometric structure of the femoral neck measured using dual-energy X-ray absorptiometry. Journal of Bone and Mineral Research 9: 1053–1064.
9. Li G-W, Chang S-X, Xu Z, Chen Y, Bao H, et al. (2013) Prediction of hip osteoporotic fractures from composite indices of femoral neck strength. Skeletal radiology 42: 195–201.
10. LaCroix A, Beck T, Cauley J, Lewis C, Bassford T, et al. (2010) Hip structural geometry and incidence of hip fracture in postmenopausal women: what does it add to conventional bone mineral density? Osteoporosis International 21: 919–929.
11. Faulkner KGK, Wacker WKW, Barden HSH, Simonelli CC, Burke PKP, et al. (2006) Femur strength index predicts hip fracture independent of bone density and hip axis length. Osteoporosis international 17: 593–599.
12. Bergot C, Bousson V, Meunier A, Laval-Jeantet M, Laredo J (2002) Hip fracture risk and proximal femur geometry from DXA scans. Osteoporosis International 13: 542–550.
13. Kaptoge S, Beck TJ, Reeve J, Stone KL, Hillier TA, et al. (2008) Prediction of incident hip fracture risk by femur geometry variables measured by hip structural analysis in the study of osteoporotic fractures. Journal of Bone and Mineral Research 23: 1892–1904.
14. Tuck S, Rawlings D, Scane A, Pande I, Summers G, et al. (2011) Femoral Neck Shaft Angle in Men with Fragility Fractures. Journal of Osteoporosis 2011.
15. Walker Harris V, Sutcliffe CG, Araujo AB, Chiu GR, Travison TG, et al. (2012) Hip bone geometry in HIV/HCV-co-infected men and healthy controls. Osteoporosis International 23: 1779–1787.
16. Macdonald H, Chu J, Nettlefold L, Maan E, Forbes J, et al. (2013) Bone geometry and strength are adapted to muscle force in children and adolescents

perinatally infected with HIV. Journal of musculoskeletal & neuronal interactions 13: 53–65.
17. Martin A, Bloch M, Amin J, Baker D, Cooper DA, et al. (2009) Simplification of antiretroviral therapy with tenofovir-emtricitabine or abacavir-Lamivudine: a randomized, 96-week trial. Clinical Infectious Diseases 49: 1591.
18. Haskelberg H, Hoy JF, Amin J, Ebeling PR, Emery S, et al. (2012) Changes in Bone Turnover and Bone Loss in HIV-Infected Patients Changing Treatment to Tenofovir-Emtricitabine or Abacavir-Lamivudine. PLoS One 7: e38377.
19. McComsey GA, Kitch D, Daar ES, Tierney C, Jahed NC, et al. (2011) Bone Mineral Density and Fractures in Antiretroviral-Naive Persons Randomized to Receive Abacavir-Lamivudine or Tenofovir Disoproxil Fumarate-Emtricitabine Along With Efavirenz or Atazanavir-Ritonavir: AIDS Clinical Trials Group A5224s, a Substudy of ACTG A5202. Journal of Infectious Diseases 203: 1791.
20. Lewiecki EM, Keaveny TM, Kopperdahl DL, Genant HK, Engelke K, et al. (2009) Once-monthly oral ibandronate improves biomechanical determinants of bone strength in women with postmenopausal osteoporosis. Journal of Clinical Endocrinology & Metabolism 94: 171–180.
21. Bonnick S, Beck T, Cosman F, Hochberg M, Wang H, et al. (2009) DXA-based hip structural analysis of once-weekly bisphosphonate-treated postmenopausal women with low bone mass. Osteoporosis international 20: 911–921.
22. Alwis G, Karlsson C, Stenevi-Lundgren S, Rosengren BE, Karlsson MK (2012) Femoral Neck Bone Strength Estimated by Hip Structural Analysis (HSA) in Swedish Caucasians Aged 6–90 Years. Calcified Tissue International 90: 174.
23. Hofbauer LC, Schoppet M (2004) Clinical implications of the osteoprotegerin/RANKL/RANK system for bone and vascular diseases. JAMA: The Journal of the American Medical Association 292: 490–495.
24. Samelson EJ, Broe KE, Demissie S, Beck TJ, Karasik D, et al. (2008) Increased Plasma Osteoprotegerin Concentrations Are Associated with Indices of Bone Strength of the Hip. Journal of Clinical Endocrinology & Metabolism 93: 1789–1795.
25. Szulc P, Hawa G, Boutroy S, Vilayphiou N, Schoppet M, et al. (2011) Cortical Bone Status Is Associated with Serum Osteoprotegerin Concentration in Men: The STRAMBO Study. Journal of Clinical Endocrinology & Metabolism 96: 2216–2226.
26. Gaudio A, Pennisi P, Muratore F, Bertino G, Ardiri A, et al. (2012) Reduction of volumetric bone mineral density in postmenopausal women with hepatitis C virus-correlated chronic liver disease: A peripheral quantitative computed tomography (pQCT) study. European Journal of Internal Medicine 23: 656–660.
27. Bloch M, Tong W, Hoy J, Richardson R, Baker D, et al. (2012) Improved Low Bone Mineral Density and Bone Turnover Markers with Switch from Tenofovir to Raltegravir in Virologically Suppressed HIV-1+ Adults at 48 Weeks: The TROP Study. Conference of Retrovirus and Opportunistic Infection. Washington.
28. Stellbrink HJ, Orkin C, Arribas JR, Compston J, Gerstoft J, et al. (2010) Comparison of changes in bone density and turnover with abacavir-lamivudine versus tenofovir-emtricitabine in HIV-infected adults: 48-week results from the ASSERT study. Clinical Infectious Diseases 51: 963.

5

Variation in the *MC4R* Gene Is Associated with Bone Phenotypes in Elderly Swedish Women

Gaurav Garg[1,9], **Jitender Kumar**[2,9], **Fiona E. McGuigan**[1,9], **Martin Ridderstråle**[3], **Paul Gerdhem**[4], **Holger Luthman**[5], **Kristina Åkesson**[1]*

1 Clinical and Molecular Osteoporosis Research Unit, Department of Clinical Sciences, Lund University and Department of Orthopaedics, Skåne University Hospital, Malmö, Sweden, 2 Department of Medical Sciences, Molecular Epidemiology and Science for Life Laboratory, Uppsala University, Uppsala, Sweden, 3 Clinical Obesity Research, Department of Endocrinology, Skåne University Hospital, Malmö, Sweden, 4 Department of Clinical Science, Intervention and Technology, Karolinska Institutet, Department of Orthopaedics, Karolinska University Hospital, Stockholm, Sweden, 5 Medical Genetics Unit, Department of Clinical Sciences, Lund University, Malmö, Sweden

Abstract

Osteoporosis is characterized by reduced bone mineral density (BMD) and increased fracture risk. Fat mass is a determinant of bone strength and both phenotypes have a strong genetic component. In this study, we examined the association between obesity associated polymorphisms (SNPs) with body composition, BMD, Ultrasound (QUS), fracture and biomarkers (Homocysteine (Hcy), folate, Vitamin D and Vitamin B12) for obesity and osteoporosis. Five common variants: rs17782313 and rs1770633 (melanocortin 4 receptor *(MC4R)*; rs7566605 (insulin induced gene 2 *(INSIG2)*; rs9939609 and rs1121980 (fat mass and obesity associated *(FTO)* were genotyped in 2 cohorts of Swedish women: PEAK-25 (age 25, n = 1061) and OPRA (age 75, n = 1044). Body mass index (BMI), total body fat and lean mass were strongly positively correlated with QUS and BMD in both cohorts ($r^2 = 0.2–0.6$). *MC4R* rs17782313 was associated with QUS in the OPRA cohort and individuals with the minor C-allele had higher values compared to T-allele homozygotes (TT vs. CT vs. CC: BUA: 100 vs. 103 vs. 103; p = 0.002); (SOS: 1521 vs. 1526 vs. 1524; p = 0.008); (Stiffness index: 69 vs. 73 vs. 74; p = 0.0006) after adjustment for confounders. They also had low folate (18 vs. 17 vs. 16; p = 0.03) and vitamin D (93 vs. 91 vs. 90; p = 0.03) and high Hcy levels (13.7 vs 14.4 vs. 14.5; p = 0.06). Fracture incidence was lower among women with the C-allele, (52% vs. 58%; p = 0.067). Variation in *MC4R* was not associated with BMD or body composition in either OPRA or PEAK-25. SNPs close to *FTO* and *INSIG2* were not associated with any bone phenotypes in either cohort and *FTO* SNPs were only associated with body composition in PEAK-25 (p≤0.001). Our results suggest that genetic variation close to *MC4R* is associated with quantitative ultrasound and risk of fracture.

Editor: Joseph Devaney, Children's National Medical Center, Washington, United States of America

Funding: The funders had no role in study design, data collection and analysis, decision to publish, or preparation of the manuscript. Financial support for the study was received from the Swedish Research Council (Grant K2009-53X-14691-07-3)(www.vr.se), Greta and Johan Kock Foundation, A Påhlsson Foundation, A Österlund Foundation, Herman Järnhardt Foundation, King Gustav V and Queen Victoria Foundation, Malmö University Hospital Research Foundation, Research and Development Council of Region Skåne, Sweden and the Swedish Medical Society.

Competing Interests: The authors have declared that no competing interests exist.

* E-mail: Kristina.Akesson@med.lu.se

9 These authors contributed equally to this work.

Introduction

Osteoporosis and obesity are both multifactorial disorders that in recent years have become major public health problems. At one time considered to be mutually exclusive, it is now recognized that these conditions share many genetic and environmental risk factors and are linked to each other through a number of complex regulatory pathways [1,2]. Epidemiological studies have shown that increased body weight is positively associated with bone mass, while low body weight is a risk factor for bone loss and osteoporosis [3]. The positive effect of body weight on bone mass may be attributable to a number of factors: increased mechanical load which has an anabolic effect on bone [4]; conversion of steroid precursors to estrogen in peripheral adipose tissue [5] or through the secretion of bone active hormones from β-cells in the pancreas and adipocytes themselves [6]. Homocysteine (Hcy), vitamin B12, vitamin D and folate are biomarkers for a number of pathologies including

cardiovascular disease and diabetes and a strong correlation between these biomarkers with BMI has been reported [7–10]. Elevated levels of Hcy and low levels of vitamin D are strong and independent risk factors for osteoporotic fracture risk [11,12].

Studies have shown that variation in diet and life style modulate Hcy, folate and vitamin B12 [13,14], all of which are important components in intermediary metabolism. Elevated Hcy levels have been associated with detrimental effects on bone metabolism, however, whether Hcy and other biochemical parameters play a causal role or act as markers for other mechanisms underlying these pathologies is unclear [15].

The complex relationship between fat cells and bone has been under intense scrutiny. Adipocytes and osteoblasts share a common progenitor, the pluripotent mesenchymal stem cell, and there is a degree of plasticity between the two cell types [16–19]. Differentiation to a particular lineage is regulated by numerous transcription factors and with increasing age there is a shift away from osteoblast towards adipocyte production [19] which in conjunction with increased osteoclast function may lead to osteoporosis [20].

At the genetic level a number of association studies have identified single nucleotide polymorphisms (SNPs) close to genes contributing to both osteoporosis and body composition [21–30]. To date, few bivariate genome-wide association studies (GWAS) for osteoporosis and obesity have been performed [31] although GWAS for obesity and its associated pathological outcomes have identified a number of SNPs close to genes expected to also play an important role in bone metabolism [31]. In the current study, we selected five SNPs identified through GWAS: rs17782313_MC4R; rs1770633_MC4R; rs7566605_INSIG2; rs9939609_FTO and rs1121980_FTO.

The FTO gene is highly expressed in the hypothalamus and is involved in energy homeostasis through the control of energy expenditure [32]. Located on chromosome 16, the FTO gene has nine exons and spans more than 400 kb. The SNPs associated with BMI in the GWAS lie in the first intron that harbors a region highly conserved across different species [33]. Individuals with the rs9939609 variant allele were shown to have a 31% increased risk per variant allele, of developing obesity [34,35]. Variation in the FTO gene has been analyzed for association with BMD in a number of populations including children and adults [36] and in a mouse knockout model, BMD was lower in the FTO knockout compared to controls [37].

The MC4R gene on chromosome 18 encodes the MC4 protein, a G-protein coupled receptor that plays a major role in the central regulation of body weight through maintaining energy homeostasis and the suppression of food intake [38]. Genetic variation in the MC4R gene has been identified as responsible for monogenic forms of obesity [39]. In a GWAS by Loos et al., SNPs present in the intergenic region upstream of MC4R were associated with BMI [33]. Patients deficient in MC4R have been reported to have increased BMD and decreased bone resorption [40], while genetic variation has been evaluated for association with bone mass, but only in children [41].

The INSIG2 gene has been reported to be associated with increased risk of obesity [42]. SNP rs7566605, located 10 kb upstream of the INSIG2 gene transcription start site, was associated with fat mass. INSIG2 is a candidate gene for increased BMI; it binds to the sterol regulatory element-binding protein complex (SREBP) and reduces the activity of cholesterol and fatty acid synthesis in the endoplasmic reticulum [43]. Although variation in the INSIG2 gene has recently identified in a GWAS for BMD [44], it has not been yet fully explored.

The rationale for our study was to comprehensively evaluate the association between selected obesity associated polymorphisms and aspects of bone strength, a complex trait not captured by BMD alone. Since the skeletal fragility associated with osteoporosis reflects reduced bone quality as well as quantity, we have assessed micro-architectural properties of bone, bone geometry and long-term fracture risk in addition to BMD and body composition. Furthermore, in order to understand the mechanisms underlying these associations, we have also evaluated the association between these polymorphisms and biomarkers for obesity and bone mass. By studying two differently aged cohorts we have evaluated age-related differences in the contribution of obesity associated polymorphisms with bone phenotypes.

Materials and Methods

Subjects

Two population based cohorts of Swedish women were studied; the OPRA cohort consisting of 1044 elderly women all aged exactly 75 and prospectively followed for 10 years and the PEAK-25 cohort consisting of 1061 women all aged exactly 25. Details of the two cohorts have been published [45,46]. Participants gave written informed consent and the study was approved by the Regional Ethical Review Board in Lund according to the Helsinki agreement.

Measurement of Bone Phenotypes and Body Composition Using DXA

Bone mineral density (g/cm^2) at the femoral neck (FN), lumbar spine (LS) and total body (TB) was measured using dual-energy x-ray absorptiometry (Lunar Prodigy: PEAK-25; Lunar DPX-L: OPRA (Lunar Corporation, Madison, WI, USA)). Fat and lean mass for total body (TB) and trunk were also measured using the same instrument. Calibrations were performed daily using a phantom supplied by the manufacturer. Precision error (coefficient of variation) for DXA scanning was 0.94%, 1.45%, 4.01% for TB, LS and FN respectively in the OPRA cohort [47] and 0.90% and 0.65% for FN and LS respectively in PEAK-25 [48]. For the OPRA cohort, all measurements at baseline were performed using the same instrument, while analyses of scans were made with software versions 1.33 and 1.35.

Hip geometry was assessed only in the OPRA cohort by employing the software provided by Lunar® (Lunar Corporation, WI, USA) for the DPX-L scanner. The following phenotypes were analyzed: Hip Axis Length (mm); femoral neck width (mm); Cross Sectional Moment of Inertia [CSMI] (Cm^4) and Section Modulus [SM] (Cm^3). To minimize variability, all variables were analyzed by a single operator. The coefficient of variation for these measurements was between 0.6 and 3.7% [49].

Ultrasound measurements (Speed of Sound (SOS) (m/s)), Broadband Ultrasound Attenuation ((BUA) (dB/MHz)) and Stiffness Index (SI)) were performed on the right calcaneus using the Lunar Achilles $^{(R)}$ system (Lunar Corporation Madison, WI, USA) to assess bone quality in both cohorts. The precision was 1.5% for derivatives of BUA and SOS [50]. Daily calibrations were made to control the long-term stability of the apparatus.

Fracture Ascertainment

In the PEAK-25 cohort the fracture incidence is low, therefore fracture data was analyzed only in the OPRA cohort. Self-reported fractures sustained between age 20 and 75 were recorded and verified from the radiological files [51]. The majority of fractures (>99%) occurring in the elderly women were attributable to low energy trauma.

Blood Sample Collection and Biochemical Phenotypes Measurements

Non-fasting blood samples were collected before noon for DNA isolation (PEAK-25 and OPRA) and to assay serum concentration of biochemical markers (OPRA). Samples were stored at −80°C until analysis. Assays were performed at the Department of Clinical Chemistry, Malmö, Skåne University Hospital according to accredited methods. Biochemical phenotypes, available only in the OPRA cohort, were assayed using standardized analytical protocols. Total serum Hcy (μmol/L) was measured using HPLC. Serum vitamin B12 (pmol/L) and folate (nmol/L) were measured using Elecsys assays (Roche Diagnostics, Mannheim, Germany) and serum 25-hydroxy vitamin D (25OHD) (nmol/L) was assessed by liquid chromatography mass spectrophotometry (LC-MS) [52].

Genotyping and Statistical Analysis

Five obesity associated SNPs from three genes were genotyped in both cohorts (Table S1) [33,42]. Sequenom's iPlex Gold system (Sequenom, San Diego, CA) was employed to score the genotypes. A total of 993 women from the OPRA and 1001 women from the PEAK-25 cohort were genotyped successfully. Approximately 3% of the samples from each cohort were genotyped in duplicate with 100% concordance. Departures from Hardy-Weinberg equilibrium were tested using the χ^2 test with one degree of freedom (HWE Program, Jurg Ott and Rockefeller University, New York). Linkage disequilibrium (LD) between SNPs from the same gene was tested using Haploview (http://www.broad.mit.edu/mpg/haploview/). Statistical analysis was performed using SPSS (version 20.0, SPSS Inc., Chicago, IL).

Using a co-dominant model (comparing the three genotypes, under the assumption that neither of the alleles is dominant), genotype specific differences between the phenotypes were analyzed with the Kruskal-Wallis test and to determine association adjusting for confounding factors (height, and smoking) regression analysis was performed. Gene interaction with Hcy was analyzed comparing the lowest and highest quartiles of serum Hcy levels, where quartile 1 was considered 'Normal' (<11.6 µmol/L) and quartile 4 'High' (>17.5 µmol/L). The $\chi2$ test was used to analyze association between genotypes and categorical variables. Multiple statistical tests were performed, however since most of the phenotypes are dependent, we report uncorrected p-values (two-tailed) and associations were considered nominally significant at the level $p<0.05$.

Results

The general and clinical characteristics of the women from the two differently aged cohorts are reported in **Table 1**. Genotype and allele frequencies did not differ between cohorts (**Table 2**). All SNPs conformed to HWE ($p>0.05$). Both SNPs from the *FTO* gene were in strong LD (OPRA, $D' = 0.98$, $r^2 = 0.84$; PEAK-25, $D' = 0.99$, $r^2 = 0.87$) therefore only rs9939609 was used for further analysis. No LD was observed for the *MC4R* SNPs ($D' = 0.45$, $r^2 = 0.13$).

The PEAK-25 participants had lower BMI and fat mass and higher lean mass compared to the elderly individuals from OPRA (**Table 1**). As previously reported, fat and lean mass were strongly positively associated with BMD [26,53], with lean mass making a greater contribution than fat mass to BMD in young women (data not shown). For QUS phenotypes, the positive association with fat and lean mass was very similar in the elderly women, while in the young women the contribution from lean mass was stronger (**Table 3**).

Association between Obesity Associated Polymorphisms and Body Composition

SNP rs9939609_*FTO* was associated with a number of body composition measurements including weight, BMI, and fat mass in PEAK-25 (**Table 4**). Individuals carrying the minor allele had higher BMI, fat mass (TB and trunk) but no association was found with lean mass (**Table 4**). The association with rs9939609_*FTO* remained after adjusting for smoking status and height ($p = 0.001$ to $p<0.0001$) (**Table 4**). We observed trends for BMI, TB fat mass and percentage trunk-fat in the same direction in the OPRA cohort, but these did not reach statistical significance. After adjustment for height and smoking status an association with percentage of trunk-fat was observed with rs9939609_*FTO* ($p = 0.007$). No association between *MC4R* or *INSIG2* polymor-

Table 1. Cohort Baseline Details.

Variable	PEAK-25	OPRA
Age (years)	25.5 (25.3–25.7)	75.2 (75.1–75.3)
Weight (kg)	63.0 (57.1–70.0)	67 (60–75)
Height (cm)	168 (163–172)	160 (157–164)
BMI (kg/m²)	22.4 (20.5–24.6)	26.0 (23.4–28.7)
Smokers#	440 (44%)	354 (34%)
Adult Fracture*	–	534 (51.1%)
Body Composition		
Total Body Fat mass (kg)	19.6 (15.2–25.1)	26.0 (20.8–31.3)
Trunk Fat mass (kg)	9.3 (6.9–12.2)	12.7 (9.8–15.4)
% Fat mass- Total Body	31.7 (26.5–36.4)	39.2 (34.1–43.1)
% Fat mass- Trunk	32.5 (26.2–38.9)	40.1 (35.3–44.1)
BMD (g/cm²)		
Total Body	1.17 (1.12–1.22)	1.00 (0.94–1.07)
Femoral Neck	1.04 (0.97–1.13)	0.75 (0.66–0.85)
Lumbar Spine	1.05 (0.99–1.13)	0.97 (0.86–1.10)
Quantitative Ultrasound		
BUA (dB/MHz)	116 (110–124)	102 (96–109)
SOS (m/s)	1571 (1551–1595)	1522 (1505–1540)
Stiffness Index	98 (88–109)	71 (62–80)
Hip Geometry		
Hip Axis Length (mm)	–	105 (102–109)
Femoral Neck Width (mm)	–	34 (32–36)
Cross-Sectional Area (cm²)	–	131 (114–155)
CSMI (cm⁴)	–	10281 (8253–13188)
Femoral Neck Shaft Angle (°)	–	129 (126–131)
Biochemistry		
Homocysteine (µmol/L)	–	14.1 (11.6–17.5)
Vitamin B12 (pmol/L)	–	308 (238–409)
Folate (nmol/L)	–	18.0 (14.0–27.0)
Vitamin D (nmol/L)	–	92.1 (74.3–112.2)

Median (Interquartile Range) reported for continuous variables; Number (%) for discrete variables. #Current or former smokers; BUA- Broadband Ultrasound Attenuation; SOS- Speed of Sound; CSMI- Cross Sectional Moment of Inertia; *Fracture of any type sustained after age 20 and before baseline.

phisms and body composition were observed in the OPRA and PEAK-25 cohorts (data not shown).

Obesity Associated Polymorphisms and Association with BMD, QUS and Geometry

SNP rs1121980 from the *FTO* gene was excluded from analysis. The remaining four SNPs were analyzed for association with bone density, but no significant genotype related differences in BMD at any skeletal site were observed in either cohort (data not shown).

Polymorphisms were also analyzed for association with bone quantitative ultrasound in both cohorts. The rs17782313_*MC4R* showed association with BUA, SOS and SI in OPRA ($p = 0.007$–0.001) (**Table 5**) and individuals carrying the minor C-allele had higher values compared to homozygotes for the common allele. The association remained even after adjustment for height and smoking ($p = 0.02$–0.0004) (**Table 5**) and additional adjustment

Table 2. Genotype and Allele Frequencies.

SNP_Gene Symbol	OPRA				PEAK-25			
	Major Allele Homozygotes No. (%)	Heterozygotes No. (%)	Minor Allele Homozygotes No. (%)	MAF	Major Allele Homozygotes No. (%)	Heterozygotes No. (%)	Minor Allele Homozygotes No. (%)	MAF
rs9939609_FTO	354 (36)	499 (50)	139 (14)	0.39	319 (32)	499 (50)	182 (18)	0.43
rs1121980_FTO	312 (32)	500 (51)	170 (17)	0.43	282 (29)	492 (50)	211 (21)	0.47
rs7566605_INSIG2	448 (46)	424 (43)	111 (11)	0.33	449 (45)	421 (43)	116 (12)	0.33
rs17782313_MC4R	550 (57)	362 (38)	53 (5)	0.24	564 (57)	363 (37)	59 (6)	0.24
rs17700633_MC4R	456 (46)	439 (44)	98 (10)	0.32	482 (48)	414 (42)	98 (10)	0.31

MAF- Minor allele frequency.

Table 3. Effect Sizes of Lean and Fat Mass on Bone Quantitative Ultrasound (QUS) Phenotypes.

OPRA	BUA	QUS Variable	
		SOS	Stiffness
Total Body Fat mass	0.30	0.21	0.28
Total Body Lean mass	0.32	0.22	0.28
Trunk Fat mass	0.32	0.23	0.31
Trunk Lean mass	0.31	0.21	0.30
PEAK-25			
Total Body Fat mass	0.14	−0.03[a]	0.05[a]
Total Body Lean mass	0.34	0.20	0.28
Trunk Fat mass	0.14	−0.02[a]	0.06[a]
Trunk Lean mass	0.27	0.14	0.22

Reported values are standardized β-coefficients; covariates are adjusted for height and smoking status.
All coefficients are significant at p<0.01 except for those marked [a] which are non-significant.

for weight (p = 0.015 to 0.007). Similar trends were observed in the PEAK-25 cohort but were not statistically significant. Polymorphisms close to *FTO* and *INSIG2* were not associated with ultrasound phenotypes in either cohort.

Femoral neck geometry is an important component of hip fracture risk and we evaluated SNP-phenotype associations in the OPRA cohort. The rs7566605_*INSIG2* showed association with FN width (p = 0.03), with individuals carrying the minor allele having a lower mean value compared to subjects homozygous for the major allele (34.1 vs. 34.5 mm), but this did not withstand adjustment for height and weight. Polymorphisms from *FTO* and *MC4R* did not show any association with bone geometry (data not shown).

Obesity Associated Polymorphisms and Association with Biomarkers and Fracture

The association between obesity associated polymorphisms, biochemical risk factors and fracture was evaluated in the OPRA cohort. Carriers of rs17782313_*MC4R* C-allele had high Hcy (p = 0.06), low serum folate (p = 0.03) and low vitamin D (p = 0.03) (**Table 5**). After adjustment for smoking and height, the association remained for folate (p = 0.01) and vitamin D (p = 0.02).

We wanted to determine whether the association between *MC4R* SNPs and QUS was influenced in relation to normal (<11.6 μmol/L) and high (>17.5 μmol/L) levels of Hcy. Only in the high Hcy group was rs17782313_*MC4R* associated with QUS (p = 0.03 to p = 0.005) and this association remained even after adjustment for height and smoking (p = 0.007 to p = 0.001) (**Table 6**) and additionally adjusted for weight the association remained significant (p = 0.01 to 0.002). Interestingly, in the high Hcy group, vitamin D levels decreased with number of C-alleles, in direct contrast with the observation in the normal Hcy group (**Table 6**). As expected, proportionally fewer women fractured prior to baseline in the lowest (BMI<23.4; 63.9%) compared to the highest BMI quartile (BMI >28.7; 52.3%); p = 0.009).

Variation in *FTO* and *INSIG2* did not appear to make an important contribution to fracture risk, even when smoking, TB-BMD and any one of body weight, BMI or fat mass were

Table 4. Association of rs9939609_FTO with Bone and Body Composition Phenotypes in the PEAK-25 Cohort.

Phenotypes	TT	TA	AA	β-Value (Adjusted)	P-value[a]	P- value[b]
	(n = 319)	(n = 499)	(n = 182)	Co-Dominant#		
Weight	61.5 (57.0–68.7)	63.0 (57.0–69.2)	64.3 (58.0–72.3)	1.57 (0.69 to 2.44)	0.038	0.0004
BMI	22.1 (20.2–24.2)	22.2 (20.5–24.5)	23.0 (21.1–25.4)	0.550 (0.24 to 0.86)	0.004	0.001
Total Body Fat mass	19.0 (14.5–23.9)	19.4 (15.2–24.8)	21.1 (16.5–26.9)	1.36 (0.67 to 2.05)	0.004	0.0001
Total Body Lean mass	40.3 (37.4–43.3)	40.0 (37.1–43.1)	40.1 (37.1–43.5)	0.15 (−0.17 to 0.46)	0.63	0.36
% Fat mass - Total Body	30.5 (25.7–35.2)	31.7 (26.3–36.4)	32.9 (28.0–38.4)	1.17 (0.56 to 1.78)	0.002	0.0001
Trunk Fat mass	8.9 (6.6–11.6)	9.3 (6.9–12.1)	10.3 (7.7–13.5)	0.764 (0.39 to 1.14)	0.004	0.00007
% Fat mass - Trunk	31.2 (25.3–37.9)	32.5 (26.1–38.4)	34.12 (28.1–41.0)	1.36 (0.78 to 1.85)	0.002	0.0001
Total Body BMD	1.16 (1.12–1.22)	1.17 (1.12–1.23)	1.18 (1.13–1.22)	0.003 (−0.003 to 0.009)	0.52	0.38
Femoral neck BMD	1.04 (0.97–1.12)	1.04 (0.97–1.14)	1.06 (0.97–1.12)	0.003 (−0.007 to 0.014)	0.86	0.53
Lumbar Spine BMD	1.23 (1.15–1.31)	1.24 (1.14–1.33)	1.24 (1.14–1.33)	−0.001 (−0.012 to 0.010)	0.93	0.85
BUA	116 (109–124)	117 (117–123)	117 (110–124)	−0.015 (−0.977 to 0.946)	0.87	0.97
SOS	1569 (1552–1594)	1573 (1551–1596)	1572 (1550–1593)	−0.881 (−3.871 to 2.109)	0.60	0.56
Stiffness Index	96.5 (87.3–108.0)	98.0 (88.9–109.6)	99.0 (87.6–107.4)	−0.254 (−1.604 to 1.096)	0.65	0.71

Reported values are median (interquartile range); #(TT vs. TA vs. AA) [a]Kruskal-Wallis; [b]Linear regression - after adjustment for height and smoking.

included in the regression model. Women carrying the MC4R_rs17782313 C-allele showed a non-significant trend towards fewer fractures although there was no allele dose effect (52.1% vs. 58.5%). As expected, compared to women without a baseline fracture, QUS values were lower in those with a fracture regardless of genotype (data not shown), however, within the fracture category women with the rs17782313_MC4R C-allele had higher QUS values ((BUA: 97 vs. 100 vs. 103; p = 0.04); (SOS: 1516 vs. 1517 vs. 1517; p = 0.18); (SI: 67 vs. 70 vs. 72; p = 0.021)) consistent with a lower fracture incidence.

Discussion

Obesity is an established risk factor for a number of complex disorders including cardiovascular complications, diabetes mellitus and hypertension, but it has been suggested to be protective against osteoporosis [54]. A complex, differential influence from lean and fat mass on bone strength is suggested [54,55] and the current study supports the supposition that lean mass makes a larger contribution to BMD during young age while fat mass plays a major role for BMD in later stages of life [54,55].

Table 5. Association of rs17782313_MC4R with Body Composition, Bone and Biochemistry phenotypes in the OPRA Cohort.

Phenotypes	TT	TC	CC	β-value (Adjusted)	P-value[a]	P-value[b]
	(n = 550)	(n = 362)	(n = 53)	Co-Dominant#		
Weight	66 (60–75)	68 (59–76)	67 (62–75)	0.419 (−0.703 to 1.542)	0.65	0.46
BMI	26.0 (23.3–28.4)	26.0 (23.5–29.1)	26.2 (23.4–27.8)	0.157 (−0.283 to 0.596)	0.58	0.49
Total Body Fat mass	25.8 (20.5–31.1)	26.0 (20.9–31.9)	27.1 (22.4–30.4)	0.431 (−0.419 to 1.281)	0.70	0.32
% Fat mass Total Body	38.5 (34.0–42.7)	39.1 (34.4–42.2)	40.0 (35.4–41.7)	0.485 (−0.276 to 1.247)	0.72	0.21
Trunk Fat mass	12.5 (9.8–15.3)	13.0 (9.7–15.7)	13.0 (10.4–14.8)	0.144 (−.280 to 0.568)	0.69	0.50
% Fat mass- Trunk	39.1 (34.2–42.7)	39.6 (34.5–43.0)	39.4 (35.8–41.9)	0.52 (−0.266 to 1.237)	0.55	0.26
Total Body BMD	0.997 (0.941–1.061)	1.011 (0.944–1.073)	1.003 (0.934–1.062)	0.004 (−0.006 to 0.015)	0.52	0.44
Femoral Neck BMD	0.752 (0.660–0.848)	0.751 (0.680–0.846)	0.724 (0.628–0.825)	−0.005 (−0.019 to 0.009)	0.33	0.52
Lumbar Spine BMD	0.97 (0.86–1.10)	0.98 (0.87–1.09)	0.95 (0.84–1.12)	0.009 (−0.044 to 0.061)	0.83	0.75
BUA	100 (95–108)	103 (97–109)	103 (95–108)	1.72 (0.606 to 2.833)	0.007	0.002
SOS	1521 (1504–1539)	1526 (1509–1544)	1524 (1506–1540)	4.227 (1.119 to 7.335)	0.024	0.008
Stiffness Index	69.0 (61.0–79.0)	73.4 (65.0–82.5)	74.0 (61.0–81.3)	2.59 (1.11 to 4.07)	0.001	0.0006
Homocysteine	13.7 (11.6–16.9)	14.4 (11.6–17.7)	14.5 (11.6–18.3)	0.337 (−0.355 to 1.028)	0.06	0.34
Folate	18.0 (15.0–28.0)	17.0 (14.0–24.0)	16.0 (14.0–22.0)	−1.544 (−2.734 to −0.353)	0.028	0.013
Vitamin D	92.6 (76.7–115.5)	91.1 (72.5–109.2)	90.2 (70.3–110.5)	−3.744 (−6.914 to −0.573)	0.027	0.018

Values are median (Interquartile Range); #(TT vs. TC vs. CC); [a]Kruskal-Wallis; [b]Linear regression after adjustment for height and smoking; Units: folate and vitamin D (nmol/L), homocysteine (μmol/L).

Table 6. SNP *rs17782313_MC4R* Interacts with Homocysteine to Influence Bone Quality.

'Normal' homocysteine levels (<11.6 μmol/L) (n = 237)

Phenotype	TT	TC	CC	β-Value (Adjusted)	p value[a]	p value[b]
	(130)	(79)	(13)	Co-Dominant#		
Total Body Fatmass	24.3 (18.7–29.2)	25.9 (21.1–30.4)	22.6 (19.4–28.7)	0.749 (−0.809 to 2.309)	0.35	0.35
Folate	32 (19–44)	29 (20–44)	32 (20–35)	−0.931 (−3.547 to 1.686)	0.76	0.48
Vitamin D	91.8 (77.2–115.5)	96.8 (73.7–111.0)	104 (72.3–134.0)	4.421 (−2.398 to 11.24)	0.46	0.21
BUA	101.4 (95.1–108.7)	102 (98–109.7)	104.3 (93.0–108.7)	1.504 (−0.5546 to 3.563)	0.34	0.15
SOS	1522 (1505–1541)	1529 (1510–1547)	1538 (1508–1554)	3.893 (−2.348 to 10.13)	0.26	0.22
Stiffness Index	71 (62–80.6)	74 (65.5–83)	79 (57.6–84.7)	2.791 (−0.1968 to 5.779)	0.16	0.06

'High' homocysteine levels (>17.5 μmol/L) (n = 246)

Phenotype	TT	TC	CC	β-Value (Adjusted)	p value[a]	p value[b]
	(111)	(90)	(16)	Co-Dominant#		
Total Body Fatmass	26.1 (19.6–31.4)	24.5 (19.2–33.2)	28.8 (24.9–30.7)	0.759 (−1.319 to 2.838)	0.49	0.48
Folate	14 (12–17)	14 (12–16)	14 (12–15)	−0.201 (−1.44 to 1.038)	0.87	0.75
Vitamin D	93.6 (75.6–116.9)	85.7 (68.9–106.7)	80.3 (64.2–104.3)	−7.394 (−13.9 to −0.8903)	0.08	0.026
BUA	98.7 (93.0–107.7)	103.5 (97–109)	106 (95.1–107.7)	4.356 (1.732 to 6.979)	0.006	0.001
SOS	1510 (1502–1535.9)	1519 (1508.2–1543)	1524 (1501–1539.9)	9.316 (2.572 to 16.06)	0.028	0.007
Stiffness Index	67 (59.9–77.9)	72 (64–82.5)	77 (64–76.8)	5.445 (2.188 to 8.702)	0.005	0.001

Values are median (Interquartile Range);
#(TT vs. TC vs. CC);
[a]Kruskal-Wallis;
[b]Linear regression after adjustment for height and smoking.

FTO has been well described in relation to body composition and obesity phenotypes [33,34,36,37]. In our study, we observed higher BMI and fat mass in relation to the rs9939609_*FTO* C-allele; however it is interesting that the association was only seen in the young women. This is consistent with suggestions that the effect size of obesity susceptibility genes varies with age [56]. Although the underlying mechanisms are unclear, data from a mouse model has shown that mRNA expression of *FTO* is regulated by nutritional intake and expression levels vary according to feeding and fasting behavior [32] and we might speculate that food intake patterns differ between young and elderly individuals. We did not find any association with BMD or other bone phenotypes in either the young or elderly cohort of women. An age-specific effect has been reported in at least one study alongside suggestions that *FTO* could be a genetic marker for peak bone mass [36] due to the potential role of *FTO* in postnatal growth [37]. Our results do not support this however since the women in the PEAK-25 cohort are at an age where peak bone mass is assumed to have been reached. Nonetheless this does not rule out the possibility that *FTO* variants could be associated with skeletal growth trajectory in childhood and adolescence. Although we found no direct association between variations in the vicinity of *FTO* and BMD or QUS parameters, it is likely that any effect of the gene on bone is indirect, through BMI and fat mass.

MC4R is crucial in the regulation of body weight and monogenic forms of obesity commonly result from mutations in its gene. Although we observed a trend for higher BMI and fat mass in both cohorts with the C-allele, the association with *MC4R*

did not reach significance, which contrasts with the findings reported in GWAS [33] and other association studies [57]. In the current study, we have shown for the first time that variation in the *MC4R* gene is associated with QUS phenotypes. A trend towards better bone quality with carriage of the variant *MC4R* rs17782313 C-allele was observed in the young women, but was more pronounced in the elderly women. Furthermore this association appeared to be mediated by both direct and indirect mechanisms which may explain in part the age specific effect observed, since a higher BMI, as displayed by the older women, is positively associated with bone strength. Although a genetic association between *MC4R* gene polymorphism and bone mass has been reported, albeit in children [41], we found no association with BMD or bone structural traits (femoral neck geometry) in our study.

One of the novel findings of our study is that *MC4R* is associated with altered vitamin D, folate and Hcy levels, which are associated with obesity. Vitamin D deficiency associated with obesity has been shown at all ages and independent of sex in a recent meta-analysis [58]. The results from our study indicates that a gene environment interaction has the potential to improve bone quality through increased fat mass in elderly women, demonstrated by the fact that the strongest association between *MC4R* and QUS was in the elevated Hcy group. This finding is in keeping with what is known about *MC4R* expression, i.e. that it is altered in response to environmental stimuli through hypothalamic neuronal networks, and recent studies suggest this has an important role in bone homeostasis [59].

Although in a meta-analysis of GWAS [39] variation in *INSIG2* was associated with femoral neck BMD, in our cohorts *INSIG2* was not associated with BMD, body composition or bone quality, although this is unsurprising since we have analyzed a BMI associated SNP which is not in LD ($r^2 = 0.01$; $D' = 0.39$) with the SNP identified in the BMD GWAS. In our study, although width at the femoral neck was narrower in elderly women with the variant allele, the association was attenuated after adjustment for height and weight and furthermore indices of bone strength and hip fracture rates were not different. To date, none of the GWAS for bone geometry have shown evidence of association within or near the *INSIG2* gene [60–63].

The strengths of this study include the extensive data collected on body composition, bone related phenotypes and biochemical risk factors for obesity and osteoporosis. By including two differently aged cohorts we have the possibility to distinguish age related effects of genetic variation on these phenotypes. The cohorts studied are well-characterized, large, of identical age within each cohort and the majority of women were of Swedish origin. Whether the findings are applicable to other ethnic groups requires replication in other populations. A limitation of the study is that biomarker data was not available in the PEAK-25 cohort, which would have enabled us to identify if there are age related effects associated with the homocysteine-*MC4R*-obesity relationship.

In summary, our data provides novel evidence that variation in the obesity associated gene *MC4R* is associated with improved quantitative ultrasound phenotypes, an important component of bone strength.

Acknowledgments

The authors acknowledge the participants of the study. Thanks are also extended to Dr Mattias Callréus for data collection, Åsa Almgren, Siv Braun and Lisa Quensell for data management, Jan-Åke Nilsson for statistical advice, Lisa Jansson for genotyping and the research nurses at the Clinical and Molecular Osteoporosis Research Unit.

Author Contributions

Conceived and designed the experiments: KÅ PG FM JK HL. Performed the experiments: GG JK. Analyzed the data: GG JK. Contributed reagents/materials/analysis tools: KÅ FM HL GG JK. Wrote the paper: GG JK FM. Revising and Approving manuscript: GG JK FM HL PG MR KÅ.

References

1. Deng FY, Lei SF, Li MX, Jiang C, Dvornyk V, et al. (2006) Genetic determination and correlation of body mass index and bone mineral density at the spine and hip in Chinese Han ethnicity. Osteoporos Int 17: 119–124.

2. Sun X, Lei SF, Deng FY, Wu S, Papacian C, et al. (2006) Genetic and environmental correlations between bone geometric parameters and body compositions. Calcif Tissue Int 79: 43–49.

3. Wardlaw GM (1996) Putting body weight and osteoporosis into perspective. Am J Clin Nutr 63: 433S–436S.

4. Skerry TM, Suva LJ (2003) Investigation of the regulation of bone mass by mechanical loading: from quantitative cytochemistry to gene array. Cell Biochem Funct 21: 223–229.

5. Horowitz MC (1993) Cytokines and estrogen in bone: anti-osteoporotic effects. Science 260: 626–627.

6. Reid IR (2002) Relationships among body mass, its components, and bone. Bone 31: 547–555.

7. Nakazato M, Maeda T, Takamura N, Wada M, Yamasaki H, et al. (2011) Relation of body mass index to blood folate and total homocysteine concentrations in Japanese adults. Eur J Nutr 50: 581–585.

8. Vaya A, Ejarque I, Tembl J, Corella D, Laiz B (2011) Hyperhomocysteinemia, obesity and cryptogenic stroke. Clin Hemorheol Microcirc 47: 53–58.

9. Vaya A, Rivera L, Hernandez-Mijares A, de la Fuente M, Sola E, et al. (2012) Homocysteine levels in morbidly obese patients: its association with waist circumference and insulin resistance. Clin Hemorheol Microcirc 52: 49–56.

10. Jungert A, Roth HJ, Neuhauser-Berthold M (2012) Serum 25-hydroxyvitamin D3 and body composition in an elderly cohort from Germany: a cross-sectional study. Nutr Metab (Lond) 9: 42.

11. Ensrud KE, Ewing SK, Fredman L, Hochberg MC, Cauley JA, et al. (2010) Circulating 25-hydroxyvitamin D levels and frailty status in older women. J Clin Endocrinol Metab 95: 5266–5273.

12. van Meurs JB, Dhonukshe-Rutten RA, Pluijm SM, van der Klift M, de Jonge R, et al. (2004) Homocysteine levels and the risk of osteoporotic fracture. N Engl J Med 350: 2033–2041.

13. McLean RR, Jacques PF, Selhub J, Tucker KL, Samelson EJ, et al. (2004) Homocysteine as a predictive factor for hip fracture in older persons. N Engl J Med 350: 2042–2049.

14. Morris MS, Jacques PF, Selhub J (2005) Relation between homocysteine and B-vitamin status indicators and bone mineral density in older Americans. Bone 37: 234–242.

15. Vacek TP, Kalani A, Voor MJ, Tyagi SC, Tyagi N (2013) The role of homocysteine in bone remodeling. Clin Chem Lab Med 51: 579–590.

16. Bellows CG, Heersche JN (2001) The frequency of common progenitors for adipocytes and osteoblasts and of committed and restricted adipocyte and osteoblast progenitors in fetal rat calvaria cell populations. J Bone Miner Res 16: 1983–1993.

17. Beresford JN, Bennett JH, Devlin C, Leboy PS, Owen ME (1992) Evidence for an inverse relationship between the differentiation of adipocytic and osteogenic cells in rat marrow stromal cell cultures. J Cell Sci 102 (Pt 2): 341–351.

18. Carnevale V, Romagnoli E, Del Fiacco R, Pepe J, Cipriani C, et al. (2010) Relationship between bone metabolism and adipogenesis. J Endocrinol Invest 33: 4–8.

19. Gimble JM, Robinson CE, Wu X, Kelly KA (1996) The function of adipocytes in the bone marrow stroma: an update. Bone 19: 421–428.

20. Rosen CJ, Bouxsein ML (2006) Mechanisms of disease: is osteoporosis the obesity of bone? Nat Clin Pract Rheumatol 2: 35–43.

21. Ackert-Bicknell CL, Demissie S, Marin de Evsikova C, Hsu YH, DeMambro VE, et al. (2008) PPARG by dietary fat interaction influences bone mass in mice and humans. J Bone Miner Res 23: 1398–1408.

22. Bustamante M, Nogues X, Mellibovsky L, Agueda L, Jurado S, et al. (2007) Polymorphisms in the interleukin-6 receptor gene are associated with bone mineral density and body mass index in Spanish postmenopausal women. Eur J Endocrinol 157: 677–684.

23. Cha S, Yu H, Kim JY (2012) Bone mineral density-associated polymorphisms are associated with obesity-related traits in Korean adults in a sex-dependent manner. PLoS One 7: e53013.

24. Fairbrother UL, Tanko LB, Walley AJ, Christiansen C, Froguel P, et al. (2007) Leptin receptor genotype at Gln223Arg is associated with body composition, BMD, and vertebral fracture in postmenopausal Danish women. J Bone Miner Res 22: 544–550.

25. McGuigan F, Larzenius E, Callreus M, Gerdhem P, Luthman H, et al. (2008) Variation in the bone morphogenetic protein-2 gene: effects on fat and lean body mass in young and elderly women. Eur J Endocrinol 158: 661–668.

26. McGuigan FE, Larzenius E, Callreus M, Gerdhem P, Luthman H, et al. (2007) Variation in the BMP2 gene: bone mineral density and ultrasound in young adult and elderly women. Calcif Tissue Int 81: 254–262.

27. Piters E, de Freitas F, Nielsen TL, Andersen M, Brixen K, et al. (2012) Association study of polymorphisms in the SOST gene region and parameters of bone strength and body composition in both young and elderly men: data from the Odense Androgen Study. Calcif Tissue Int 90: 30–39.

28. Xiao WJ, He JW, Zhang H, Hu WW, Gu JM, et al. (2011) ALOX12 polymorphisms are associated with fat mass but not peak bone mineral density in Chinese nuclear families. Int J Obes (Lond) 35: 378–386.

29. Zhao J, Bradfield JP, Li M, Zhang H, Mentch FD, et al. (2011) BMD-associated variation at the Osterix locus is correlated with childhood obesity in females. Obesity (Silver Spring) 19: 1311–1314.

30. Zhao LJ, Guo YF, Xiong DH, Xiao P, Recker RR, et al. (2006) Is a gene important for bone resorption a candidate for obesity? An association and linkage study on the RANK (receptor activator of nuclear factor-kappaB) gene in a large Caucasian sample. Hum Genet 120: 561–570.

31. Liu YZ, Pei YF, Liu JF, Yang F, Guo Y, et al. (2009) Powerful bivariate genome-wide association analyses suggest the SOX6 gene influencing both obesity and osteoporosis phenotypes in males. PLoS One 4: e6827.

32. Gerken T, Girard CA, Tung YC, Webby CJ, Saudek V, et al. (2007) The obesity-associated FTO gene encodes a 2-oxoglutarate-dependent nucleic acid demethylase. Science 318: 1469–1472.

33. Loos RJ, Lindgren CM, Li S, Wheeler E, Zhao JH, et al. (2008) Common variants near MC4R are associated with fat mass, weight and risk of obesity. Nat Genet 40: 768–775.

34. Frayling TM, Timpson NJ, Weedon MN, Zeggini E, Freathy RM, et al. (2007) A common variant in the FTO gene is associated with body mass index and predisposes to childhood and adult obesity. Science 316: 889–894.

35. Rouskas K, Kouvatsi A, Paletas K, Papazoglou D, Tsapas A, et al. (2012) Common variants in FTO, MC4R, TMEM18, PRL, AIF1, and PCSK1 show evidence of association with adult obesity in the Greek population. Obesity (Silver Spring) 20: 389–395.

36. Guo Y, Liu H, Yang TL, Li SM, Li SK, et al. (2011) The fat mass and obesity associated gene, FTO, is also associated with osteoporosis phenotypes. PLoS One 6: e27312.

37. Gao X, Shin YH, Li M, Wang F, Tong Q, et al. (2010) The fat mass and obesity associated gene FTO functions in the brain to regulate postnatal growth in mice. PLoS One 5: e14005.

38. Tao YX (2010) The melanocortin-4 receptor: physiology, pharmacology, and pathophysiology. Endocr Rev 31: 506–543.

39. Willer CJ, Speliotes EK, Loos RJ, Li S, Lindgren CM, et al. (2009) Six new loci associated with body mass index highlight a neuronal influence on body weight regulation. Nat Genet 41: 25–34.

40. Ahn JD, Dubern B, Lubrano-Berthelier C, Clement K, Karsenty G (2006) Cart overexpression is the only identifiable cause of high bone mass in melanocortin 4 receptor deficiency. Endocrinology 147: 3196–3202.

41. Timpson NJ, Sayers A, Davey-Smith G, Tobias JH (2009) How does body fat influence bone mass in childhood? A Mendelian randomization approach. J Bone Miner Res 24: 522–533.

42. Herbert A, Gerry NP, McQueen MB, Heid IM, Pfeufer A, et al. (2006) A common genetic variant is associated with adult and childhood obesity. Science 312: 279–283.

43. Gong Y, Lee JN, Brown MS, Goldstein JL, Ye J (2006) Juxtamembranous aspartic acid in Insig-1 and Insig-2 is required for cholesterol homeostasis. Proc Natl Acad Sci U S A 103: 6154–6159.

44. Estrada K, Styrkarsdottir U, Evangelou E, Hsu YH, Duncan EL, et al. (2012) Genome-wide meta-analysis identifies 56 bone mineral density loci and reveals 14 loci associated with risk of fracture. Nat Genet 44: 491–501.

45. Gerdhem P, Brandstrom H, Stiger F, Obrant K, Melhus H, et al. (2004) Association of the collagen type 1 (COL1A 1) Sp1 binding site polymorphism to femoral neck bone mineral density and wrist fracture in 1044 elderly Swedish women. Calcif Tissue Int 74: 264–269.

46. Kumar J, Swanberg M, McGuigan F, Callreus M, Gerdhem P, et al. (2011) LRP4 association to bone properties and fracture and interaction with genes in the Wnt- and BMP signaling pathways. Bone 49: 343–348.

47. Lenora J, Akesson K, Gerdhem P (2010) Effect of precision on longitudinal follow-up of bone mineral density measurements in elderly women and men. J Clin Densitom 13: 407–412.

48. Callreus M, McGuigan F, Ringsberg K, Akesson K (2012) Self-reported recreational exercise combining regularity and impact is necessary to maximize bone mineral density in young adult women: a population-based study of 1,061 women 25 years of age. Osteoporos Int 23: 2517–2526.

49. Tenne M, McGuigan FE, Ahlborg H, Gerdhem P, Akesson K (2010) Variation in the PTH gene, hip fracture, and femoral neck geometry in elderly women. Calcif Tissue Int 86: 359–366.

50. Karlsson MK, Obrant KJ, Nilsson BE, Johnell O (1998) Bone mineral density assessed by quantitative ultrasound and dual energy X-ray absorptiometry. Normative data in Malmo, Sweden. Acta Orthop Scand 69: 189–193.

51. Gerdhem P, Akesson K (2007) Rates of fracture in participants and non-participants in the Osteoporosis Prospective Risk Assessment study. J Bone Joint Surg Br 89: 1627–1631.

52. Gerdhem P, Ivaska KK, Isaksson A, Pettersson K, Vaananen HK, et al. (2007) Associations between homocysteine, bone turnover, BMD, mortality, and fracture risk in elderly women. J Bone Miner Res 22: 127–134.

53. Gerdhem P, Ringsberg KA, Akesson K, Obrant KJ (2003) Influence of muscle strength, physical activity and weight on bone mass in a population-based sample of 1004 elderly women. Osteoporos Int 14: 768–772.

54. Namwongprom S, Rojanasthien S, Mangklabruks A, Soontrapa S, Wongboontan C, et al. (2013) Effect of fat mass and lean mass on bone mineral density in postmenopausal and perimenopausal Thai women. Int J Womens Health 5: 87–92.

55. Hawamdeh ZM, Sheikh-Ali RF, Alsharif A, Otom AH, Ibrahim AI, et al. (2013) The Influence of Aging on the Association Between Adiposity and Bone Mineral Density in Jordanian Postmenopausal Women. J Clin Densitom. [Epub ahead of print].

56. Kvaloy K, Kulle B, Romundstad P, Holmen TL (2013) Sex-specific effects of weight-affecting gene variants in a life course perspective-The HUNT Study, Norway. Int J Obes (Lond) 9: 1221–9.

57. Liem ET, Vonk JM, Sauer PJ, van der Steege G, Oosterom E, et al. (2010) Influence of common variants near INSIG2, in FTO, and near MC4R genes on overweight and the metabolic profile in adolescence: the TRAILS (TRacking Adolescents' Individual Lives Survey) Study. Am J Clin Nutr 91: 321–328.

58. Vimaleswaran KS, Berry DJ, Lu C, Tikkanen E, Pilz S, et al. (2013) Causal relationship between obesity and vitamin D status: bi-directional Mendelian randomization analysis of multiple cohorts. PLoS Med 10: e1001383.

59. Patel MS, Elefteriou F (2007) The new field of neuroskeletal biology. Calcif Tissue Int 80: 337–347.

60. Chen Y, Xiong DH, Guo YF, Pan F, Zhou Q, et al. (2010) Pathway-based genome-wide association analysis identified the importance of EphrinA-EphR pathway for femoral neck bone geometry. Bone 46: 129–136.

61. Hsu YH, Zillikens MC, Wilson SG, Farber CR, Demissie S, et al. (2010) An integration of genome-wide association study and gene expression profiling to prioritize the discovery of novel susceptibility Loci for osteoporosis-related traits. PLoS Genet 6: e1000977.

62. Liu YZ, Wilson SG, Wang L, Liu XG, Guo YF, et al. (2008) Identification of PLCL1 gene for hip bone size variation in females in a genome-wide association study. PLoS One 3: e3160.

63. Zhao LJ, Liu XG, Liu YZ, Liu YJ, Papasian CJ, et al. (2010) Genome-wide association study for femoral neck bone geometry. J Bone Miner Res 25: 320–329.

6

Blood Clot Formation Does Not Affect Metastasis Formation or Tumor Growth in a Murine Model of Breast Cancer

Stephanie Rossnagl[1,2], Anja von Au[1,2], Matthaeus Vasel[1,2], arco G. Cecchini[3], Inaam A. Nakchbandi[1,2]*

1 Max-Planck Institute of Biochemistry, Martinsried, Germany, 2 Institute of Immunology, University of Heidelberg, Heidelberg, Germany, 3 Department of Urology, University of Bern, Bern, Switzerland

Abstract

Cancer is associated with increased fracture risk, due either to metastasis or associated osteoporosis. After a fracture, blood clots form. Because proteins of the coagulation cascade and activated platelets promote cancer development, a fracture in patients with cancer often raises the question whether it is a pathologic fracture or whether the fracture itself might promote the formation of metastatic lesions. We therefore examined whether blood clot formation results in increased metastasis in a murine model of experimental breast cancer metastasis. For this purpose, a clot was surgically induced in the bone marrow of the left tibia of immundeficient mice. Either one minute prior to or five minutes after clot induction, human cancer cells were introduced in the circulation by intracardiac injection. The number of cancer cells that homed to the intervention site was determined by quantitative real-time PCR and flow cytometry. Metastasis formation and longitudinal growth were evaluated by bioluminescence imaging. The number of cancer cells that homed to the intervention site after 24 hours was similar to the number of cells in the opposite tibia that did not undergo clot induction. This effect was confirmed using two more cancer cell lines. Furthermore, no difference in the number of macroscopic lesions or their growth could be detected. In the control group 72% developed a lesion in the left tibia. In the experimental groups with clot formation 79% and 65% developed lesions in the left tibia (p = ns when comparing each experimental group with the controls). Survival was similar too. In summary, the growth factors accumulating in a clot/hematoma are neither enough to promote cancer cell homing nor support growth in an experimental model of breast cancer bone metastasis. This suggests that blood clot formation, as occurs in traumatic fractures, surgical interventions, and bruises, does not increase the risk of metastasis formation.

Editor: Rajeev Samant, University of Alabama at Birmingham, United States of America

Funding: Funding was provided by the Max-Planck Society and the University of Heidelberg. The funders had no role in study design, data collection and analysis, decision to publish, or preparation of the manuscript.

Competing Interests: The authors have declared that no competing interests exist.

* E-mail: inaam.nakchbandi@immu.uni-heidelberg.de

Introduction

Breast and prostate cancer represent the most common solid tumors in adults associated with bone metastasis [1]. These metastases originate from circulating cancer cells that hijack the hematopoietic stem cell niches in the bone marrow taking advantage of its unique richness in cytokines [2–4]. The growth of a metastatic lesion in the bone often increases the risk of a pathologic fracture [5,6]. These fractures are mostly predictable [7] and largely contribute to a worsened quality of life in patients with metastatic bone disease [5]. While most fractures occur in the presence of a metastatic lesion, cancer is often associated with osteoporosis and hence an increase in fracture risk [8]. Occasionally, a fracture site is later found to contain metastatic disease. Therefore the question occasionally arises as to whether the occurrence of a fracture in a patient with cancer is a reflection of the presence of a metastatic lesion at the fracture site or whether the pathologic processes that take place in the event of a fracture increase the risk of establishment of tumor cells at the site of the fracture.

One of the first events that take place after a fracture is the development of a hematoma, in which the coagulation cascade is activated. Blood clots include a number of proteins that have been shown to directly affect tumor development. Thrombin, a terminal clotting protein, supports cancer implantation and growth [9]. Factor XIII stabilizes thrombi and supports metastasis formation by interfering with natural-killer mediated cancer cell removal [10]. Fibrinogen, another molecule involved in the clotting cascade was shown to support cancer cell adhesion and survival [11]. Other participants in the coagulation cascade such as tissue factor have been associated with metastatic disease in correlative studies and a causative role is presumed albeit not proven [12,13]. Furthermore, the platelets themselves produce SDF-1 (stromal-cell derived factor-1), which can act as a chemotactic agent for cancer cells [14]. Thus, molecules upregulated in the early stages of clot formation or in fracture hematomas and proteins concentrated there as a result of coagulation activation that support infiltration by inflammatory cells can also be involved in tumor development. Indeed, interfering with some of these events seems to negatively affect cancer development [15,16].

Based on these and other studies one might be inclined to conclude that the formation of a blood clot as might occur in fractures is associated with the development of metastatic disease. We therefore aimed to test whether the development of a blood clot can be directly responsible for the formation of a metastatic lesion. This seems particularly relevant in view of observational studies suggesting that events associated with tooth extraction are enough to increase the rate of metastasis formation [17]. To achieve this aim, we used an experimental model, in which a blood clot is induced in the left tibia. Cancer cells selected to home to the bone marrow were then introduced in the circulation by means of intracardiac injection to ensure the presence of large numbers of circulating cancer cells at the time of clot formation [18]. Using this model we examined the homing of cancer cells to the blood clot in the bone marrow in the left tibia in comparison to the opposite side that did not undergo clot induction. We also compared the development of metastatic lesions in these mice to control mice that did not undergo clot induction. We found neither an increase in the number of cancer cells localized to the clot nor an increase in the number of metastatic lesions developing in the injured left tibia. This suggests that the formation of clots/ hematomas, albeit rich in growth factors does not provide optimal conditions for cancer growth. Thus there is currently no evidence to support fear of increased metastasis formation after clot formation as might occur in fractures and surgical interventions.

Methods

Mice

CD1 nu/nu animals were obtained from Charles River Laboratories (Kissleg, Germany). These mice carry a *foxn* mutation that results in their inability to produce functional T cells and therefore these animals are suited for a xenotransplant model. In addition, hair follicle development is impaired, and hence these mice are nude, allowing for bioluminescence imaging without shaving.

The studies in mice were approved by the animal protection committee of the University of Heidelberg and Regierungspräsidium Karlsruhe #G48/08, #G120/11, #G73/13 and #G136/ 13, thus, all animal work was conducted according to relevant national and international guidelines. All surgery was performed under anesthesia, and all efforts were made to minimize suffering.

Cancer cells

MDA-MB-231B/luc$^+$ or PC-3M-Pro4/luc$^+$ were cultured in DMEM/10%FCS with 800 and 500 µg/ml geneticine respectively [18]. Huh-7 hepatoma cells were obtained from Cell Bank, Japan: JCRB0403) and cultured in DMEM/10% FCS. Cells were counted using an automated cell counter (CASY-TT, Innovatis).

Intracardiac injection of cancer cells

For intracardiac injection of cancer cells, mice were anesthetized (Ketamine 120 mg/kg/xylazine 16 mg/kg). A cancer cell suspension (10^5/100 µl PBS) (MDA-MB-231 selected to home to the bone marrow and establish bone metastases), PC3 or Huh-7 was injected into the left heart ventricle [18]. Tumor growth was evaluated weekly starting 3 weeks after intracardiac injection by bioluminescence reporter imaging.

Induction of blood clot

Intratibial bone marrow flushing was performed as described [18], but without injecting cancer cells intratibially. Briefly, mice were anesthetized [18,19], skin and muscle were cut and pushed aside from over the left tibia, two holes, 3–4 mm apart with a

diameter of ~0.35 mm each, were drilled with a dental drill (Bredent) through bone cortex. Bone marrow was flushed out with 0.5 ml phosphate buffered saline injected in the upper hole, which was then sealed with surgical bone wax (Ethicon; Johnson and Johnson) together with the lower hole. Lastly, the cutaneous wound was sutured. In the homing experiment, the opposite side was not operated upon to maximize the difference, but in the growth experiment the control group underwent sham operations without drilling or flushing.

Bioluminescence imaging

For bioluminescent reporter imaging that allows following bone metastasis growth longitudinally, mice were anesthetized with isofluran and injected with d-luciferin (150 mg/kg body weight)(-Synchem). Exactly 5 minutes after injection, photon signal was detected using an "IVIS-100" imaging system, and evaluated using the analysis software "Living Image" (version 2.50).

X-ray analysis

Lytic lesions were detected by radiography using a Faxitron. Lytic lesions on x-rays were analyzed using "Image J" (Wayne Rasband, NIH).

Staining protocols, histomorphometry and determination of clot area

Bones were fixed in 3.7% neutral-buffered formalin (NBF), embedded in polymethylmethacrylate, sectioned and stained per Masson Goldner with hematoxilin (Gill II, Carl Roth, Karlsruhe, Germany), acid fuchsin-ponceau xylidine, and phosphomolybdic acid-orange G and light green [20]. For dynamic histomorphometry, calcein was administered twice, once immediately after clot induction and then 48 hours later intraperitoneally at 30 mg/kg (Sigma-Aldrich, Munich, Germany), and mice euthanized 24 hours later. Primary cancellous bone was defined as the 120 µm band below the growth plate. Cancellous bone was defined as the remaining trabecular area that extends down 2 mm [21]. The same sections were used for dynamic and static histomorphometry, and data obtained from evaluation of the cancellous bone area defined above are presented. The ASBMR nomenclature was used [22]. The following measurements are mentioned: osteoid surface (OS), bone surface (BS), osteoblast number (Ob.N), bone formation rate (BFR = MS*MAR/BS, mm2/mm/.yr.), number of osteoclasts (Oc.N), and erosion surface (ES). ImageJ was used (Wayne Rasband, NIH). Staining for thrombin was performed on plastic sections using a polyclonal antibody directed against thrombin (Abcam 92621) for one hour. The secondary antibody used was a goat anti-rabbit antibody labeled with Alexa 647 (Abcam 150079). Blood clot size was determined after initial screening of the sections to determine the section with the largest clot size. The selected sections were stained per Masson-Goldner. The apparent hematoma area after 5 min, 24 h and 48 h of clot induction was analyzed using ImageJ (Wayne Rasband, NIH). To perform enzymatic stains 5 µm cryosections of 3.7% neutral-buffered-formalin-fixed bones were performed using adhesive film (SECTION-LAB Co. Ltd.) as described [23]. Until further use the sections were stored at −80°C. TRAcP (tartrate-resistant acid phosphatase) to detect osteoclasts was stained as described [24]. Briefly: the slides were placed in dH2O and the following solution was prepared: 16 mg Naphthol ASTR phosphate (Sigma) was dissolved in 1 ml dimethylformamide. The Naphthol ASTR phosphate was added to 10 ml 0.1 M acetate buffer with Pararosaniline and the pH adjusted to 5.0. Finally 3 drops of Manganese sulfate were added.

The wet slides were incubated 4 mins with the staining solution and after gently rinsed with dH2O and mounted with Mowiol. Alkaline phosphatase staining to detect osteoblasts was performed as described [25]. Briefly, slides were placed in Tris buffer. And the following staining solution prepared: 40 mg Naphthol ASBI phosphate (Sigma) was dissolved in 2 mL of dimethylformamide (Merck). 40 mg of Fast Blue RR salt (Sigma) was dissolved in 2 mL of dimethylformamide. To prepare the final staining solution, 2 mL of naphthol ASBI solution was combined with 2 mL of Fast Blue RR salt solution. This was then added to 35 mL of Tris buffer (pH 9.4, Roth). The solution was filtered before use and was prepared fresh as the substrate deteriorates over time. The slides were incubated for 2 min in the staining solution. After incubation in stain, slides were rinsed in dH2O and mounted with Mowiol. Alkaline phosphatase–rich structures are stained a dark blue color. The number of TRAcP osteoclasts was counted and the surface of alkaline phosphatase stain was measured and adjusted to total bone surface as described [26]. Sections were photographed using a Keyence microscope and processed using ImageJ. Quantification was performed in at least three mice per group or more as noted in the figure legends.

DNA analysis

For evaluating the homing of circulating tumor cells mice were sacrificed 1 h, 4 h, 24 h and 48 h after intracardiac injection and bones and bone marrow taken for further analysis.

Genomic DNA was isolated from bone marrow using DNeasy Blood and Tissue kit (Qiagen). Quantitative real-time polymerase chain reaction (qPCR) was performed using a light cycler 2.0 Instrument (Roche) using the following primers and probes that detect resistance towards Geneticin in the construct introduced in the MDA and PC3 cell lines to allow bioluminescence imaging in a method similar to the use of the alu sequence described by other groups [27]. These primers however overcome the problem with contamination by human DNA and are as follows: forward 5'-3': ACTGTTCGCCAGGCTCAAGGC, reverse 5'-3' GCGAATCGGGAGCGGCGAT and probe #31. Huh-7 cells were detected using the following primers and probe: forward: 5'CAT GGT GAA ACC CCG TCT CTA 3'; reverse: 5'GCC TCA GCC TCC CGA GTA G 3'; probe: 5' ATT AGC CGG GCG TGG TGG CG 3'. Results were normalized to mouse bone marrow cells using probe #64 and primers for β-actin (Universal probe library, Roche). An external standard curve using known numbers of human and mouse specific cells was created for Geneticin (for MDA and PC3), alu (for Huh-7) and β-actin (for murine bone marrow). Performing qPCR on bone and bone marrow DNA and comparing the results with a standard curve for tumor cells in mouse marrow we were able to detect as few as 0.2–0.5 human cancer cells/10^6 murine bone marrow cells.

Flow cytometry

Bone marrow was flushed from the upper third of the tibiae with 100 μl PBS/tibia, red cells lysed, and cancer cells stained with an APC-conjugated antibody directed against human CD49e, which is the integrin α5 subunit. This antibody does not bind to murine cells and detects 96% of MDA cancer cells (Clone NKI-SAM-1, Biolegend). The antibody was used at a final concentration of 0.25 μg/ml. Flow cytometry was performed using LSR-2 (BD-Biosciences), and at least 3 million cells were counted per sample.

Statistical analyses

Analyses were performed using SPSS (V14.0). Comparisons between two groups were performed using Student's t-test or Wilcoxon paired test as appropriate. In the analysis for homing of cancer cells after different time periods from clot induction a one way ANOVA was first performed. Analysis of occurrence of tibial lesions was performed using Fisher's exact test. Calculations for sample size ahead of experiments to detect a difference with a power of 0.80 as well as post-hoc power analysis were performed using the PS program available online (http://biostat.mc.vanderbilt.edu/wiki/Main/PowerSampleSize). A test was defined as significant if p<0.05. Results are presented as mean±standard-error-of-the-mean (M±SEM).

Results

Intratibial hematoma and clot formation

In order to determine whether the model we contemplated using indeed resulted in the development of a blood clot within the bone marrow, we performed the procedure of intratibial bone marrow flushing in mice and examined the tibiae 5 and 60 minutes, as well as 24, 48 and 72 hours after the end of the procedure. Sections within the tibia showed the formation of a clot already within 5 minutes after end of the procedure as seen with Masson Goldner staining (figure 1 A and inset below). Smaller clots were still detectable after 24 hours (figure 1B and inset), but by 72 hours the clot had almost completely resolved (figure 1C). The presence of the clot was further confirmed by thrombin staining (figure 1D). Quantification confirmed the decrease in size of the clot over time (figure 1E).

Effect of blood clot induction on bone histomorphometry

Cancer growth increases whenever there is an increase in bone turnover [28]. In order to determine whether flushing of the bone marrow and the development of a blood clot resulted in increased turnover we compared the flushed tibia with the opposite side tibia. The time point used was three days after the procedure to allow for cell changes to take place. As shown in figure 2, no obvious differences could be detected in bone sections. Both dynamic and static histomorphometric analyses were performed. Despite a trend to increased osteoblast numbers (p = 0.09), bone formation rate remained similar. Bone resorption was not affected as evidenced by similar osteoclast numbers and erosion surface on static histomorphometry. Using enzymatic staining we confirmed the absence of an effect on both osteoblasts (by measuring the surface of alkaline phosphatase staining) (figure 3A) and on osteoclasts (by counting the number of tartrate-resistant acid phosphatase-stained osteoclasts) (figure 3B).

Thus, induction of a blood clot does not affect bone turnover by the time the clot resolved.

Intratibial hematoma formation is not associated with increased homing of cancer cells

We then sought to examine whether the presence of a blood clot was associated with increased number of cancer cells arriving to the clot. We used three different cell lines, one that was selected to home to the bone marrow and form breast cancer metastases (MDA-MB-231B/luc+), one that forms prostate metastases in the bone (PC3/luc+) and a hepatoma cell line not reported to form bone metastases. Since these are human cell lines, they have to be used in immune-deficient mice lacking mature T-cells to avoid destruction of the human cells. Mice underwent intracardial injection of cancer cells followed one minute later by flushing of bone marrow in the left tibia. Twenty-four hours later the upper half of the left tibia (site of intratibial clot induction) was isolated and the number of tumor cells arriving at the site was evaluated

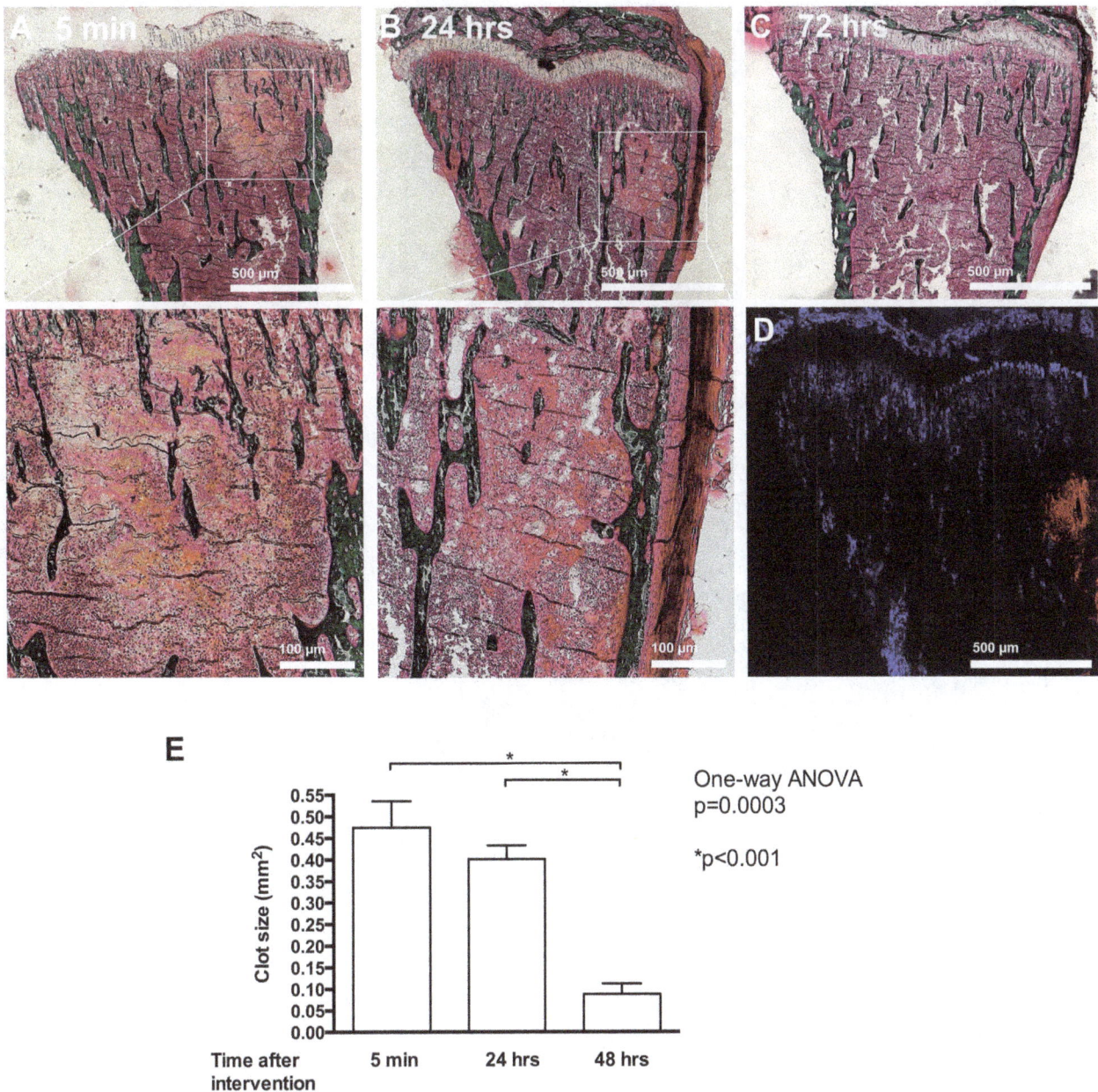

Figure 1. Induction of hematoma and clot formation in the bone marrow. (A) Induction of bleeding results in clot formation within 5 minutes as evidenced by Masson-Goldner staining. *Bar represents 500 μm*. The enlarged inset below shows the blood clot. *Bar represents 100 μm*. (B) The clot is still present, albeit partially reorganized at 24 hours after bleeding induction. *Bar represents 500 μm*. Enlarged inset is shown below. *Bar represents 100 μm*. (C) After 72 hours the clot resolved. (D) Thrombin staining of the bone shown in B confirms the presence of thrombin (in red) in the clot area. (E) Quantification of the change in hematoma size at different time points. After induction of bleeding in the bone marrow, mice were euthanized at the times mentioned, and tibiae examined. n = 3–4 mice/time point.

using quantitative real time polymerase chain reaction (qPCR) to determine the number of cancer cells, whereby the frequency of a specific sequence found exclusively in the cancer cell line corrected to murine β-actin reflecting the number of murine bone marrow cells was used. As a control, the right tibia (site without clot induction) was evaluated. Injecting these cell lines intracardially one minute before clot induction was not associated with a change in cancer cells homing to the bone marrow (figure 4A). Using flow cytometry we were able to confirm the absence of a difference in the breast cancer cells (MDA-MB-231B/luc+) cells (figure 4B). We then asked whether the use of surgical wax might have any

inhibitory effect on homing of cancer cells. This was not the case, because injecting MDA cancer cells 1 minute before clot induction did not affect the total number of cancer cells at the site of the clot both in the presence or absence of wax (figure 4C). We next evaluated whether injecting cancer cells at different time points has any effect on homing, and injected cancer cells 15 minutes before, 1 minute before and 5 minutes after clot induction. Here too, there was no difference in the number of cancer cells homing to the bone marrow (figure 4D). We then wondered, whether homing was affected by the length of time since injections. Therefore the number of cancer cells that homed to the clot was evaluated at

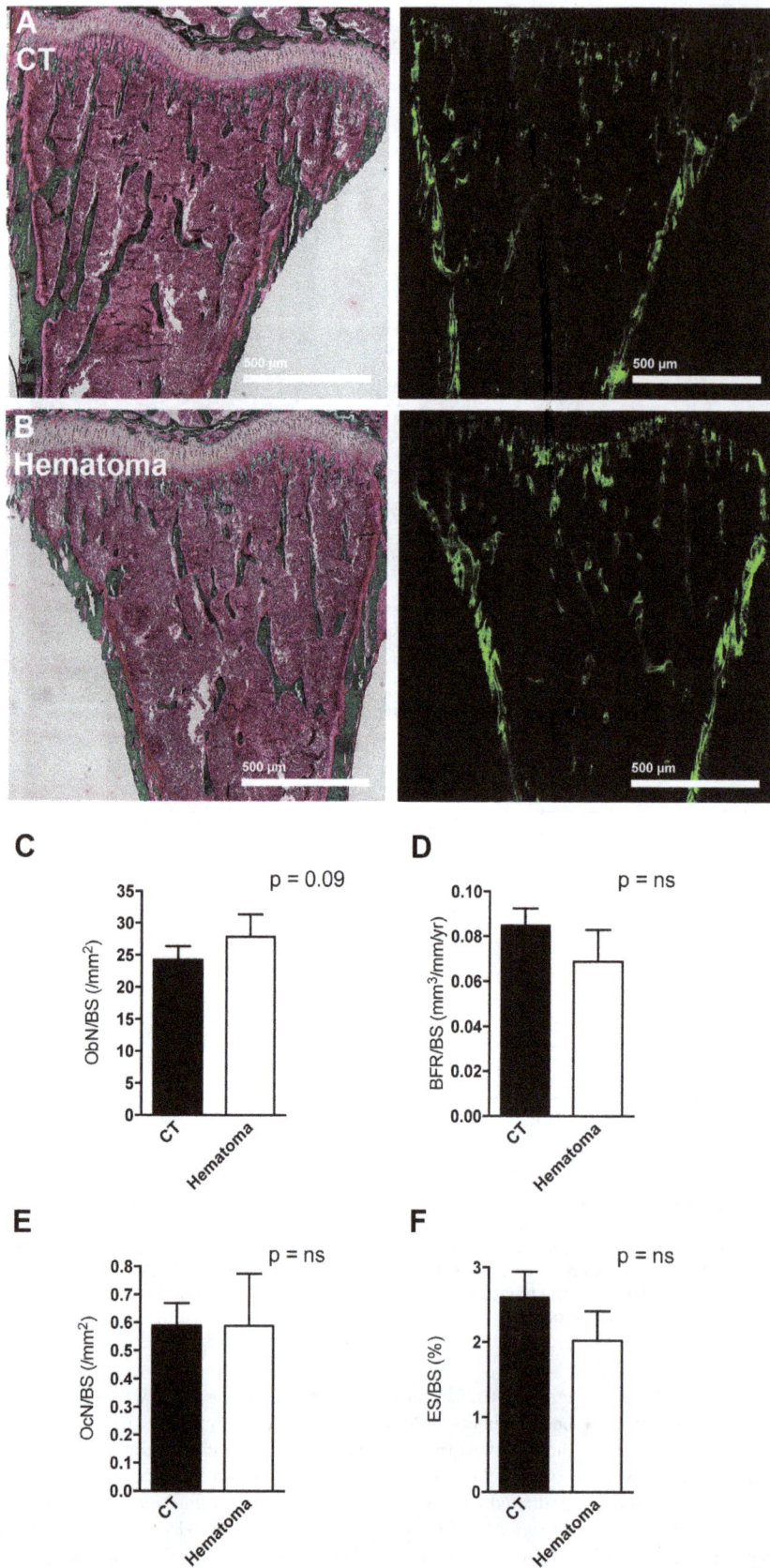

Figure 2. Bone histomorphometry after clot induction. (A–B) After three days from the time of induction of a blood clot Masson-Goldner staining (on the left) and calcein labeling (on the right) showed no difference between control (CT) in panel A and hematoma induction in panel B in the same mouse. Neither osteoblast number (C), nor bone formation rate (D), nor osteoclast number (E), nor erosion surface (F) were different

between the two tibiae. CT represents the right tibia without clot induction and hematoma represents the left tibia in which bone marrow was flushed and a blood clot was induced. Tibiae were obtained three days after clot induction in the left tibia, embedded in polymethylmethacrylate and stained using Masson-Goldner. n = 4 mice.

different time points after clot induction followed by injection of cancer cells. There was no difference in the number of human cancer cells arriving at the site of intervention compared to the opposite side after one, four, 24 and 48 hours in a one-way ANOVA (figure 4E in the − 1 min group). A similar experiment was performed, whereby cancer cells were injected after clot induction (+5 min group). At 1 hour, less cancer cells were detected in the hematoma, but this effect was lost at later time points (figure 4F). This suggests that the presence of a blood clot does not offer a permissive environment for homing of cancer cells.

Metastasis development in the presence of hematoma

We next examined whether the formation of a blood clot was associated with an increase in the chance of metastatic lesion formation. Two experimental mice groups were evaluated. In the

first group (− 1 min), the mice underwent intracardial cancer cell injection followed 1 minute later by the procedure to induce intratibial clot formation. In the second group (+5 min), the mice underwent the procedure to induce intratibial clot formation, followed by injection of cancer cells into the left ventricle five minutes later. Tumor cells injected intracardially circulate for approximately one hour after which time most cells are cleared from the circulation. Twenty-four hours later no bioluminescence signal can be detected (data not shown). The control sham-operated group received only intracardiac cancer cell injections without clot induction in the left tibia.

Weekly bioluminescence measurements starting three weeks after cancer cell injection were performed. This was possible because the cancer line used contained a luciferase construct [18]. Since the cancer cell line has been selected to only home to the

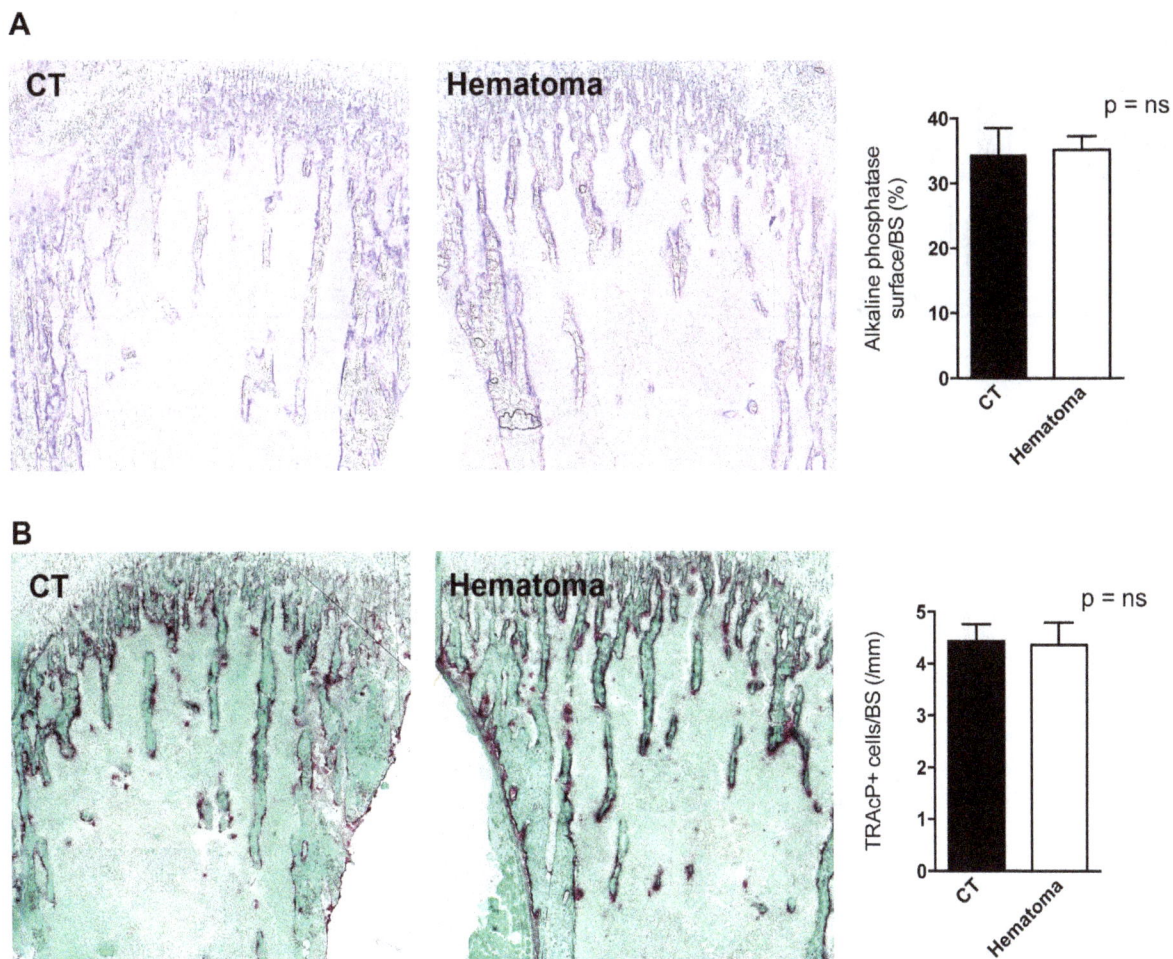

Figure 3. Enzymatic staining of bone sections. (A) Osteoblast surface as evidenced by evaluating the surface stained positive for alkaline phosphatase did not differ between CT and hematoma bones. A representative stained pair of tibiae is shown on the left and quantification is shown on the right. (B) The number of osteoclasts as evidenced by counting the cells that stained positive for tartrate-resistant acid phosphatase and correcting to bone surface was not affected by clot induction. A representative stained pair of tibiae is shown on the left and quantification is shown on the right. CT represents the right tibia without clot induction and hematoma represents the left tibia in which bone marrow was flushed and a blood clot was induced. Tibiae were obtained three days after clot induction in the left tibia, fixed in 3,7% PFA, cryo-sectioned using adhesive film and stained as outlined in the methods. n = 4 mice.

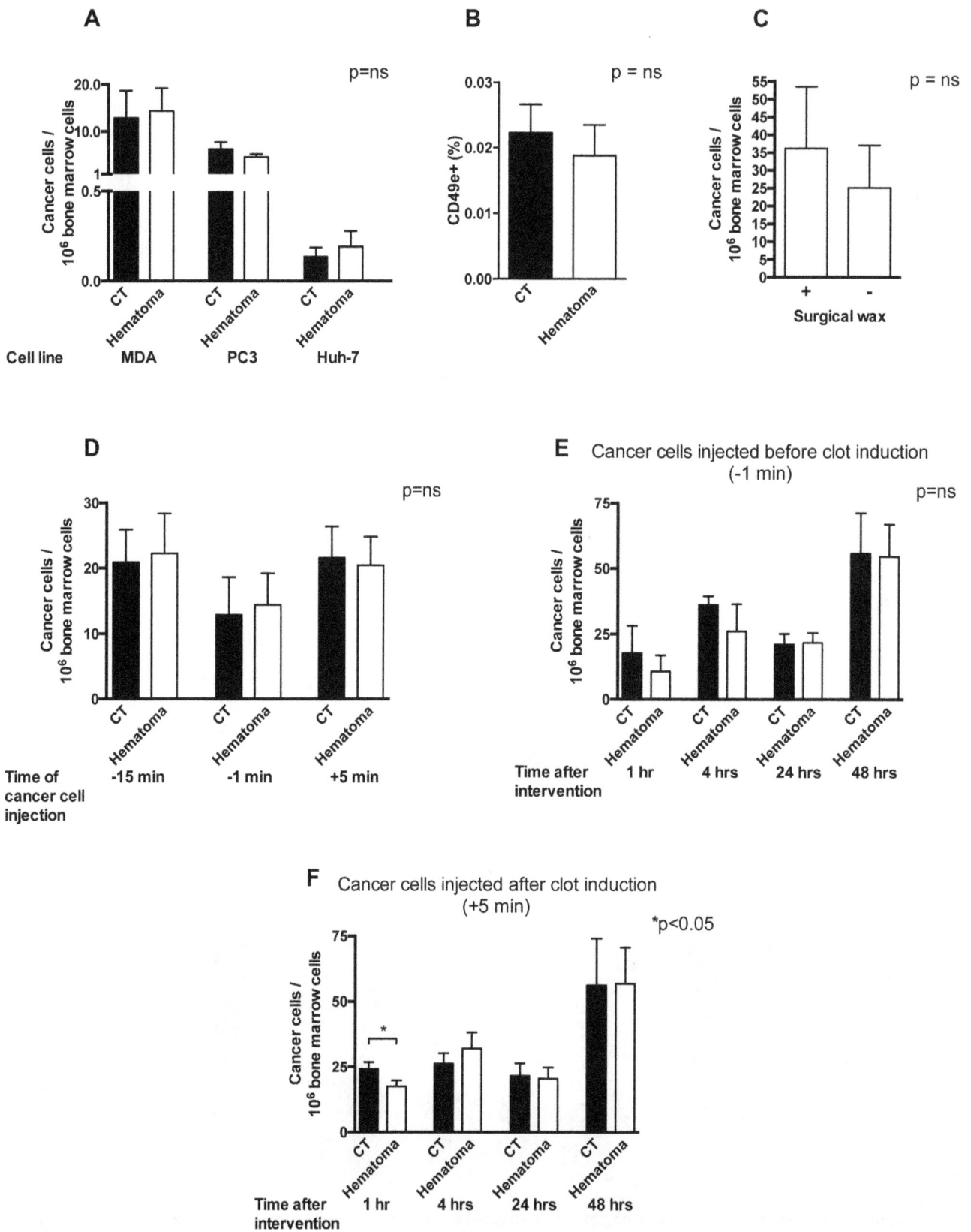

Figure 4. Infiltration of blood clots by cancer cells. (A) Induction of a blood clot in the left tibia does not result in an increase in the number of infiltrating cancer cells compared to the right control tibia (CT) in the same mouse when cancer cells are injected 1 minute before blood clot induction using three cell lines (Breast cancer selected to home to the bone marrow: MDA-MB-231B/luc+; prostate cancer able to form bone metastases: PC3/luc+; and hepatoma cells not reported to form bone metastases: Huh-7). Cancer cells were injected 1 minute before clot induction. 24 hours later the bone marrow was isolated from the upper third of both tibiae and the number of cancer cells was evaluated by quantitative PCR of

a cancer cell specific sequence and corrected to the total number of murine cells in the sample. n = 4–5/group. (B) The number of MDA cancer cells evaluated by flow cytometry was similar between the CT and hematoma group. MDA cancer cells were injected 1 minute before clot induction. 24 hours later the bone marrow was isolated from the upper third of both tibiae, red cells lysed, stained with a labeled human-specific CD49e (integrin α5) antibody and at least 3 million bone marrow cells were counted. n = 10 mice. (C) The use of surgical wax in the tibia following clot induction does not affect homing of cancer cells. 1 minute before clot induction MDA cancer cells were injected. The hole performed in the tibia in order to induce the blood clot in the bone marrow was either closed with surgical wax or left until bleeding stopped spontaneously (3–5 minutes) before closing the wound. n = 4 pairs. (D) Injection of MDA cancer cells 15 minutes before, 1 minute before and 5 minutes after clot induction did not affect the number of cancer cells in the bone marrow detected after 24 hours. Samples were prepared as in A. p = ns for each time point. (E) Evaluation of cancer cell numbers when injected 1 minute before clot induction did not reveal a difference in the number of cancer cells detected in the bone marrow at different time points (1, 4, 24 and 48 hours after clot induction). p = ns and n = 4–5 per time point. (F) Evaluation of cancer cell numbers when injected 5 minutes after clot induction showed a significant decrease in the number of cancer cells detected in the bone marrow at 1 hour after clot induction (p<0.05) but not at later time points (4, 24 and 48 hours after clot induction) (p = ns). n = 4–8 per time point.

bone marrow, no lesions outside the skeleton could be detected. Examples from 5 pairs of bioluminescence and x-ray pictures obtained from CT and the +5 min group are presented in figure 5.

Seven weeks after cancer cell injection 13 out of 18 mice (72%) of the mice in the control group developed lesions in the left tibia. Intracardiac cancer cell injection prior to clot induction (−1 min) resulted in 11 affected in the left tibia (out of 14 mice) (79%). Similarly, injection of cancer cells 5 minutes after clot induction

resulted in 11 mice affected with left tibia lesions (out of 17 mice) (65%) (figure 6A). Examined differently, a total of 115 lesions had developed in the control group, out of which 13 (11%) were localized in the left tibia and 17 in the right tibia. Intracardiac cancer cell injection prior to intratibial flushing (−1 min) resulted in 85 bone metastatic lesions, out of which 11 (13%) were localized to the left tibia, and 11 in the right tibia (n = 18 and 14 mice, p = ns), while injection of cancer cells 5 minutes after clot induction resulted in 89 bone metastatic lesions, out of which 11 (12%) were localized to the left tibia, and 11 in the right tibia (n = 18 and 17 mice, p = ns) (figure 6B). The summary of the lesion numbers and their locations at 7 weeks after cancer cell injection (including mice that died prior to seven weeks) are presented in Table 1 (sample size was calculated a priori for a power of 0.80). This suggests that with a post hoc power of 0.89 (−1 min group) and 0.92 (+5 min group) the presence of a blood clot does not affect the development of a macroscopic lesion. Tumor burden was not affected since the total bioluminescence signal per mouse (figure 6C), and per lesion (figure 6D) did not differ between the experimental and the control group. In support of these findings, analysis of x-ray films obtained at seven weeks after cancer cell injection revealed comparable sizes of lytic lesions between the groups (figure 6E). In line with these findings, median survival did not differ between all three groups (CT 7.5 weeks; −1 min group 8.0 weeks; +5min group 8.5 weeks; p = ns for the CT and experimental pairs) (figure 6F).

Based on these findings, we conclude that the presence of a blood clot does not affect the development of a macroscopic lesion or the growth characteristics of bone metastases in a murine model of breast cancer metastasis.

Discussion

The principal finding of our study is that the formation of a clot and hematoma in the bone marrow neither increases the chance that a cancer cell becomes incorporated in the clot, nor is it associated with an increase in the chance that a metastatic lesion develops in the area of the clot, nor does it affect the later growth of tumors.

With experimental evidence emerging in 1990s the seed and soil theory that implies that homing and growth of cancer cells is facilitated in locations that provide the right microenvironment, has gained much ground among scientists working on metastasis formation [29]. The accumulation of blood outside a blood vessel results in the activation of the coagulation cascade associated with the formation of a blood clot, with the ensuing accumulation of thrombin and various other proteins that support tumor establishment and growth [9–11]. Clot formation is also associated with activation of platelet aggregation, which release SDF-1, VEGF (Vascular endothelial growth factor) and PDGF (platelet-derived growth factor) [14,30,31]. These three molecules were shown to exert pro cancerous effects. While SDF-1 normally serves as a

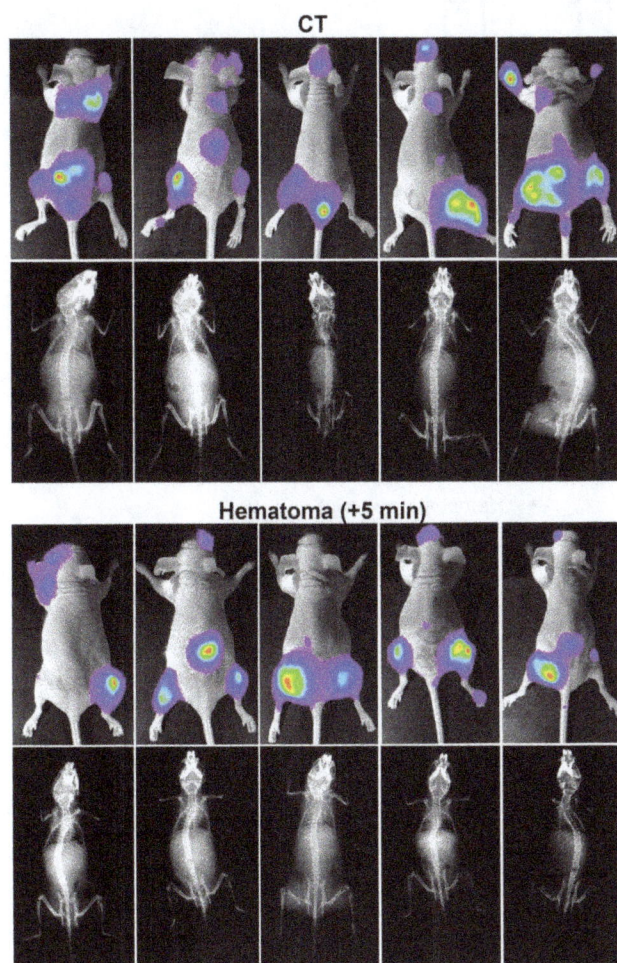

Figure 5. Bioluminescence and x-ray imaging *in vivo*. Representative bioluminescence images from the last measurements before death and x-ray images at the time of death from 5 CT and 5 experimental mice in the group injected with cancer cells 5 minutes after clot induction. Upper panel represents the paired pictures from the CT group and the lower panel represents the paired pictures from the experimental group.

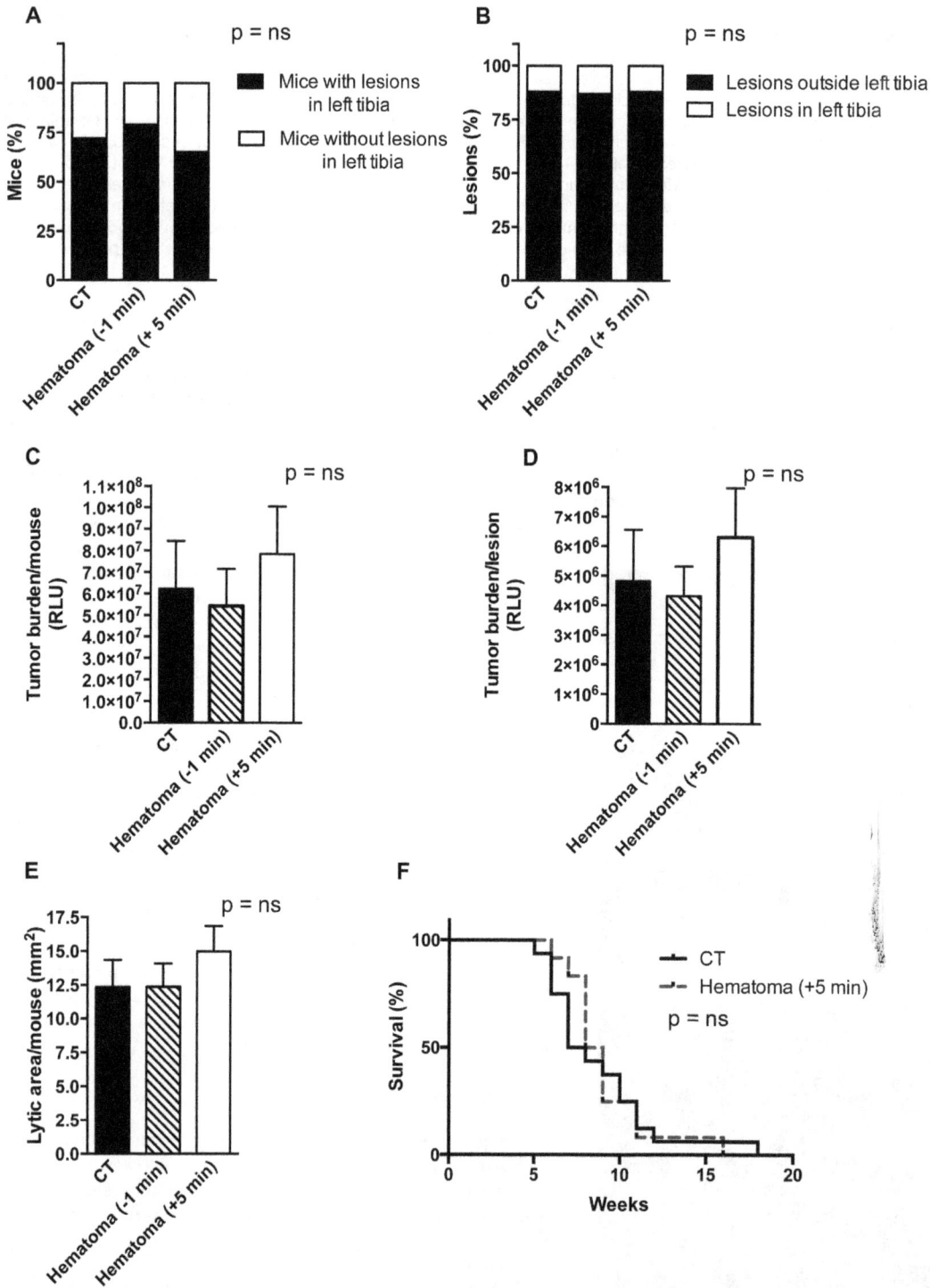

Figure 6. Comparison of control and experimental groups. (A) In the control group 13 lesions developed in the left tibia while in both experimental groups 11 developed in the left tibia. The percentages of mice with lesions in the left tibia is shown. n = 18, 14 and 17 mice. (B) The percentage of left tibia lesions in comparison to the total number of lesions is similar in both CT-experimental group pairs. n as in A. (C) Total bioluminescence signal per mouse expressed in relative light units (RLU) was similar between the control and the experimental groups at 7 weeks. n = 12, 11 and 15 mice. (D) Total bioluminescence signal per lesion was similar too. n as in C. (E) The size of the lytic lesions at 7 weeks was comparable. n as in A. (F) Survival curves of the control group (CT) and the experimental +5 min hematoma group shows that there is no difference in median survival (7.5 vs. 8.5 weeks, p = ns). n as in A. For ease of presentation CT was compared with the group with the seemingly larger median survival only.

Table 1. Comparison of control and experimental groups.

Number of lesions and their locations (confirmed by bioluminescence and x-ray)	Control group n = 18 (%)*	Hematoma group -1 min n = 14 (%)*	Hematoma group +5 min n = 17 (%)*
Total number of bone lesions	115	85	89
Left tibia (Control or hematoma)	13 (11)	11 (13)	11 (12)
Right tibia	17 (15)	11 (13)	11 (12)
Cranium and jaw	17 (16)	12 (14)	17 (19)
Spine	16 (14)	12 (14)	14 (16)
Ribs	1 (1)	3 (4)	3 (3)
Shoulder	6 (5)	8 (9)	5 (5)
Hip	6 (5)	7 (8)	2 (2)
Femur	7 (6)	4 (5)	8 (9)
Humerus	15 (13)	5 (6)	8 (9)
Forelimb foot	9 (8)	6 (7)	5 (5)
Hindlimb foot	8 (7)	6 (7)	8 (9)
Number of lesions/mouse	**6.4**	**6.1**	**5.3**

The number of macroscopic lesions detectable by bioluminescence imaging in the left tibia was similar between control animals that did not undergo clot induction and experimental animals with a blood clot in which cancer cells were injected 1 minute prior to (−1 min), or 5 minutes after clot induction (+5 min). Data from all mice (including those that already died) 7 weeks after cancer cell injection are shown. Data were analyzed using Fisher's exact test and no significant differences were detected in the CT/experimental group pairs.
*The percentage presented is calculated as follows: number of lesions at a specific site/total number of lesions in the group.

chemotaxis signal for platelets and inflammatory cells to initiate the wound healing process [14,32], it is similarly chemotactic for cancer cells and was shown to stimulate cancer cell migration and establishment in the bone marrow [33]. Therefore, in its presence, cancer cells in the circulation would be expected to proceed to the site of clot formation. Both PDGF and VEGF support angiogenesis [34–36]. However angiogenesis is only required at a later time point when the lesion is already about 1 mm^3 in size [37] indicating that this effect should influence only tumor growth and development but not the homing of circulating cancer cells. Lastly, platelets promote cancer development by impairing the function of natural killer cells [38]. Thus the accumulation of platelets in a blood clot should be permissive to cancer cell homing and may promote growth.

Associated with the flushing of the bone marrow, shear forces on the blood vessels and the sinusoids result in leakage of blood with all its components into the bone marrow cavity. Nevertheless no increase in the number of cancer cells trapped in the clot could be detected. It thus seems that the prometastatic roles of various members of the coagulation cascade and the platelets in the cytokine rich environment of the bone marrow are not critical at physiologic concentrations for the early development of cancer lesions or for their later growth. The lack of effect on growth starting after 3 weeks could however be due to recovery and resolution of the blood clot by then. Lastly, an inhibitory role due to the presence of megakaryocytes cannot be excluded, because megakaryocytes in the bone marrow have been shown to induce apoptosis and decrease proliferation of prostate cancer cells [39].

Bone marrow disruption is associated with the formation of a mineralizing trabecular network and an increase in osteoblasts [40]. Untreated osteoblasts *in vitro* and osteoblasts lining the bone marrow *in vivo* release a variety of cancer promoting cytokines such as interleukin-6 (IL-6) and monocyte chemotactic protein-1 (MCP-1) [4,41], both of which have also been shown to promote cancer cell migration and invasion [4,42,43]. We therefore performed histomorphometric analyses of the bone after clot induction [41].

However, flushing the bone marrow in our model did not induce significant changes in bone formation as shown in figures 2 and 3. This contrasts to histologic changes shown with disruption of the bone marrow and reported before [40], and is in line with the lack of a difference in cancer development between the flushed tibia and the opposite sides. The clot induction was not associated with an increase in bone resorption either. Therefore, the release of growth factors from the bone matrix in our model of clot induction is limited [44]. Thus, our model stands in contrast to fracture models where the broken bone results in the formation of a blood clot followed by infiltration by inflammatory cells, formation of the fibrocartilagenous callus, and finally bone remodeling resulting in normal bone structure in the area of the fracture. Even though inflammation is associated with the release of some cytokines that affect bone cells, and hence a low level of bone remodeling with release of growth factors from the matrix might ensue during the early stages after fracture formation [45–47], the major remodeling step during fracture healing takes place after the blood clot had resolved [48]. Our experimental clot induction model examines the effect of blood clot formation within the cytokine-rich environment of the bone marrow. Because of the absence of measurable bone remodeling it thus does not include the role of the growth factors released from the matrix during remodeling. However, the bone marrow itself is a microenvironment already rich with cytokines that can promote cancer cell homing and growth [49], whereby the same cytokines required for hematopoiesis seem to be beneficial for homing of cancer cells to the bone marrow and tumor growth. One such cytokine is SDF-1 that is involved in hematopoiesis and chemotaxis [14,50]. Furthermore, osteoblasts release a variety of cancer promoting cytokines that support cancer development as discussed [4,42,43]. The similar homing and cancer growth between the flushed side and the opposite side in our model therefore suggests that blood clots even in a cancer-promoting environment do not necessarily support cancer formation.

The decision to introduce cancer cells by intracardiac injection was based on the need to provide for a large number of circulating cancer cells looking for a home during clot induction [51]. This model thus seems better suited to examine the role of clot proteins in supporting cancer cell homing and growth than introducing a cancer, from which the cells would first need to move out and roam in the blood stream before migrating into the clot [27]. By using two different time points for the injection of cancer cells in relationship to induction of blood clotting we evaluated both the role of the initial thrombin surge and acute release of clotting factors on already circulating cancer cells (in the −1 min model) and the role of the presence of a clot prior to the surge in circulating cancer cells (in the +5 min model). In the case of introduction of the cancer cells 5 minutes after clot induction (+5 min) the decrease in the number of cancer cells that homed to the bone marrow one hour after clot induction was surprising. In particular since we had expected an increase in homing of cancer cells to the clot driven by the availability of the various clotting factors. This decrease could be explained by the volume taken up by the blood clot that results in a decrease in the volume of circulating blood in the bone marrow and hence a decrease in the number of cancer cells [51]. A related possible explanation is that the blood clot does not allow infiltration by cancer cells due to the accumulation of matrix. This early effect however does not bear any relevance to the number of cancer cells at the site of clot after 24 hours or affect the development of cancerous lesions. While our data do not allow for a conclusion with regard to whether a larger clot might have caused an increase in the homing of cancer cells, it seems reasonable to conclude, based on our findings, that the formation of a 0.5 mm^2 clot (as shown in figure 1E) is not associated with increased homing of cancer cells to the clot after 24 hours.

Even though this experimental model compares favorably to other cancer models because it is based on a human cancer cell line and shares the ability to induce bone metastatic lesions with the clinical human counterpart, other cancer types might be more responsive to various cancer-promoting effects of physiologic concentrations of blood clot components. Nevertheless, it seems safe to predict that the effect in other models is probably limited in particular since two further cell lines failed to show an increase in homing of cancer cells to the blood clot.

Conclusions

Based on our findings we therefore conclude that, in a mouse model of human breast cancer, induction of a hematoma/clot did not promote bone metastasis formation or growth. Accordingly, there is currently no experimental evidence to support the possibility of metastasis formation in freshly injured areas in patients with cancer. It seems more likely that the coincidence of metastasis at sites of surgical interventions or trauma is due exclusively to chance.

Acknowledgments

We thank Reinhard Fässler for his invaluable input, Günther Hämmerling and Bernd Arnold for permission to use the bioluminescence imaging system, Justo Lorenzo Bermejo for statistical advice, and Stefan Meuer for his continued support.

Author Contributions

Conceived and designed the experiments: IAN. Performed the experiments: SR MV AvA. Analyzed the data: SR MV AvA IAN. Contributed reagents/materials/analysis tools: MC. Wrote the paper: IAN.

References

1. Coleman RE (2001) Metastatic bone disease: clinical features, pathophysiology and treatment strategies. Cancer Treat Rev 27: 165–176.
2. Benoy IH, Elst H, Philips M, Wuyts H, Van Dam P, et al. (2006) Real-time RT-PCR detection of disseminated tumour cells in bone marrow has superior prognostic significance in comparison with circulating tumour cells in patients with breast cancer. Br J Cancer 94: 672–680.
3. Wood DP Jr, Banks ER, Humphreys S, McRoberts JW, Rangnekar VM (1994) Identification of bone marrow micrometastases in patients with prostate cancer. Cancer 74: 2533–2540.
4. Bussard KM, Gay CV, Mastro AM (2008) The bone microenvironment in metastasis; what is special about bone? Cancer Metastasis Rev 27: 41–55.
5. Lipton A (2010) Bone continuum of cancer. Am J Clin Oncol 33: S1–7.
6. Melton LJ 3rd, Hartmann LC, Achenbach SJ, Atkinson EJ, Therneau TM, et al. (2012) Fracture risk in women with breast cancer: A population-based study. J Bone Miner Res.
7. Snell W, Beals RK (1964) Femoral Metastases and Fractures from Breast Cancer. Surg Gynecol Obstet 119: 22–24.
8. Body JJ (2011) Increased fracture rate in women with breast cancer: a review of the hidden risk. BMC Cancer 11: 384.
9. Green D, Karpatkin S (2010) Role of thrombin as a tumor growth factor. Cell Cycle 9: 656–661.
10. Palumbo JS, Barney KA, Blevins EA, Shaw MA, Mishra A, et al. (2008) Factor XIII transglutaminase supports hematogenous tumor cell metastasis through a mechanism dependent on natural killer cell function. J Thromb Haemost 6: 812–819.
11. Palumbo JS, Kombrinck KW, Drew AF, Grimes TS, Kiser JH, et al. (2000) Fibrinogen is an important determinant of the metastatic potential of circulating tumor cells. Blood 96: 3302–3309.
12. Rak J, Milsom C, May L, Klement P, Yu J (2006) Tissue factor in cancer and angiogenesis: the molecular link between genetic tumor progression, tumor neovascularization, and cancer coagulopathy. Semin Thromb Hemost 32: 54–70.
13. Garnier D, Milsom C, Magnus N, Meehan B, Weitz J, et al. (2010) Role of the tissue factor pathway in the biology of tumor initiating cells. Thromb Res 125 Suppl 2: S44–50.
14. Massberg S, Konrad I, Schurzinger K, Lorenz M, Schneider S, et al. (2006) Platelets secrete stromal cell-derived factor 1alpha and recruit bone marrow-derived progenitor cells to arterial thrombi in vivo. J Exp Med 203: 1221–1233.

15. Nakchbandi W, Muller H, Singer MV, Lohr JM, Nakchbandi IA (2008) Prospective study on warfarin and regional chemotherapy in patients with pancreatic carcinoma. J Gastrointestin Liver Dis 17: 285–290.
16. Nakchbandi IA, Lohr JM (2008) Coagulation, anticoagulation and pancreatic carcinoma. Nat Clin Pract Gastroenterol Hepatol 5: 445–455.
17. Hirshberg A, Leibovich P, Horowitz I, Buchner A (1993) Metastatic tumors to postextraction sites. J Oral Maxillofac Surg 51: 1334–1337.
18. Wetterwald A, van der Pluijm G, Que I, Sijmons B, Buijs J, et al. (2002) Optical imaging of cancer metastasis to bone marrow: a mouse model of minimal residual disease. Am J Pathol 160: 1143–1153.
19. von Au A, Vasel M, Kraft S, Sens C, Hackl N, et al. (2013) Circulating fibronectin controls tumor growth. Neoplasia 15: in press.
20. Bentmann A, Kawelke N, Moss D, Zentgraf H, Bala Y, et al. (2010) Circulating fibronectin affects bone matrix, whereas osteoblast fibronectin modulates osteoblast function. J Bone Miner Res 25: 706–715.
21. Kawelke N, Bentmann A, Hackl N, Hager HD, Feick P, et al. (2008) Isoform of fibronectin mediates bone loss in patients with primary biliary cirrhosis by suppressing bone formation. J Bone Miner Res 23: 1278–1286.
22. Parfitt AM, Drezner MK, Glorieux FH, Kanis JA, Malluche H, et al. (1987) Bone histomorphometry: standardization of nomenclature, symbols, and units. Report of the ASBMR Histomorphometry Nomenclature Committee. J Bone Miner Res 2: 595–610.
23. Kawamoto T (2003) Use of a new adhesive film for the preparation of multi-purpose fresh-frozen sections from hard tissues, whole-animals, insects and plants. Arch Histol Cytol 66: 123–143.
24. Baron R, Vignery A, Neff L, Silvergate A, Santa Maria A (1983) Processing of undecalcified bone specimens for bone histomorphometry. In: Recker R, editor. Bone Histomorphometry: Techniques and Interpretations Boca Raton, FL, USA: CRC Press Inc.
25. Cosby CN, Troiano NW, Kacena MA (2008) The Effects of Storage Conditions on the Preservation of Enzymatic Activity in Bone. J Histotechnol 31: 169–173.
26. Xue Y, Xiao Y, Liu J, Karaplis AC, Pollak MR, et al. (2012) The calcium-sensing receptor complements parathyroid hormone-induced bone turnover in discrete skeletal compartments in mice. Am J Physiol Endocrinol Metab 302: E841–851.
27. Havens AM, Pedersen EA, Shiozawa Y, Ying C, Jung Y, et al. (2008) An in vivo mouse model for human prostate cancer metastasis. Neoplasia 10: 371–380.

28. van der Pluijm G, Que I, Sijmons B, Buijs JT, Lowik CW, et al. (2005) Interference with the microenvironmental support impairs the de novo formation of bone metastases in vivo. Cancer Res 65: 7682–7690.

29. Mundy GR (2002) Metastasis to bone: causes, consequences and therapeutic opportunities. Nat Rev Cancer 2: 584–593.

30. Hannink M, Donoghue DJ (1989) Structure and function of platelet-derived growth factor (PDGF) and related proteins. Biochim Biophys Acta 989: 1–10.

31. Wartiovaara U, Salven P, Mikkola H, Lassila R, Kaukonen J, et al. (1998) Peripheral blood platelets express VEGF-C and VEGF which are released during platelet activation. Thromb Haemost 80: 171–175.

32. Kowalska MA, Ratajczak MZ, Majka M, Jin J, Kunapuli S, et al. (2000) Stromal cell-derived factor-1 and macrophage-derived chemokine: 2 chemokines that activate platelets. Blood 96: 50–57.

33. Gazitt Y (2004) Homing and mobilization of hematopoietic stem cells and hematopoietic cancer cells are mirror image processes, utilizing similar signaling pathways and occurring concurrently: circulating cancer cells constitute an ideal target for concurrent treatment with chemotherapy and antilineage-specific antibodies. Leukemia 18: 1–10.

34. Battegay EJ, Rupp J, Iruela-Arispe L, Sage EH, Pech M (1994) PDGF-BB modulates endothelial proliferation and angiogenesis in vitro via PDGF beta-receptors. J Cell Biol 125: 917–928.

35. Nor JE, Christensen J, Mooney DJ, Polverini PJ (1999) Vascular endothelial growth factor (VEGF)-mediated angiogenesis is associated with enhanced endothelial cell survival and induction of Bcl-2 expression. Am J Pathol 154: 375–384.

36. Fradet A, Sorel H, Bouazza L, Goehrig D, Depalle B, et al. (2011) Dual function of ERRalpha in breast cancer and bone metastasis formation: implication of VEGF and osteoprotegerin. Cancer Res 71: 5728–5738.

37. Gimbrone MA Jr, Leapman SB, Cotran RS, Folkman J (1972) Tumor dormancy in vivo by prevention of neovascularization. J Exp Med 136: 261–276.

38. Nieswandt B, Hafner M, Echtenacher B, Mannel DN (1999) Lysis of tumor cells by natural killer cells in mice is impeded by platelets. Cancer Res 59: 1295–1300.

39. Li X, Koh AJ, Wang Z, Soki FN, Park SI, et al. (2011) Inhibitory effects of megakaryocytic cells in prostate cancer skeletal metastasis. J Bone Miner Res 26: 125–134.

40. Suva LJ, Seedor JG, Endo N, Quartuccio HA, Thompson DD, et al. (1993) Pattern of gene expression following rat tibial marrow ablation. J Bone Miner Res 8: 379–388.

41. Bussard KM, Venzon DJ, Mastro AM (2010) Osteoblasts are a major source of inflammatory cytokines in the tumor microenvironment of bone metastatic breast cancer. J Cell Biochem 111: 1138–1148.

42. Obata NH, Tamakoshi K, Shibata K, Kikkawa F, Tomoda Y (1997) Effects of interleukin-6 on in vitro cell attachment, migration and invasion of human ovarian carcinoma. Anticancer Res 17: 337–342.

43. Salcedo R, Ponce ML, Young HA, Wasserman K, Ward JM, et al. (2000) Human endothelial cells express CCR2 and respond to MCP-1: direct role of MCP-1 in angiogenesis and tumor progression. Blood 96: 34–40.

44. Buijs JT, Stayrook KR, Guise TA (2011) TGF-beta in the Bone Microenvironment: Role in Breast Cancer Metastases. Cancer Microenviron 4: 261–281.

45. Nakchbandi IA, Mitnick MA, Masiukiewicz US, Sun BH, Insogna KL (2001) IL-6 negatively regulates IL-11 production in vitro and in vivo. Endocrinology 142: 3850–3856.

46. Horwood NJ, Kartsogiannis V, Quinn JM, Romas E, Martin TJ, et al. (1999) Activated T lymphocytes support osteoclast formation in vitro. Biochem Biophys Res Commun 265: 144–150.

47. Pfeilschifter J, Chenu C, Bird A, Mundy GR, Roodman GD (1989) Interleukin-1 and tumor necrosis factor stimulate the formation of human osteoclastlike cells in vitro. J Bone Miner Res 4: 113–118.

48. Nunamaker DM (1998) Experimental models of fracture repair. Clin Orthop Relat Res: S56–65.

49. Shiozawa Y, Pedersen EA, Havens AM, Jung Y, Mishra A, et al. (2011) Human prostate cancer metastases target the hematopoietic stem cell niche to establish footholds in mouse bone marrow. J Clin Invest 121: 1298–1312.

50. Sugiyama T, Kohara H, Noda M, Nagasawa T (2006) Maintenance of the hematopoietic stem cell pool by CXCL12-CXCR4 chemokine signaling in bone marrow stromal cell niches. Immunity 25: 977–988.

51. Phadke PA, Mercer RR, Harms JF, Jia Y, Frost AR, et al. (2006) Kinetics of metastatic breast cancer cell trafficking in bone. Clin Cancer Res 12: 1431–1440.

7

Bivariate Genome-Wide Association Analyses Identified Genes with Pleiotropic Effects for Femoral Neck Bone Geometry and Age at Menarche

Shu Ran[2], Yu-Fang Pei[2], Yong-Jun Liu[1], Lei Zhang[2], Ying-Ying Han[2], Rong Hai[3], Qing Tian[1], Yong Lin[2], Tie-Lin Yang[4], Yan-Fang Guo[5], Hui Shen[1], Inderpal S. Thethi[1], Xue-Zhen Zhu[2], Hong-Wen Deng[1,2]*

1 School of Public Health and Tropical Medicine, Tulane University, New Orleans, Louisiana, United States of America, **2** Center of System Biomedical Sciences, School of Medical Instrument and Food Engineering, University of Shanghai for Science and Technology, Shanghai, P. R. China, **3** Inner Mongolia People's Hospital, Hohhot, P. R. China, **4** School of Life Science and Technology, Xi'an Jiaotong University, Xi'an, Shanxi, P. R. China, **5** School of Basic Medical Science, Institute of Bioinformatics, Southern Medical University, Guangzhou, Guangdong, P. R. China

Abstract

Femoral neck geometric parameters (FNGPs), which include cortical thickness (CT), periosteal diameter (W), buckling ratio (BR), cross-sectional area (CSA), and section modulus (Z), contribute to bone strength and may predict hip fracture risk. Age at menarche (AAM) is an important risk factor for osteoporosis and bone fractures in women. Some FNGPs are genetically correlated with AAM. In this study, we performed a bivariate genome-wide association study (GWAS) to identify new candidate genes responsible for both FNGPs and AAM. In the discovery stage, we tested 760,794 SNPs in 1,728 unrelated Caucasian subject, followed by replication analyses in independent samples of US Caucasians (with 501 subjects) and Chinese (with 826 subjects). We found six SNPs that were associated with FNGPs and AAM. These SNPs are located in three genes (i.e. NRCAM, IDS and LOC148145), suggesting these three genes may co-regulate FNGPs and AAM. Our findings may help improve the understanding of genetic architecture and pathophysiological mechanisms underlying both osteoporosis and AAM.

Editor: Yi-Hsiang Hsu, Harvard Medical School, United States of America

Funding: The study was partially supported by startup funds from Shanghai University of Science and Technology and Shanghai Leading Academic Discipline Project (S30501). The investigators of this work were partially supported by grants from NIH (R01AG026564, RC2DE020756, R01AR057049, R01AR050496 and R03TW008221), a SCOR (Specialized Center of Research) grant (P50AR055081) supported by National Institute of Arthritis and Musculoskeletal and Skin Diseases (NIAMS) and the Office of Research on Women's Health (ORWH), and the Edward G. Schlieder Endowment and the Franklin D. Dickson/Missouri Endowment. Lei Zhang was also supported by the National Natural Science Foundation of China project (31100902). The funders had no role in study design, data collection and analysis, decision to publish, or preparation of the manuscript.

Competing Interests: The authors have declared that no competing interests exist.

* E-mail: hdeng2@tulane.edu

Introduction

Bone strength at the hip is directly related to the risk of hip fracture, the most serious and disabling type of osteoporotic fractures [1]. Femoral neck geometry is a major determinant of the mechanical resistance of the hip and plays an important role, independent of bone mineral density (BMD), in determining bone strength and osteoporotic fractures [2]. Femoral neck geometric parameters (FNGPs) measure bone structural properties (such as shape, size, and microarchitecture) and are believed to be as good as BMD in predicting hip fracture risk [3]. FNGPs, including cortical thickness (CT), periosteal diameter (W), buckling ratio (BR), cross-sectional area (CSA), and section modulus (Z), can be conveniently and accurately inferred from dual energy X-ray absorptiometry (DXA) measurements.

FNGPs have strong genetic determination with heritability ranging from 40–50% [4–7]. Earlier studies, including ours in Caucasians and Chinese, have identified some promising candidate genes associated with FNGPs [8–12].

Menarche is the first menstrual cycle in female human beings, which occurs when thickened endometrial tissue undergoes a

sudden death because of fluctuations of estrogen levels. Age at menarche (AAM) is an important factor that affects women's health. Late AAM is related with higher risk of osteoporosis in women, which may partially due to the less exposure to estrogen [13,14]. It has been shown that AAM is under strong genetic control and heritability of AAM is as high as 50–70% [15,16].

Since FNGPs and AAM are heritable traits highly related to risk of osteoporosis and women's health, it would be interesting to investigate whether there are pleiotropic genes that influence variation in both FNGPs and AAM. Previous studies were largely conducted on FNGPs or AAM separately using univariate analysis method which does not consider potential correlations between them [7,17]. This problem could be addressed by performing multivariate analysis which analyzes correlated traits simultaneously. Compared to univariate analysis, multivariate analysis has an advantage in detecting pleiotropic genes by considering the correlations between traits in the model. In addition, the multiple testing problems caused by testing different traits separately in univariate analysis can be alleviated in multivariate analysis.

Here we report the first bivariate genome-wide association study (GWAS) for FNGPs and AAM in a sample of 1,728 unrelated US

Table 1. Basic characteristics of the study subjects.

Traits	Discovery Caucasians (n = 1728)	Replication Caucasians (n = 501)	Replication Chinese (n = 826)
Age (years)	51.58 (12.92)	50.15 (17.69)	37.46 (13.77)
Height (cm)	163.28 (6.27)	163.85 (6.51)	158.38 (5.22)
Weight (kg)	71.45 (16.04)	71.32 (15.92)	54.63 (8.09)
AAM (years)	12.92 (1.58)	12.90 (1.49)	13.91 (1.61)
CT (cm)	0.15 (0.02)	0.15 (0.03)	0.14 (0.02)
W (cm)	3.30 (0.34)	3.36 (0.25)	3.11 (0.35)
BR	11.46 (2.42)	11.61 (2.74)	11.07 (2.76)
CSA (cm^2)	2.45 (0.48)	2.48 (0.45)	2.24 (0.38)
Z (cm^3)	1.45 (0.36)	1.49 (0.31)	1.26 (0.29)

Note:
All the values are presented as mean (standard deviation).

Caucasian female subjects followed by replication analyses in independent Caucasians and Chinese samples. We identified three genes (i.e. NRCAM, IDS and LOC148145) that were associated with both FNGPs and AAM, suggesting their roles in co-regulating FNGPs and AAM. Our findings may help improve the understanding of genetic architecture and pathophysiological mechanisms underlying both osteoporosis and AAM.

Table 2. Results of bivariate GWAS for AAM and three FNGPs ($p<10^{-5}$ in the discovery sample).

Traits pair	SNP	Chr	Position	Gene	P value in discovery sample	P value in replication Caucasian	P value in replication Chinese	Combined p value[1]	Combined p value[2]
AAM-CT									
	rs8113142	19	33704761	LOC148145	3.87×10^{-7}	–	0.73	–	4.54×10^{-6}
	rs4141232	**19**	**33727396**	**LOC148145**	**4.12×10^{-7}**	**0.03**	0.89	2.37×10^{-7}	5.80×10^{-6}
	rs4805257	19	33822305	LOC148145	1.62×10^{-6}	–	0.58	–	1.40×10^{-5}
	rs6578985	11	2094715	IGF2	1.06×10^{-6}	0.36	0.18	6.02×10^{-6}	3.14×10^{-6}
	rs6578987	11	2098162	IGF2	1.28×10^{-6}	–	0.14	–	2.96×10^{-6}
	rs6578986	11	2094728	IGF2	1.28×10^{-6}	–	0.34	–	6.81×10^{-6}
	rs4929957	11	2084885	IGF2	4.97×10^{-6}	–	0.08	–	6.26×10^{-6}
AAM-W									
	rs7929583	11	86904123	RAB38	4.35×10^{-6}	0.85	0.85	5.00×10^{-5}	5.00×10^{-5}
	rs12146626	11	86907172	RAB38	4.25×10^{-6}	0.92	0.84	5.26×10^{-5}	4.83×10^{-5}
	rs10898723	11	86904392	RAB38	8.58×10^{-6}	0.84	0.87	9.25×10^{-5}	9.56×10^{-5}
	rs6975557	**7**	**107760533**	**NRCAM**	**2.82×10^{-5}**	**8.33×10^{-5}**	0.45	**4.84×10^{-8}**	1.56×10^{-4}
	rs13230316	**7**	**107778803**	**NRCAM**	**5.58×10^{-5}**	**1.10×10^{-4}**	0.58	1.22×10^{-7}	3.67×10^{-4}
	rs5980450	**X**	**148285691**	**IDS**	**6.76×10^{-5}**	–	**0.05**	–	4.60×10^{-5}
	rs4844014	**X**	**148212344**	**IDS**	**7.31×10^{-5}**	**0.39**	**0.05**	3.27×10^{-4}	4.94×10^{-5}
	rs7064959	**X**	**148294515**	**IDS**	**8.64×10^{-5}**	–	**0.05**	–	5.77×10^{-5}
AAM-BR									
	rs4141232	19	33727396	LOC148145	6.99×10^{-7}	0.96	0.87	1.02×10^{-5}	9.31×10^{-6}
	rs7929583	11	86904123	RAB38	3.54×10^{-6}	0.84	0.58	4.08×10^{-5}	2.89×10^{-5}
	rs12146626	11	86907172	RAB38	4.36×10^{-6}	0.44	0.58	2.72×10^{-5}	3.51×10^{-5}
	rs10898723	11	86904392	RAB38	7.43×10^{-6}	0.35	0.62	3.69×10^{-5}	6.12×10^{-5}

Note:
Combined p value[1]: Combined p values by joint analyses of the Caucasian discovery and the Caucasian replication samples.
Combined p value[2]: Combined p values by joint analyses of the Caucasian discovery and the Chinese replication samples.
–: p value not available.
Bold: SNPs that were replicated in the replication samples.

Table 3. Characteristics of SNPs bivariately associated with FNGPs and AAM.

SNP	Chr	Position	Gene	Role	Allele[a]	MAF[b]	MAF[c]	MAF[d]	MAF[e]	MAF[f]	AAM-CT	AAM-W	AAM-BR
rs4141232	19	33727396	LOC148145	upstream	C/T	0.16	0.15	0.18	0.20	0.23	4.12×10^{-7}	1.09×10^{-3}	6.99×10^{-7}
rs6975557	7	107760533	NRCAM	intron	G/A	0.28	0.26	0.26	0.45	0.41	6.29×10^{-3}	2.82×10^{-5}	5.31×10^{-4}
rs13230316	7	107778803	NRCAM	intron	G/C	0.27	0.26	0.25	0.45	0.38	7.14×10^{-3}	5.58×10^{-5}	6.63×10^{-4}
rs5980450	X	148285691	IDS	downstream	A/G	0.06	–	0.03	0.15	0.15	0.44	6.76×10^{-5}	6.07×10^{-3}
rs4844014	X	148212344	IDS	downstream	C/A	0.06	0.06	0.03	0.14	0.15	0.55	7.31×10^{-5}	6.91×10^{-3}
rs7064959	X	148294515	IDS	downstream	G/A	0.06	–	0.04	0.13	0.15	0.75	8.64×10^{-5}	0.01

Note:
[a]The first allele represents the minor allele of each locus.
[b]Minor allele frequency calculated in our discovery Caucasian sample (n = 1728).
[c]Minor allele frequency calculated in our replication Caucasian sample (n = 501).
[d]Minor allele frequency reported for Caucasians in the public database of HapMap CEU.
[e]Minor allele frequency calculated in our replication Chinese subjects.
[f]Minor allele frequency reported for Chinese in the public database of HapMap.
–: MAF not available.

Methods

Subjects

The discovery sample contained 1,728 unrelated Caucasian female subjects recruited in Midwestern US (Kansas City, MO, and Omaha, NE) for studies of osteoporosis and related health problems. All the identified subjects were US Caucasians of European origin. The replication samples included Caucasians and Chinese. The Caucasian replication sample included 501 unrelated female subjects living in Omaha, NE, USA, and its surrounding areas. There was no overlap between the discovery and replication Caucasian samples. The Chinese replication sample included 826 unrelated female subjects living in Changsha or Xi'an, China.

The study was approved by Institutional Review Boards of Creighton University, University of Missouri-Kansas City, Hunan Normal University of China and Xi'an Jiaotong University of China. All the subjects signed informed-consent documents and completed structured questionnaires. The exclusion criteria were detailed in our previous publications [18]. Briefly, subjects with chronic diseases and conditions that might affect bone metabolism and AAM were excluded from this study.

Areal BMD (g/cm^2) and region area (cm^2) of FN were measured using dual-energy X-ray absorptiometry scanners Hologic QDR 4500 W (Hologic Inc., Bedford, MA, USA). The machines were calibrated daily. The coefficient of variation (CV) values obtained from the DXA measurements for FN bone size and FN BMD were 1.94% and 1.87%. Bone geometric parameters were calculated using the DXA-derived FN BMD and bone size. The methods for calculating these variables were detailed elsewhere [7,19,20]. The five estimated FNGPs are CT, W, BR, CSA, and Z. CT is an estimate of mean cortical thickness, W is the outer diameter of the bone, BR is an index of cortical instability indicating the risk of fracture by buckling, CSA is an indicator of bone axial compression strength, and Z is an index of bone bending strength indicating the bending resistance of a tube.

Genotyping

For each study subject, we extracted genomic DNA from peripheral blood leukocytes using standard protocols, and genotyping experiments were performed strictly following the standard protocol recommended by related manufacturer. The subjects of the discovery sample and the Chinese replication sample were genotyped using Affymetrix Genome-wide Human SNP 6.0 genotyping arrays (Affymetrix, Santa Clara, CA, USA) which include 909,622 SNPs [21]. The Caucasian replication sample was genotyped using Affymetrix Human Mapping 500 K arrays which included 500,567 SNPs.

Quality Control

In order to obtain high quality genotyping data, we followed strict quality control procedures. Samples with a minimum call rate of 95% were included in the analyses. For the Caucasian sample, the final mean call rate reached a level of 98.93%. We discarded SNPs that deviated from Hardy-Weinberg equilibrium $(p<0.0001)$ and those with a minor allele frequency (MAF) <0.01. After quality control, the numbers of SNPs available for association analysis were 760,794 in the discovery sample, 702,413 in the Chinese replication sample, and 407,192 in the Caucasian replication sample.

Statistical Analyses

The five FNGPs were adjusted by age, height and weight [22], while AAM was adjusted by height and weight [23,24] using Minitab (Minitab Inc., State College, PA, USA). The covariates-adjusted phenotypic values were used in subsequent association analyses. We tested the phenotypic correlation between FNGPs and AAM using bivariate correlation analysis in Minitab.

The association analyses between genotype and the covariates-adjusted traits were performed using a bivariate linear regression

Table 4. Proportions of phenotype correlation explain correlations coefficients of three trait pairs.

	AAM-CT	AAM-W	AAM-BR
corr1	−0.05	0.04	0.08
corr2	−0.04	0.03	0.07
corrp	18.52%	25.26%	12.99%

Note:
Corr1: The original phenotype correlation coefficients.
Corr2: The phenotype correlation coefficients after adjusted by the SNPs.
Corrp: The proportion of correlations between each trait pairs explained by the reported SNPs, which is calculated by $corrp = (corr1 - corr2)/corr1$.

Table 5. Results of univariate association analyses for the six SNPs in the discovery sample and the replication samples.

SNP	Univariate p value discovery sample (n = 1728)				Univariate p value Replication Chinese sample (n = 826)				Univariate p value Replication Caucasian sample (n = 501)			
	AAM	CT	W	BR	AAM	CT	W	BR	AAM	CT	W	BR
rs4141232	3.48×10^{-3}	7.70×10^{-6}	6.67×10^{-3}	5.88×10^{-6}	0.82	0.95	0.63	0.81	0.46	0.01	0.96	0.66
rs6975557	0.02	0.03	8.62×10^{-5}	7.57×10^{-4}	0.28	7.57×10^{-4}	0.53	7.57×10^{-4}	0.63	0.66	2.09×10^{-5}	0.57
rs13230316	0.03	0.02	1.25×10^{-4}	6.30×10^{-4}	0.36	6.30×10^{-4}	0.65	6.30×10^{-4}	0.75	0.59	2.49×10^{-5}	0.68
rs5980450	0.47	0.40	2.36×10^{-5}	3.70×10^{-3}	0.02	3.70×10^{-3}	0.39	3.70×10^{-3}	–	–	–	–
rs4844014	0.77	0.39	1.91×10^{-5}	3.13×10^{-3}	0.02	3.13×10^{-3}	0.43	3.13×10^{-3}	0.17	0.40	0.93	0.91
rs7064959	0.86	0.51	1.79×10^{-5}	5.00×10^{-3}	0.03	0.42	0.33	0.32	–	–	–	–

Note:
–: p value not available.

model. The model is represented by $\mathbf{y}_{1i} = \mathbf{\mu} + \mathbf{\beta} x_i + \mathbf{\varepsilon}_i$, where $\mathbf{y}_i$ is the vector of the two traits for individual i; $\mathbf{\mu}$ is the vector of grand means; $\mathbf{\beta}$ is the vector of its effects, and x_i is the genotype score for individual i. $\mathbf{\varepsilon}_i$ is the vector of residues following a multivariate normal distribution with mean zero. The genotype x_i was encoded with an additive mode of inheritance. The association was examined by testing the significance of $\mathbf{\beta}$, and the test was performed with R package lm. Individual p values achieved in the three studied samples were then combined by fisher's method [25]. Genomic control approach was used to evaluate population effect and control potential population stratification that may lead to spurious association results. The p value of 5×10^{-8} was used as the threshold to claim significant associations at the genome-wide level, after accounting for multiple-testing by applying Bonferroni correction. Since Bonferroni correction is quite conservative, we reported SNPs that achieved a p value of 10^{-5} or less in the discovery stage. For replication, due to the prior evidence of association, we used a threshold of the nominal p level of 0.05.

We evaluated the proportion of phenotype correlations between each trait pairs explained by the reported SNPs. We define corr1 as the original phenotype correlation coefficients and corr2 as the phenotype correlation coefficients after adjusted by the SNPs. The proportion of correlations between each trait pairs explained by the reported SNPs (corrp) was calculated by the formula: $corrp = (corr1 - corr2)/_{corr1}$.

For the SNPs showing potential pleiotropic effects, we further investigated the effect direction and causal relationship. The effect direction of the SNPs was evaluated using a linear regression model implemented in PLINK [26]. The causal relationship of the SNPs was examined by comparing adjusted/conditional models in bivariate linear regression analyses, in which the genotype of each of the reported SNPs was adjusted as a covariate in turn.

For comparison purpose, we also performed univariate association analyses for each trait using a univariate linear regression model with the R package lm. To compare statistical power between univariate and bivariate association analyses, we performed power analyses using the GEE (Generalized Estimation Equation) implemented in R. The power analyses were based on the sample sizes of 1,728, 826, and 501 unrelated subjects as used in the present study for discovery and replication analyses. Simulation analysis was performed to calculate the power.

The coefficient of linkage disequilibrium (LD) between specific SNPs was obtained from the Haploview system [27]. We used the FASTSNP program (http://fastsnp.ibms.sinica.edu.tw) to explore potential functions of the reported SNPs [28].

Results

The basic characteristics of the discovery and replication samples are summarized in Table 1. Correlation analysis of the study traits showed that AAM was significantly correlated with FNGPs. In the discovery sample, significant correlations were observed between AAM and three FNGPs (CT, W, and BR), and the correlation coefficients were -0.054 ($p = 0.028$) for AAM and CT, 0.043 ($p = 0.082$) for AAM and W, 0.077 ($p = 0.002$) for AAM and BR, respectively. The significant correlations observed here are consistent with previous findings of others [29,30]. We subsequently focused biviarate analyses on AAM and these three FNGPs.

We identified six SNPs that were associated with both FNGPs and AAM in the discovery sample ($p < 10^{-5}$). These SNPs were replicated in independent Caucasian and/or Chinese replication samples (Table 2). Among them, rs4141232 is located in the upstream of the LOC148145 gene ($p = 4.12 \times 10^{-7}$ for AAM-CT), rs6975557 and rs13230316 are located in the intron of the NRCAM (neuronal cell adhesion molecule isoform A) gene ($p = 2.82 \times 10^{-5}$ and 5.58×10^{-5} for AAM-W, respectively), and the other three SNPs, rs5980450, rs4844014, and rs7064959, are located in the downstream of the IDS (Iduronate-2-sulfatase) gene ($p = 6.76 \times 10^{-5}$, 7.31×10^{-5} and 8.64×10^{-5} for AAM-W, respectively). Three SNPs (rs4141232, rs6975557 and rs13230316) were replicated in the Caucasian sample ($p = 0.03$, 8.33×10^{-5} and 1.10×10^{-4}, respectively). The other three SNPs (rs5980450, rs4844014, and rs7064959) near the IDS gene were replicated in the Chinese sample ($p = 0.05$) (Table 2). Combined p values of meta-analyses are also shown in Table 2.

The characteristics of the six SNPs bivariately associated with FNGPs and AAM are shown in Table 3. The proportions of phenotype correlation explained by the six SNPs were 18.52% for AAM-CT, 25.26% for AAM-W, and 12.99% for AAM-BR, respectively (Table 4).

Based on SNPs genotyped in GWAS, we estimated inflation factor (λ) which is a measure of population stratification. Generally, for a homogenous population with no stratification the value of λ should be equal or close to 1. In our GWAS cohorts, the estimated λ values for AAM, CT, W, and BR were 0.938, 0.982, 0.934, and 0.936, respectively, suggesting no or very modest population stratification, if any.

We performed univariate association analyses for the six identified SNPs in the three studied samples. As presented in Table 5, p values of univariate association analyses were less

Sample size=1728

Sample size=826

Sample size=501

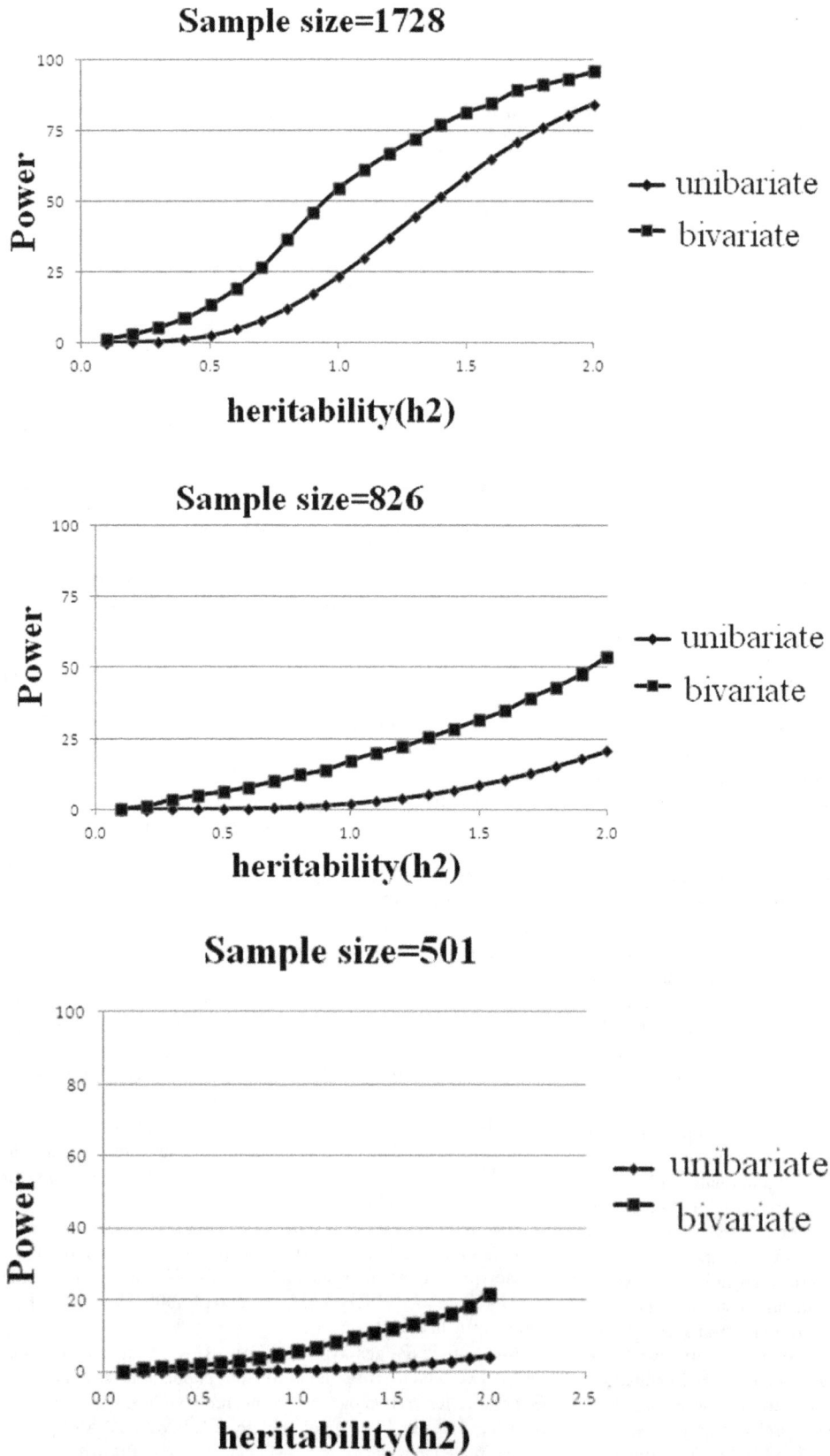

Figure 1. Comparison of statistical power of bivariate vs. univariate association analyses in three samples of this study. The Y axis shows the expected power, and the X axis shows the heritability. Type 1 error was set at 0.05 and minor allele frequency (MAF) was set at 0.1. The sample sizes were 1728 (discovery Caucasians), 826 (replication Chinese) and 501 (replication Caucasians), respectively.

Table 6. The effect direction of the SNPs in discovery and replication samples.

	Gene	Discovery Caucasian sample (n = 1728)				Minor allele	Replication Chinese sample (n = 826)			
		β/AAM	β/CT	β/W	β/BR		β/AAM	β/CT	β/W	β/BR
rs4141232	LOC148145	−0.13	0.20	−0.13	−0.21	C	0.02	−0.004	0.02	0.01
rs6975557	NRCAM	0.10	−0.09	0.16	0.13	G	−0.05	−0.04	0.03	0.07
rs13230316	NRCAM	0.09	−0.09	0.16	0.13	G	−0.03	−0.04	0.02	0.06
rs5980450	IDS	−0.07	−0.06	0.30	0.21	A	0.21	0.04	−0.06	−0.07
rs4844014	IDS	−0.06	−0.06	0.30	0.22	C	0.19	0.03	−0.05	−0.06
rs7064959	IDS	−0.03	−0.05	0.32	0.21	G	0.21	0.06	−0.06	−0.07

Note:
The effect direction was assessed using a linear regression model. A positive/negative regression coefficients (β) value means that the minor allele is associated with a higher/lower trait value. The three FNGP phenotypes were adjusted by age, height and weight while AAM was adjusted by height and weight.

significant than those of bivariate analyses. Power calculation showed that bivariate analysis exhibited consistently higher statistical power than univariate analysis did for any of the three samples (Fig. 1).

The effect directions of these SNPs are presented in Table 6. A positive beta value means that the minor allele is associated with a higher trait value. Since these SNPs were not included in the SNP arrays scanned in the Caucasian replication sample, their effect directions are not available for this sample. The effect direction for AAM was contrary between discovery and Chinese replication samples. For CT, W and BR, two SNPs of the NRCAM gene had the same effect direction in both samples, while three SNPs near the IDS gene had contrary effect directions between the two samples.

We examined the causal relationships of the six SNPs (Table 7). It can be seen that for the SNPs located in the same gene, using the genotype of one SNP as a covariate, the association signals disappeared, suggesting these SNPs are in linkage disequilibrium.

Table 7. The causal relationship of the six SNPs for three trait pairs in the discovery sample.

	Covariate	Gene	rs4141232	rs6975557	rs13230316	rs5980450	rs4844014	rs7064959
AAM-CT								
	rs4141232	LOC148145	–	4.67×10^{-3}	4.63×10^{-3}	0.54	0.67	0.85
	rs6975557	NRCAM	4.26×10^{-7}	–	0.96	0.55	0.64	0.77
	rs13230316	NRCAM	2.90×10^{-7}	0.91	–	0.56	0.41	0.64
	rs5980450	IDS	8.10×10^{-7}	9.09×10^{-3}	8.89×10^{-3}	–	0.84	0.83
	rs4844014	IDS	1.02×10^{-6}	7.95×10^{-3}	9.05×10^{-3}	0.88	–	0.98
	rs7064959	IDS	1.38×10^{-6}	8.69×10^{-3}	9.90×10^{-3}	0.91	0.99	–
AAM-W								
	rs4141232	LOC148145	–	2.43×10^{-5}	4.39×10^{-5}	9.03×10^{-5}	9.33×10^{-5}	1.30×10^{-4}
	rs6975557	NRCAM	4.04×10^{-4}	–	1.00	7.64×10^{-5}	5.60×10^{-5}	5.87×10^{-5}
	rs13230316	NRCAM	2.76×10^{-4}	0.94	–	6.98×10^{-5}	8.78×10^{-5}	9.29×10^{-5}
	rs5980450	IDS	7.82×10^{-4}	4.83×10^{-5}	1.02×10^{-4}	–	0.82	0.81
	rs4844014	IDS	7.76×10^{-4}	5.00×10^{-5}	1.15×10^{-4}	0.86	–	0.91
	rs7064959	IDS	1.20×10^{-3}	4.57×10^{-5}	1.07×10^{-4}	0.88	0.90	–
AAM-BR								
	rs4141232	LOC148145	–	2.58×10^{-4}	2.81×10^{-4}	8.40×10^{-3}	8.94×10^{-3}	0.02
	rs6975557	NRCAM	3.66×10^{-7}	–	0.97	7.67×10^{-3}	6.17×10^{-3}	0.01
	rs13230316	NRCAM	2.74×10^{-7}	0.92	–	6.42×10^{-3}	2.43×10^{-3}	6.94×10^{-3}
	rs5980450	IDS	1.21×10^{-6}	8.43×10^{-4}	9.51×10^{-4}	–	0.77	0.83
	rs4844014	IDS	1.34×10^{-6}	7.92×10^{-4}	1.07×10^{-3}	0.83	–	0.97
	rs7064959	IDS	2.37×10^{-6}	7.78×10^{-4}	1.06×10^{-3}	0.88	0.93	–

Note:
The causal relationship of the SNPs was examined by comparing adjusted/conditional models in bivariate linear regression analyses, in which the genotype of each of the six SNPs was adjusted as a covariate in turn. P values of the analyses are shown in the table.

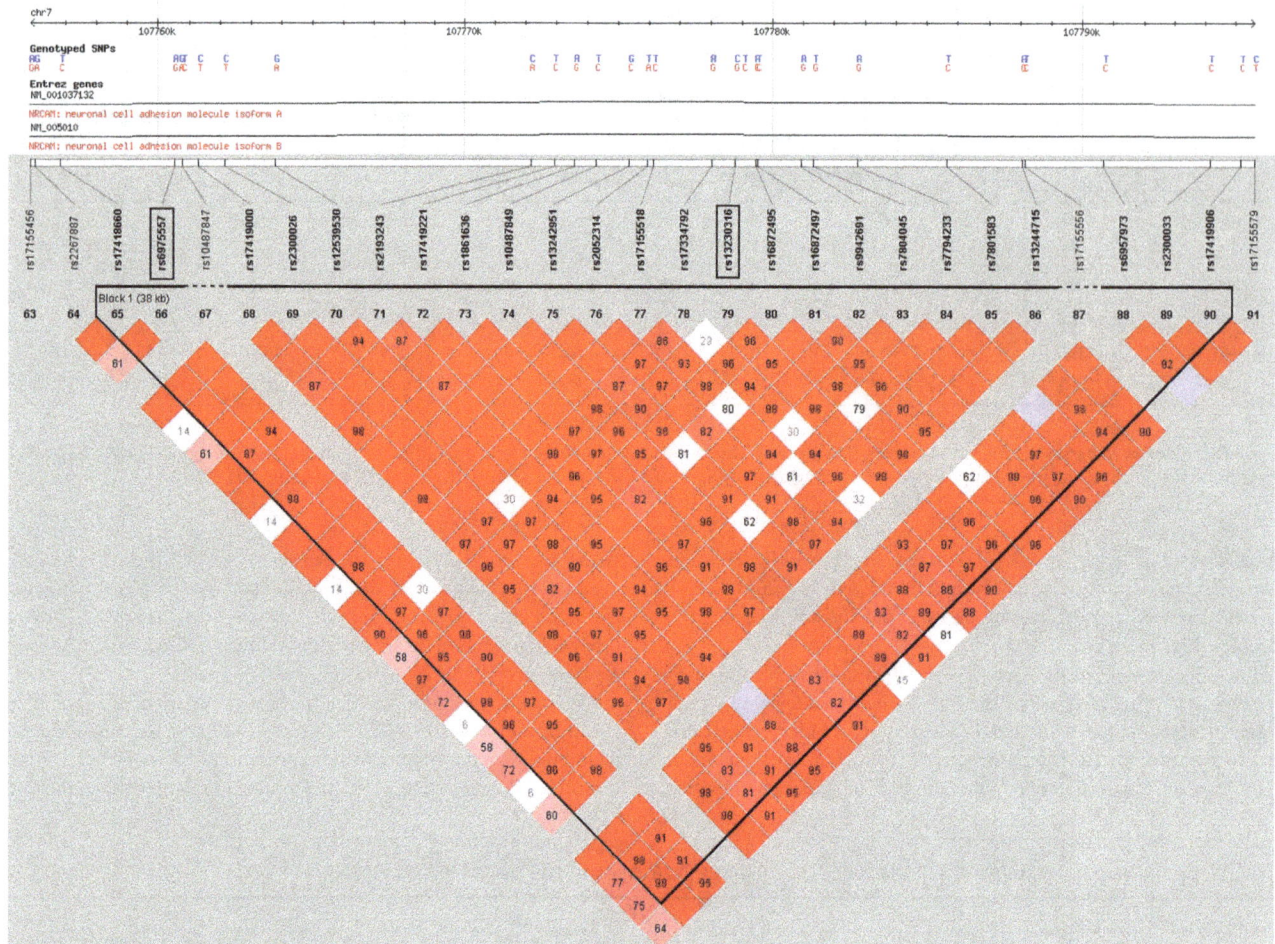

Figure 2. LD structure of the NRCAM gene in the discovery Caucasian sample. The region demarcated in red indicates that $r^2>0.9$. The region includes only one LD block as indicated by triangle with black lines. SNP rs6975557 and rs13230316 are located within one block.

When the genotypes of the SNPs located in different genes were used as a covariate, the association signals remained, suggesting they are independent. From biology point of view, the concept of causality is more complex than comparison of adjusted/conditional models as used here. The causal effects of the variants need to be further explored and validated via deep re-sequencing of the gene locus and subsequent molecular functional studies.

Analysis using the software Haploview in the Caucasian sample showed that SNPs rs6975557 and rs13230316 located in the NRCAM gene are in the same LD block ($r^2 \geq 0.97$) (Fig. 2). The SNPs rs8113142, rs4141232, and rs4805257 near the LOC148145 gene are in two LD blocks ($r^2 = 0.93$, and 0.88, respectively) (Fig. 3). The SNPs rs5980450, rs4844014, and rs7064959 near the IDS gene are not available in the Haploview.

Using the FASTSNP program, we investigated the potential functions of these six SNPs. The SNPs rs6975557 and rs13230316 are located at potential transcription factor-binding sites and thus may have a role in transcription regulation. A G→A change at rs6975557 may result in the elimination of the binding sites for transcription factor GATA-1, while a G→C change at rs13230316 may produce a change in the binding sites of S8 and OCT-1. The other four SNPs (i.e., rs4141232, rs5980450, rs4844014, and rs7064959) did not show known functions according to the FASTSNP program.

Discussion

To the best of our knowledge, this is the first bivariate GWAS for FNGPs and AAM, which identified three novel genes (i.e., NRCAM, IDS and LOC148145) which may contribute to covariation of FNGPs and AAM. GWAS were largely performed by analyzing individual traits separately in a univariate framework. Although univariate analysis is effective for discovering novel genes responsible for a specific disease or trait, the approach generally ignores the potential genetic co-predisposition to human diseases. Bivariate analysis considers the correlation between traits and has an advantage in identifying genes with pleiotropic effects. The approach may help reveal the interconnected pathophysiological networks for a spectrum of common human diseases [31,32].

The gene NRCAM encodes a neuronal cell adhesion molecule [33]. Early studies showed that NRCAM gene expression increased during osteogenic and chondrogenic differentiation [34], suggesting it may function in osteoblasts and chondrocytes and probably be master control gene. The NRCAM gene is located on the chromosome 7q31, a region showed significant association with BMD in a published GWAS [35]. NRCAM is also a gene involved in regulation of estrogen. As one of the oocyte-specific genes, the NRCAM possess embryogenesis cellular growth and differentiation identified from the human primordial follicles cDNA library [36].

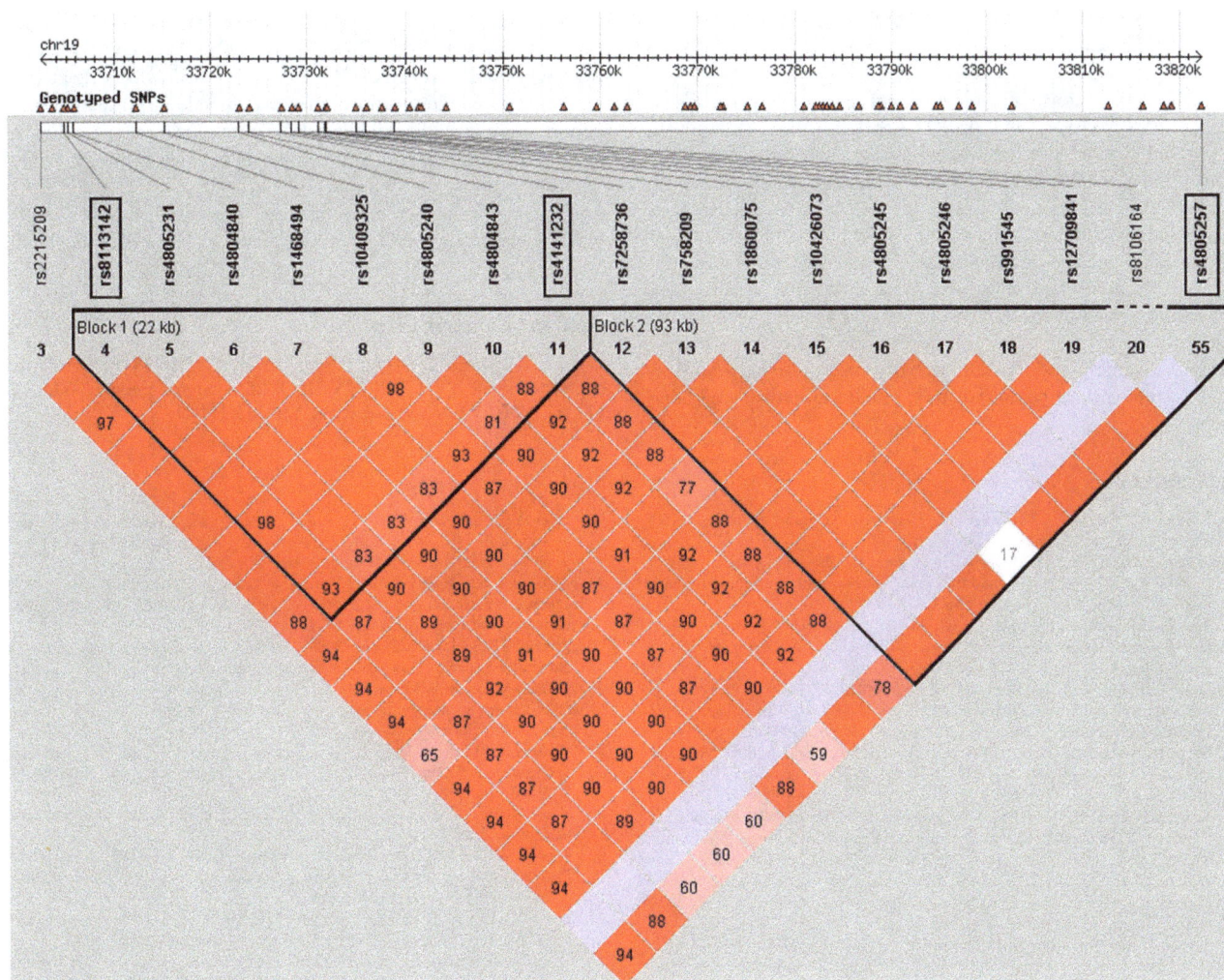

Figure 3. LD structure of the upstream of LOC148145 gene in the discovery Caucasian sample. The region demarcated in red indicates that $r^2>0.9$. The region includes two LD blocks (Block1 and Block2) marked by triangles with black lines. SNPs rs8113142 and rs4141232 are located in Block1, and the SNP rs4805257 is located in Block 2.

The IDS gene encodes Iduronate-2-sulfatase which is required for the lysosomal degradation of heparan sulfate and dermatan sulfate [37]. Mutations in the gene that result in enzymatic deficiency may lead to the sex-linked Mucopolysaccharidosis Type II [38]. Since glycosaminoglycans are fundamental in connective tissue structure and function, mucopolysaccharidosis disorders are characterized by severe skeletal abnormality including abnormal bone structure, growth failure and severe articular cartilage and joint problems [39]. The IDS gene also has relationship to AAM. IDS plays an important role in metabolism of steroid hormones such as estrone and estradiol [40]. Significant declines in activity of IDS was observed in the mammary cell lines MCF7 and T47D with estrogen exposure, with higher doses of estradiol associated with more significant declines [41]. The collective evidence suggests that IDS is important for both bone metabolism and AAM.

The LOC148145 gene locates on the chromosome 19q12. It is the non-coding RNA gene. The biological function of this gene is currently unclear and thus the exact mechanisms by which LOC148145 is involved in co-regulation of bone and AAM await discovery.

For the six SNPs associated with FNGPs and AAM, the effect directions were not completely consistent in the discovery and replication studies. The inconsistency could be explained by several reasons. First, it may be caused by genetic heterogeneity. For instance, allele frequencies of genetic variants could be different among diverse populations due to different evolution histories, which results in different genotype phenotype associations [42]. Recent studies showed that replicable findings in specific populations might be more generalizable in other populations, and such variants are more likely to be causal in nature [43]. Second, GWAS is an indirect association method based on linkage disequilibrium between SNP markers. Significant associations may be found at genetic markers that are in linkage disequilibrium with causal variants, rather than the causal variants *per se*. Therefore, inconsistency of the effect directions could be a result of different patterns of linkage disequilibrium in different populations.

Interestingly, there was an overlap between the results of this study and those of some published studies. Elks et al. reported the largest meta-analysis of GWAS for AAM in 87,802 women of European ancestry [44]. In that study, the SNP rs6589964 was strongly associated with AAM ($p = 1.9 \times 10^{-12}$). In our study, this

SNP achieved p values of 6.64×10^{-4} to 8.79×10^{-4} for three trait pairs in the Caucasian discovery sample and p values of 2.86×10^{-3} to 6.27×10^{-3} in the Chinese replication sample.

In the current study, FNGPs were calculated based on DXA-derived FN BMD and bone size. This is a convenient method to obtain bone geometric indices using the areal BMD with the assumption that the mineral in the cross section is confined to an annular cortical region. However, the DXA measured BMD is restricted to two dimensions, and the resolution and accuracy of the structural parameters are affected. Despite this, studies showed that the geometry of femoral neck cross sections was reasonably well characterized by DXA compares to a more rigorous 3D finite element technique [45]. In particular, due to the wide availability of DXA scanners and the low radiation exposure of scanning, DXA is still the most popular method in clinical settings and bone research.

In summary, by performing a bivariate GWAS, we identified three novel genes (NRCAM, IDS and LOC148145) that may co-regulate FNGPs and AAM. Our findings need to be validated in different populations and molecular functional studies. Once confirmed, our findings may help improve our understanding of genetic architecture and pathophysiological mechanisms underlying osteoporosis and fracture risk. Our findings also furnish a foundation for further molecular and functional analyses of the genes in regulating timing of menarche and women's health in general.

Author Contributions

Conceived and designed the experiments: HWD YJL HS. Performed the experiments: SR YYH RH TLY HS XZZ. Analyzed the data: YFP LZ QT YL YFG. Wrote the paper: SR YJL IST HWD.

References

1. Kannus P, Parkkari J, Sievanen H, Heinonen A, Vuori I, et al. (1996) Epidemiology of hip fractures. Bone 18: 57S–63S.
2. Turner CH, Hsieh YF, Muller R, Bouxsein ML, Baylink DJ, et al. (2000) Genetic regulation of cortical and trabecular bone strength and microstructure in inbred strains of mice. J Bone Miner Res 15 (6): 1126–1131.
3. Melton LJ, Beck TJ, Amin S, Khosla S, Achenbach SJ, et al. (2005) Contributions of bone density and structure to fracture risk assessment in men and women. Osteoporos Int 16 (5): 460–467.
4. Demissie S, Dupuis J, Cupples LA, Beck TJ, Kiel DP, et al. (2007) Proximal hip geometry is linked to several chromosomal regions: genome-wide linkage results from the Framingham Osteoporosis Study. Bone 40 (3): 743–750.
5. Shen H, Long JR, Xiong DH, Liu YJ, Liu YZ, et al. (2005) Mapping quantitative trait loci for cross-sectional geometry at the femoral neck. J Bone Miner Res 20 (11): 1973–1982.
6. Xiong DH, Shen H, Xiao P, Guo YF, Long JR, et al. (2006) Genome-wide scan identified QTLs underlying femoral neck cross-sectional geometry that are novel studied risk factors of osteoporosis. J Bone Miner Res 21 (3): 424–437.
7. Zhao LJ, Liu XG, Liu YZ, Liu YJ, Papasian CJ, et al. (2010) Genome-wide association study for femoral neck bone geometry. J Bone Miner Res 25 (2): 320–329.
8. Qureshi AM, McGuigan FE, Seymour DG, Hutchison JD, Reid DM, et al. (2001) Association between COLIA1 Sp1 alleles and femoral neck geometry. Calcif Tissue Int 69 (2): 67–72.
9. Rivadeneira F, Houwing-Duistermaat JJ, Beck TJ, Janssen JA, Hofman A, et al. (2004) The influence of an insulin-like growth factor I gene promoter polymorphism on hip bone geometry and the risk of nonvertebral fracture in the elderly: the Rotterdam Study. J Bone Miner Res 19 (8): 1280–1290.
10. Moffett SP, Zmuda JM, Oakley JI, Beck TJ, Cauley JA, et al. (2005) Tumor necrosis factor-alpha polymorphism, bone strength phenotypes, and the risk of fracture in older women. J Clin Endocrinol Metab 90 (6): 3491–3497.
11. Xiong DH, Liu YZ, Peng YL, Zhao LJ, Deng HW (2005) Association analysis of estrogen receptor alpha gene polymorphisms with cross-sectional geometry of the femoral neck in Caucasian nuclear families. Osteoporos Int 16 (12): 2113–2122.
12. Jiang H, Lei SF, Xiao SM, Chen Y, Sun X, et al. (2007) Association and linkage analysis of COL1A1 and AHSG gene polymorphisms with femoral neck bone geometric parameters in both Caucasian and Chinese nuclear families. Acta Pharmacol Sin 28 (3): 375–381.
13. Roy DK, O'Neill TW, Finn JD, Lunt M, Silman AJ, et al. (2003) Determinants of incident vertebral fracture in men and women: results from the European Prospective Osteoporosis Study (EPOS). Osteoporos Int 14 (1): 19–26.
14. Silman A J (2003) Risk factors for Colles' fracture in men and women: results from the European Prospective Osteoporosis Study. Osteoporos Int 14 (3): 213–218.
15. Anderson CA, Duffy DL, Martin NG, Visscher PM (2007) Estimation of variance components for age at menarche in twin families. Behav Genet. 37 (5): 668–677.
16. van den Berg SM, Boomsma DI (2007) The familial clustering of age at menarche in extended twin families. Behav Genet 37 (5): 661–667.
17. Liu YZ, Guo YF, Wang L, Tan LJ, Liu XG, et al. (2009) Genome-wide association analyses identify SPOCK as a key novel gene underlying age at menarche. PLoS Genet 5: e1000420.
18. Deng HW, Deng HY, Liu YJ, Liu YZ, Xu FH, et al. (2002) A genomewide linkage scan for quantitative-trait loci for obesity phenotypes. Am J Hum Genet 70 (5): 1138–1151.
19. Beck T. (2003) Measuring the structural strength of bones with dual-energy X-ray absorptiometry: principles, technical limitations, and future possibilities. Osteoporos Int 14 Suppl 5: S81–S88.
20. Chen Y, Xiong DH, Guo YF, Pan F, Zhou Q, et al. (2010) Pathway-based genome-wide association analysis identified the importance of EphrinA-EphR pathway for femoral neck bone geometry. Bone 46 (1): 129–136.
21. McCarroll SA, Kuruvilla FG, Korn JM, Cawley S, Nemesh J, et al. (2008) Integrated detection and population-genetic analysis of SNPs and copy number variation. Nat Genet 40: 1166–1174.
22. Zhang F, Tan LJ, Lei SF, et al. (2009) The differences of femoral neck geometric parameters: effects of age, gender and race. Osteoporos Int 21: 1205–1214.
23. Onland-Moret NC, Peeters PH, van Gils CH, Clavel-Chapelon F, Key T, et al. (2005) Age at menarche in relation to adult height: The EPIC study. Am J Epidemiol 162: 623–632.
24. Wellens R, Malina RM, Roche AF, Chumlea WC, Guo S, et al. (1992) Body size and fatness in young adults in relation to age at menarche. Am J Hum Biol 4: 783–787.
25. RA F (1948) Combining independent tests of significance. The American Statistician 2: 30.
26. Purcell S, Neale B, Todd-Brown K, Thomas L, Ferreira MA, et al. (2007) PLINK: a tool set for whole-genome association and population-based linkage analyses. Am J Hum Genet 81: 559–575.
27. Barrett JC, Fry B, Maller J, Daly MJ (2005) Haploview: analysis and visualization of LD and haplotype maps. Bioinformatics 21: 263–265.
28. Yuan HY, Chiou JJ, Tseng WH, Liu CH, Liu CK, et al. (2006) FASTSNP: an always up-to-date and extendable service for SNP function analysis and prioritization. Nucleic Acids Res 34: W635–W641.
29. Rauch F, Klein K, Allolio B, Schonau E (1999) Age at menarche and cortical bone geometry in premenopausal women. Bone 25 (1): 69–73.
30. Petit MA, Beck TJ, Lin HM, Bentley C, Legro RS, et al. (2004) Femoral bone structural geometry adapts to mechanical loading and is influenced by sex steroids: the Penn State Young Women's Health Study. Bone 35 (3): 750–759.
31. Liu YZ, Pei YF, Liu JF, Yang F, Guo Y, et al. (2009) Powerful bivariate genome-wide association analyses suggest the SOX6 gene influencing both obesity and osteoporosis phenotypes in males. PLoS One 4 (8): e6827.
32. Liu J, Pei Y, Papasian CJ, Deng HW (2009) Bivariate association analyses for the mixture of continuous and binary traits with the use of extended generalized estimating equations. Genet Epidemiol 33: 217–227.
33. Marui T, Funatogawa I, Koishi S, Yamamoto K, Matsumoto H, et al. (2009) Association of the neuronal cell adhesion molecule (NRCAM) gene variants with autism. Int J Neuropsychopharmacol 12: 1–10.
34. Baksh D, Song L, Tuan RS (2004) Adult mesenchymal stem cells: characterization, differentiation, and application in cell and gene therapy. J Cell Mol Med 8 (3): 301–316.
35. Hsu YS, Nandakumar K, and Karasik D (2011) Musculoskeletal Genetics and -Omics: Meeting Report from the 32nd Annual Meeting of the American Society for Bone and Mineral Research. IBMS BoneKEy 8 (2): 112–122.
36. Serafica MD, Goto T, Trounson AO (2005) Transcripts from a human primordial follicle cDNA library. Hum Reprod 20 (8): 2074–2091.
37. Tuschl K, Gal A, Paschke E, Kircher S, Bodamer OA (2005) Mucopolysaccharidosis type II in females: case report and review of literature. Pediatr Neurol 32: 270–272.
38. Morini SR, Steiner CE, Gerson LB (2010) Mucopolysaccharidosis type II: skeletal-muscle system involvement. J Pediatr Orthop B 19 (4): 313–317.
39. Marucha J, Jurecka A, Syczewska M, Rozdzynska-Swiatkowska A, Tylki-Szymanska A. (2011) Restricted joint range of motion in patients with MPS II: correlation with height, age and functional status. Acta Paediatr 101 (4): e183–e188.
40. Bhattacharyya S, Tobacman JK (2007) Steroid sulfatase, arylsulfatases A and B, galactose-6-sulfatase, and iduronate sulfatase in mammary cells and effects of sulfated and non-sulfated estrogens on sulfatase activity. J Steroid Biochem Mol Biol 103 (1): 20–34.

41. Tobacman JK, Bhattacharyya S (2005) Sulfatase enzyme activity in MCF-7 and MCF-10a cells following exposure to estrogenic hormones. AACR Meeting Abstracts.

42. Economou M, Trikalinos TA, Loizou KT, Tsianos EV, Ioannidis JP (2004) Differential effects of NOD2 variants on Crohn's disease risk and phenotype in diverse populations: a metaanalysis. Am J Gastroenterol 99: 2393–2404.

43. Zuo L, Gelernter J, Zhang CK, Zhao H, Lu L, et al. (2012) Genome-Wide Association Study of Alcohol Dependence Implicates KIAA0040 on Chromosome 1q. Neuropsychopharmacology 37: 557–566.

44. Elks CE, Perry JR, Sulem P, Chasman DI, Franceschini N, et al. (2010) Thirty new loci for age at menarche identified by a meta-analysis of genome-wide association studies. Nat Genet 42: 1077–1085.

45. Danielson ME, Beck TJ, Karlamangla AS, Greendale GA, Atkinson EJ, et al. (2012) A comparison of DXA and CT based methods for estimating the strength of the femoral neck in post-menopausal women. Osteoporos Int. Jul 19.

8

Association between Secreted Phosphoprotein-1 (*SPP1*) Polymorphisms and Low Bone Mineral Density in Women

Jen-Hau Chen[1,2,3], **Yen-Ching Chen**[3], **Chien-Lin Mao**[3], **Jeng-Min Chiou**[4], **Chwen Keng Tsao**[5], **Keh-Sung Tsai**[1,2,6]*

1 Department of Geriatrics and Gerontology, National Taiwan University Hospital, No. 1, Taipei, Taiwan, **2** Department of Internal Medicine, National Taiwan University Hospital, No. 7, Taipei, Taiwan, **3** Institute of Epidemiology and Preventive Medicine, College of Public Health, National Taiwan University, Taipei, Taiwan, **4** Institute of Statistical Science, Academia Sinica, Nankang, Taipei, Taiwan, **5** MJ Health Management Institution, 12F., No. 413, Section 4, Taipei, Taiwan, **6** Department of Laboratory Medicine, National Taiwan University Hospital, No. 7, Taipei, Taiwan,

Abstract

Background: A recent meta-analysis found that secreted phosphoprotein-1 (SPP1) can predict the risk of both osteoporosis and fracture. No study has explored the association of *SPP1* haplotype-tagging single nucleotide polymorphisms (htSNPs) and haplotypes with bone mineral density (BMD).

Methods: This is a cross-sectional study. A total of 1,313 healthy Taiwanese women aged 40 to 55 years were recruited from MJ Health Management Institute from 2009 to 2010. BMD was dichotomized into high and low BMD groups. Three common (allele frequency ≥5%) htSNPs were selected to examine the association between sequence variants of *SPP1* and BMD.

Results: Homozygosity for the T allele of rs4754 were protective from low BMD [TT vs. CC: adjusted OR (AOR) = 0.58, 95% confidence interval (CI) = 0.83–0.89]. A protective effect was also found for women carrying 2 copies of Hap3 TCT (AOR = 0.57, 95% CI = 0.34–0.95). Menopausal status marginally interacted with *SPP1* rs6839524 on BMD ($p = 0.049$). Postmenopausal women carrying variant rs6839524 (GG+GC vs. CC: AOR = 2.35, 95% CI = 1.06–5.20) or Hap1 TGC (AOR = 2.36, 95% CI = 1.06–5.24) were associated with 2.4-fold risk of low BMD. For women with low BMI (<18.5 kg/m^2), variant rs6839524 (AOR = 7.64) and Hap1 (AOR = 6.42) were associated with increased risk of low BMD. These findings did not reach statistical significance after correction for multiple tests.

Conclusions: *SPP1* htSNP protected against low BMD in middle-aged women. *SPP1* genetic markers may be important for the prediction of osteoporosis at an early age.

Editor: Maria Eugenia Saez, CAEBi, Spain

Funding: Funding for the study was provided by National Science Council grants 98-2314-B-002-081, 99-2314-B-002-128, and 101-2118-M-001-011-MY3. The funders had no role in study design, data collection and analysis, decision to publish, or preparation of the manuscript.

Competing Interests: The authors have declared that no competing interests exist.

* E-mail: kstsaimd1128@ntuh.gov.tw

Introduction

Osteoporosis, characterized by low bone mass and propensity to fracture, has become a global health issue as the rapid growth of aging population [1,2]. About 21% of women aged 50 to 84 years has osteoporosis, which is three times higher than that in men [3]. In the US (1988–1994), the prevalence of osteoporosis was highest among white (19%), followed by Mexican American (16%) and black (7%) [4], which in part correspondence to the levels of bone mineral density (BMD) ranged from lowest in Asian, followed by native Americans, Hispanic, and then African American [5]. This may be explained by different lifestyle in the East and West. Compared with other Asian countries, Japanese and Korean, but not Taiwanese, women showed clear age-dependent loss of BMD [6]. Osteoporosis is a "silent disease" until a sudden strain, twist, fall, or fracture, which is associated with increased mortality in later life [1]. Therefore, it is important to identify osteoporosis risk at an early age to prevent fall and fracture risk in late life.

Secreted phosphoprotein-1 (SPP1) is known as osteopontin. It is a glycoprotein related to bone formation and anchoring of osteoclasts to the bone remodeling matrix via binding with vitronectin receptor [7,8]. SPP1 exists in osteoblasts and mineralized bone matrix and intramembranous ossification [7], which enhances osteoblastic differentiation and proliferation [9,10]. SPP1 modulates both bone formation and resorption [11]. As compared to wildtype mice, *SPP1* gene knockout mice are resistant to bone resorption [12]. A Chinese study found that the heritability of BMD was quite high (0.6 to 0.9, vary by body site and sex) [13], therefore, genetic difference may pay a role on BMD level. Because SPP1 is involved in osteogenesis and bone remodeling, *SPP1* polymorphisms may play an important role in the pathogenesis of osteoporosis. Variation on functional single nucleotide polymorphisms (SNPs) may affect the production of *SPP1* protein and then bone formation; intronic SNPs may affect BMD via regulating the alternative splicing and the subsequent protein production [14,15].

Few epidemiologic studies have explored the association between *SPP1* polymorphisms and osteoporosis or BMD. One study found that increased plasma SPP1 level was associated with low BMD [16]. The other candidate-gene study including white and African Americans reported no difference between average hip or spine BMD level by genotypes of *SPP1* rs11730582 or rs4754 [17]. However, the selection of these two SNPs only captured limited genetic information in *SPP1* gene ($r^2 = 0.62$). In addition, these studies did not assess the association between *SPP1* genetic polymorphisms and low BMD or osteoporosis. A meta-analysis study, included 5 genome-wide association studies [GWASs, using data mining approach to explore a massive number of SNPs for specific outcome(s)] on BMD and fracture, found that polymorphisms of 9 genes (*ESR1*, *LRP4*, *ITGA1*, *LRP5*, *SOST*, *SPP1*, *TNFRSF11A*, *TNFRSF11B*, and *TNFSF11*) were significantly associated with BMD level; and *SPP1*, *SOST*, *LRP5*, and *TNFRSF11A* were also related to elevated risk of fracture [18]. Another recent meta-analysis, included 17 GWASs on BMD, found that polymorphisms of *FAM210A*, *SLC25A13*, *LRP5*, *MEPE/SPP1*, *SPTBN1*, and *DKK1* were significantly associated with both BMD and fracture risk [19]. Among the genes that can predict both BMD and fracture risk, *SPP1* is the only one that modulates both osteoblast and bone resorption [8], and associated with the risk of both vertebral and non-vertebral fracture [18]. In addition, no studies have explored how *SPP1* genetic polymorphisms affect the risk of low BMD by using representative haplotype-tagging single nucleotide polymorphisms (htSNPs) and haplotypes. Data in Asian is also lacking.

Because of the above research gap, this study was aimed to explore the association between *SPP1* polymorphisms and the risk of low BMD in middle-aged women. A systematic approach was used to select representative htSNPs in *SPP1* to capture sufficient genetic information and to identify SNPs representative for Asian population. We also evaluated the interactions between *SPP1* polymorphisms and menopausal status or body mass index (BMI) on BMD, which has not been explored previously.

Materials and Methods

Study population

This is a cross-sectional study. A total of 1,567 healthy Taiwanese (Chinese ethnicity) women, aged 40 to 55 years, were recruited from MJ Health Management Institution from October 2009 to August 2010. The outcome of this study is spinal BMD (g/cm^2). Spinal BMD is the major site measured at the MJ Health Management Institute. Participants with the following conditions or diseases were excluded (n = 254): (1) diseases known to affect BMD levels (e.g., hyperparathyroidism, hyperthyroidism, type 1 diabetes, inflammatory bowel disease, chronic active hepatitis, liver cirrhosis, chronic cholestatic diseases, and multiple myeloma), (2) took medications for osteoporosis (e.g., raloxifene), (3) received hormone replacement therapy or other medications (e.g., steroid, oral contraceptive agents) that may affect BMD, (4) lack of BMD at lumbar spine, (5) lack of blood samples or genotyping data. A total of 1,313 women were included for data analyses.

A questionnaire was administered to collect information on demography, lifestyle (e.g., smoking status, alcohol consumption, and exercise), and disease history, etc. A blood sample was collected in an 8 ml EDTA tube from each participant. Genomic DNA was extracted by using QuickGene-Mini80 kit (Fujifilm, Tokyo, Japan). Participants with the following conditions were excluded: BMD was measured at sites other than spine (n = 85), lack of blood sample (n = 113), or genotyping data (n = 2), and had

steroid or hormone therapy (n = 70). Some participants may lack of two or more information above.

Ethics Statement

The study protocol has been approved by the Institutional Review Boards of National Taiwan University and MJ Health Management Institution. Written informed consent was obtained from each study participant. The consent from the legal guardian/next of kin was obtained when patients had serious cognitive impairment. This research carried out with human subjects complies with the World Medical Association Declaration of Helsinki - Ethical Principles for Medical Research Involving Human Subjects.

Measurement of bone mineral density

The BMD (g/cm^2) of the lumbar spine (L1-L4) was measured by a dual-energy X-ray absorptiometry densitometer (DXA, General Electric Lunar Health Care, DPX-L, USA). Calibration of BMD measurement was performed daily. The long-term coefficient of variation in BMD was around 1%. This healthy population included few participants with osteoporosis (<1%). Instead of using osteoporosis as the outcome variable, BMD was tertiled (i.e. T1, T2, and T3) on the basis of the data of the whole population in order to identify the subgroup with an elevated risk of low BMD. Previous studies [20,21] and our recent study [22] have used similar approaches that involve BMD tertiles. The high BMD group comprised participants in T2 plus T3 (i.e., the reference group) and the low BMD group comprised participants in T1 (i.e., the comparison group) with a BMD cut-off point of 1.27 g/cm^2.

SNP selection and genotyping assays

Common (frequency ≥0.05) SNPs in *SPP1* were identified from genotyping data of Han Chinese in Beijing, China (CHB) of the International HapMap Project (http://hapmap.ncbi.nlm.nih.gov). Haplotype block was defined by Haploview program (http://www.broadinstitute.org/haploview/haploview) using modified Gabriel algorithm [23,24]. Three representative htSNPs [rs11730582 in 5′untranslated region (UTR), rs6839524 in intron, and rs4754 in exon] were selected from 12 common SNPs using tagSNP program [25] based on the common disease/common variant hypothesis [26]. TaqMan Assay was used to determine genotypes using HT7900 (Applied Biosystems Inc., CA, USA). Genotyping success rate was greater than 95% for each SNP. Quality control samples were replicates of 5% study participants and the concordance rate was 100%.

Statistical analyses

Hardy-Weinberg equilibrium (HWE) test was performed for each SNP to check genotyping error. The expectation-maximization algorithm was used to estimate haplotype frequencies in the haplotype block using tagSNP program [25]. High and low BMD was defined as above. Power analysis was performed by using QUANTO program (http://hydra.usc.edu/GxE/).

Logistic regression model was used to estimate the adjusted odds ratio (AOR) and 95% confidence interval (CI) for the risk of low BMD in participants carrying either 1 or 2 versus 0 copies of minor allele of each SNP and each multilocus haplotype. Haplotype trend regression [27] was used to test the global association between *SPP1* haplotypes and low BMD. Given a significant global test, haplotype-specific tests can provide some guidance as to which variant(s) contributes to the significant global test. The association between *SPP1* genetic polymorphisms and continuous BMD were also assessed by using general linear model (GLM). After stepwise model selection and the inclusion of variables with biological importance, age, menopausal status (yes/no), BMI (kg/m^2), alkaline phosphatase (ALP, IU/L), uric acid (UA, mg/dL), low-density lipoprotein (LDL, mg/dL), and exercise (frequency × duration × intensity) were adjusted in the models. All participants had normal creatinine level (<1.3 mg/dL) and thus this variable was not explored in this study.

A likelihood ratio test was used to evaluate how menopausal status (pre- and post-menopause) and BMI groups (<18.5, 18.5 to <24, ≥24 kg/m^2) modified the association between *SPP1* polymorphisms and risk of low BMD. Stratified analyses were performed by menopausal status and BMI groups. Correction for multiple tests was performed by false discovery rate (FDR) using method of Benjamini and Hochberg (1995) [28]. Statistical analyses were performed by using SAS 9.2 (SAS Institute, Cary, NC) and all statistical tests were two-sided.

Results

Characteristics of the study population

This study included 1,313 participants. The differences between participants with low and high BMD are summarized in Table 1

SPP1 polymorphisms and BMD

Three *SPP1* htSNPs [rs11730582 (5′ UTR), rs6829524 (intron), and rs4754 (exon)] were genotyped. The minor allele frequencies (MAFs) of these SNPs ranged from 31% to 42%, which were similar to the MAFs of CHB data from International HapMap Project (29 to 38%). All *SPP1* SNPs were in HWE among participants with low BMD, high BMD, or the whole population. Power analysis showed that given 881 and 432 participants with low and high BMD, respectively, rs4754 (MAF = 0.31) has over 0.99 of power to detect an OR at 0.58. Because of the modest effect and high MAF, the power is low (<0.7) for rs11730582 (MAF = 0.33) and rs6829524 (MAF = 0.42) to detect an OR at 1.14 and 0.91, respectively.

Homozygosity for the T allele of rs4754 were protective from low BMD (TT vs. CC: AOR = 0.58, 95% CI = 0.83–0.89, *p* = 0.005, Table 2). This association did not reach statistical significance after correction for multiple tests. The other two htSNPs did not show significant relationship with the outcome.

Three common htSNPs (rs11730582, rs6839524, and rs4754) spanning *SPP1* gene formed one block using the modified Gabriel algorithm [23,24]. Four common (frequency ≥0.05) haplotypes were identified (cumulative frequency, 97.9%); the global test for the association between *SPP1* haplotypes and low BMD was significant (*p*<0.0001, Table 2). Two copies of Hap3 TCT were protective from low BMD (AOR = 0.57, 95% CI = 0.34–0.95, *p* = 0.03, Table 2). Other haplotypes were not associated with the outcome. The conditional haplotype analysis was performed conditioning on other haplotypes and the results did not reach statistical significance (Hap1: ref; Hap2: AOR = 1.14, 95% CI = 0.90–1.44; Hap3: AOR = 0.93, 95% CI = 0.74–1.17; Hap4: AOR = 0.85, 95% CI = 0.59–1.24). These findings did not remain significant after correction for multiple tests.

We also kept only participants with the lowest and the highest BMD tertile and compared them for the same analyses above. Because of removing one-third of the study population (the 2nd tertile), the statistical power decreased and the protective effect for rs4754 and Hap3 no longer reached statistical significance.

Interactions between menopausal status and SPP1 polymorphisms

Menopausal status has known as an important modifier for BMD. Interaction between menopausal status and *SPP1* htSNPs or haplotypes for low BMD did not reach statistical significance. After stratification by menopausal status, postmenopausal women carrying variant rs6839524 were associated with low BMD (GG+GC vs. CC: AOR = 2.35, 95% CI = 1.06–5.20, *p* = 0.03). Postmenopausal women carrying Hap1 TGC was associated with low BMD (AOR = 2.36, 95% CI = 1.06–5.24, *p* = 0.03). These findings did not reach statistical significance after correction for multiple tests. No significant association was found in other subgroups or for other *SPP1* htSNPs/haplotypes after stratification by menopausal status.

Interaction between BMI and SPP1 polymorphisms

No significant interaction was observed between *SPP1* SNPs or haplotypes and low BMD. After stratification by BMI groups (< 18.5, 18.5 to <24, ≥24 kg/m^2), women with low BMI (<18.5 kg/m^2) carrying rs6839524 variant were associated with low BMD (GG+GC vs. CC: AOR = 7.64, 95% CI = 1.42–40.97, *p* = 0.02). Women with low BMI (<18.5 kg/m^2) carrying Hap1 TGC were associated with low BMD (AOR = 6.42, 95% CI = 1.23–33.60, *p* = 0.03). These findings did not reach statistical significance after correction for multiple tests.

The power for assessing interaction between *SPP1* SNPs and menopausal status or BMI is low because of the smaller sample size in subgroup analysis and the results should be interpreted with caution.

Discussion

To the best of our knowledge, this is the first study exploring the association between *SPP1* polymorphisms and low BMD using htSNPs in Asian population. We found that homozygosity for the T allele of *SPP1* rs4754 (TT) and Hap3 TCT were associated with low BMD; the former result remained significant after correction for multiple tests for SNP analysis but lost significance after correction for multiple tests for SNP and haplotype analysis. The only candidate-gene study [17], which included white and black populations, only compared mean BMD by *SPP1* genotypes of 2 SNPs (i.e., no estimation of multivariable OR and 95% CI) and no significant difference was observed. Previous GWASs and meta-analysis [18,19,29–33] for BMD or fracture risk mainly focused on white population. In addition, haplotype analysis, which offers more information than single-locus SNPs, has not been performed previously. Therefore, our results provide important information because of the estimation of outcome risk by using multivariable OR, large sample size (n>1,300), selection of representative htSNP, and performing haplotype analysis.

Among 3 htSNPs genotyped in this study, rs4754 is a synonymous SNP. That is, rs4754 does not lead to the change of amino acid but may affect BMD level via its influence on translational efficiency. Interestingly, C allele is the major allele of rs4754 in Chinese (MAF: C = 0.66, T = 0.34) but the minor allele in white (MAF: C = 0.23, T = 0.77, http://hapmap.ncbi.nlm.nih.gov). Therefore, the inconsistent findings were observed between this Asian study and previous studies focused on whites [18,19,29–33]. Hap3 TCT also showed significant association with high BMD, which may be attributable to the only SNP rs4754 with the minor allele in Hap3. Three htSNPs were in one haplotype block and strong linkage disequilibrium (LD) were observed between rs11730582 and rs6839524 (|D′| = 0.98) as well as between rs6839524 and rs4754 (|D′| = 0.96). However, the pairwise r^2 for

Table 1. Characteristics of the study population.

Variables	Low BMD (<1.27 g/cm²)	High BMD (≥1.27 g/cm²)	p
	n=881	n=432	
	Mean ± SE		
Age	46.8±0.2	45.6±0.2	**<0.001**
Alkaline phosphatase (IU/L)	61.5±0.6	55.5±0.7	**<0.001**
	n (%)		
Menopause			**<0.001**
Yes	227 (26)	45 (11)	
No	647 (74)	381 (89)	
Cigarette smoking			0.45
Yes	63 (8)	39 (9)	
No	777 (92)	378 (91)	
Alcohol consumption			0.84
Yes	50 (6)	27 (7)	
No	775 (94)	379 (93)	
Body mass index (kg/m²)			**<0.0001**
<18.5	56 (6)	15 (3)	
≥18.5 to <24	652 (74)	279 (65)	
≥24	172 (20)	137 (32)	
High-density lipoprotein (mg/dL)			0.71
≥50	808 (92)	396 (92)	
<50	73 (8)	33 (8)	
Low-density lipoprotein (mg/dL)			**0.0001**
<130	670 (76)	366 (85)	
≥130	211 (24)	63 (15)	
Triglyceride (mg/dL)			0.28
<150	794 (90)	381 (88)	
≥150	87 (10)	51 (12)	
Uric acid (mg/dL)			**0.006**
<6	806 (91)	374 (87)	
≥6	75 (9)	58 (13)	
Hypertension			0.48
Yes	88 (10)	49 (11)	
No	793 (90)	382 (89)	
Diabetes			0.05
Yes	262 (30)	151 (35)	
No	619 (70)	281 (65)	
Regular exercise			0.39
Yes	368 (47)	194 (50)	
No	412 (53)	195 (50)	

Abbreviations: BMD, bone mineral density; BMI, body mass index; hypertension, systolic blood pressure >140 mmHg or diastolic blood pressure >90 mmHg or had medication for controlling blood pressure; diabetes, fasting glucose ≥126 mg/dl or using medication for diabetes; regular exercise: walking or hiking ≥30 mins/2 to 3 days.
Numbers in bold indicate significant findings ($p<0.05$).

any two SNPs were low (0.02 to 0.34). Especially, both D′ (0.30) and r^2 (0.02) were low between rs11730582 and rs4754, this may explain the non-significant association between *SPP1* rs11730582 and BMD.

SPP1 plays a role in a wide spectrum of physiologic and pathologic processes [34–37]. First, it mediates the attachment of osteoclasts to bone matrix and then regulates bone resorption and normal bone development [37]. The polymorphisms of *SPP1* gene may regulate SPP1 structure, decrease serum SPP1 level, change or reduce SPP1 protein, which may affect bone formation, resorption and the osteoclastic process. The downgrading of osteoclastic process may slow BMD decline and thus prevent

Table 2. Association of *SPP1* common htSNPs and haplotypes with low BMD.

	Freq.	0 copies		1 copy			2 copies		
	(%)	BMD (L/H)	AOR	BMD (L/H)	AOR (95% CI)	*p*	BMD (L/H)	AOR (95% CI)	*p*
SNP									
rs11730582		394/206	1.00	385/177	1.17 (0.89–1.53)	0.54	102/49	1.13 (0.73–1.74)	0.83
rs6839524		295/157	1.00	429/197	1.25 (0.94–1.67)	0.05	158/78	0.91 (0.63–1.32)	0.22
rs4754		439/195	1.00	368/179	1.07 (0.81–1.41)	0.02	74/57	**0.58 (0.83–0.89)**	**0.005**
Haplotype (Global test *P*<0.0001)									
Hap1 TGC	41.2	299/162	1.00	431/193	1.30 (0.97–1.73)	0.08	151/77	0.90 (0.62–1.31)	0.58
Hap2 CCC	26.3	466/248	1.00	351/160	1.18 (0.90–1.55)	0.24	64/24	1.45 (0.83–2.53)	0.20
Hap3 TCT̲	23.9	522/243	1.00	317/153	1.08 (0.82–1.43)	0.60	42/36	**0.57 (0.34–0.95)**	**0.03**
Hap4 C̲C̲T̲	6.5	782/371	1.00	92/59	0.73 (0.49–1.09)	0.13	7/2	1.81 (0.35–9.34)	0.48
Total	97.9								

Abbreviations: SNP, single nucleotide polymorphism; Freq., haplotype frequency; BMD, bone mineral density; AOR, adjusted odds ratio; CI, confidence interval; L, low BMD; H, high BMD.
All models were adjusted for age, menopausal status, BMI (kg/m²), serum ALP (IU/L), UA (mg/dL), LDL (mg/dL), and exercise (frequency × duration × intensity).
The SNPs with underscore indicate variant allele.
Numbers in bold indicated significant findings (*p*<0.05).

osteoporosis. Second, SPP1 plays an important role in regulating immune response [38]. Therefore, polymorphisms of SPP1 may block or reduce the inflammation responses and thus showed increased BMD. In addition, SPP1 polymorphisms may also interact with two important modifiers, menopausal status or BMI, on BMD as detailed below.

It has been known that sex hormone plays an important role in maintaining bone strength [39]. For most of women, BMD decreases rapidly during the first few years after menopause [40] as a result of excessive osteoclastic activities via unopposed osteoclastic activation after rapid declination of estrogen. Because SPP1 modulates osteoclast and thus sequence variants of SPP1 may affect bone resorption. This may explain our finding that postmenopausal women carrying 1 or 2 copies of variant rs6839524 were associated with low BMD (AOR = 2.35), which did not reach statistical significance after correction of multiple tests. An association was also observed for Hap1, which rs6839524 is the only SNP with minor allele. It is possible that variant rs6839524 affects bone formation and this effect becomes more evident after menopause. In addition, rs6839524 is an intronic SNP and its variation may affect the alternative splicing, e.g., altering mRNA folding or the stability of mRNA structure, and then the subsequent protein production [14,15]. All these may explain the associations, which did not reach statistical significance after correction of multiple tests, between rs6839524 or Hap1 and low BMD in postmenopausal women.

BMI has been related to BMD previously. Low BMI has been associated with increased risk of osteoporosis and fracture [41] and the association varied by ethnic groups, e.g., positive association between one unit increase of BMI and BMD in white women but negative association was observed in African American women [42]. Because of different diet and lifestyle, body shape can be quite different between people in Western and Eastern countries. However, relevant data and research in Asian population are sparse. Our research, for the first time, explored that among women with low BMI (<18.5 kg/m^2), variant carriers of rs6839524 (AOR = 7.64) or Hap1 TGC (AOR = 6.42) were associated with low BMD, which did not reach statistical significance after correction for multiple tests. The application of these polymorphisms will help us to identify women with low BMD.

This study has several strengths. First, the selections of a set of representative htSNPs for Asian captured the majority of genetic

information of SPP1 ($r^2 = 0.82$, estimated by tagSNP program) as compared with that ($r^2 = 0.65$) of the only candidate-gene study [17]. Second, haplotypes capture unknown variants via LD between these SNPs and thus provide more information than single SNP. In addition, unlike most previous studies, this study included premenopausal women (n~1000) that allowed us to assess how menopausal status interacted with SPP1 polymorphisms on BMD and, importantly, to predict outcome risk at an early age.

This study had some limitations. First, this is a cross-sectional study, which causal inference is usually not available. Functional analysis will be needed to unravel the underlying mechanism between SPP1 polymorphisms and BMD. In addition, the original questionnaire did not collect fracture information. Because this population is healthy, fracture frequency is low. We also assessed the association between SPP1 genetic polymorphisms and continuous BMD by using GLM and no significant findings were observed. Because the aim of this study is to identify a high-risk population of low BMD, no further analyses were performed by using continuous BMD as outcome.

SPP1 plays a role in bone formation and resorption. This study has some first findings. Homozygosity for the T allele of rs4754 and Hap3 TCT in SPP1 were significantly associated with low BMD in this Asian population. rs6839524 and haplotypes in SPP1 have not been explored before. Variant carriers of rs6839524 and Hap 1 TGC were associated with low BMD in menopausal women or women with low BMI. These findings did not reach statistical significance after correction for multiple tests. Because of the complex role of SPP1 in bone physiology, functional and larger studies are warranted to confirm our findings.

Acknowledgments

The authors gratefully acknowledge Dr. Wen-Chung Lee for epidemiological consultation.

Author Contributions

Conceived and designed the experiments: KST YCC JHC. Performed the experiments: CLM. Analyzed the data: CLM JMC YCC JHC. Contributed reagents/materials/analysis tools: JHC YCC KST. Wrote the paper: CLM JHC JMC YCC CKT KST. Approval of the final version of the manuscript: CLM JHC JMC YCC CKT KST.

References

1. Sànchez-Riera L, Wilson N, Kamalaraj N, Nolla JM, Kok C, et al. (2010) Osteoporosis and fragility fractures. Best Pract Res Clin Rheumatol 24: 793–810.
2. Vestergaard P, Rejnmark L, Mosekilde L (2007) Increased mortality in patients with a hip fracture-effect of pre-morbid conditions and post-fracture complications. Osteoporos Int 18: 1583–1593.
3. Kanis JA, Johnell O, Oden A, Jonsson B, De Laet C, et al. (2000) Risk of hip fracture according to the World Health Organization criteria for osteopenia and osteoporosis. Bone 27: 585–590.
4. Dawson-Hughes B, Looker AC, Tosteson ANA, Johansson H, Kanis JA, et al. (2011) The potential impact of the National Osteoporosis Foundation guidance on treatment eligibility in the USA: an update in NHANES 2005–2008. Osteoporos Int.
5. Barrett-Connor E, Siris ES, Wehren LE, Miller PD, Abbott TA, et al. (2005) Osteoporosis and fracture risk in women of different ethnic groups. J Bone Miner Res 20: 185–194.
6. Sugimoto T, Tsutsumi M, Fujii Y, Kawakatsu M, Negishi H, et al. (1992) Comparison of bone mineral content among Japanese, Koreans, and Taiwanese assessed by dual-photon absorptiometry. Journal of Bone and Mineral Research 7: 153–159.
7. Denhardt D, Noda M (1998) Osteopontin expression and function: Role in bone remodeling. J Cell Biochem: 92–102.
8. Choi ST, Kim JH, Kang E-J, Lee S-W, Park M-C, et al. (2008) Osteopontin might be involved in bone remodelling rather than in inflammation in ankylosing spondylitis. Rheumatology (Oxford) 47: 1775–1779.
9. Moore M, Gotoh Y, Rafidi K (1991) Characterization of a cDNA for chicken osteopontin: expression during bone development, osteoblast differentiation, and tissue distribution. Biochemistry.
10. Zohar R, Cheifetz S, McCulloch C (1998) Analysis of intracellular osteopontin as a marker of osteoblastic cell differentiation and mesenchymal cell migration. European Journal of Oral Sciences 106: 401–407.
11. Standal T, Borset M, Sundan A (2004) Role of osteopontin in adhesion, migration, cell survival and bone remodeling. Exp Oncol 26: 179–184.
12. Rittling SR, Matsumoto HN, Mckee MD, Nanci A, An X-R, et al. (1998) Mice Lacking Osteopontin Show Normal Development and Bone Structure but Display Altered Osteoclast Formation In Vitro. J Bone Miner Res 13: 1101–1111.
13. Feng Y, Hsu Y, Terwedow H, Chen C, Xu X, et al. (2005) Familial aggregation of bone mineral density and bone mineral content in a Chinese population. Osteoporos Int 16: 1917–1923.
14. Moyer RA, Wang D, Papp AC, Smith RM, Duque L, et al. (2011) Intronic polymorphisms affecting alternative splicing of human dopamine D2 receptor are associated with cocaine abuse. Neuropsychopharmacology 36: 753–762.
15. Kawase T, Akatsuka Y, Torikai H, Morishima S, Oka A, et al. (2007) Alternative splicing due to an intronic SNP in HMSD generates a novel minor histocompatibility antigen. Blood 110: 1055–1063.

16. Chang IC, Chiang TI, Yeh KT, Lee H, Cheng YW (2010) Increased serum osteopontin is a risk factor for osteoporosis in menopausal women. Osteoporos Int 21: 1401–1409.

17. Taylor BC, Schreiner PJ, Doherty TM, Fornage M, Carr JJ, et al. (2005) Matrix Gla protein and osteopontin genetic associations with coronary artery calcification and bone density: the CARDIA study. Hum Genet 116: 525–528.

18. Richards JB, Kavvoura FK, Rivadeneira F, Styrkarsdottir U, Estrada K, et al. (2009) Collaborative meta-analysis: associations of 150 candidate genes with osteoporosis and osteoporotic fracture. Ann Intern Med 151: 528–537.

19. Estrada K, Styrkarsdottir U, Evangelou E, Hsu YH, Duncan EL, et al. (2012) Genome-wide meta-analysis identifies 56 bone mineral density loci and reveals 14 loci associated with risk of fracture. Nat Genet 44: 491–501.

20. Bidoli E, Schinella D, Franceschi S (1998) Physical activity and bone mineral density in Italian middle-aged women. Eur J Epidemiol 14: 153–157.

21. Nock NL, Patrick-Melin A, Cook M, Thompson C, Kirwan JP, et al. (2011) Higher bone mineral density is associated with a decreased risk of colorectal adenomas. Int J Cancer 129: 956–964.

22. You YS, Lin CY, Liang HJ, Lee S, Tsai KS, et al (2013(Epub ahead of Print)) Association between Metabolome and Low Bone Mineral Density in Taiwanese Women Determined by 1H NMR Spectroscopy. Journal of Bone and Mineral Research.

23. Chen YC, Giovannucci E, Lazarus R, Kraft P, Ketkar S, et al. (2005) Sequence variants of Toll-like receptor 4 and susceptibility to prostate cancer. Cancer Res 65: 11771–11778.

24. Gabriel SB, Schaffner SF, Nguyen H, Moore JM, Roy J, et al. (2002) The structure of haplotype blocks in the human genome. Science 296: 2225–2229.

25. Stram DO, Leigh Pearce C, Bretsky P, Freedman M, Hirschhorn JN, et al. (2003) Modeling and E-M Estimation of Haplotype-Specific Relative Risks from Genotype Data for a Case-Control Study of Unrelated Individuals. Hum Hered 55: 179–190.

26. (2001) Challenges for the 21st century. Nat Genet 29: 353–354.

27. Zaykin DV, Westfall PH, Young SS, Karnoub MA, Wagner MJ, et al. (2002) Testing association of statistically inferred haplotypes with discrete and continuous traits in samples of unrelated individuals. Hum Hered 53: 79–91.

28. Benjamini Y, Hochberg Y (1995) Controlling the false discovery rate: a practical and powerful approach to multiple testing. J R Statist Soc B 57: 289–300.

29. Hofman A, Breteler MMB, van Duijn CM, Krestin GP, Pols HA, et al. (2007) The Rotterdam Study: objectives and design update. Eur J Epidemiol 22: 819–829.

30. Sayed-Tabatabaei FA, van Rijn MJE, Schut AFC, Aulchenko YS, Croes EA, et al. (2005) Heritability of the function and structure of the arterial wall: findings of the Erasmus Rucphen Family (ERF) study. Stroke 36: 2351–2356.

31. Richards JB, Rivadeneira F, Inouye M, Pastinen TM, Soranzo N, et al. (2008) Bone mineral density, osteoporosis, and osteoporotic fractures: a genome-wide association study. Lancet 371: 1505–1512.

32. Styrkarsdottir U, Halldorsson BV, Gretarsdottir S, Gudbjartsson DF, Walters GB, et al. (2009) New sequence variants associated with bone mineral density. Nat Genet 41: 15–17.

33. Kiel DP, Demissie S, Dupuis J, Lunetta KL, Murabito JM, et al. (2007) Genome-wide association with bone mass and geometry in the Framingham Heart Study. BMC Med Genet 8 Suppl 1: S14.

34. Gravallese EM (2003) Osteopontin: a bridge between bone and the immune system. Journal of Clinical Investigation 112: 147–149.

35. Reinholt FP, Hultenby K, Oldberg A, Heinegard D (1990) Osteopontin—a possible anchor of osteoclasts to bone. Proceedings of the National Academy of Sciences of the United States of America 87: 4473–4475.

36. Denhardt D (1993) Osteopontin: a protein with diverse functions. The FASEB journal.

37. O'Regan AW, Chupp GL, Lowry JA, Goetschkes M, Mulligan N, et al. (1999) Osteopontin is associated with T cells in sarcoid granulomas and has T cell adhesive and cytokine-like properties in vitro. Journal of Immunology 162: 1024–1031.

38. Denhardt DT, Noda M, O'Regan AW, Pavlin D, Berman JS (2001) Osteopontin as a means to cope with environmental insults: regulation of inflammation, tissue remodeling, and cell survival. Journal of Clinical Investigation 107: 1055–1061.

39. Satoh Y, Soeda Y, Dokou S (1995) Analysis of Relationships Between Sex-Hormone Dynamics and Bone Metabolism and Changes in Bone Mass in Surgically Induced Menopause. Calcif Tissue Int 57: 258–266.

40. Saarelainen J, Kiviniemi V, Kröger H, Tuppurainen M, Niskanen L, et al. (2011) Body mass index and bone loss among postmenopausal women: the 10-year follow-up of the OSTPRE cohort. J Bone Miner Metab.

41. Morin S, Tsang JF, Leslie WD (2009) Weight and body mass index predict bone mineral density and fractures in women aged 40 to 59 years. Osteoporosis International 20: 363–370.

42. Castro JP, Joseph LA, Shin JJ, Arora SK, Nicasio J, et al. (2005) Differential effect of obesity on bone mineral density in White, Hispanic and African American women: a cross sectional study. Nutr Metab (Lond) 2: 9.

9

Earliest Cranio-Encephalic Trauma from the Levantine Middle Palaeolithic: 3D Reappraisal of the Qafzeh 11 Skull, Consequences of Pediatric Brain Damage on Individual Life Condition and Social Care

Hélène Coqueugniot[1,2*], Olivier Dutour[1,3,4], Baruch Arensburg[5], Henri Duday[1,3], Bernard Vandermeersch[1], Anne-marie Tillier[1,6]

1 Unité Mixte de Recherche 5199 – De la Préhistoire à l'Actuel: Culture, Environnement et Anthropologie (PACEA), Centre National de la Recherche Scientifique (CNRS) – Université de Bordeaux, Pessac, France, 2 Department of Human Evolution, Max Planck Institute for Evolutionary Anthropology, Leipzig, Germany, 3 Laboratoire d'Anthropologie biologique Paul Broca, Ecole Pratique des Hautes Etudes (EPHE), Paris, France, 4 Department of Anthropology, University of Western Ontario, London, Ontario, Canada, 5 Department of Anatomy and Anthropology, Sackler School of Medicine, Tel Aviv University, Ramat Aviv, Israel, 6 Museum of Archaeology and Anthropology, University of Pennsylvania, Philadelphia, Pennsylvania, United States of America

Abstract

The Qafzeh site (Lower Galilee, Israel) has yielded the largest Levantine hominin collection from Middle Palaeolithic layers which were dated to *circa* 90–100 kyrs BP or to marine isotope stage 5b–c. Within the hominin sample, Qafzeh 11, *circa* 12–13 yrs old at death, presents a skull lesion previously attributed to a healed trauma. Three dimensional imaging methods allowed us to better explore this lesion which appeared as being a frontal bone depressed fracture, associated with brain damage. Furthermore the endocranial volume, smaller than expected for dental age, supports the hypothesis of a growth delay due to traumatic brain injury. This trauma did not affect the typical human brain morphology pattern of the right frontal and left occipital petalia. It is highly probable that this young individual suffered from personality and neurological troubles directly related to focal cerebral damage. Interestingly this young individual benefited of a unique funerary practice among the south-western Asian burials dated to Middle Palaeolithic.

Editor: David Frayer, University of Kansas, United States of America

Funding: This research has been financially supported by the Irene Levi Sala Care Archaeological Foundation (http://prehistory.org.il/?page_id=894). The funder had no role in study design, data collection and analysis, decision to publish, or preparation of the manuscript.

Competing Interests: The authors have declared that no competing interests exist.

* Email: helene.coqueugniot@u-bordeaux.fr

Introduction

Relevant information about Middle Palaeolithic societies can be obtained from paleopathological investigations. Identification of skeletal abnormalities and degenerative joint disease, as well as evidence for bone lesions caused by trauma, can provide insights into the adaptation patterns and social behavior of these early nomadic hunter-gatherers. With regard to south-western Asia, the first pathological data, to our knowledge, were those brought in 1939 by McCown and Keith's original description of the Mount Carmel people. During the last three decades, new attempts emerged in the studies of near eastern fossil record, related to enrichment in the fossil hominin sample. In this perspective, fossil specimens have benefited from new paleopathological investigations.

Among Levantine Middle Palaeolithic hominins, evidence of cranial traumatic lesions was provided by McCown and Keith [1] in their description of the partial skeletons from the Skhul Cave. According to these authors, the Skhul 1 child exhibits a depressed area in the mid-line of the frontal bone nearby the glabellar region which was interpreted [1] (pp 309–310) as consequence of a blow.

These authors also mentioned the presence of a perforation and fracture of the right temporal in the roof of the ear which could result from an impact. However, the paleopathological condition of these two cranial lesions remains unclear as the authors themselves concluded [1] that both injuries ".. were inflicted at death or not unlikely at some time soon after death". In an unpublished study, three of us (AmT, HD and BA) were not able to conclude if frontal and temporal changes observed on this fossil were pathological or taphonomical. McCown and Keith [1] (p 281) also drew attention to the presence of an injury "caused by a glancing blow at, or soon after death" in the left parieto-occipital area of the Skhul IX adult skull.

Later, in his original study of the Shanidar hominins from Iraqi Kurdistan, Trinkaus [2] provided a description of several pathological conditions displayed by one of the individuals, Shanidar 1. This adult individual sustained, among several skeletal lesions, a crushing skull fracture which involved the frontal process of the left zygomatic bone and the lateral margin of the left orbit. This ante-mortem traumatic injury most probably caused blindness of the left eye [2].

Within the Qafzeh hominin sample from lower Galilee, the skull of the adult Qafzeh 6 shows a concave indentation of the outer table of the frontal bone, without a fracture, in the area of the left supra-orbital region [3]. Such a condition can result from either trauma due to an accidental self-hurt or a blow to the head due to inter-personal violence. One of the immature individuals from the site, Qafzeh 11, presents a skull lesion previously attributed to healed trauma [4–6]. The goal of this study is to reappraise the Qafzeh 11 impact wound using 3D imaging methods, to better understand the pathological condition that affected this young individual. Indeed, 3D reconstructions applied to paleopathology allow us to better explore inner bone lesions, to evaluate their impact on soft tissues and to estimate volumetric data contributing to fossil reconstruction and preservation [7–9].

Material

The Qafzeh site has yielded the largest hominin collection (N = 27, including partial eight skeletons, isolated bones and teeth) from Middle Palaeolithic layers in south-western Asia (e.g. [6,10–11]). The Middle Palaeolithic sequence (units XVII to XXIII) was dated by a combination of electron spin resonance and thermoluminescence methods to circa 90–100 kyrs BP or to marine isotope stage 5b–c [12–13]. Human remains were discovered at the front of the cave's entrance in layers that contain a low density of lithic artifacts, a huge assemblage of micromammals and a few hearths. Within the Mousterian lithic assemblage [14–16], centripetal and/or bi-directional preparations prevail and the typical products are side scrapers, large oval flakes and quadrangular Levallois flakes. The makers of the Mousterian lithic industries at Qafzeh are identified as early anatomically modern humans [6,10,17].

A majority of the Qafzeh individuals fails to attain reproductive adulthood and among them, Qafzeh 11 is of special interest. It represents a single specimen recovered from layer XXIII, at the bottom of the Mousterian sequence, while most of the fossil human sample originates from layer XVII. A large stone damaged the trunk, pelvic area and lower limbs. Age at death of Qafzeh 11 was estimated circa 12–13 yrs while the sex remains unknown [5]. The partial skeleton of Qafzeh 11 is characterized by a combination of morphological traits in which modern features prevail, in comparisons with other Palaeolithic children [5–6]. Cranial morphology shows changes affecting the vault symmetry and base angulation; however their interpretation in terms of peri- or post-mortem changes remains unclear [6].

Besides these changes, Qafzeh 11 presents a cranial lesion previously attributed to a healed trauma [4–5]. This lesion is characterized by an anterior depression on the right side of the frontal squama. It is limited forwards by a healed fracture line, which ends up to an oval shaped hole. The latter has been attributed to a taphonomical change [4–5]. Healing process led to small thin bone remodelling, the frailty of it explaining its post-mortem loss (figure 1). Regarding the overall shape of the bone lesion and x-ray examination, the diagnosis of traumatic skeletal injury indeed prevails over that of an epidermoid bone cyst [3]. Surprisingly, comparative analysis between Qafzeh 11 and another child from same site, Qafzeh 10 younger in individual age (circa 6 years old), reveals that Qafzeh 11 had the smallest endocranial volume, respectively 1273±48 cc and 1251±48 cc [6].

Methods

Specimen number
Q11

Repository information
Department of Anatomy and Anthropology, Faculty of Medicine, Sackler School of Medicine building Tel Aviv University, Ramat Aviv, Israel.

Authority giving permission of study
Professor Israel Hershkovitz, curator of the collection, head of the Department. Last author (Am.T.) obtained his authorization for studying all the immature individuals from the Qafzeh site. The curator of this collection does agree the publication. There is no permit number.

Endocranial volume (EV) was estimated to set Qafzeh 11 within a normal modern variability of brain size growth, using two methods. EV was firstly calculated using equations recently proposed [18]; then an attempt of direct EV measurement on virtual endocast (see below) was performed although the skull base is damaged. For comparison, we used a modern data set issued from a digital bone library of immature skulls [18]. This sample comes from the identified osteological collection of Strasbourg University, France [19]. The EV values of Qafzeh 11 were compared to those available for other specimens (adult and immature) from the same site based upon cranial dimensions of Qafzeh 6, 9 and 10 [6,10].

Following advances provided by digital 3D reconstructions, CT-scans of the Qafzeh 11 skull were carried out to reassess the traumatic condition which affected the adolescent during his/her life. These 3D reconstructions of Qafzeh 11 allow: (i) to precisely visualize 3D aspects of the internal and external surfaces of the cranial vault and of inner structures in the area of the pathological condition, (ii) to evaluate the potential impact of skull damage on the brain and (iii) to localize this impact on the brain surface.

Qafzeh 11 skull was CT scanned at the Carmel Medical Center, Haifa, Israel on a Brillance iCT 256, Philips Medical system (Cleveland, Ohio) with an isometric voxel size of 0.67 mm. Other acquisition parameters are 120 kV for voltage and 298 mA for current.

3D reconstructions of skull and endocast were performed using TIVMI software program [20] that is based on HMH (Half Maximum Height) algorithm [21] and applied to bone 3D reconstructions [22]. It has proved to be more precise and reliable for 3D measurements than other software programs currently implementing different algorithms for 3D reconstructions [23]. Besides providing additional estimation of the endocranial volume, virtual reconstruction allowed us to localize the impact of the cranial lesion on the brain surface, taking as a reference a 3D reconstruction of extant human brain [24] and checking the accurate correspondences of their anatomical landmarks [25].

Measurements of the endocast were taken using these landmarks and metric tools implemented in TIVMI. The cranium was horizontally oriented according to the "mean transverse plane" adapted from the original Frankfurt plane to study morphometry on digitalized skulls [26]; mean sagittal and coronal planes were drawn according to this method.

Results

The endocranial volume of Qafzeh 11 ranges from 1283.44 to 1333.18 cc using updated formulas [18]. Previously, values ranging from 1251±48 cc to 1303±46 cc [6] were obtained

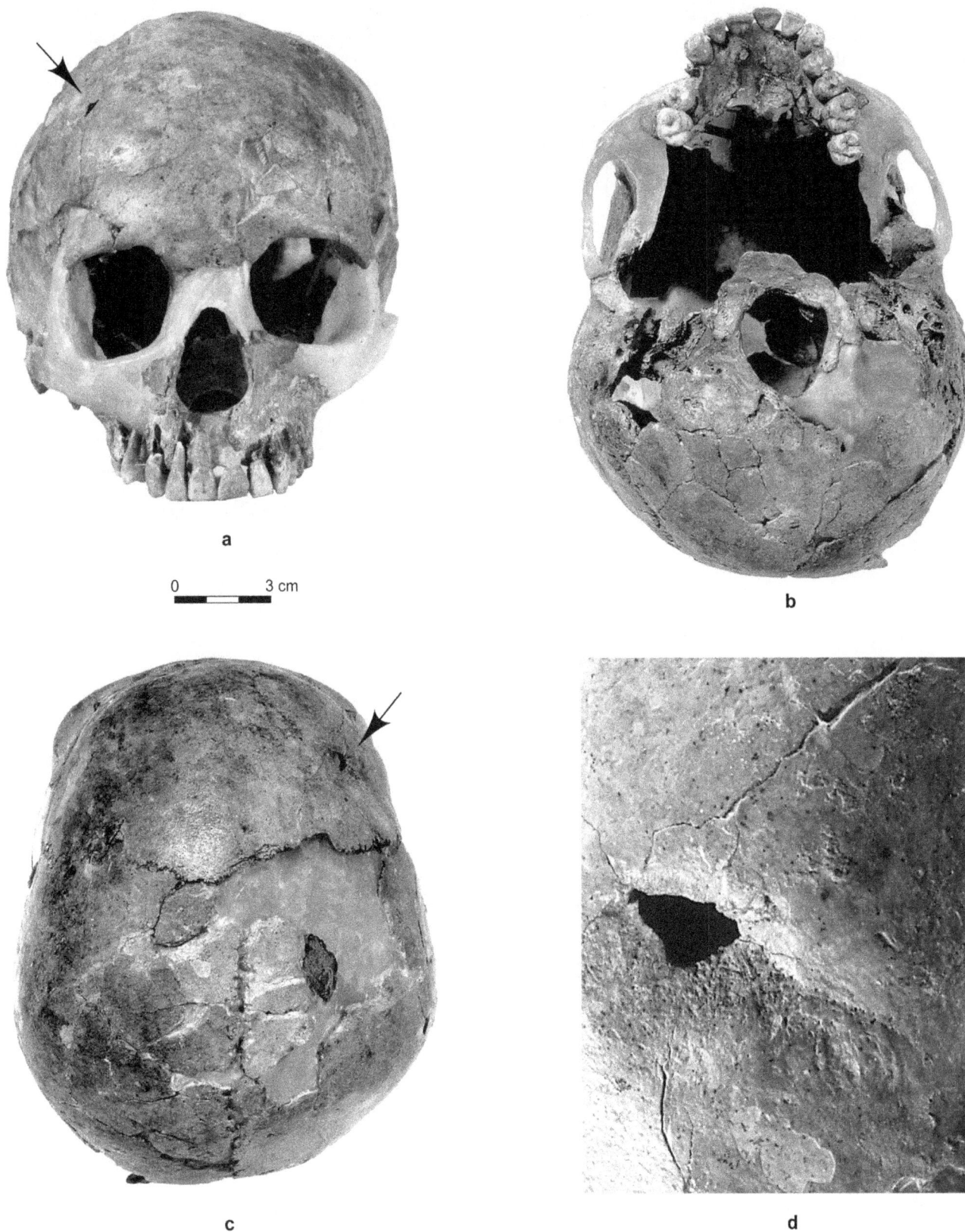

Figure 1. The Qafzeh 11 skull. a: norma facialis. b: norma inferior. c: norma superior. d: close-up view of the frontal lesion (healed fracture line is visible on the right side of the hole while fracturing lines above and below the hole are corresponding to post-mortem alteration). Black arrows on a and c indicate location of the lesion.

using other equations [27]. EV value obtained from virtual endocast is slightly lower (1200 cc), but as anterior part of the skull base is missing, the endocranial virtual reconstruction is not complete.

The proportional endocranial volume (PEV) of Qafzeh 11, based upon EV values calculated from recent formulas, corresponds to 81–86% of the EV values of mature individuals from the site (Qafzeh 6 and 9). When considering dental maturation of this individual (giving an age estimation of about 12–13 years), this PEV value is smaller than expected in comparison with modern endocranial growth pattern defined by Coqueugniot and Hublin [18]. PEV value of Qafzeh 11 actually corresponds to values from younger children (4–6 years). For the same site, the PEV value of Qafzeh 10 child (estimated to be 6 years old from dental maturation) falls within the present modern range (86–88%) for the corresponding age (figure 2). Therefore, it appears that the small endocranial volume of Qafzeh 11 cannot be considered as normal relative to its dental age. Growth retardation in cranio-encephalic development can be proposed from this result.

The 3D reconstructed calvaria clearly evidenced a depressed skull fracture of the right part of the frontal bone in the process of healing (figure 3A). It is located on the right part of the frontal squama just above the pterionic area. The depressed fragment of the frontal bone has a quadrangular shape (size:

29.7×23.4×26.5×11.7 mm); the posterior face is delineated by the coronal suture, the anterior face is near the frontal boss as well as the upper face which lies at 31.8 mm from the frontal midline. The fractured fragment is depressed forwards. Its anterior face penetrates endocranially whereas the posterior face is shifted outwards, dislocating the coronal suture and causing a sutural separation (figure 3B). Other fracture lines, different from taphonomic fracturing, can be identified although they are less obviously visible due to the bone remodelling of healing process. This is shown by a star-like aspect of fracture lines radiating from the impact area. This type of fracture, that can be related to a blunt force trauma, clinically corresponds to cranio-encephalic wound and raises the question of its impact on the brain.

Anatomical structures can be identified on the virtual endocast of Qafzeh 11 reconstructed by one of us (HC), despite missing parts, taphonomic fragmentation and post-mortem skull deformation (figures 3, 4). Normal cerebral hemispheres display an asymmetric development (figures 4A,B,E) characterized by a differential protrusion of one hemisphere relative to the other, known as petalia [25,28]. The right frontal lobe protrudes in front of the left by 1.71 mm. In addition the right frontal bec is more extended downwards than the left one. By contrast, the left occipital lobe projects 1.79 mm behind the right one. Yet, the occipital asymmetry known as Yakovlevian torque [28–29] cannot

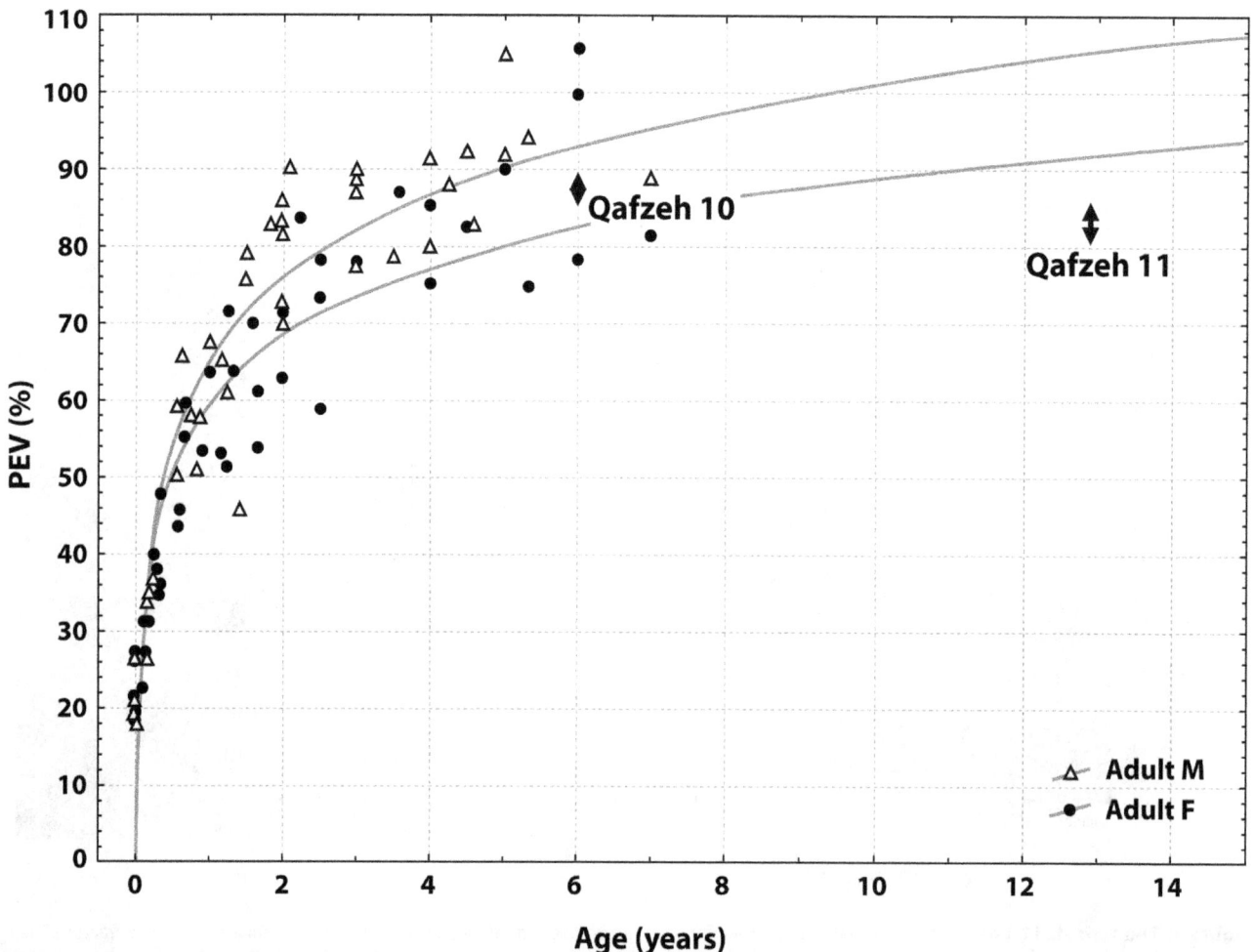

Figure 2. Proportional endocranial volume (PEV) of specimens Qafzeh 11 and 10 plotted on modern PEV from identified immature osteological collection (Coqueugniot and Hublin, 2012). Arrows represent PEV variation range.

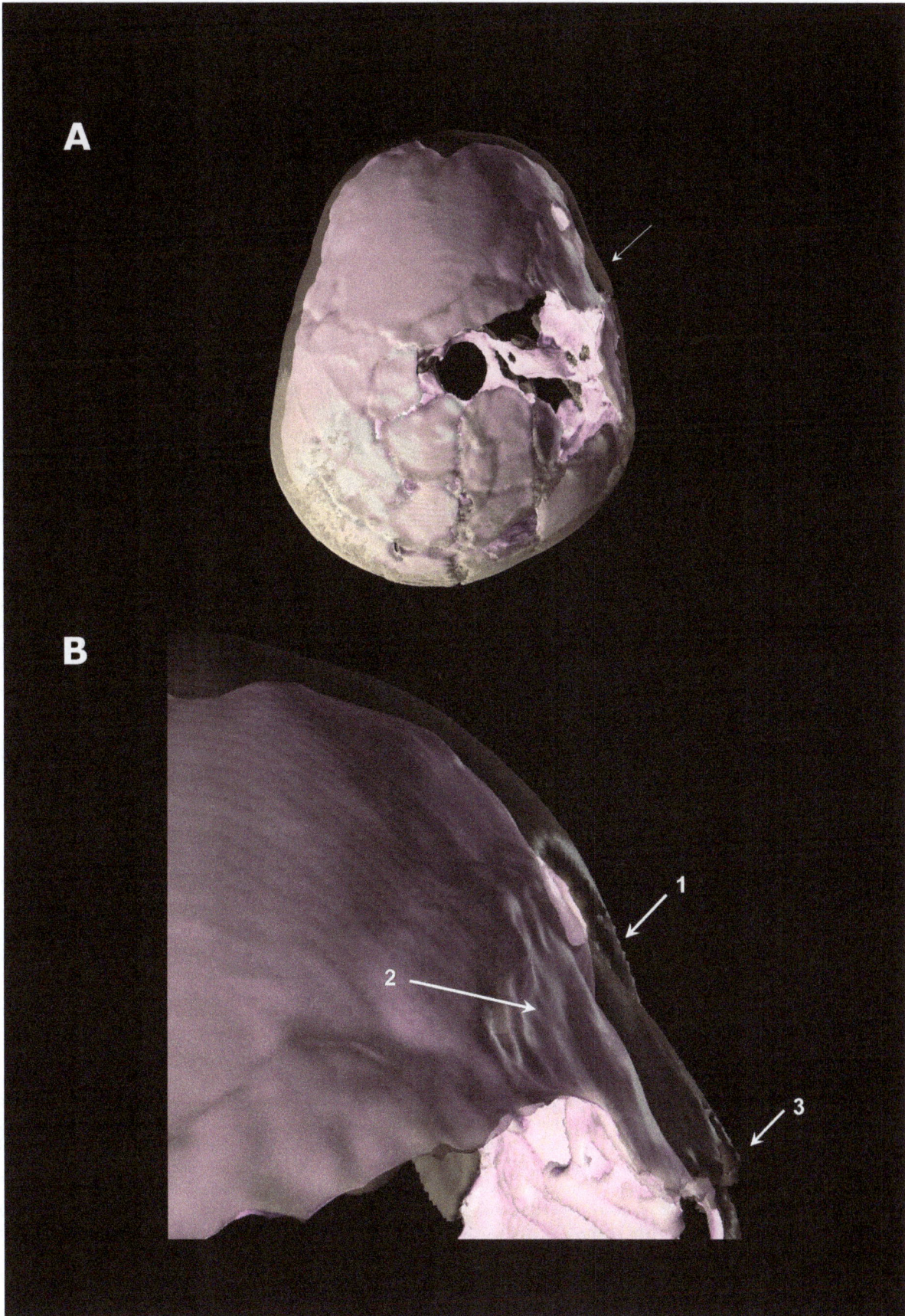

Figure 3. Superior view of Qafzeh 11 3D reconstructed skull showing the depressed fracture on the frontal's right side. The skull vault appears in transparency and the virtual endocranial cast in pink. A: general view. B: close up view of the trauma area. 1: anterior part of the frontal bone depressed fracture penetrating the endocranial volume. 2: irregular shape of virtual endocranial surface indicating brain damage. 3: diastasis of the right coronal suture.

be assessed here. Besides the right frontal petalia and left occipital one, the right frontal lobe is wider than the left and the left occipital lobe wider than the right. Interestingly, the two hemispheres are similar in length (153.7 mm at left and 153.6 mm at right).

Middle meningeal artery imprints are clearly visible on the left side of Qafzeh 11 endocast, showing the prevalence of the anterior branches (bregmatic and obelic) and lack of anastomosis (figure 4C), as previously described [6]. The imprint of the inferior frontal gyrus is visible on both sides. On the left it is possible to distinguish its reliefs (pars triangularis, pars opercularis and pars orbitalis) as well as those of the middle frontal gyrus and anterior central gyrus. On the right side, the imprint of the depressed fracture is localized upwards to the imprint of the inferior frontal gyrus. It may involve the posterior part of the middle frontal gyrus and the anterior part of the anterior central gyrus.

Comparison of the fossil virtual endocast with 3D reconstruction of digitized brain [24], confirms that the cranial depressed fracture observed on Qafzeh 11 (figures 3, 4D) only corresponds to the frontal area of the brain, forward to the central sulcus (Rolandic fissure) and upwards from the Sylvian fissure. The depressed skull fracture is localized forward to the precentral gyrus (primary motor cortex) and slightly behind the prefrontal cortex. The depressed fragment stretches over the middle part of the three frontal gyri. The corresponding brain areas are responsible for psychomotricity i.e. Brodmann areas 6 and 8 [30]. These areas control movement, rules for performing specific tasks, management of uncertainty, visual attention and eye movements [31]. The lesion may have affected the orbital part of inferior frontal gyrus (area 44) that is involved in speech language production on the left side (Broca's area), but seems to be involved in social communications on both sides.

Discussion

When a pathological condition is recognized in skeletal remains, the nature of the bone damage or injury is sometimes not easy to determine precisely. Peri-mortem trauma can be difficult to differentiate from skeletal post-mortem changes due to taphonomic processes (e.g. [32]). Cases of serious cranial trauma are seldom documented in the human Upper Pleistocene fossil record from south-western Asia (e.g. [2–5]) and Western Europe [33–34]. Zollikoffer et al. [33] asserted that the cranial injury displayed by the Neanderthal St-Césaire 1 resulted from an act "of intragroup, interpersonal violence" but did not cause the immediate death. Examining the pathological condition of Krapina 34.7 parietal fragment, Mann and Monge shared the same statement, i.e. the serious trauma "was not a mortal wound"; however they concluded that its cause "appears to one of an accident associated with life style of living and sleeping in caves" [34].

In his original description of the healed trauma which affected Qafzeh 11, Dastugue [4] mentioned that the skull fracture was not lethal, related to a minor trauma and only localized on the skull vault. According to him, this so-called "benign fracture" did not have significant repercussions and occurred when Qafzeh 11 was young. Furthermore, the healing response had probably not

undergone its complete trajectory before the death of the adolescent [4]. Dastugue concluded that the cause of death was unknown.

3D reconstructions clearly show that the Qafzeh 11 skull fracture was not a simple one. Indeed, this frontal bone fracture appears to be compound, with a broken piece of frontal squama that is depressed, isolated forwards by a linear fracture and backwards by sutural diastasis. As previously mentioned [4], this fracture type generally results from a blunt force trauma (getting struck or kicked in the head by heavy and blunt material, accidentally or intentionally with weapon). This type of trauma can be interpreted as resulting from interpersonal violence, but as has been demonstrated by paediatricians, complex cranial fractures like this one can also occur accidentally [35]. Contrary to the assumption of a non-serious wound made previously [4], the depressed fracture of Qafzeh 11 skull that can be considered as at least a moderate traumatic brain injury (TBI) [36], actually presents a high level of risk for brain damages (intra-cranial haemorrhages, diverse types of central nervous system lesions such as concussion, contusion, laceration, which can lead to destruction of brain tissue or cerebral scar). Besides the neurological damages due to focal brain lesion in the right frontal area, more precisely the areas 6 and 8. These areas are responsible for psychomotricity which may have led to troubles for controlling movement, difficulties for performing specific tasks, managing uncertainty, visual attention and eye movements and possibly the right area 44 (that seems also to be involved in oral communication as the left Broca's area, that is specialized in speech production). It is highly probable this young individual suffered also from personality changes due to traumatic brain injury. This personality disturbance is thought to be directly related to brain trauma and appears to be very frequent: 65% in severe to mild/moderate TBI, according to Max et al. [36]) but according to McAllister [37] "virtually all individuals who survive moderate and severe TBI are left with significant long-term neurobehavioral sequelae". These troubles are characterized by a "distress or impairment in social, occupational, or other important areas of functioning" and manifested in children as a "marked deviation from normal development" [36].

Two methods have confirmed the small endocranial volume of Qafzeh 11. The virtual reconstructed endocranial volume provides an underestimated value due to the lack of anterior part of skull base which technically limits endocast segmentation and therefore makes its complete virtual reconstruction speculative. Recently, Kondo et al. [38] proposed a semi-virtual reconstruction of the Qafzeh 9 endocast. They obtained a EV value of 1411–1477 cc that is smaller than the initial estimation of 1508–1554 cc [10] and the mean value of 1531 cc provided by Holloway et al. [25]. Considering that (i) EV virtual values appear to be smaller than calculated ones for the base- damaged Qafzeh 9 and 11 skulls, (ii) virtual EV are not available for other specimens of the site (Qafzeh 10 and 6), we prefer using estimated EV value calculated from formulae.

As for Qafzeh 11, EV values are nevertheless consistent each other and corroborate a small endocranial volume related to individual age whatever the method used. This can be interpreted as growth retardation due to the trauma. Indeed, generalized

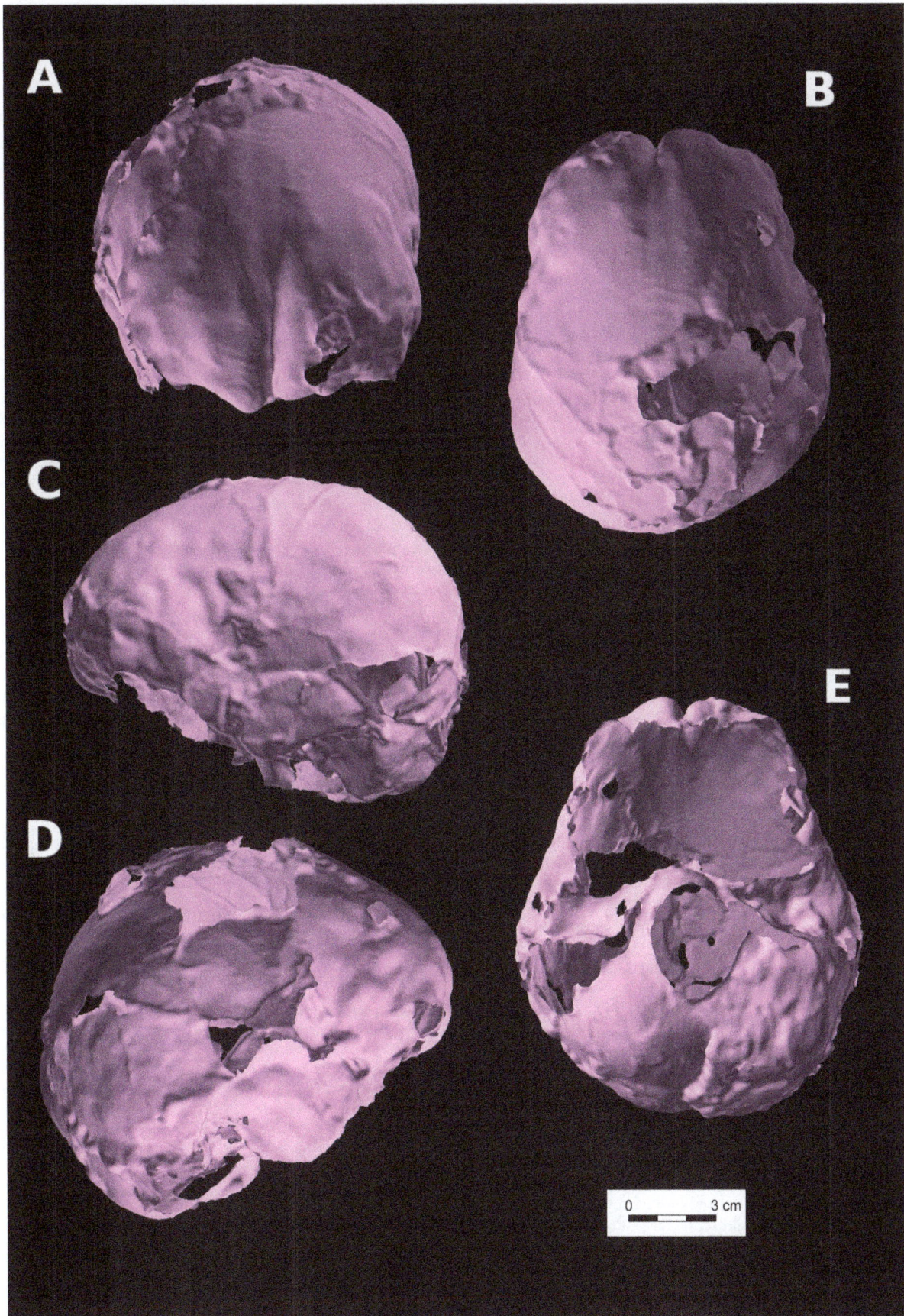

Figure 4. Virtual endocast of Qafzeh 11. A: norma frontalis. B: norma superior. C: left norma lateralis. D: right norma lateralis. E: norma basilaris.

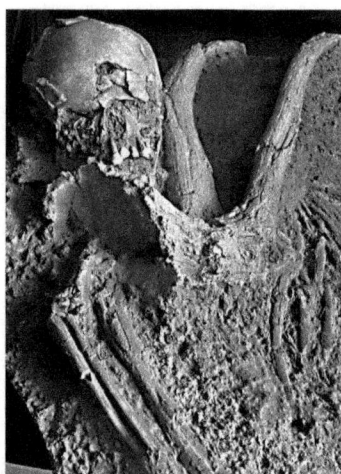

Figure 5. Partial view of the Qafzeh 11 burial showing the deposit of the red deer antlers in close contact with the child skeleton (cast).

atrophic changes resulting in reduced overall brain volume has been documented in moderate-to-severe pediatric traumatic brain injury [39–40]. In addition to this focal effect on brain, a general growth retardation due to post-traumatic endocrine disturbance [41] could be raised here.

Hemispheric asymmetry is present on Qafzeh 11. This feature has already been described on fossil hominins (e.g. [25,29,42–43]) including Qafzeh 9 [38] and among extant populations (e.g. [28,44]). Therefore, despite the depressed frontal fracture that had probably impacted the underlying brain tissue of Qafzeh 11 frontal lobe, the physiological hemispheric asymmetric pattern was not affected.

As Qafzeh 11 has a PEV corresponding to a 4–6 years old modern child, we hypothesize that the trauma occurred at or before this age. Among skeletal indicators of growth disturbance and stress during childhood, is the manifestation of growth arrest lines (Harris lines) in the metaphyseal region of the long bones. These non-specific stress indicators usually vanish during life. Unfortunately, the preservation state of long bones does not allow any kind of investigation in the case of Qafzeh 11. Pathological alterations of the dental enamel, such as transverse linear enamel hypoplasia (LEH), are also employed in the assessment of physiological stress events and growth disturbances during childhood (e.g. [45–48]). Presence of enamel hypoplasia on three lower teeth of Qafzeh 11 (right and left first molars, right second molar) was previously described by Skinner [49]. However, data collected on the specimen by one of us (AmT) point to the lack of LEH on the permanent upper and lower teeth and on the isolated germs of upper third molars as well [3]. Both lower right M1 and M2 indeed present a different enamel coloration above the cervix, located at the same height of the two crowns. This alteration is most probably of taphonomic origin and we suggest that the skull trauma didn't impact M1 and M2 complete crown formation, indicating that it probably occurred around 6 years of age.

In sum, the Qafzeh 11 child represents, to our knowledge, the oldest documented human case of severe cranial trauma available from south-western Asia, dated to 90–100 kyrs BP. The adult Shanidar 1 skull exhibits an indisputable evidence of trauma, that was sometimes interpreted as a consequence of interpersonal violence [2,50] but the specimen is probably more recent [51]. For Qafzeh 11, the exact circumstances surrounding the injury remain unknown, although this kind of injury generally results from a blunt force trauma.

Whatever the origin and severity of a given pathological condition observed on human Middle Palaeolithic hominins, speculations were made with regard to its consequences on individual life conditions and social status, in terms of disability, impairment and social care. Consequently, these questions are widening the debate introducing notions of altruism and compassion in prehistoric human communities and their possible role in human life history (e.g. [2,52–58]).

In this respect, it is crucial to assemble biological and pathological data with cultural observations and their subsequent interpretations. For the Qafzeh 11 subadult, it is now clear that severe cranio-encephalic trauma experienced during childhood, deeply impacted his/her cognitive and social communication skills. Interestingly Qafzeh 11 benefited from special social attention at his/her death, as shown from archaeological details. The Qafzeh 11 skeleton, recovered at the bottom of the Mousterian sequence in front of the entrance of the cave, revealed that the corpse was originally lying in a pit on its back, the head turned to the right with upper limbs flexed [59]. The hands maintained their anatomical configuration and were lying together near the face western-oriented. The pelvic region and the lower limbs extended to the south from the skull, were post-deposition-ally damaged by a large stone. Besides this, there was a complete lack of mixing or bone displacement with an absence of animal scavenging traces. Furthermore, two deer antlers were lying on the upper part of the adolescent's chest, near his/her face and they were in close contact with the palmar side of the hand bones (figure 5). Such a hand location, within the original body spatial arrangement, attested a funerary offering and not an accidental incorporation. All these observations strongly support the inter-pretation of a deliberate, ceremonial burial for Qafzeh 11.

At Qafzeh several other burials occur [59–62], but Qafzeh 11 represents a unique case of differential treatment with convincing evidence for ritual behavior. We interpret the Qafzeh 11 burial as resulting from a ritual practice applied to a young individual who experienced a severe cranial trauma most probably followed by significant neurological and psychological disorders, including troubles in social communication. These biological and archaeo-logical evidences reflect an elaborate social behavior among the Qafzeh Middle Palaeolithic people.

Acknowledgments

This study was made possible by the field work done at Qafzeh Cave by a team led by one of us (B.V.) and supported by the French Ministry of Foreign Affairs. We are deeply grateful to Professor I. Hershkovitz (Tel Aviv University), for access to the fossil, and technical assistance. We thank Professor N. Peled (Carmel Medical Center, Haifa, Israel) for providing helpful technical support for access to the medical scanner. Thanks are also due to V. Slon (Tel Aviv University) for help in collecting digital data. The authors are greatly indebted to B. Dutailly (UMR 5199 PACEA) who has developed TIVMI software program for anthropology, helped and advised us constantly throughout the development of this work.

Author Contributions

Conceived and designed the experiments: HC OD BA HD BV AmT. Performed the experiments: HC. Analyzed the data: HC OD AmT. Contributed reagents/materials/analysis tools: HC BA BV AmT. Wrote the paper: HC OD AmT.

References

1. McCown TD, Keith A (1939) The Stone Age of Mount Carmel. vol. II. Oxford: Clarendon University Press. 390 p.

2. Trinkaus E (1983) The Shanidar Neandertals. New York: Academic Press. 502 p.

3. Tillier AM, Arensburg B, Duday H, Vandermeersch B (2004) Dental Pathology, Stressful Events and Disease in Levantine Early Anatomically Modern Humans: Evidence from Qafzeh. In: Goren Inbar N, Speth JD, editors. Human Paleoecology in the Levantine Corridor. Oxbow Book. pp. 135–148.

4. Dastugue J (1981) Pièces pathologiques de la nécropole moustérienne de Qafzeh. Paléorient 7: 135–140.

5. Tillier AM (1984) L'enfant Homo 11 de Qafzeh (Israël) et son apport à la compréhension des modalités de la croissance des squelettes moustériens. Paléorient 10: 7–48.

6. Tillier AM (1999) Les enfants moustériens de Qafzeh. Interprétation phylogénétique et paléoauxologique. Paris: Cahiers de Paléoanthropologie, CNRS Editions. 239 p.

7. Coqueugniot H, Desbarats P, Dutailly B, Panuel M, Dutour O (2010) Les outils de l'imagerie médicale et de la 3D au service des maladies du passé. In: Vergnieux R, Delevoie C, editors. Virtual Retrospect 2009. Ausonius Editions: Collection Archéovision, volume 4. pp. 177–180.

8. Coqueugniot H, Dutailly B, Desbarats P, Dutour O (2012) VIRCOPAL (VIRtual COllection of PALeo-specimens): 3D ressources for teaching and research in Paleopathology. 19th European Meeting of the Paleopathology Association, Lille, France, abstract volume: 41.

9. Dutour O, Coqueugniot H, Naji S, Colombo A, Herrscher E, et al. (2012) Contribution of 3D imaging to identify paleopathological processes. 39th Annual Meeting of the Paleopathology Association Portland, Oregon, abstract volume: 13–14.

10. Vandermeersch B (1981) Les hommes fossiles de Qafzeh. Paris: Cahiers de Paléoanthropologie, CNRS Editions. 319 p.

11. Tillier AM (in press) New Middle Palaeolithic hominin Dental Remains from Qafzeh (Israel). Paléorient.

12. Schwarcz H, Grün R, Vandermeersch B, Bar-Yosef O, Valladas H, et al. (1988) ESR dates for the Hominid Burial site of Qafzeh in Israel. J Hum Evol 17: 733–737.

13. Valladas H, Reyss J.L, Joron JL, Valladas G, Bar Yosef O, et al. (1988) Thermoluminescence dating of Mousterian "Proto-cro-magnon" remains from Israel and the origin of Modern man. Nature 331: 614–616.

14. Boutié P (1989). Etude technologique de l'industrie moustérienne de la grotte de Qafzeh (près de Nazareth, Israël). In: Bar-Yosef O, Vandermeersch B., editors. Investigations in South Levantine Prehistory. Oxford: British Archaeological Reports International Series 497. pp. 213–229.

15. Hovers E (1997) Variability of Levantine Mousterian Assemblages and Settlement patterns. Implications for the Development of Human Behavior. PhD Dissertation, Hebrew University, Jerusalem. 385 p.

16. Hovers E (2009) The Lithic assemblages of Qafzeh Cave. Oxford: Oxford University Press. 320 p.

17. Howell FC (1958) Upper Pleistocene Men of Southwestern Asian Mousterian. In: Hundert Jahre Neanderthaler Neandertal Centenary 1856–1956. Böhlau Verlag Köln-Graz. pp. 185–198.

18. Coqueugniot H, Hublin JJ (2012) Age-related changes in digital endocranial volume during human ontogeny: Results from an osteological reference collection. Am J Phys Anthropol 147: 312–318.

19. Rampont M (1994) Les squelettes, os et dents de foetus, nouveau-nés et enfants du Musée Anatomique de Strasbourg. Aspects historiques et catalogue. Ph.D. Dissertation, University of Louis Pasteur, Medicine Faculty, Strasbourg. 170 p.

20. Dutailly B, Coqueugniot H, Desbarats P, Gueorguieva S, Synave R (2009) 3D surface reconstruction using HMH algorithm. Proceedings of IEEE International Conference on Image Processing: 2505–2508.

21. Spoor CF, Zonneveld FW, Macho GA (1993) Linear measurements of cortical bone and dental enamel by computed tomography: applications and problems. Am J Phys Anthrop 91: 469–484.

22. Coqueugniot H, Dutailly B, Desbarats P, Dutour O (2013) Procédé de modélisation d'une pièce formée de tissu osseux. Bordeaux and Aix-Marseille Universities, France. French patent n°1151284.

23. Guyomarc'h P, Santos F, Dutailly B, Desbarats P, Bou C, et al. (2012) Three-dimensional computer-assisted craniometrics: a comparison of the uncertainty in measurement induced by surface reconstruction performed by two computer programs. Forensic Sci Int 219: 221–227.

24. Amunts K, Lepage C, Borgeat L, Mohlberg H, Dickscheid T, et al. (2013) BigBrain: An Ultrahigh-Resolution 3D Human Brain Model. Science 340: 1472–1475.

25. Holloway RL, Broadfield DC, Yuan MS (2004) The human fossil record. Volume Three: Brain endocasts - The Paleoneurological Evidence. Wiley-Liss, Hoboken. 315 p.

26. Guyomarc'h P, Santos F, Dutailly B, Coqueugniot H (2013) Facial soft tissue depths in French adults: Variability, specificity and estimation. Forensic Sci Int 231: 411.e1–411.510.

27. Coqueugniot H (1994) Équations d'estimation de la capacité crânienne chez l'enfant: application paléoanthropologique. Anthropologie (Brno) 32: 243–250.

28. Toga AW, Thompson PM (2003) Mapping brain asymmetry. Nature Neuroscience 4: 37–48.

29. LeMay M (1976) Morphological cerebral asymmetries of modern man, fossil man and non human primate. Ann NY Acad Sci 280: 349–366.

30. Brodmann K (1909) Vergleichende Lokalisationslehre der Grosshirnrinde. Leipzig: Johann Ambrosius Barth. Translated by L. Garey as Localisation in the cerebral cortex. Springer 2006. 298 p.

31. Lloyd D (2007) What do Brodmann areas do?, Or: Scanning the Neurocracy. Hartford, CT: Program in Neuroscience. Available: http://www.trincoll.edu/~dlloyd/brodmann.html

32. Waldron T (2009) Palaeopathology. Cambridge manuals in Archaeology, Cambridge University Press. 279 p.

33. Zollikoffer CPE, Ponce de Leon MS, Vandermeersch B, Levêque F (2002) Evidence for interpersonal violence in the St-Cesaire Neanderthal. Proc Natl Acad Sci USA 99: 6444–6448.

34. Mann A, Monge J (2008) A Neandertal parietal fragment from Krapina (Croatia) with a serious cranial trauma. In: Monge J, Mann A, Frayer DW, Radovčic J, editors. New insights on the Krapina Neandertals. Zagreb: Croatian Natural History Museum. pp. 261–268.

35. Wood JN, Christian CW, Adams CM, Rubin DM (2009) Skeletal Surveys in Infants With Isolated Skull Fractures. Pediatrics 123: e247–e252.

36. Max JE, Marie Robertson BA, Lansing AE (2001) The Phenomenology of Personality Change Due to Traumatic Brain Injury in Children and Adolescents. J Neuropsychiatry Clin Neurosci 13: 161–170.

37. McAllister TW (2008) Neurobehavioral sequelae of traumatic brain injury: evaluation and management. World Psychiatry 7: 3–10.

38. Kondo O, Kubo D, Suzuki H, Ogihara N (2014) Virtual endocast of Qafzeh 9: a preliminary assessment of right-left asymmetry. In: Akazawa T, Ogihara NC, Tanabe H, Terashima H, editors. Dynamics of learning in Neanderthals and Modern Humans, volume 2: Cognitive and Physical Perspectives. Springer Japan. pp. 183–190.

39. Levine B, Kovacevic N, Nica EI, Cheung G, Gao F, et al. (2008) The Toronto Traumatic Brain Injury Study: injury severity and quantified MRI. Neurology 70: 771–778.

40. Merkley TL, Bigler ED, Wilde EA, McCauley SR, Hunter JV, et al. (2008) Diffuse changes in cortical thickness in pediatric moderate-to-severe traumatic brain injury. J Neurotrauma 25: 1343–1345.

41. Garcia-Segura LM (2009) Hormones and brain plasticity. New York: Oxford University Press. 496 p.

42. Grimaud-Hervé D (1997) L'évolution de l'encéphale chez Homo erectus et Homo sapiens. Exemples de l'Asie et de l'Europe. Paris: Cahiers de Paléoanthropologie, CNRS éditions. 405 p.

43. Balzeau A, Grimaud-Hervé D, Détroit F, Holloway RL, Cobes B, et al. (2013) First description of the Cro-Magnon 1 endocast and study of brain variation and evolution in anatomically modern Homo sapiens. Bull Mém Soc Anthropol Paris 25: 1–18.

44. Chang Chui H, Damasio AR (1980) Human cerebral asymmetries evaluated by computed tomography. J Neurol Neurosurg Psychiatry 43: 873–878.

45. Goodman H, Rose JC (1990) Assessment of systemic physiological perturbations from dental enamel hypoplasia and associated histological structures. Yearb Phys Anthropol 33: 59–110.

46. Neiburger E (1990) Enamel hypoplasias: poor indications of dietary stress. Am J Phys Anthropol 82: 231–232.

47. Berti PR, Mahaney MC (1992) Quantification of the confidence interval of linear enamel hypoplasia chronologies. In: Capasso LL, Goodman AH, editors. Recent Contributions to the study of Enamel Developmental defects. Chieti Italy: Journal of Paleopathology Monogr Publ.2. pp. 19–30.

48. Schultz M, Carli-Thiele P, Schmidt-Schultz TH, Kiedorf U, Kiedorf H, et al. (1998) Enamel Hypoplasias in Archaeological Skeletal remains. In: Alt KW, Rösing FW, Teschler-Nicola M, editors. Dental Anthropology. Fundamentals, Limits and Prospects. Wien, New York: Springer. pp. 293–312.

49. Skinner M (1996) Developmental Stress in Immature Hominines from Late Pleistocene Eurasia: Evidence from enamel Hypoplasia. J Archaeol Sci 23: 833–852.

50. Churchill SE, Franciscus RG, McKean-Peraza H, Daniel JA, Warren BR (2009) Shanidar 3 Neandertal rib puncture wound and paleolithic weaponry. J Hum Evol 57: 163–178.

51. Cowgill LW, Trinkaus E, Zeder MA (2007) Shanidar 10: a Middle Paleolithic immature distal lower limb from Shanidar Cave, Iraqi Kurdistan. J Hum Evol 53: 213–223.

52. Lebel S, Trinkaus E, Faure M, Fernandez P, Guérin C, et al. (2001) Comparative morphology and paleobiology of Middle Pleistocene human remains from the Bau de l'Aubesier, Vaucluse, France. Proc Natl Acad Sci USA 98: 11097–11102.

53. Trinkaus E (1985) Pathology and posture of the La Chapelle-aux-Saints Neanderthal. Am J Phys Anthrop 67: 19–41.

54. DeGusta D (2002) Comparative skeletal pathology and the case for conspecific care in Middle Pleistocene Hominins. J Archaeol Sci 29: 1435–1438.

55. Tillier AM, Arensburg B, Duday H, Vandermeersch B (2001) An early case of hydrocephalus: the Middle Paleolithic Qafzeh 12 child (Israel). Am J Phys Anthrop 114: 166–170.

56. Lordkipanidze D, Vekua A, Ferring R, Rightmire GP, Agusti J, et al. (2005) The earliest toothless hominin skull. Nature 434: 717–718.

57. Gracia A, Arsuaga JL, Martinez I, Lorenzo C, Carretero JM, et al. (2009) Craniosynostosis in the Middle Pleistocene human Cranium 14 from the Sima de los Huesos, Atapuerca, Spain. Proc Natl Acad Sci USA 106: 6573–6578.

58. Hublin JJ (2009) The prehistory of compassion. Proc Natl Acad Sci USA 106: 6429–6430.

59. Vandermeersch B (1970) Une sépulture moustérienne avec offrandes découverte dans la grotte de Qafzeh. C R Acad Sc Paris 270 D: 298–301.

60. Vandermeersch B (1969) Les nouveaux squelettes moustériens découverts à Qafzeh (Israël) et leur signification. C R Acad Sc Paris 268 D: 2562–2565.

61. Tillier AM (1995) Paléoanthropologie et pratiques funéraires au Levant méditerranéen durant le Paléolithique moyen: le cas des sujets non adultes. Anthropologie du Proche-Orient, Données récentes. Volume coordonné par B. Vandermeersch. Paléorient 21/2: 63–76.

62. Tillier AM (2009) L'homme et la mort. L'émergence du geste funéraire en Préhistoire. Paris: CNRS Editions. 186 p.

10

The Spatiotemporal Role of COX-2 in Osteogenic and Chondrogenic Differentiation of Periosteum-Derived Mesenchymal Progenitors in Fracture Repair

Chunlan Huang[1]**, Ming Xue**[1]**, Hongli Chen**[1]**, Jing Jiao**[2]**, Harvey R. Herschman**[2]**, Regis J. O'Keefe**[1]**, Xinping Zhang**[1]*

1 Center for Musculoskeletal Research, University of Rochester, School of Medicine and Dentistry, Rochester, New York, United States of America, **2** Department of Molecular and Medical Pharmacology, David Geffen School of Medicine, University of California Los Angeles, Los Angeles, California, United States of America

Abstract

Periosteum provides a major source of mesenchymal progenitor cells for bone fracture repair. Combining cell-specific targeted *Cox-2* gene deletion approaches with *in vitro* analyses of the differentiation of periosteum-derived mesenchymal progenitor cells (PDMPCs), here we demonstrate a spatial and temporal role for Cox-2 function in the modulation of osteogenic and chondrogenic differentiation of periosteal progenitors in fracture repair. *Prx1Cre*-targeted *Cox-2* gene deletion in mesenchyme resulted in marked reduction of intramembraneous and endochondral bone repair, leading to accumulation of poorly differentiated mesenchyme and immature cartilage in periosteal callus. In contrast, *Col2Cre*-targeted *Cox-2* gene deletion in cartilage resulted in a deficiency primarily in cartilage conversion into bone. Further cell culture analyses using *Cox-2* deficient PDMPCs demonstrated reduced osteogenic differentiation in monolayer cultures, blocked chondrocyte differentiation and hypertrophy in high density micromass cultures. Gene expression microarray analyses demonstrated downregulation of a key set of genes associated with bone/cartilage formation and remodeling, namely *Sox9*, *Runx2*, *Osx*, *MMP9*, *VDR* and *RANKL*. Pathway analyses demonstrated dysregulation of the HIF-1, PI3K-AKT and Wnt pathways in Cox-2 deficient cells. Collectively, our data highlight a crucial role for Cox-2 from cells of mesenchymal lineages in modulating key pathways that control periosteal progenitor cell growth, differentiation, and angiogenesis in fracture repair.

Editor: Xing-Ming Shi, Georgia Regents University, United States of America

Funding: This study is supported by grants from the Musculoskeletal Transplant Foundation (XPZ), NYSTEM N08G-495 (XPZ) and N09G346 (XPZ), and the National Institutes of Health (R21 DE021513 to XPZ, RC1 AR058435 to XPZ, AR R01 AR048681 to XPZ and RJO, P50 AR054041 to RJO). The funders had no role in study design, data collection and analysis, decision to publish, or preparation of the manuscript.

Competing Interests: The authors have declared that no competing interests exist.

* Email: Xinping_Zhang@URMC.rochester.edu

Introduction

Fracture healing is a unique postnatal bone regeneration process that occurs as a cascade of well-orchestrated biological events leading to the restoration of bone tissue. Fracture healing requires the formation of an external bone callus, which is initiated primarily by the progenitor cells residing in the periosteum [1–4]. Analogous to embryonic skeletal development, periosteum-initiated fracture repair implicates endochondral and intramembranous bone formation, which proceed in a sequential and organized manner [5,6]. While adult bone repair recapitulates some essential regulatory mechanisms that occur in early skeletal development, repair is a unique bone morphogenetic process, orchestrated by an ensemble of genes distinct from early skeletal development [7]. Due to an inability to directly target the periosteum, the molecular mechanisms and the implicated molecular pathway(s) that control the differentiation program of periosteal mesenchymal progenitor cells in bone fracture repair remains poorly understood. Identifying the critical genes in periosteum-initiated bone repair, establishing their spatiotemporal expression, and elucidating their integrated roles will be essential to understand bone regeneration and to develop useful therapeutics to improve skeletal repair and reconstruction.

Cox-2 is the inducible isoform of cyclooxygenase, the enzyme responsible for a major control step in prostanoid biosynthesis pathway. Cox-2 plays an important role in cancer biology, in vascular pathophysiology, and in a variety of inflammatory disorders [8,9]. Global deletion of the *Cox-2* gene in mice does not affect overall skeletal development [10,11]. However, global absence of Cox-2 markedly impairs fracture healing [12,13]. An important role for Cox-2 in fracture healing has been shown in aged animals. Older mice have a marked reduction of *Cox-2* expression in the fracture callus, exhibiting delayed neovascularization and endochondral bone formation [14]. *In-situ* hybridization analyses demonstrate that *Cox-2* expression peaks at the early stage of intramembranous and endochondral stage of bone healing [15]. Elevated *Cox-2* expression is detected in chondroprogenitors and proliferating chondrocytes at days 5 and 7 post-fracture. Cox-2 expression is subsequently reduced in hypertrophic chondrocytes during the remodeling phase of healing, suggesting that Cox-2 expression is tightly regulated during fracture repair. In contrast to loss of Cox-2 function, Cox-2 gain of function by overexpression at the healing site accelerates fracture healing in animal models [16].

While an essential role of Cox-2 in fracture repair has been established, targeted tissues and implicated pathways remain unclear. Here we utilize two tissue-specific promoter driven-Cre transgenic mouse lines to delete the *Cox-2* gene in limb mesenchymal lineages (with Prx1Cre) and in chondrocytes (with Col2Cre), respectively. To determine the mechanistic involvement of Cox-2 in control of osteogenic and chondrogenic differentiation of periosteal mesenchymal progenitors, we further performed differentiation and gene expression profile analysis using periosteum-derived mesenchymal progenitor cells (PDMPCs) isolated from the healing periosteum of the mutant and control mice [17,18]. Our study established a critical role for Cox-2 in the differentiation paradigm of periosteal mesenchymal progenitor cell in fracture repair, underscoring the importance of spatial and temporal regulation of Cox-2 in bone repair and regeneration.

Materials and Methods

Animal models

To determine the gene recombination efficiency of Prx1Cre and Col2Cre lines in fracture callus, *Col2Cre; RosaR* and *Prx1Cre; RosaR* mice were generated and characterized for beta-galactosidase expression. Cox-2 conditional deletion (*Cox-2^{f/f}*) mice [19] were crossed with *Prx1-1Cre* or *Col2Cre* transgenic mice to produce *Cox-2^{f/f}; Prx1Cre* and *Cox-2^{f/f}; Col2Cre* mice. All studies and procedures were approved by the Institutional Animal Care and Use Committee at the University of Rochester. Littermates were used for analysis.

Fracture healing model

Closed stabilized femoral fractures were created in two month-old mice [14,15]. Mice were anesthetized with a mix of Ketamine and Xylazine. The skin and the underlying soft tissues over the knee were incised lateral to the patellar tendon. The tendon was displaced medially, and a small hole was drilled into the distal femur using a 26-gauge needle. A stylus pin from a 25G Type spinal needle (BD Medical Systems, Franklin Lakes, NJ) was inserted into the intramedullary canal and clipped. The wound was closed by suturing. Fractures were created at the diaphyseal region of mouse femurs using a three-point bending Einhorn device, as previously described [20]. Fracture healing was examined in gender and age-matched littermates. *Cox-2^{f/f}; Col2Cre* and *Cox-2^{f/f}; Prx1Cre* were compared with their respective Cre-negative *Cox-2^{f/f}* littermate controls for analyses.

Micro-CT Imaging Analyses

Femurs were harvested at indicated time points and scanned using a Viva micro-CT system (Scanco Medical, Switzerland) at a voxel size of 10.5 μm to image bone. New bone formation was measured as previously described [21]. The threshold was chosen using 2D evaluation of several slices in the transverse anatomical plane. In this way, mineralized callus was identified while surrounding soft tissue was excluded. An average threshold of 220 was optimal and was used uniformly for all samples. Each sample was contoured around the external callus and along the edge of the cortical bone, excluding the marrow cavity. New bone volume was measured on the surface of fracture samples as previously described [15]. Gender and age matched littermates were used for analyses. Indices of cortical bone morphology from the diaphyseal tibia were assessed by micro-CT imaging as described previously [11]. Cortical bone morphology in male and female mice were analyzed separately and presented as gender-matched groups as indicated.

Histology and histomorphometric Analyses

Fractured femurs were harvested and processed for histological analyses as previously described [12]. Femurs were disarticulated from the hip and trimmed to remove excess muscle and skin. Specimens were stored in 10% neutral buffered formalin for 3 days. The tissues were infiltrated and embedded in paraffin. Sections were prepared and stained with Alcian blue/Hematoxylin as previously described [12]. Histomorphometric analyses were performed using Osteometrics software to determine the area of bone, cartilage, and mesenchyme (a subtraction of total callus from bone and cartilage tissue) by manual tracing. Pre-existing cortical bone was excluded from the analyses. The percent areas of bone, cartilage, and mesenchyme were used to illustrate the composition of the fracture callus. At least three nonconsecutive sections from each sample were used for histomorphometric analyses. The means of ten samples from each group were used for statistical analyses.

Isolation of periosteum-derived mesenchymal progenitors (PDMPCs) from autograft periosteum

We have previously devised a method which allows isolation of sufficient numbers of periosteum-derived mesenchymal progenitors (PDMPCs) from day 5 periosteum callus of autografts to perform *in vitro* differentiation analyses [17,18]. Briefly, autograft transplantations were performed in *Cox-2^{f/f}; Prx1Cre* mice and their Cre-negative control mice. Mice were anesthetized by peritoneal injection of a mix of Ketamine and Xylazine. A 7–8 mm long incision was made in hind limb, and the mid-shaft femur was exposed by blunt dissection of muscles without disturbing the periosteum. A 4-mm mid-diaphyseal segment was removed from the femur of the donor mice using a sharp diamond-cutting wheel attached to a cordless dremel. The same 4 mm cortical bone graft was then inserted back into the segmental defect and stabilized by a 22-gauge metal pin placed through the intramedullary marrow cavity (autograft transplantation). Donor bone autografts were collected at day 5 post-transplantation. Bone marrow inside the bone graft was removed and discarded by repeated flushing of the marrow cavities with serum-free α-MEM medium. Periosteum tissues were scraped off and pooled in a Petri dish. After digestion with Collagenase D (Roche Applied Science, Indianapolis, IN) at a concentration of 1 mg/ml for 1 hour, cells released from periosteal tissues were pooled and cultured in α-MEM medium containing 1% penicillin and streptomycin, 1% glutamine, and 20% fetal bovine serum (FBS). Once confluent, cells were trypsinized and further expanded in α-MEM medium containing 10% FBS. Periosteal cells from second and third passage were collected and used for all experiments.

For osteogenesis assays, cells isolated from Cox-2^{f/f}; Prx1Cre mice and their Cre-negative control mice were cultured as monolayers in fresh α-MEM media containing 1% penicillin and streptomycin, 1% glutamine, and 10% fetal bovine serum (FBS). Since PDMPCs can spontaneously differentiated into osteoblastic cells in regular media following 7 day culture, the basal level of differentiation was examined in control and KO cells in regular media. To examine osteogenic differentiation in response to BMP-2, identical amount of BMP-2 (100 ng/ml) was added to the control and KO culture. Cells were harvested on day 7 for Alkaline Phosphatase staining (ALP) staining and RNA analyses as previously described [17,18]. For chondrogenesis assays, 2×10^5 cells per well were seeded as micromass in a 24-well plate and cultured in DMEM media with 10% fetal bovine serum with or without identical amount of BMP-2 (100 ng/ml). Cell pellets were harvested on day 1 and 7 for Alcian Blue staining and gene expression analyses.

Real-Time PCR Analyses

Total RNA was prepared using a Qiagen RNA extraction kit. Exactly 0.5 μg of mRNA from 4 different samples was pooled and reverse transcribed to make single-strand cDNA, using a commercial first strand cDNA synthesis kit (Invitrogen). Quantitative RT-PCR reaction was performed using SyberGreen (ABgene, Rochester, NY) in a RotorGene real time PCR machine (Corbett Research, Carlsbad, CA). All genes were compared to a standard β-actin control. Data were assessed quantitatively using analysis of variance, comparing relative levels of transcript expression as a function of time. All primers used for the assessment can be found in previous publications [15,17,18] or listed in Table S2. Data are expressed as the means ± SEM. Statistical significance between experimental groups was determined using one-way ANOVA and a Tukey's posthoc test (GraphPad Prism, San Diego, CA). A P value <0.05 was considered statistically significant.

Western blot analyses

Cells were lysed in Golden lysis buffer supplemented with protease inhibitor (Roche Applied Science). The protein extracts (10 μg) were separated using NuPAGE BisTris gels (Invitrogen). Gels were transferred to a polyvinylidene difluoride membrane (PerkinElmer Life Sciences Waltham, MA) and probed with anti–Cox-2 (Cayman Chemical Inc, Ann Arbor, MI) and anti–β-actin monoclonal antibody (Sigma, St. Louis, MO).

Microarray analyses

For microarray analysis, a total of 24 RNA samples in 8 indicated groups (n = 3 per group) were prepared from micromass cultures of Cox-2$^{f/f}$; Prx1Cre or Cox-2$^{f/f}$ PDPMCs, with or without BMP-2 treatment, at day 1 and day 7. Total RNA from each sample was isolated using an RNeasy Mini extraction kit. RNA quality and purity were determined using a NanoDrop ND-1000 spectrophotometer (NanoDrop Technologies, Wilmington, DE, USA). RNA integrity was determined by the Agilent 2100 bioanalyser (Agilent Technologies, Palo Alto, CA, USA). Whole mouse gene expression microarrays (Ilumina, BD-202-0202), containing over 25,600 unique probes and over 19,100 unique genes, were used to detect the gene expression profile each sample. The raw data obtained from all 24 samples were normalized by applying a background correction (using the 'normexp' algorithm) followed by normalization of intensity distributions within and between arrays (using the 'quantile' algorithm). The resulting data were imported into Partek Genomics Suite (Partek Inc., St. Louis, MO) and log2 transformed for statistical processing and hierarchical clustering analyses. Differential gene expression and hierarchical clustering were generated from comparison between 8 different groups, using one-way ANOVA. Differentially expressed genes were selected with a p value less than 0.01 and a fold of change of more than 2 when comparing between groups. Heat maps were generated by Partek Genomics Suite software. All raw and processed data files have been deposited in the National Center for Biotechnology Information Gene Expression Omnibus dataset.

Biological processes, functional classifications and gene annotations were analyzed using Partek Genomics Suite associated with Kyoto Encyclopedia of Genes and Genomes (KEGG) pathway database (updated December 2013), as well as database for Annotation, Visualization and Integrated Discovery (DAVID) (http://david.abcc.ncifcrf.gov). To identify biological processes with significant enrichment, the distribution of genes from our data was compared with a reference annotation gene list for each gene ontology (GO) category. Fisher exact P values were used for gene enrichment analysis. The value ranges from 0 to 1, where value equal to zero represents perfect enrichment. P value less than or equal to 0.05 is considered significantly enriched in the annotation categories.

Results

Targeted Cox-2 gene deletion in cartilage or mesenchyme results in impaired fracture healing

To establish Cre-recombinase mediated gene targeting efficiency and specificity, femoral fractures were created in two-month-old Prx1Cre; RosaR and Col2Cre; RosaR mice. Prior to fracture in intact bone, intense LacZ staining was identified in all limb mesenchymal lineages, including strong staining in the periosteum of Prx1Cre; RosaR mice (Fig. 1A&B). Bone marrow and muscle were largely negative for LacZ staining. Following fracture, LacZ staining was observed in mesenchyme, chondrocytes and osteoblasts throughout the fracture callus in Prx1Cre; RosaR mice at day 7, indicating efficient gene recombination in all limb mesenchymal lineages (Fig. 1C–F). In Col2Cre; RosaR fracture callus, strong LacZ staining was observed as early as day 5 post-fracture, primarily in chondrocytes along the periosteal surface and within the bone marrow cavity, where endochondral bone formation takes place (Fig. 1G&H). Mesenchymal progenitors (Fig. 1I) at the fracture junctions and osteoblasts (Fig. 1J) at the distal flanking region of the callus remained negative for LacZ staining.

Long bone length and cortical bone morphology were examined in Cox-2$^{f/f}$; Prx1Cre mice and their littermate controls. No significant differences in long bone length or cortical bone thickness could be determined between Cox-2$^{f/f}$ and Cox-2$^{f/f}$; Prx1Cre mice (Fig. S1), consistent with our previous findings in global Cox-2$^{-/-}$ mice [11]. Fracture healing was examined in both Cox-2$^{f/f}$; Prx1Cre and Cox-2$^{f/f}$; Col2Cre mice, along with gender and age-matched control Cre-negative Cox-2$^{f/f}$ mice. Micro-CT analyses showed delayed bony union in both Cox-2$^{f/f}$; Prx1Cre and Cox-2$^{f/f}$; Col2Cre mice at day 14 post-fracture (Fig. 2A–F). Quantitative and volumetric analyses demonstrated a 47% and a 25% reduction of new bone callus in Cox-2$^{f/f}$; Prx1Cre and Cox-2$^{f/f}$; Col2Cre mice, respectively (Fig. 2G). Evaluation of new bone callus from individual micro-CT-images suggested that 80% of Cre negative mice demonstrated mature union with formation of a complete bridging callus on day 14. In contrast, only 10% of Cox-2$^{f/f}$; Col2Cre mice showed mature union and none of the Cox-2$^{f/f}$; Prx1Cre mice showed any evidence of bony union at day 14 post-fracture.

Histologic analyses showed mature bridging callus at day 14 in the Cox-2$^{f/f}$ control mice of both groups, with only a small amount of residue cartilage present in the callus (Fig. 2H). In contrast, substantial amounts of cartilaginous tissue remained in the fracture callus of Cox-2$^{f/f}$; Col2Cre mice at day 14 (Fig. 2I). Cartilage conversion into bone was markedly reduced, yet intramembranous bone formation flanking the cartilaginous tissue (arrows in Fig. 2I) remained largely intact in these mice. Careful examination of the cartilaginous tissue showed that they were mostly mature chondrocytes (Fig. 2J) or less differentiated chondrocytes (Fig. 2K). In Cox-2$^{f/f}$; Prx1Cre fracture callus, where Cox-2 is deleted in mesenchymal progenitors, severe reduction of bone formation at the periosteal sites was evident (Fig. 2L). Extensive mesenchyme (Fig. 2M) and poorly differentiated cartilage tissue (Fig. 2N) were observed throughout the fracture callus. Histomorphometric analyses revealed marked differences in callus composition among the three groups of mice at day 14 post-fracture (Fig. 2K). Compared to the Cre-negative controls which contained 8% mesenchyme, 9.9% mature cartilage and 0% immature

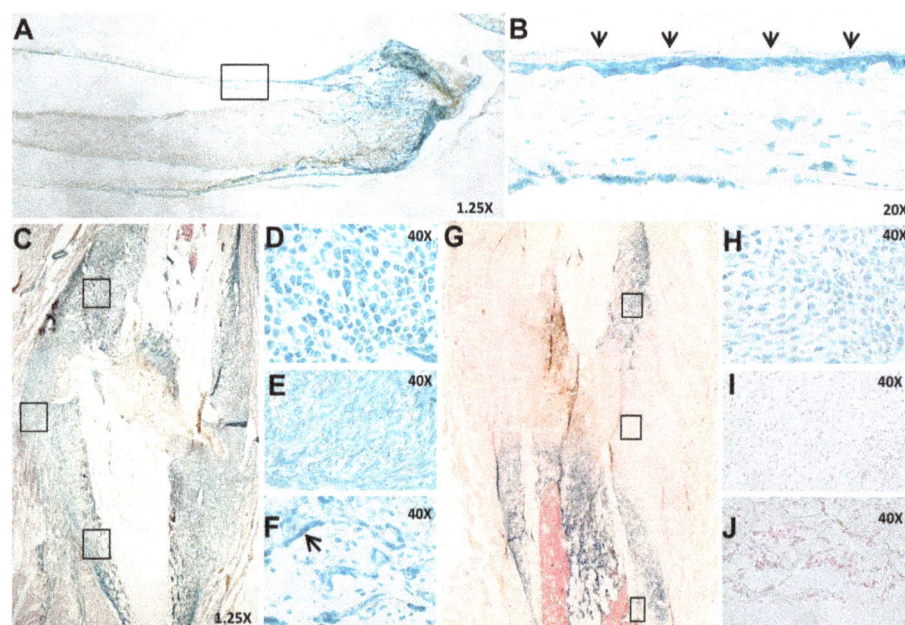

Figure 1. Efficient Prx1Cre- and Col2Cre-mediated targeted gene recombination in fracture callus. A tissue section from long bone of *Prx1Cre; RosaR* mice show intense LacZ staining in bone and cartilage, but not in bone marrow (A). The boxed region in A, shown at a higher magnification (20×), demonstrates LacZ staining in periosteum (arrows in B). Fracture callus at day 7 from *Prx1Cre; RosaR* shows intense LacZ staining throughout the callus region at the cortical bone junction (C). Boxed regions in C (from top to bottom), shown at a higher magnification (20×), illustrate effective gene recombination in chondrocytes (D), mesenchyme (E) and osteoblasts (arrows in F). *Col2Cre; RosaR* fracture callus at day 5 shows effective gene recombination in chondroprogenitors and chondrocytes, but not mesenchymal cells (G). Higher magnification images (20×) in the boxed region (from top to bottom) show positive LacZ staining in chondrocytes (H) but not in mesenchyme cells (I) or osteoblasts (J).

cartilage in the fracture callus, *Cox-2^{f/f}; Prx1Cre* mice had an average of 52% mesenchyme and 12% immature cartilage in the fracture callus (Fig. 2K, open bar, n = 10, p<0.05). As a result, the percentage of new bone formation in *Cox-2^{f/f}; Prx1Cre* mice was reduced by nearly 3-fold as compared to their Cre-negative controls. In *Cox-2^{f/f}; Col2Cre* callus, the percentage area of mesenchyme was increased to 25% of the total callus. However, unlike *Cox-2^{f/f}; Prx1Cre* callus, which was primarily occupied by mesenchyme and poorly differentiated cartilage, the *Cox-2^{f/f}; Col2Cre* callus had an average of 23% mature cartilage and 3% immature cartilage at the cortical bone junctions, leading to a 1.8-fold reduction of new bone formation in the fracture callus (Fig. 2K, gray bar, n = 10, p<0.05).

Cox-2 deficient periosteal progenitors exhibit impaired osteogenic and chondrogenic differentiation in cell culture

To further understand the role of Cox-2 in periosteum-mediated repair, PDMPCs were isolated from the periosteum of *Cox-2^{f/f}; Prx1Cre* mice and their Cre-negative littermate controls. Cox-2-deficient PDMPCs exhibited reduced ALP staining both at the basal level and following BMP-2 stimulation (Fig. 3A). Prx1Cre-mediated *Cox-2* gene deletion also markedly reduced *ALP, RUNX2, OSX* and *OCN* gene expression, both in untreated cultures and upon BMP-2 treatment (Fig. 3B). Western blot analyses demonstrated a modest, but statistically significant, induction of Cox-2 protein by BMP-2 treatment in control cells and the absence of Cox-2 protein in PDMPCs isolated from *Cox-2^{f/f}; Prx1Cre* mice (Fig. 3C). Quantification of Western blot data from three experiments demonstrates an average of ~1.5 fold induction of Cox-2 by BMP-2 in monolayer cultures from COX-

2^{ff} (wild type) mice and ~95% reduction of Cox-2 protein in the Cox-2^{f/f}; Prx1Cre cells (Fig. 3D).

Chondrogenesis and chondrocyte differentiation were examined in PDMPC micromass cultures (Fig. 4). Two time points that reflect chondrogenesis onset (day 1) and chondrocyte maturation (day7) were examined [22,23], in the presence and absence of BMP-2 treatment (n = 3 per group). In contrast to monolayer culture, Western blot analyses demonstrated that Cox-2 protein was markedly induced by BMP-2 in the high-density micromass cultures (Fig. 4A), suggesting Cox-2 as a BMP-2 responsive gene in chondrogenic conditions. The induction of Cox-2 expression by BMP-2 was further confirmed by RT-PCR analyses (Fig. S2); these data demonstrate robust induction of *Cox-2* mRNA expression in both day 1 and day 7 BMP-2 treated cultures. Prx1Cre-mediated *Cox-2* gene deletion decreased chondrogenesis and chondrocyte differentiation induced by BMP-2, as evidenced by reduced Alcian Blue staining (Fig. 4B), suppressed *SOX-9* expression at day 1 and further reduced expression of a set of chondrocyte marker gene expression at day 7 (Fig. 4C). Of note is that *Cox-2* gene deletion reduced BMP-2-induced *Col2a1* expression by 50%, but blocked the expression of BMP-2-induced chondrocyte maturation genes, namely *Col10a1, Ihh, MMP13* and *Col11a1* at day 7 (Fig. 3C), suggesting that mesenchymal cell-specific Cox-2 expression is required for both chondrogenesis and chondrocyte maturation and hypertrophy. Consistently, *ALP* and *OCN*, the bone marker genes associated with endochondral ossification, were similarly reduced in BMP-2-treated culture at day 7, demonstrating a key role of Cox-2 in mesenchymal differentiation.

To obtain a deeper understanding of the molecular regulation of osteogenic and chondrogenic differentiation of PDMPCs, gene expression microarray analyses were performed. These differential

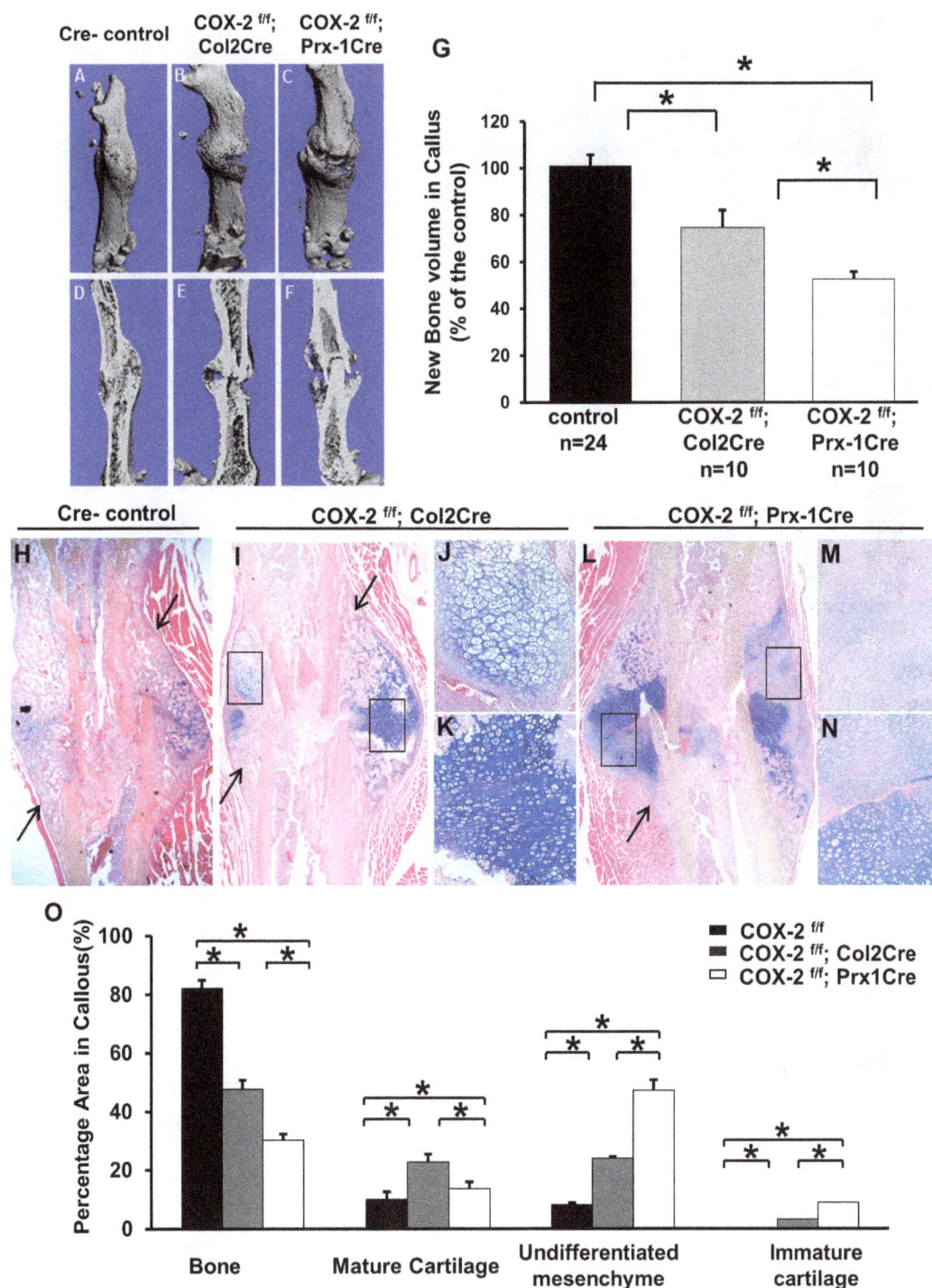

Figure 2. Targeted *Cox-2* gene deletion via Prx1Cre and Col2Cre impaired fracture healing. Representative micro-CT images of fracture callus at day 14 post-fracture in control *Cox-2^{f/f}* (A and D), *Cox-2^{f/f}; Col2Cre* (B and E) and *Cox-2^{f/f}; Prx1Cre* (C and F). Volumetric analyses demonstrate marked reduction of new bone formation in *Cox-2^{f/f}; Prx1Cre* and *Cox-2^{f/f}; Col2Cre* fracture callus (G). Representative histology sections of fracture callus at day 14 from control *Cox-2^{f/f}* (H), *Cox-2^{f/f}; Col2Cre* (I–K), and *Cox-2^{f/f}; Prx1Cre* (L–N) mice. Boxed regions in I show presence of mature (J) and under-differentiated chondrocytes (K) in *Cox-2^{f/f}; Col2Cre* fracture callus. Boxed regions in L show poorly differentiated mesenchyme (M) and immature cartilage (N) in *Cox-2^{f/f}; Prx1Cre* fracture callus. Arrows indicate regions of intramembraneous bone formation in H, I and L. Quantitative histomorphometric analyses show the composition of bone, cartilage and mesenchyme tissue in periosteal callus (K). Data are presented as means ± SEM, * p<0.05. n = 10.

gene profiling studies are directed at identifying Cox-2 mediated differences in gene expression in micromass cultures of *Cox-2^{f/f}; Prx1Cre* and *Cox-2^{f/f}* PDMPCs. In the absence of BMP-2 at day 1,

143 genes were found to be suppressed by 2-fold or more in the Cox-2 deficient cells as compared to the control PDMPCs. Biological GO enrichment analyses show functional cluster

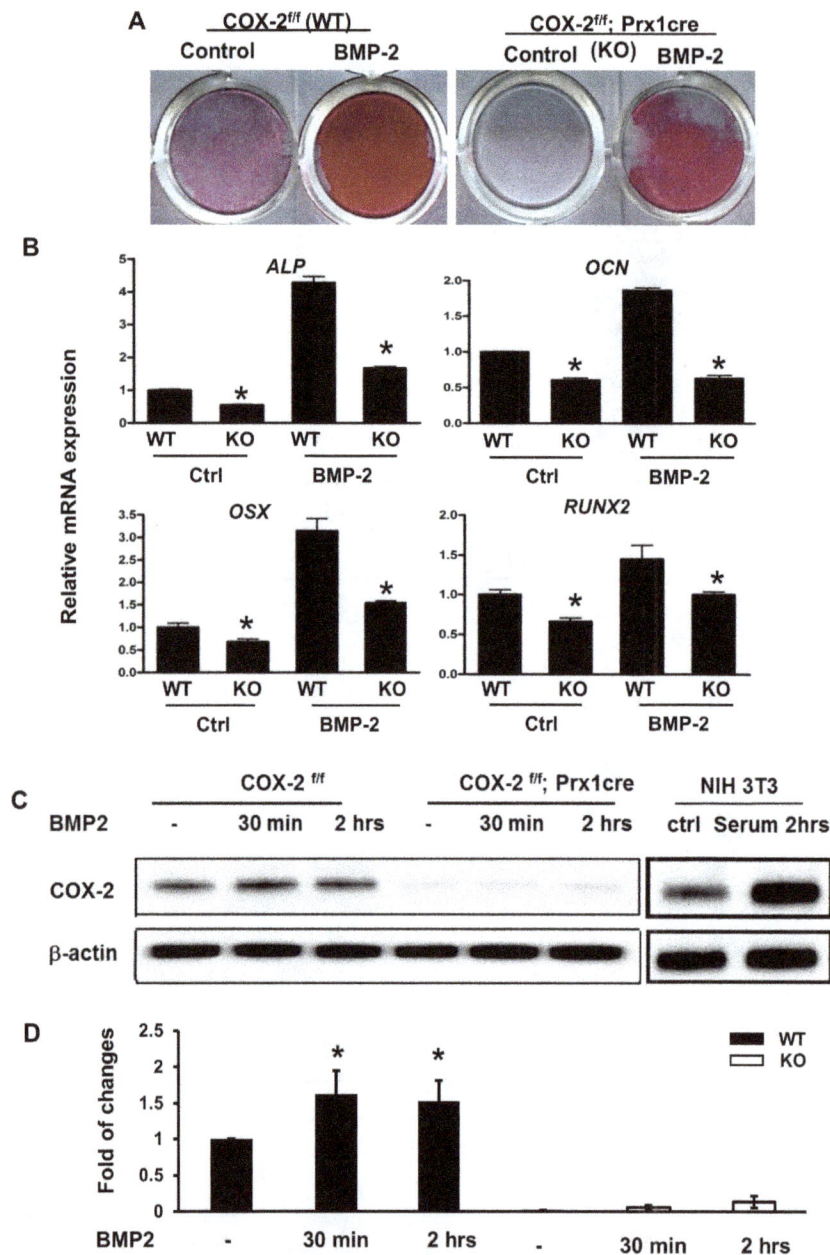

Figure 3. Osteogenic differentiation was impaired in Cox-2 deficient PDMPCs. Periosteal progenitors were isolated from *Cox-2^{f/f}* (WT) and *Cox-2^{f/f}; Prx1Cre* (KO) mice. Monolayer cultures demonstrate reduced differentiation of *Cox-2* deficient cells, both under basal conditions and in response to BMP-2 stimulation, as evidenced by reduced ALP staining (A) and decreased osteogenic gene expression at day 7 (B). * indicates p<0.05, as compared to the control. Western blot analyses demonstrate a modest induction of Cox-2 protein in WT cells and ablation of Cox-2 protein in Cox-2 deficient cells (C). Quantification of western blot analyses from three separate experiments shows induction of Cox-2 protein in WT cells and near absence of Cox-2 protein in the Prx-1Cre-mediated conditional KO cells (*, p<0.05).

categories of genes involved in bone development and ossification process (11 genes, p<4.0E-5), immune/inflammatory response (21 genes, p<8.2E-5), growth factor activity (7 genes, p<3.3E-4), Wnt pathway (6 genes, p<0.001) and morphogenesis of a branching structure (7 genes, p<0.005) (Table S1). Several known key regulators associated with bone/cartilage ossification and remodeling were significantly suppressed in the Cox-2 deficient cells, namely *Sox9* (2.7-fold), *Sp7 (OSX)* (2.2-fold), *MMP13* (4.5-fold), *MMP9* (4.8-fold), *RANKL (3.7-fold) and Vitamin D receptor (VDR)* (4.8-fold), suggesting reduced osteogenic/chondrogenic potential and bone/cartilage remodeling activity in Cox-2 deficient cells.

Following micromass culture for 7 days, PDMPCs underwent spontaneous differentiation to induce a series of genes critical for bone formation, namely *SP7* (5.1-fold), *BMP4* (23.5-fold), and *FGFR3* (4.3-fold), and *Osteocalcin* (4-fold). Among the genes associated with bone/cartilage development and ossification, we identified 25 genes that were significantly suppressed at day 7 in the Cox-2 deficient cells (Fig. S3B), providing further evidence to show the disruption of bone morphogenetic pathway in micromass culture as a consequence of targeted *Cox-2* gene deletion in PDMPCs.

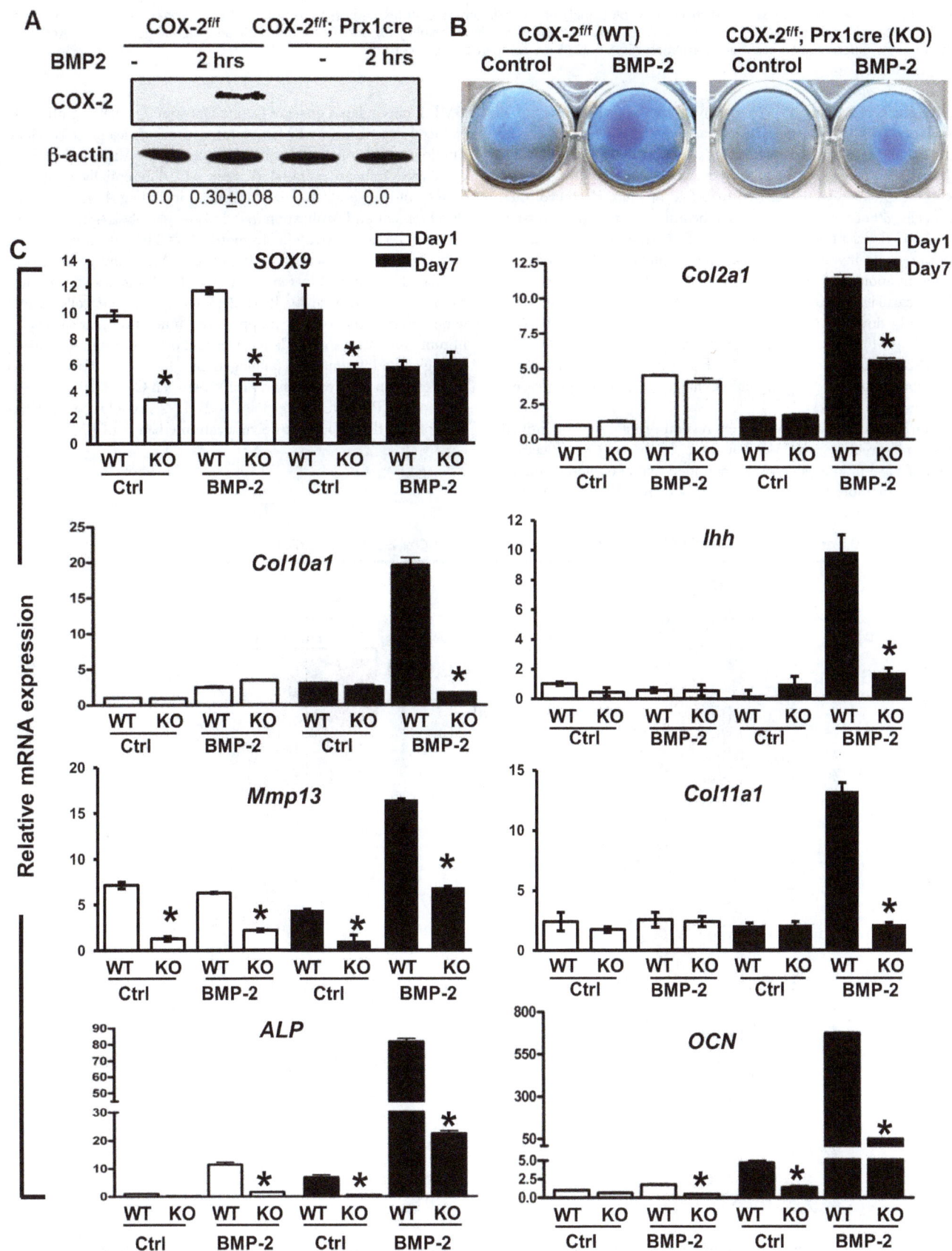

Figure 4. Chondrogenic differentiation was impaired in periosteal progenitors from mice with a targeted *Cox-2* gene deletion. Periosteal mesenchymal progenitors were isolated from *Cox-2^{f/f}* (WT) and *Cox-2^{f/f}; Prx1Cre* (KO) periosteum. Western blot analyses demonstrated marked Cox-2 induction by BMP-2 in WT cells and absence of Cox-2 protein in Cox-2 deficient cells. Numbers at the bottom of the image show

normalized density ratio of each lane in western blot analyses (A). Micromass cultures demonstrate impaired chondrogenesis and chondrocyte differentiation in KO cells at day 1 and day 7, as indicated by Alcian Blue staining (B) and Real Time PCR analyses of genes associated with chondrocyte differentiation and bone formation (C). * p<0.05, as compared to the control.

To further identify BMP responsive genes whose expression is mediated by COX-2, we separately analyzed the gene profiling in control and Cox-2 deficient PDMPCs at day 1 and day 7 following BMP-2 treatment. At day 1, among 193 BMP-2-responsive genes whose expression were changed by 2-fold or more in control *Cox-2^{f/f}* cells, 30 of these genes had significantly suppressed expression in Cox-2 deficient cells in response to BMP-2. These 30 genes are known to be involved in regulation of cellular proliferation and differentiation and in developmental process associated with bone/cartilage formation (Fig. 5A). Among genes that were markedly down-regulated by one day of exposure to BMP-2 in *Cox-2^{f/f}* (WT) cells, 20 of those genes were less down-regulated by BMP-2 in *Cox-2* deficient cells (Fig. 5B). These genes were functionally mapped to annotation categories of immune process and response to stress.

Markedly differences in gene expression profiles were identified in samples treated with BMP-2 at day 7. In control *Cox-2^{f/f}* cells, a total of 1183 unique genes were identified that exhibited a change of 2-fold or more following BMP-2 treatment (Fig. S4A). Among

BMP-2 upregulated genes, 447 unique transcripts had significantly reduced expression in BMP-2-treated *Cox-2* deficient cells. Gene ontology (GO) enrichment analyses using DAVID and Partek-associated software annotated these 449 differentially expressed genes into several major categories, including bone/cartilage development and ossification (p = 2.0E-8), glycolysis/gluconeogenesis (p = 7.1E-7), extracellular matrix (p = 3.0E-10), angiogenesis and vessel development (p<0.01) (Table 1). Among genes downregulated by BMP-2 in *Cox-2^{f/f}* WT cells, 208 genes showed less suppressed expression by BMP-2 in *Cox-2* deficient cells. These genes were functionally mapped to annotation categories of immune system response, leukocytes and osteoclast differentiation, biological adhesion, and angiogenesis (Table 1). The marked differences in gene expression profile between Cox-2 deficient cells and control PDMPCs in response to BMP-2 strongly suggest Cox-2 as one of the important downstream mediators of BMP-2.

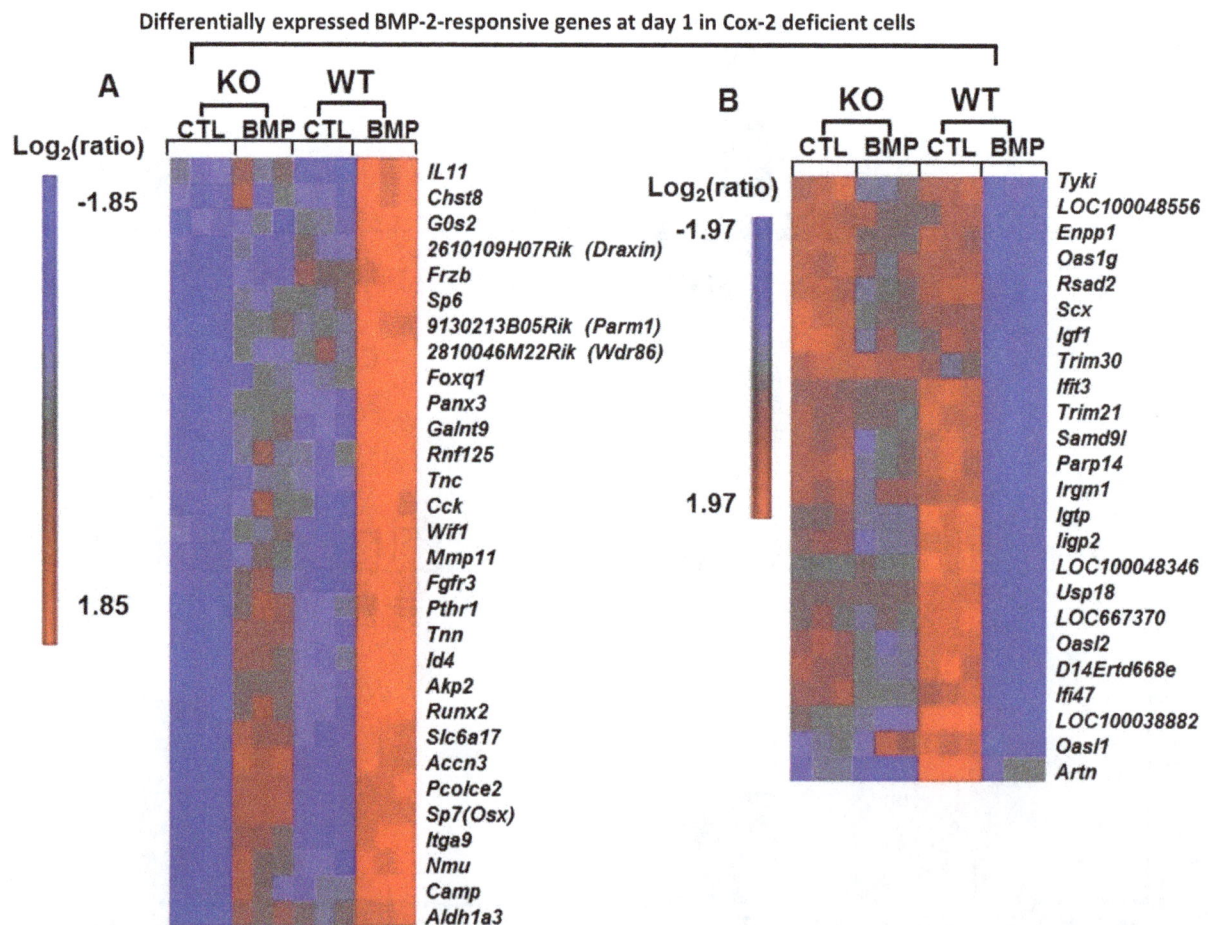

Figure 5. Differentially down- and up-regulated genes in *Cox-2^{f/f}* and *Cox-2^{f/f}; Prx1Cre* PDMPCs in response to BMP-2. Heat map showing differential expression of 30 BMP-2-upregulated genes (A) and 24 BMP-2-downregulated genes (B) in Cox-2^{f/f} (WT) in micromass cultures at day 1 and their corresponding expression levels in BMP-2 treated *Cox-2^{f/f}; Prx1Cre* (KO) micromass cultures. Each column shows the relative gene expression of a sample for the indicated pathway-associated genes. Gene up-regulation is presented in red and gene down-regulation is in blue.

Table 1. Go classification of the differentially expressed genes in Cox-2 deficient cells at day 7 in response to BMP-2.

Functional classification	Fisher exact p value	Genes included in the group
Upregulated by BMP-2 in WT, significantly suppressed in KO (447 genes)		
Bone/cartilage development process (ossification)	2.0E-8	39
Glycolysis/gluconeogenesis	7.1E-7	14
Extracellular matrix	3.0E-10	27
Angiogenesis and vessel development	<0.01	24
Down-regulated by BMP-2 in WT, significantly less regulated in KO (208 genes)		
Immune system response	3.0E-5	42
Leukocytes and osteoclasts differentiation	9.6E-4	13
Biological adhesion	6.3E-3	15
angiogenesis	<0.01	14

The table lists major functional categories enriched by DAVID using differentially expressed, BMP-2 up-regulated or down-regulated genes following seven days of culture in the presence or absence of BMP-2. Fisher exact P values for the gene-enrichment categories were generated by DAVID. "Genes included in the group" indicate the number of genes enriched for that category from the input gene list.

Enriched biological pathway analyses demonstrate dysregulation of the HIF1, PI3K-AKT and Wnt pathways in Cox-2 deficient PDMPCs

The genes differentially expressed in *Cox-2$^{f/f}$* and *Cox-2$^{f/f}$; Prx1Cre* PDMPCs at day 1 and day 7 in the presence and absence of BMP-2 were further analyzed using the KEGG pathway database available in the Partek Genomic Suite. The main signaling pathways dysregulated by the absence of Cox-2 are the PI3K-AKT, HIF-1 and Wnt pathways. At day 1, genes annotated to the PI3K-AKT pathway, whose expression were suppressed in *Cox-2* deficient cells in the presence of BMP-2, include *FGFR2* (1.4-fold, p<0.01), *FGFR3* (2.6-fold, p<0.01), *Itga9 (1.6fold, p< 0.01), Tnc (2.4-fold, p<0.01), Tnn (2.2fold, p<0.01)*. At day 7, 34 of the annotated PI3K-AKT pathway genes had significantly altered expression in *Cox-2* deficient cells; eight of these genes were down-regulated, relative to wild-type cells, in the absence of any treatment and 26 of these genes were down-regulated, relative to wild type cells, following BMP-2 treatment (Fig. 6, top panel A).

Additional remarkable changes identified in Cox-2 deficient PDMPCs were the altered gene expressions annotated to the hypoxia inducible factor 1 (HIF-1) pathway. Among 41 HIF-1 pathway genes identified from control *Cox-2$^{f/f}$* cells at day 7, 24 genes showed altered expression in the Cox-2 deficient cells (Fig. 6. top panel B). Real-time PCR analyses further confirmed the suppressed expression of several key genes of the HIF-1 pathway, namely *EGLN1, EGLN3, VEGFA, ANGPT4* and *HIF-1a* in Cox-2 deficient cells day 7 (Fig. 6C). These data indicate strongly a key role for Cox-2 in modulating HIF-1 pathway activation in PDMPCs.

Wnt pathway genes were also enriched among the genes differentially expressed between *Cox-2$^{f/f}$* and *Cox-2$^{f/f}$; Prx1Cre* PDMPCs at days 1 and 7. Several well-documented Wnt pathway inhibitory genes involved in bone metabolism were significantly suppressed at basal level in Cox-2$^{f/f}$; Prx1Cre PDMPCs at day 1 in micromass culture, including *Prickle1, Cdh2, Frzb, Sfrp1 and 2* (Fig. 7A). At day 7, 28 Wnt pathway-associated genes were suppressed in untreated cultures or following BMP-2 treatment. The altered genes included Wnt pathway receptors, as well as positive and negative regulators of the Wnt signaling pathway (Fig. 7B). Real-time PCR analyses further confirmed the altered expression of several key Wnt pathway associated genes in Cox-2$^{f/f}$;

Prx1Cre PDMPCs, namely, *Wif-1, N-cadherin, LRP4, FRZB, and TCF7* (Fig. 7C).

Discussion

During fracture healing mesenchymal progenitors residing in periosteum undergo osteogenic and chondrogenic differentiation to induce intramembranous and endochondral bone formation. To understand the spatiotemporal control of periosteal mesenchymal progenitor cell differentiation during repair and regeneration, we specifically deleted the *Cox2* gene in mesenchyme via Prx1cre or in cartilage via Col2Cre. Our studies show that Cox-2 acts at the early mesenchyme differentiation stage and mediates both osteogenic and chondrogenic differentiation of PDMPC during repair. Targeted *Cox-2* deletion via Prx1Cre in mesenchyme disrupted the entire differentiation program of mesenchyme progenitors, leading to reduction of bone formation and accretion of mesenchyme and immature cartilage in the callus (Figure 1). By contrast, targeted *Cox-2* deletion via *Col2Cre* expression in cartilage impaired fracture healing primarily by disrupting chondrocyte maturation, vascular invasion and endochondral bone formation. Consistent with the *in vivo* observation, cell differentiation and gene profiling analyses showed that *Prx1Cre*-mediated *Cox-2* deletion blunted osteogenic PDMPC differentiation, attenuated chondrogenesis and blocked BMP-2-induced chondrocyte maturation and terminal differentiation. Our data are consistent with the previous observation which demonstrates a marked induction of *Cox-2* mRNA at the onset of endochondral and intramembranous repair in early fracture callus [14,15], further providing direct evidence for a unique spatiotemporal role of Cox-2 in osteogenic and chondrogenic differentiation of periosteal progenitor cells in bone repair and regeneration.

To obtain mechanistic information underlying impaired fracture healing in Cox-2 deficient mice, we utilized a previously established method which allows isolation and *in vitro* analyses of mesenchymal progenitors derived from autografted periosteal callus (PDMPCs) [17,18,24]. This procedure permits robust isolation and recovery of otherwise limiting cell populations for biochemical and molecular analyses. By analyzing the differentiation potential and gene profiling of PDMPCs obtained directly from the healing site, we demonstrated that Cox-2 deficient cells exhibited decreased osteogenic and chondrogenic differentiation

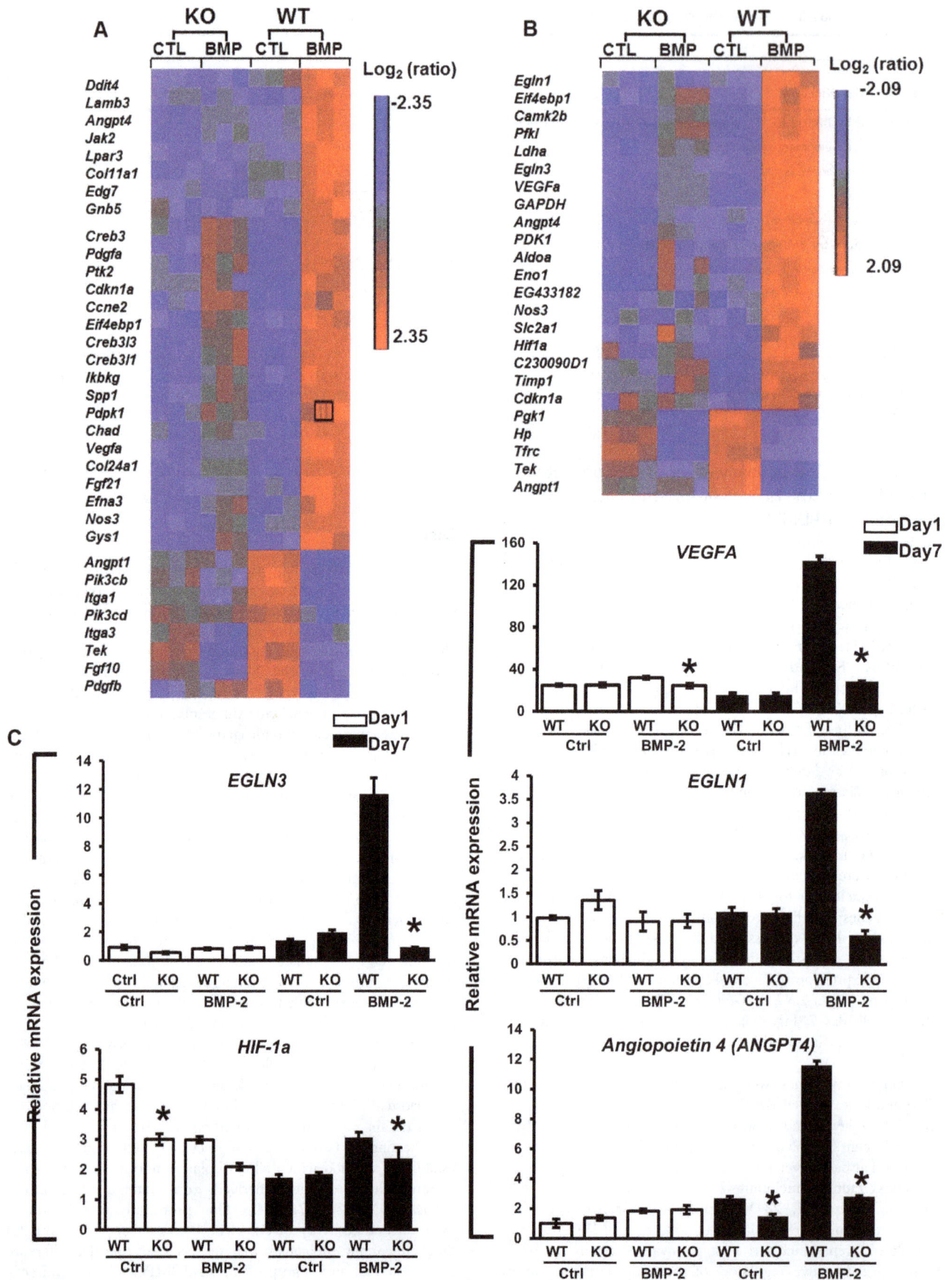

Figure 6. Dysregulation of the PI3K/AKT and HIF-1pathways in Cox-2 deficient PDMPCs. Heat maps showing differentially expressed genes associated with the PI3K/AKT (A) and the HIF-1 pathway (B) in micromass cultures in the presence and absence of BMP-2 for seven days. Each column shows the relative gene expression of a sample for the indicated pathway-associated genes. RT-PCR analyses further quantitate the values for the key genes in the HIF-1 pathway at day 1 (white bars) and day 7 (black bars) (C), namely VEGFA, EGLN1, EGLN3, HIF-1α and ANGPT4. * p<0.05, as compared to the control.

potential under basal culture conditions, for both monolayer and micromass culture. Gene profiling analyses revealed significant down-regulation in Cox-2 deficient cells of a set of key genes that control bone/cartilage ossification and remodeling as compared to the wild type controls; the genes Sox9, Sp7 (OSX), MMP13, MMP9, RANKL and VDR. The reduced expression of this key set of genes in Cox-2 deficient mesenchymal progenitors is likely to explain the impaired bone formation and delayed cartilage remodeling observed in the Cox-2 mutant mice at the onset of fracture healing, indicating that the differentiation of the mesenchymal progenitors depends on Cox-2 expression during initiation of healing. The data are consistent with the anabolic effects of prostaglandins, e.g. prostaglandin E2 (PGE2) in stimulating bone formation and bone/cartilage remodeling in repair [15,25–27], underscoring a direct role of Cox-2 from cells of mesenchymal lineages in modulating expression of this key set of genes in repair and regeneration. In addition to the altered gene expression associated with bone formation, GO analyses also identified functional gene clusters (Table S1) that regulate immune and inflammatory responses, suggesting that Cox-2 deletion in mesenchymal progenitors could further modify immune response and change local inflammatory microenvironments at the onset of bone healing [28,29].

By analyzing PDMPC differentiation in response to BMP-2 treatment, our study demonstrated a key role of Cox-2 in BMP-2-induced mesenchymal differentiation. BMP-2 is known for its strong osteo-inductive and chondro-inductive actions on mesenchymal progenitors in vivo and in vitro [30]. Recent studies have further established BMP-2 as a critical gene in the initiation of bone fracture repair [31]. Similar to Cox-2, BMP-2 deletion via Prx1Cre produces minimal effects on embryonic long bone development (23). However, postnatal deletion of the BMP-2 gene in periosteum impairs chondrogenic and osteogenic differentiation of mesenchymal progenitor cells and impedes periosteum-mediated endochondral and intramembranous bone formation [17,32]. While we observed modest Cox-2 protein induction in monolayer cultures, both Cox-2 protein and mRNA were markedly induced by BMP-2 in micromass cultures, suggesting a key role of Cox-2 in BMP-2 mediated chondrogenic differentiation of PDMPCs. Prx1Cre-mediated Cox-2 deletion further attenuated BMP-2-induced osteogenic differentiation in monolayer culture and completely blocked chondrocyte maturation and terminal differentiation in micromass culture. These data speak directly to the mechanism by which BMP-2 mediates bone differentiation, and establishes Cox-2 as a critical downstream mediator of BMP-2 action, demonstrating an important role of the BMP-2/Cox-2 axis in control of chondrogenic and osteogenic differentiation of mesenchymal progenitors in postnatal bone tissue repair.

By using GO pathway enrichment analyses, we identified the phosphoinositide 3-kinase/protein kinase B (PI3K/AKT), Hypoxia Inducible Factor-1 (HIF-1) and the Wnt pathway as key signaling pathways targeted by Cox-2 in BMP-2-induced PDMPC differentiation. The PI3K/AKT pathway crosstalks with a number of signaling pathways, including BMP/TGFβ signaling pathway, mTOR, NF-κb, JAK/STAT, MAPK, CREB, P53 and VEGF, which are known for their roles in stem/progenitor cell proliferation, osteoblast and chondrocyte differentiation, apoptosis

and angiogenesis [33–35]. The PI3K/AKT pathway also plays a role in regulating glycolysis and gluconeogenesis processes [36,37], which are markedly affected by Cox-2 deletion (Table 1). A link between Cox-2 and the PI3K/AKT pathway has recently been reported in mouse and human osteoblasts [38]. Downregulation of COX-2 via gene silencing suppresses phosphorylation of AKT and PTEN. Interestingly, PGE2, one of the potential downstream products resulting from cyclooxygenase activity, failed to reverse COX-2-dependent AKT phosphorylation, suggesting a potential PGE2 independent mechanism(s) in BMP-2/COX-2/PI3K/AKT-mediated regulation of cell differentiation.

The HIF-1 pathway plays a central role in cellular response to hypoxic condition and is essential for bone/cartilage development and chondrocyte survival [39]. The HIF-1 pathway is also critically important in bone repair and regeneration [40,41]. While a direct link between HIF-1 pathway and Cox-2-mediated repair remains to be established, hypoxia regulates PGE2 release in osteoblasts [42,43] and COX-2/PGE2 signalling is involved in a hypoxia-induced angiogenic response in endothelial cells [44].The central player of HIF-1 pathway is HIF-1α, which is regulated at the post-transcriptional level by the HIF prolyl-hydroxylase domain enzymes (PHDs) (gene name: Egl nine homologs, Eglns). Eglns hydroxylate the α-subunit of HIF-1α, enabling binding of the von Hippel-Lindau (VHL) protein for poly-ubiquitination, which ultimately leads to proteolytic proteasomal degradation of HIF-1α [45,46]. In our current study, HIF-1α expression was only modest regulated during chondrogenic differentiation. However, the HIF prolyl-hydroxylase domain enzymes Egln1 and Egln3 were markedly induced by BMP-2 in PDMPCs at day 7, and this induction was abolished in the Cox-2 deficient cells. The data suggest a requirement for Cox-2 expression in BMP-2 induction of Egln1 and 3, and their likely subsequent involvement in chondrocyte differentiation, vascular invasion and endochondral bone formation. In addition to Egln1 and Egln3, a subset of genes associated with hypoxia, angiogenesis and vasculogenesis, namely VEGFA and Angiopoietin 4 (ANGPT4), Ddit4, Eif4ebp1, Camk2b, Pfkl, Ldha, Aldoa, PDK1, Slc2a1 were also markedly suppressed in Cox-2 deficient PDMPCs (Fig. 6B). These data suggest a central role for Cox-2 from mesenchymal lineage in coordinating osteogenesis and angiogenesis in response to hypoxia during endochondral bone repair.

The Wnt pathway is known to play key roles in bone and cartilage development [47]. Canonical Wnt pathway activation favors osteoblastic differentiation, but inhibits chondrogenesis [48,49]. Activation of β-catenin signaling further stimulates chondrocyte hypertrophy and vascular invasion [50]. Although detailed molecular actions of the Wnt pathway on different phases of endochondral bone repair remain to be determined, genetic manipulation of Wnt signaling in mice demonstrates that inhibition of Wnt/β-catenin expression suppresses early chondrogenesis but favors osteogenesis, leading to accelerated but reduced fracture repair [51–53]. In our current study, we noted that Cox-2 inactivation in PDMPCs down regulated a group of genes that are classified as negative regulators of the canonical Wnt pathway; e.g., N-cadherin, FRZB and Sfrps, along with Sox9 at day 1 (Fig. 7A) Contrary to accelerated repair observed in a Wnt/β-catenin gain-of-function mouse model, Cox-2 deficiency is associated with a

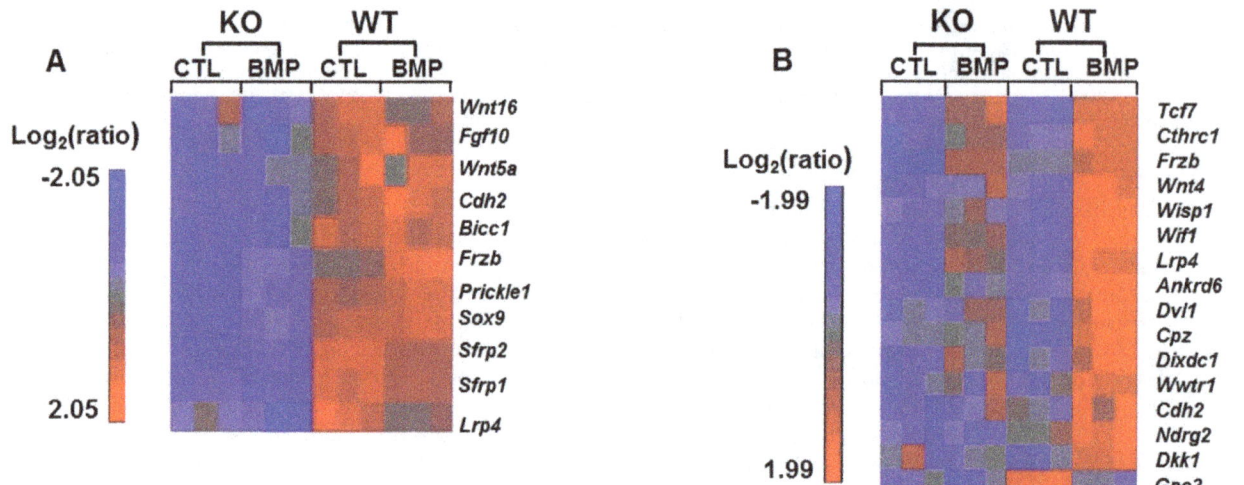

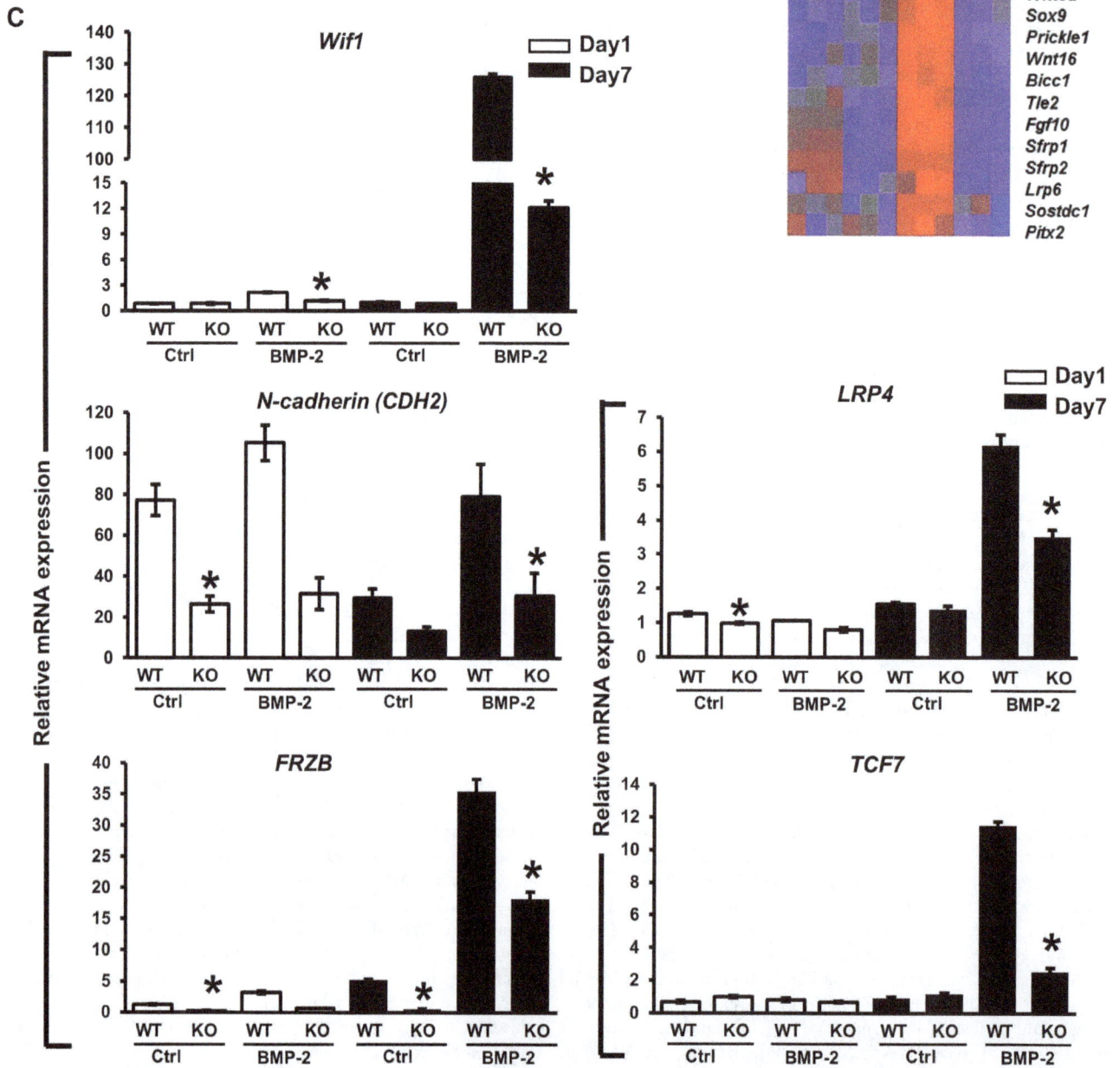

Figure 7. Deferentially expressed genes associated with the Wnt pathway in Cox-2$^{f/f}$ and Cox-2$^{f/f}$; Prx1Cre PDMPCs. Heat maps showing differentially expressed genes associated with the Wnt pathway at day 1 (A) and day 7 (B) micromass cultures. Each column shows the relative gene expression of a sample for the indicated Wnt pathway-associated genes. RT-PCR demonstrates expression of key genes in the Wnt pathway at day 1 (white bars) and day 7 (black bars) in cells with a targeted *Cox-2* gene deletion and in their littermate controls (C), namely *Wif1*, *N-cadherin (CDH2)*, *LRP4*, *FRZB*, and *TCF7*. * p<0.05, as compared to the control.

marked reduction of osteogenesis *in vitro* and *in vivo*, indicating that Cox-2 orchestrates a complex signaling interplay in conjunction with Wnt pathway regulators during repair and regeneration.

NSAIDs (non-steroidal anti-inflammatory drugs) which often inhibit both Cox-1 and Cox-2 are well known as having a negative effect on fracture healing in rat models [54,55]. Prolonged use of targeted Cox-2 inhibitors delays fracture healing in rats [13]. Transient inhibition of Cox-2 has small and reversible effects on fracture healing, suggesting that the adverse effect of Cox-2 inhibition may be both dosage and duration dependent [56,57]. Pharmacological inhibition of Cox-2 activity is also reported to have an inhibitory effect on differentiation of human and mouse mesenchymal stem cells [58,59]. Pharmacological studies are often confounded by dosing issue, specificity and the potential off-targeting effects of the drug. Using a gene targeting approach, our current study moves the field forward, we believe, by identifying cells that are likely to be the specific (or a specific) cell type in which COX-2 expression plays a modulatory role in fracture repair, and demonstrates the consequences of targeted Cox-2 gene deletion on fracture repair *in vivo*.

In summary, using cell-type specific *Cox-2* gene deletion, we demonstrate a spatial and temporal role for Cox-2 function in endochondral and intramembranous bone repair; targeted *Cox-2* gene deletion inhibits BMP-2-induced osteogenic, chondrogenic and angiogenic responses in periosteum-derived mesenchymal progenitors. Gene profiling analyses uncovered Cox-2-targeted pathways, e.g., the HIF-1, PI3K/AKT and Wnt pathways that modulate periosteal progenitor cell differentiation in bone fracture repair and regeneration. Identification of critical genes/targets in periosteal-derived mesenchymal progenitor cell differentiation could assist in identification of novel drug targets, facilitating development of new therapeutic solutions for bone repair and regeneration.

Supporting Information

Figure S1 Cox-2$^{f/f}$; Prx1cre mice have normal long bone length and cortical bone morphology. Quantitative measurements show identical length (A) and cortical thickness (B) in tibias of two-month-old Cox-2$^{f/f}$ and Cox-2$^{f/f}$; Prx1Cre mice. Data are presented as means ± SEM, n = 6.

Figure S2 *Cox-2* mRNA expression in day 1 and day 7 micromass cultures. Real Time PCR analyses show robust induction of Cox-2 gene expression by BMP-2 in micromass culture. Cox-2 mRNA was reduced by more than 95% in the Cox-2$^{f/f}$; Prx1Cre cells isolated from periosteal callus. * p<0.05, as compared to the control.

Figure S3 Comparison of Cox-2$^{f/f}$ (WT) and Cox-2$^{f/f}$; Prx1cre PDMPC gene expression profiles at day 1 vs. day 7 identified 1159

differentially expressed genes that exhibited a change of 2 fold or more. Hierarchical clustering analyses were used to generate the heat maps showing expression of these genes in Cox-2$^{f/f}$ (WT) and Cox-2$^{f/f}$; prx1cre (KO) cells at day 1 and 7 (A). Subsets of genes (111genes) associated with bone/cartilage formation and mineralization in Cox-2$^{f/f}$ and Cox-2$^{f/f}$; prx1cre cells at day 1 and 7 are further illustrated in the heat maps generated by hierarchical clustering analyses (B). The suppressed genes in Cox-2$^{f/f}$; prx1cre (KO) cells as compared to the Cox-2$^{f/f}$ (WT) cells at day 7 are listed in no particular order at the bottom. Gene up-regulation is presented in red and gene down-regulation is in blue.

Figure S4 Heat map showing expression of 1183 BMP-2 responsive genes in Cox-2$^{f/f}$ (WT) and Cox-2$^{f/f}$; prx1cre cells (KO) at day 7 (A). Among them, 181 unique probes associated with bone/cartilage formation and mineralization in Cox-2$^{f/f}$ (WT) and Cox-2$^{f/f}$; prx1cre (KO) cells were subjected to hierarchical clustering analyses to generate a heat map (B). Thirty-nine genes representing significantly suppressed genes in the KO cells at basal level or following BMP-2 treatment are listed at bottom without particular order. Gene up-regulation is presented in red and gene down-regulation is in blue.

Table S1 Go classification of the differentially expressed genes in Cox-2 deficient cells at day 1 without any treatment. Table S1 lists major functional categories enriched by DAVID using differentially expressed genes in Cox-2 deficient cells at day 1 without BMP-2 treatment. Genes suppressed or increased by 2 fold or more in the absence of Cox-2 were separately analyzed. Fisher exact P values for the gene-enrichment categories were generated from a reference gene list provided by Partek Genomic Suite software. "Genes included in the group" indicate the number of genes enriched for that category from the input gene list.

Table S2 Additional RT-PCR primers used for RT-PCR analyses in this study are listed.

Acknowledgments

We thank Ryan Tierry, Sarah Mack and Nehal for their assistance with histological work and Michael Thullen for microCT analyses.

Author Contributions

Conceived and designed the experiments: XPZ RJO. Performed the experiments: CH MX HC JJ. Analyzed the data: CH XPZ HRH. Contributed reagents/materials/analysis tools: HRH. Wrote the paper: XPZ HRH.

References

1. Eyre-Brook AL (1984) The periosteum: its function reassessed. Clin Orthop Relat Res: 300–307.

2. Malizos KN, Papatheodorou LK (2005) The healing potential of the periosteum molecular aspects. Injury 36 Suppl 3: S13–19.

3. McKibbin B (1978) The biology of fracture healing in long bones. J Bone Joint Surg Br 60-B: 150–162.

4. Colnot C, Zhang X, Knothe Tate ML (2012) Current insights on the regenerative potential of the periosteum: molecular, cellular, and endogenous engineering approaches. J Orthop Res 30: 1869–1878.

5. Barnes GL, Kostenuik PJ, Gerstenfeld LC, Einhorn TA (1999) Growth factor regulation of fracture repair. J Bone Miner Res 14: 1805–1815.

6. Gerstenfeld LC, Cullinane DM, Barnes GL, Graves DT, Einhorn TA (2003) Fracture healing as a post-natal developmental process: molecular, spatial, and temporal aspects of its regulation. J Cell Biochem 88: 873–884.

7. Zuscik MJ, Hilton MJ, Zhang X, Chen D, O'Keefe RJ (2008) Regulation of chondrogenesis and chondrocyte differentiation by stress. J Clin Invest 118: 429–438.

8. Smith WL, Langenbach R (2001) Why there are two cyclooxygenase isozymes. J Clin Invest 107: 1491–1495.

9. Agarwal S, Reddy GV, Reddanna P (2009) Eicosanoids in inflammation and cancer: the role of COX-2. Expert Rev Clin Immunol 5: 145–165.

10. Morham SG, Langenbach R, Loftin CD, Tiano HF, Vouloumanos N, et al. (1995) Prostaglandin synthase 2 gene disruption causes severe renal pathology in the mouse. Cell 83: 473–482.

11. Robertson G, Xie C, Chen D, Awad H, Schwarz EM, et al. (2006) Alteration of femoral bone morphology and density in COX-2–/– mice. Bone 39: 767–772.

12. Zhang X, Schwarz EM, Young DA, Puzas JE, Rosier RN, et al. (2002) Cyclooxygenase-2 regulates mesenchymal cell differentiation into the osteoblast lineage and is critically involved in bone repair. J Clin Invest 109: 1405–1415.

13. Simon AM, Manigrasso MB, O'Connor JP (2002) Cyclo-oxygenase 2 function is essential for bone fracture healing. J Bone Miner Res 17: 963–976.

14. Naik AA, Xie C, Zuscik MJ, Kingsley P, Schwarz EM, et al. (2009) Reduced COX-2 expression in aged mice is associated with impaired fracture healing. J Bone Miner Res 24: 251–264.

15. Xie C, Liang B, Xue M, Lin AS, Loiselle A, et al. (2009) Rescue of impaired fracture healing in COX-2–/– mice via activation of prostaglandin E2 receptor subtype 4. Am J Pathol 175: 772–785.

16. Lau KH, Kothari V, Das A, Zhang XB, Baylink DJ (2013) Cellular and molecular mechanisms of accelerated fracture healing by COX2 gene therapy: studies in a mouse model of multiple fractures. Bone 53: 369–381.

17. Wang Q, Huang C, Xue M, Zhang X (2011) Expression of endogenous BMP-2 in periosteal progenitor cells is essential for bone healing. Bone 48: 524–532.

18. Wang Q, Huang C, Zeng F, Xue M, Zhang X (2010) Activation of the Hh pathway in periosteum-derived mesenchymal stem cells induces bone formation in vivo: implication for postnatal bone repair. Am J Pathol 177: 3100–3111.

19. Ishikawa TO, Herschman HR (2006) Conditional knockout mouse for tissue-specific disruption of the cyclooxygenase-2 (Cox-2) gene. Genesis 44: 143–149.

20. Bonnarens F, Einhorn TA (1984) Production of a standard closed fracture in laboratory animal bone. J Orthop Res 2: 97–101.

21. Zhang X, Xie C, Lin AS, Ito H, Awad H, et al. (2005) Periosteal progenitor cell fate in segmental cortical bone graft transplantations: implications for functional tissue engineering. J Bone Miner Res 20: 2124–2137.

22. Wang Y, Belflower RM, Dong YF, Schwarz EM, O'Keefe RJ, et al. (2005) Runx1/AML1/Cbfa2 mediates onset of mesenchymal cell differentiation toward chondrogenesis. J Bone Miner Res 20: 1624–1636.

23. Zhang X, Ziran N, Goater JJ, Schwarz EM, Puzas JE, et al. (2004) Primary murine limb bud mesenchymal cells in long-term culture complete chondrocyte differentiation: TGF-beta delays hypertrophy and PGE2 inhibits terminal differentiation. Bone 34: 809–817.

24. Huang C, Tang M, Yehling E, Zhang X (2013) Overexpressing Sonic Hedgehog Peptide Restores Periosteal Bone Formation in a Murine Bone Allograft Transplantation Model. Mol Ther.

25. Paralkar VM, Borovecki F, Ke HZ, Cameron KO, Lefker B, et al. (2003) An EP2 receptor-selective prostaglandin E2 agonist induces bone healing. Proc Natl Acad Sci U S A 100: 6736–6740.

26. Ninomiya T, Hosoya A, Hiraga T, Koide M, Yamaguchi K, et al. (2011) Prostaglandin E(2) receptor EP(4)-selective agonist (ONO-4819) increases bone formation by modulating mesenchymal cell differentiation. Eur J Pharmacol 650: 396–402.

27. Li X, Pilbeam CC, Pan L, Breyer RM, Raisz LG (2002) Effects of prostaglandin E2 on gene expression in primary osteoblastic cells from prostaglandin receptor knockout mice. Bone 30: 567–573.

28. Zhang Q, Shi S, Liu Y, Uyanne J, Shi Y, et al. (2009) Mesenchymal stem cells derived from human gingiva are capable of immunomodulatory functions and ameliorate inflammation-related tissue destruction in experimental colitis. J Immunol 183: 7787–7798.

29. Yaqub S, Tasken K (2008) Role for the cAMP-protein kinase A signaling pathway in suppression of antitumor immune responses by regulatory T cells. Crit Rev Oncog 14: 57–77.

30. Riley EH, Lane JM, Urist MR, Lyons KM, Lieberman JR (1996) Bone morphogenetic protein-2: biology and applications. Clin Orthop: 39–46.

31. Tsuji K, Bandyopadhyay A, Harfe BD, Cox K, Kakar S, et al. (2006) BMP2 activity, although dispensable for bone formation, is required for the initiation of fracture healing. Nat Genet 38: 1424–1429.

32. Chappuis V, Gamer L, Cox K, Lowery JW, Bosshardt DD, et al. (2012) Periosteal BMP2 activity drives bone graft healing. Bone 51: 800–809.

33. Manning BD, Cantley LC (2007) AKT/PKB signaling: navigating downstream. Cell 129: 1261–1274.

34. Mukherjee A, Rotwein P (2009) Akt promotes BMP2-mediated osteoblast differentiation and bone development. J Cell Sci 122: 716–726.

35. Mukherjee A, Wilson EM, Rotwein P (2010) Selective signaling by Akt2 promotes bone morphogenetic protein 2-mediated osteoblast differentiation. Mol Cell Biol 30: 1018–1027.

36. DeBerardinis RJ, Lum JJ, Hatzivassiliou G, Thompson CB (2008) The biology of cancer: metabolic reprogramming fuels cell growth and proliferation. Cell Metab 7: 11–20.

37. Wallace DC (2005) Mitochondria and cancer: Warburg addressed. Cold Spring Harb Symp Quant Biol 70: 363–374.

38. Li CJ, Chang JK, Wang GJ, Ho ML (2011) Constitutively expressed COX-2 in osteoblasts positively regulates Akt signal transduction via suppression of PTEN activity. Bone 48: 286–297.

39. Schipani E, Ryan HE, Didrickson S, Kobayashi T, Knight M, et al. (2001) Hypoxia in cartilage: HIF-1alpha is essential for chondrocyte growth arrest and survival. Genes Dev 15: 2865–2876.

40. Wan C, Gilbert SR, Wang Y, Cao X, Shen X, et al. (2008) Activation of the hypoxia-inducible factor-1alpha pathway accelerates bone regeneration. Proc Natl Acad Sci U S A 105: 686–691.

41. Zou D, Zhang Z, Ye D, Tang A, Deng L, et al. (2011) Repair of critical-sized rat calvarial defects using genetically engineered bone marrow-derived mesenchymal stem cells overexpressing hypoxia-inducible factor-1alpha. Stem Cells 29: 1380–1390.

42. Lee CM, Genetos DC, Wong A, Yellowley CE (2010) Prostaglandin expression profile in hypoxic osteoblastic cells. J Bone Miner Metab 28: 8–16.

43. Lee CM, Genetos DC, You Z, Yellowley CE (2007) Hypoxia regulates PGE(2) release and EP1 receptor expression in osteoblastic cells. J Cell Physiol 212: 182–188.

44. Zhao L, Wu Y, Xu Z, Wang H, Zhao Z, et al. (2012) Involvement of COX-2/PGE2 signalling in hypoxia-induced angiogenic response in endothelial cells. J Cell Mol Med 16: 1840–1855.

45. Jaakkola P, Mole DR, Tian YM, Wilson MI, Gielbert J, et al. (2001) Targeting of HIF-alpha to the von Hippel-Lindau ubiquitylation complex by O2-regulated prolyl hydroxylation. Science 292: 468–472.

46. Ivan M, Haberberger T, Gervasi DC, Michelson KS, Gunzler V, et al. (2002) Biochemical purification and pharmacological inhibition of a mammalian prolyl hydroxylase acting on hypoxia-inducible factor. Proc Natl Acad Sci U S A 99: 13459–13464.

47. Regard JB, Zhong Z, Williams BO, Yang Y (2012) Wnt signaling in bone development and disease: making stronger bone with Wnts. Cold Spring Harb Perspect Biol 4.

48. Akiyama H, Lyons JP, Mori-Akiyama Y, Yang X, Zhang R, et al. (2004) Interactions between Sox9 and beta-catenin control chondrocyte differentiation. Genes Dev 18: 1072–1087.

49. Day TF, Guo X, Garrett-Beal L, Yang Y (2005) Wnt/beta-catenin signaling in mesenchymal progenitors controls osteoblast and chondrocyte differentiation during vertebrate skeletogenesis. Dev Cell 8: 739–750.

50. Dao DY, Jonason JH, Zhang Y, Hsu W, Chen D, et al. (2012) Cartilage-specific beta-catenin signaling regulates chondrocyte maturation, generation of ossification centers, and perichondrial bone formation during skeletal development. J Bone Miner Res 27: 1680–1694.

51. Chen Y, Alman BA (2009) Wnt pathway, an essential role in bone regeneration. J Cell Biochem 106: 353–362.

52. Chen Y, Whetstone HC, Lin AC, Nadesan P, Wei Q, et al. (2007) Beta-catenin signaling plays a disparate role in different phases of fracture repair: implications for therapy to improve bone healing. PLoS Med 4: e249.

53. Gaur T, Wixted JJ, Hussain S, O'Connell SL, Morgan EF, et al. (2009) Secreted frizzled related protein 1 is a target to improve fracture healing. J Cell Physiol 220: 174–181.

54. Altman RD, Latta LL, Keer R, Renfree K, Hornicek FJ, et al. (1995) Effect of nonsteroidal antiinflammatory drugs on fracture healing: a laboratory study in rats. J Orthop Trauma 9: 392–400.

55. Allen HL, Wase A, Bear WT (1980) Indomethacin and aspirin: effect of nonsteroidal anti-inflammatory agents on the rate of fracture repair in the rat. Acta Orthop Scand 51: 595–600.

56. Gerstenfeld LC, Einhorn TA (2004) COX inhibitors and their effects on bone healing. Expert Opin Drug Saf 3: 131–136.

57. Gerstenfeld LC, Thiede M, Seibert K, Mielke C, Phippard D, et al. (2003) Differential inhibition of fracture healing by non-selective and cyclooxygenase-2 selective non-steroidal anti-inflammatory drugs. J Orthop Res 21: 670–675.

58. Kellinsalmi M, Parikka V, Risteli J, Hentunen T, Leskela HV, et al. (2007) Inhibition of cyclooxygenase-2 down-regulates osteoclast and osteoblast differentiation and favours adipocyte formation in vitro. Eur J Pharmacol 572: 102–110.

59. Wang JH, Liu YZ, Yin LJ, Chen L, Huang J, et al. (2013) BMP9 and COX-2 form an important regulatory loop in BMP9-induced osteogenic differentiation of mesenchymal stem cells. Bone 57: 311–321.

11

Hip Fractures and Bone Mineral Density in the Elderly— Importance of Serum 25-Hydroxyvitamin D

Laufey Steingrimsdottir[1]*, Thorhallur I. Halldorsson[1], Kristin Siggeirsdottir[2], Mary Frances Cotch[4], Berglind O. Einarsdottir[2], Gudny Eiriksdottir[2], Sigurdur Sigurdsson[2], Lenore J. Launer[3], Tamara B. Harris[3], Vilmundur Gudnason[2,5], Gunnar Sigurdsson[2,5]

1 Unit for Nutrition Research, University of Iceland and Landspitali University Hospital, Reykjavik, Iceland, 2 Icelandic Heart Association Research Institute, Kopavogur, Iceland, 3 Intramural Research Program, Laboratory of Epidemiology, Demography and Biometry, National Institute of Aging, Bethesda, Maryland, United States of America, 4 Division of Epidemiology and Clinical Applications, National Eye Institute, Bethesda, Maryland, United States of America, 5 University of Iceland, Reykjavik, Iceland

Abstract

Background: The significance of serum 25-hydroxyvitamin D [25(OH)D] concentrations for hip fracture risk of the elderly is still uncertain. Difficulties reaching both frail and healthy elderly people in randomized controlled trials or large cohort studies may in part explain discordant findings. We determined hazard ratios for hip fractures of elderly men and women related to serum 25(OH)D, including both the frail and the healthy segment of the elderly population.

Methods: The AGES-Reykjavik Study is a prospective study of 5764 men and women, age 66–96 years, based on a representative sample of the population of Reykjavik, Iceland. Participation was 71.8%. Hazard ratios of incident hip fractures and baseline bone mineral density were determined according to serum concentrations of 25(OH)D at baseline.

Results: Mean follow-up was 5.4 years. Compared with referent values (50–75 nmol/L), hazard ratios for hip fractures were 2.24 (95% CI 1.63, 3.09) for serum 25(OH)D <30 nmol/L, adjusting for age, sex, body mass index, height, smoking, alcohol intake and season, and 2.08 (95% CI 1.51, 2.87), adjusting additionally for physical activity. No difference in risk was associated with 30–50 nmol/L or ≥75 nmol/L in either model compared with referent. Analyzing the sexes separately, hazard ratios were 2.61 (95% CI 1.47, 4.64) in men and 1.93 (95% CI 1.31, 2.84) in women. Values <30 nmol/L were associated with significantly lower bone mineral density of femoral neck compared with referent, z-scores -0.14 (95% CI −0.27, −0.00) in men and −0.11 (95% CI −0.22, −0.01) in women.

Conclusions: Our results lend support to the overarching importance of maintaining serum 25(OH)D above 30 nmol/L for bone health of elderly people while potential benefits of having much higher levels could not be detected.

Editor: Bin He, Baylor College of Medicine, United States of America

Funding: This study was funded by the National Institutes of Health, USA contract N01- AG-12100, and the National Institute on Aging Intramural Research Program, the National Eye Institute USA (Z01-EY000401), National Institutes of Health, Hjartavernd (The Icelandic Heart Association), and Althingi (Icelandic Parliament). The funders had no role in study design, data collection and analysis, decision to publish, or preparation of the manuscript.

Competing Interests: The authors have declared that no competing interests exist.

* E-mail: laufey@hi.is

Introduction

The importance of vitamin D for skeletal health has long been recognized, and serum 25-hydroxyvitamin D [25(OH)D] is the generally accepted indicator of vitamin D status. Still, optimal serum concentration for bone health is a subject of active debate and intensive research [1]. The Institute of Medicine recently recommended serum levels of 40–50 nmol/L for most adults, based on multiple skeletal outcomes [2], while other experts have suggested levels as high as 75 to 100 nmol/L [3,4].

Several functional indicators are used for vitamin D adequacy as it relates to bone health of the elderly, including bone mineral density and prevention of bone loss [5,6], as well as surrogate measures such as maximal calcium absorption and suppression of parathyroid hormone levels [4,7]. However, fracture prevention, and the levels of 25(OH)D associated with decreased fracture risk

may be a more relevant and clinically useful functional marker, as it relates directly to health and quality of life of the elderly. Still, associations between circulating 25(OH)D concentrations and incident fractures in old age remain uncertain [5,6,8]. While several prospective cohort studies have reported higher risk for fractures at lower 25(OH)D concentrations [3,9–14], others show no such association [15–17]. Further, the reported thresholds of significance for fracture risk are quite varied, ranging from 30–40 nmol/L (11) to a high of 90–100 nmol/L [3].

Hip fracture risk of the elderly is a function of multiple factors, including bone mineral density, muscle strength and balance, all of which have been related to vitamin D status and function [9,18]. In nine out of ten instances, hip fracture is sustained through a fall [19], and risk of falling has been related to vitamin D status [20].

Adding to this uncertainty, Randomized controlled trials (RCTs), often considered to provide the highest quality evidence, have not shown a consistent benefit from vitamin D supplements for hip bone mineral density (BMD) or fracture prevention, except possibly in the institutionalized elderly [21] or when given in combination with calcium [22]. Conversely, a recent meta-analysis of RCTs, estimating actual intake of vitamin D rather than prescribed dose, concluded that intakes ≥800 IU/day may be somewhat favorable in the prevention of hip fractures and other non-vertebral fractures in adults 65 years or older [23].

Given the social and economic burden of hip fractures in the elderly, prevention and risk reduction are of prime importance. Sufficient doses of vitamin D for skeletal health in old age need particular elucidation. However, high-risk groups, such as the frail elderly, may be difficult to reach in large cohort studies or RCTs of community-living adults, which in turn may have contributed to the discordant findings of previous studies.

Here we report on the risk of incident hip fractures in the elderly related to circulating 25(OH)D concentrations and bone mineral density in participants in the large prospective AGES-Reykjavik Study, selected at random from the general population.

Methods

Participants

The Ages Gene/Environment Susceptibility (AGES) -Reykjavik Study [24] is a follow-up of the population based Reykjavik Cohort Study, initiated in 1967.

A total of 27,281 men and women, all Caucasians, born in 1907–1935 and residing in Reykjavik and nearby communities were selected at random from the national registry. From these, 19,381 attended the study during the period 1967 to 1991 [25]. From the 11,549 cohort members still alive when AGES-Reykjavik Study examinations began in September 2002, 8,030 individuals were randomly chosen and invited to the study. From these, 5,764 participants, age 66–96 years (mean age 76 years), had enrolled in the AGES-Reykjavik Study by January 2006 (71.8% of invited), with continuous recruitment throughout the period. Participants were offered free taxi rides to the clinic at every visit and personal assistance from the drivers in order to better reach those with limited mobility.

Ethics statement

Written informed consent was obtained from all participants, and the study was approved by the Icelandic National Bioethics Committee (VSN: 00-063) and the National Institute on Aging Intramural Institutional Review Board (MedStar IRB for the Intramural Research Program, Baltimore, MD).

Clinical data collection

Extensive data were collected in the AGES-Reykjavik Study during a series of clinical examinations, according to standardized study protocols by staff of the Icelandic Health Association. Data were gathered on smoking, alcohol intake and consumption frequency of selected foods, including milk and dairy products, using a validated food frequency questionnaire [26]. Physical activity was assessed by self-reported level of physical activity during the last 12 months, where participants were asked how frequently in times per month, week or day they engaged in moderate or vigorous activity, giving examples of this level of activity for clarification. Participants got personal assistance in answering questions. Quantitative computed tomography (QCT) - scanning was performed for BMD measurements.

Of the 5,764 participants of AGES-Reykjavik, 303 did not meet the inclusion criteria, e.g., lacking serum 25(OH)D measurements, leaving 5461 individuals included in the study, all with available fracture data. Of these, 679 individuals did not undergo QCT scanning, leaving 4782 individuals for the analysis of BMD and vitamin D status.

Measurement of serum 25(OH)D

Blood was collected during the first clinic visit to AGES-study, from September 2002 to January 2006, and fasting serum samples were kept frozen at −80°C on-site in the IHA laboratory. Quantitative determination of total 25(OH) D (D_2 and D_3) was conducted by means of a direct, competitive chemiluminescence immunoassay (CLIA), using the LIAISON 25 OH Vitamin D Total assay (DiaSorin, Inc., Stillwater, Minnesota). The inter assay coefficient of variation was <6.5%, using a previously frozen serum pool as the control sample and <12.7% when the calculated data were from measurements using Liaison quality controls.

Bone mineral density measurements

During the first clinic visit, QCT measurements, providing true volumetric density, were taken on the left hip, using a 4-detector CT system (Sensation, Siemens Medical Systems, Erlangen, Germany). Using a standardized protocol, scans were obtained encompassing the proximal femur from a level 1 cm above the acetabulum to a level 5 mm inferior to the lesser trochanter with 1 mm slice thickness. To calibrate CT Hounsfield units to equivalent bone mineral concentration, all subjects were scanned with a calibration phantom (Image Analysis, Columbia, KY, USA). Further procedures and quality assessments have been described in detail elsewhere [24,27].

The variables used in the present study are volumetric integral BMD (mg/cm^3), reflecting both trabecular and cortical bone mass, of the femoral neck and trochanteric region separately. Reasons for exclusion from the QCT were inability to lie supine, body weight over 150 kg or having undergone hip replacement surgery.

Fractures

Hip fracture data were recorded, verified and confirmed from medical and radiological records as previously described [28]. Incident fractures were recorded from participants' enrollment into the study until 31st of December 2009, with a mean follow-up time of 5.4 years (SD 1.5). Hip fractures were defined according to International Classification of Diseases version 10, diagnostic codes S72.0, S72.1, S72.2 (WHO 1994). The AGES-Reykjavik Study fracture registration has been shown to have a capture rate of about 97% for hip fracture [28].

Statistical analyses

The mean and standard deviation (SD) were used to describe continuous variables and percentages were used for dichotomous variables. Serum 25(OH)D was categorized, a priori, into four groups of <30, ≥30–50, ≥50–75 and ≥75 nmol/L. The group ≥50–75 nmol/L (sufficient level) was used as referent, to establish whether beneficial effects could be detected at higher levels (≥75 nmol/L) and to compare with lower levels, (30–50 nmol/L) and (<30 nmol/L), concentrations that have been considered inadequate and depleted, according to the Institute of Medicine [2]. The absolute BMD values (in mg/cm^3) of the femoral neck and trochanteric area were transformed into a gender-specific z-score, based on the internal distribution in our study population. The z-score for femoral neck was used as the primary outcome measure when examining the association between 25(OH)D and BMD, which was performed as a secondary analysis.

Cox Proportional Hazard Model was used when examining the association between 25(OH)D and bone fractures; and linear regression when examining the association with bone mineral density. As a measure of association we used χ^2-test (Type III) for dichotomous outcomes and t-test for continuous outcomes under the null hypothesis that all 25(OH)D groups were equal (p for effect). For testing linear trend, ordinal values (0,1,2,3) for serum 25(OH)D were entered in the regression model. All of the analyses were carried out using SAS statistical software (version 9.2, SAS Institute, Cary, NC).

In our analyses we selected a priori and included the following set of covariates: age (continuous, no missing), sex (binary, no missing) height (continuous, 0.1% missing), current smoking (binary, 2.5% missing), body mass index (BMI) (<18.5, 18.5–24.9, 25–29.9, 30–34.9, 35–39.9 and 40+, 0.1% missing), current alcohol intake (0, 1–25, 26–50 and 50+ g/day, 3% missing), season (winter: Dec, Jan, Feb, spring: Mar, Apr, May, summer: June, July, Aug, autumn: Sept Oct Nov, no missing), current physical activity (never, rarely, occasionally, moderate, high, 4.0% missing). As self reported milk and dairy product intake and serum 25(OH)D at baseline were essentially uncorrelated (Spearman r = 0.06), milk and dairy product intake was not included as covariate. The proportion of subjects missing data on one or more covariate was 4.4%. Due to the relatively low number of missing values for most covariates, missing values were replaced with median (continuous) and most frequent (dichotomous) values. Two models were used for covariate adjustment: Model A adjusting for age, sex, smoking, BMI, height, alcohol intake and season of blood sample collection; and Model B, additionally adjusting for physical activity.

To check the robustness of our findings with respect to imputation for missing covariates and length of follow-up we 1) ran all analyses using complete case analyses (all subjects with missing covariates excluded); and 2) examined the association between baseline 25(OH)D with hip fractures, excluding all fractures occurring within 6 months from baseline.

Results

A total of 261 hip fractures were encountered during a mean follow-up time of 5.4 years (SD 1.5). Characteristics of the study participants by sex and serum 25(OH)D are shown in **Table 1**. Fourteen per cent of men and 19% of women had serum 25(OH)D concentrations below 30 nmol/L, and 21% and 14% had concentrations ≥75 nmol/L, men and women respectively. There were significant negative trends associated with 25(OH)D category for the following variables in both men and women: BMI, % physically inactive, % drinking no alcohol and % smoking, while positive trends were found for BMD. There was no significant association between level of serum 25(OH)D and mean age for men or women.

For males the mean (SD) integral BMD was 254 (51)mg/cm^3 for femoral neck and 250 (50)mg/cm^3 for trochanter. The corresponding values for females were 244 (50)mg/cm^3 and 226 (48)mg/cm^3. The mean (SD) serum 25(OH)D was 57 (25)nmol/L and 51 (24)nmol/L for males and females, respectively.

Table 2 shows hip fracture hazard ratios according to serum 25(OH)D categories for all participants and for men and women separately. Compared with referent values of 50–75 nmol/L, the risk for hip fractures more than doubled in all subjects with levels below 30 nmol/L, values remaining relatively stable through adjustment models. Adjusting for age, height and BMI, current smoking, season of blood sampling and alcohol intake, the hazard

ratio was 2.24 (95% CI 1.63, 3.09) and with further adjustment for physical activity it was 2.08 (95% CI 1.51, 2.87). No increase in risk was associated with serum concentrations 30–50 nmol/L compared with referent values and neither was there any difference in risk associated with values ≥75 nmol/L in either adjustment model. When the sexes were analyzed separately, hazard ratio for men was 2.61 (95% CI 1.47, 4.64), compared with 1.93 (95% CI 1.31, 2.84) for women in the fully adjusted model. Again risk ratios did not change significantly between the different adjustment models in either sex. Values between 30–50 nmol/L and values ≥75 nmol/L were not associated with changes in risk compared with referent values in either sex.

Based on the prevalence of hip fractures in the 50–75 nmol/group for all subjects (4.0%) we estimated the excess number of fractures, i.e. expected minus observed fractures, in the <30 nmol/L group. Expected fractures were 38, or 0.04*938 (number of subjects with <30 nmol/L), while 77 fractures were observed. This suggests that 15% (or 39 excess fractures out of 261 in total) may be attributable to poor (<30 nmol/L) serum 25(OH)D status.

Associations between 25(OH)D concentrations and BMD at baseline in femoral neck are shown in **Table 3**, with BMD reported as z-scores. Using the values 50–75 nmol/L as referent, values below 30 nmol/L were consistently associated with slightly lower BMD z-score. In Model A, adjusting for age, height, BMI, smoking, alcohol intake and season, the adjusted difference in z-score was −0.18 (95% CI −0.31, −0.04) in men and −0.13 (95% CI −0.23, −0.03) in women. In model B, additionally adjusting for physical activity, the corresponding values were −0.14 (95% CI −0.27, −0.00) and −0.11 (95% CI −0.22, −0.01), men and women, respectively. No significant difference in risk was associated with other categories of 25(OH)D concentrations, except for a small increase at concentrations ≥75 nmol/L. Taking both sexes together, there was an increase of 0.10 (95% CI 0.02, 0.18) in Model A, with values remaining stable through further adjustment. When sexes were analyzed separately, only BMD z-scores for males remained significantly higher in the ≥75 nmol/L group than in the referent. Comparable values were found for BMD in trochanter associated with 25(OH)D concentrations in both sexes (data not shown). A total of 679 participants in the study did not undergo QCT scanning. Associations between hip fractures and 25(OH)D concentrations in the 4782 individuals with available scanning data were found to be similar to those observed in the larger group of 5461 participants.

Figure 1 shows the percentage of incident hip fractures according to baseline values of 25(OH)D in all participants, during a mean follow-up time of 5.4 years, mean time to event 3.4 years (SD1.8). A total of 10.6% of those with values below 15 nmol/L experienced a fracture, while corresponding proportions were 7.6% and 4.4% for those with values from 15–30 nmol/L and 30–50 nmol/L, respectively. There was non-significant change in the percentage at higher 25(OH)D values. However, mean time to fracture was not significantly different between the 25(OH)D groups, 3.1 years (SD 1.8) in the lowest category, compared with 3.9 years (SD 3.9), 3.3 years (SD 1.3) and 3.5years (SD 1.6) in the higher categories.

Finally we found little evidence to suggest that imputing values for missing covariates may have contributed to residual confounding. As an example, when comparing the referent with <30 nmol/L for both sexes using model B (Table 2) the hazard ratio for hip fracture was 2.08 (1.51, 2.87) and was essentially unchanged 2.08 (1.49, 2.91) when subjects with missing covariate information were excluded. Correspondingly when all individuals with hip fracture events occurring within 6 months (n = 14) were excluded (using

Table 1. Characteristics of male and female participants at baseline according to categories of serum 25-hydroxyvitamin D (N = 5461), mean and SD.

	Serum 25-hydroxyvitamin D (nmol/L)				
	<30	30-<50	50-<75	≥75	P value[1]
Males (n = 2346)					
n (%)	337 (14%)	638 (28%)	886 (38%)	485 (21%)	
Femoral neck BMD, mg/cm^3	245 (59)	253 (51)	254 (50)	259 (53)	0.0005
Trochanter BMD, mg/cm^3	242 (51)	248 (51)	252 (47)	255 (51)	0.0002
Age in years	76.7 (5.8)	76.8 (5.5)	76.7 (5.4)	76.8 (5.4)	0.65
Height, cm	175.1 (6.2)	175.1 (6.2)	175.5 (6.2)	175.8 (6.2)	0.03
BMI, kg/m^2	27.2 (4.3)	27.3 (3.9)	26.7 (3.7)	26.3 (3.5)	<0.0001
% Physically inactive	61	46	37	34	<0.0001
% Not drinking alcohol	34	30	24	27	0.002
% Current smokers	23	12	8	9	<0.0001
Females (n = 3125)					
n (%)	601 (19%)	992 (32%)	1103 (35%)	429 (14%)	
BMD for femoral neck (mg/cm^3)	240 (50)	245 (52)	245 (49)	248 (48)	0.03
BMD for trochanter (mg/cm^3)	221 (49)	227 (50)	227 (46)	229 (45)	0.02
Age in years	76.8 (5.6)	76.7 (5.8)	76.3 (5.7)	76.7 (5.6)	0.20
Height, cm	160.3 (5.7)	160.7 (5.6)	161.1 (5.9)	160.8 (6.1)	0.006
BMI, kg/m^2	28.1 (5.5)	27.8 (4.9)	26.6 (4.4)	26.2 (4.3)	<0.0001
% Physically inactive	66	50	45	42	<0.0001
% Not drinking alcohol	54	41	35	37	<0.0001
% Current smokers	18	12	11	10	0.0001

[1]T-test for trend for continuous covariates with serum 25-hydroxyvitamin D entered as ordinal values.
Chi-square test for dichotomous covariates.

imputed covariate values), the hazard ratio was 2.10 (1.51, 2.93). There was no trend with respect to time to fracture across categories of 25(OH)D. As an example the mean time to event was 3.1 years (SD 1.8) in the lowest (<30 nmol/L) compared with 3.3 years (SD 1.3) in the referent category (50 -<75 nmol/L).

Discussion

In this prospective cohort study of 5461 elderly people experiencing a sizable number of hip fractures (n = 261), the estimated risk of hip fracture was twice as high in individuals with serum 25(OH)D concentrations below 30 nmol/L, using 50–75 nmol/L as a referent and adjusting for a series of relevant cofactors. The risk increase associated with low 25(OH)D levels was somewhat higher for men than women, but remained stable and highly significant in both sexes through various adjustments. No statistically significant difference in risk was associated with other categories of 25(OH)D concentrations, for levels either between 30 and 50 nmol/L or above 75 nmol/L, compared with the referent values.

The relevance of vitamin D status for hip fracture risk has been considered uncertain in large systematic reviews of vitamin D and bone health [5,6]. Indeed, several cohort studies have found no associations between hip fracture risk and vitamin D [15–17], while some studies have reported risk protection by quite high serum 25(OH)D concentrations, up to 100 nmol/L [3,10]. Still others show tendencies for increased risk at low levels below 30–

40 nmol/L, with no further protection at higher concentrations [9,11,13]. According to a large multi-center study from Norway [14] there is a moderate increase in risk for hip fractures among those in the lowest quartile for baseline 25(OH)D (≤42.1 nmol/L) compared with the highest ≥67.9 nmol/L), with a hazard ratio of 1.34. Also, RCTs are not unequivocal in their conclusions, regarding either the efficacy or ideal dose of vitamin D supplements for fracture prevention [21,22,29]. Elucidating the significance of vitamin D for hip fracture risk of the elderly is of great public health significance, considering the public health costs, high mortality and human suffering related to hip fractures [30]. As vitamin D of varying doses is widely used in clinical practice to lower the risk of osteoporotic fractures, it is of prime importance to determine whether relatively high 25(OH)D concentrations are needed for risk protection, concentrations which generally require larger doses of vitamin D supplementation than the 800 IU currently recommended for the elderly by the Institute of Medicine [2] and recently endorsed in a review of randomized controlled trials [31]. Even though these higher doses are not considered toxic, adverse effects, such as increased risk of kidney stones, have been indicated in studies like the Women's Health Initiative [32]. The study of Sanders et al. [33] further alerts to possible adverse outcomes associated with large doses, as they reported increased risk for falls and fractures in a group of elderly people receiving 500,000 IU of vitamin D annually for 3 to 5 years.

Table 2. Hazard ratios for hip fractures according to serum 25-hydroxyvitamin D categories among all subjects (N = 5461), and stratified by sex.

		Unadjusted	Model A[2]	Model B[3]
		HR (95% CI)	HR (95% CI)	HR (95% CI)
All Subjects	cases/n (%)			
<30 nmol/L	77/938 (8.2%)	2.14 (1.57, 2.94)	2.24 (1.63, 3.09)	2.08 (1.51, 2.87)
30–50 nmol/L	71/1620 (4.4%)	1.10 (0.80, 1.52)	1.13 (0.82, 1.56)	1.11 (0.80, 1.53)
50–75 nmol/L	80/1989 (4.0%)	1.00	1.00	1.00
≥75 nmol/L	33/914 (3.6%)	0.91 (0.61, 1.37)	0.90 (0.60, 1.35)	0.94 (0.62, 1.41)
P for effect[1]		<0.0001	<0.0001	<0.0001
Males	cases/n (%)			
<30 nmol/L	25/337 (7.4%)	2.61 (1.49, 4.58)	2.81 (1.59, 4.96)	2.61 (1.47, 4.64)
30–50 nmol/L	24/604 (3.8%)	1.35 (0.77, 2.36)	1.52 (0.86, 2,67)	1.49 (0.84, 2.63)
50–75 nmol/L	25/886 (2.8%)	1.00	1.00	1.00
≥75 nmol/L	14/485 (2.9%)	0.99 (0.51, 1.90)	0.97 (0.50, 1.88)	1.02 (0.53, 1.97)
P for effect[1]		0.003	0.001	0.006
Females	cases/n (%)			
<30 nmol/L	52/601 (8.7%)	1.89 (1.29, 2.76)	2.06 (1.40, 3.02)	1.93 (1.31, 2.84)
30–50 nmol/L	47/992 (4.7%)	0.97 (0.66, 1.44)	1.01 (0.68, 1.50)	0.99 (0.67, 1.47)
50–75 nmol/L	55/1103 (5.0%)	1.00	1.00	1.00
≥75 nmol/L	19/429 (4.4%)	0.94 (0.56, 1.58)	0.86 (0.51, 1.46)	0.89 (0.53, 1.51)
P for effect[1]		0.001	0.0002	0.001

Abbreviations: HR Hazard Ratio, CI confidence interval.
[1] Chi-square test (type 3).
[2] Adjusted for age at recruitment, sex (when all subjects are included), height, body mass index, current smoking, season of blood sampling and alcohol intake.
[3] Additionally adjusted for current physical activity.

Differences in previous study outcomes have been explained in part by the different populations under study as well as possible differences in confounder adjustments [5]. Specifically, the frail and sickly may not be included or reached in all community-based studies of the elderly, but lower vitamin D status is consistently reported among the frail compared with those more physically active and in better health [3,9]. Thus, the segment of the elderly population having the lowest 25(OH)D levels may not be included in many cohort studies and the significance of very low values thus overlooked or minimized [9,11]. In our study, which was based on a random sample from the general population, the participation rate was high, or 71.8%, and the distribution of 25(OH)D concentration was quite wide, with comparable proportions of the population having values below 30 nmol/L and above 75 nmol/L. A significant proportion of all hip fractures in our study (15%), may thus be attributed to poor or deficient (<30 nmol/L) serum 25(OH)D. Interestingly, this is a comparable proportion to that reported from combined calcium and vitamin D supplementation for reducing fracture risk [34]. Possibly the relatively high calcium intake in our population, due to widespread use of milk and dairy products, may contribute to this effect [7].

The fracture incidence observed in our study, where both sexes were taken together for improved statistical power, also strongly indicates that there is a nonlinear relationship between circulating 25(OH)D and fracture risk, with only small gains being associated with serum levels above 50 nmol/L. The highest incidence was observed in the group with 25(OH)D values below 15 nmols, with steeply decreasing proportion with increased circulating vitamin D up to 50 nmol/L, but little differences above those concentrations.

While appropriate adjustments were made for season in our analysis, seasonal variation in 25(OH)D values was less pronounced in the present study than previously reported for younger populations in Reykjavik, geographically located at 64° N [7]. The difference in mean values obtained in summer and winter was only 4 nmol/L in this elderly population. The relative lack of seasonal variation indicates that vitamin D intake may play a more important role for vitamin D status in this population compared with younger people. Indeed, cod liver oil, either as liquid or capsules, is a common supplement in Iceland, with 61% of this population reporting taking the supplement daily and 13% several times per week, according to AGES questionnaire. However, intake of milk or dairy products at baseline was not associated with vitamin D status in our study. Notably, milk or dairy products were not fortified with vitamin D during the study period.

We measured volumetric QCT-BMD rather than areal BMD, but similar associations have been shown between fractures and BMD using these two measures [35,36]. Similar to many previous studies [3,12] we found a slight but significant positive trend between BMD in femoral neck and serum concentrations of 25(OH)D in both sexes. Again, only levels below 30 nmol/L were consistently significantly different from the referent, which is in concordance with our results regarding increases in hip fracture risk below 30 nmol/L. However, according to earlier studies the observed difference of 0.10-0.16 BMD z-scores might be expected to be associated with only modest increases in fracture risk [37,38]. The two-fold increase in risk associated with low 25(OH)D in our study supports the contention that the relationship between vitamin D and fracture risk may indeed be non-linear [1]. It has been suggested that vitamin D may reduce fracture rates through

Table 3. Differences in z-score (number of SD from age corrected mean) of femoral neck bone mineral density according to serum 25-hydroxyvitamin D categories at baseline (N = 4782).

	Unadjusted	Model A[2]	Model B[3]
	Δ(95% CI)	Δ (95% CI)	Δ (95% CI)
Femoral neck BMD(z-score)			
All (N = 4782)			
<30 nmol/L	−0.13 (−0.21, −0.04)	−0.15 (−0.23, −0.07)	−0.13 (−0.21, −0.05)
30–50 nmol/L	−0.02 (−0.09, 0.05)	−0.04 (−0.11, 0.03)	−0.03 (−0.10, 0.03)
50–75 nmol/L	Referent	Referent	Referent
≥75 nmol/L	0.08 (−0.01, 0.16)	0.10 (0.02, 0.18)	0.09 (0.01, 0.17)
P for effect[1]	0.0006	<0.0001	0.0001
Males (n = 2104)			
<30 nmol/L	−0.18 (−0.31, −0.04)	−0.18 (−0.31, −0.04)	−0.14 (−0.27, −0.00)
30–50 nmol/L	−0.02 (−0.13, 0.08)	−0.04 (−0.15, 0.07)	−0.03 (−0.13, 0.08)
50–75 nmol/L	Referent	Referent	Referent
≥75 nmol/L	0.10 (−0.02, 0.21)	0.12 (0.01, 0.24)	0.11 (−0.01, 0.22)
P for effect[1]	0.004	0.0009	0.01
Females (n = 2678)			
<30 nmol/L	−0.10 (−0.21, 0.01)	−0.13 (−0.23, −0.03)	−0.11 (−0.22, −0.01)
30–50 nmol/L	−0.01 (−0.11, 0.08)	−0.04 (−0.12, 0.05)	−0.03 (−0.12, 0.05)
50–75 nmol/L	Referent	Referent	Referent
≥75 nmol/L	0.06 (−0.06, 0.18)	0.07 (−0.04, 0.19)	0.07 (−0.04, 0.18)
P for effect[1]	0.14	0.01	0.03

Abbreviations: CI confidence interval.
[1]F-test (type 3).
[2]Adjusted for age at recruitment, sex (when all subjects are included), height, body mass index, current smoking, season of blood sampling and alcohol intake.
[3]Additionally adjusted for current physical activity.

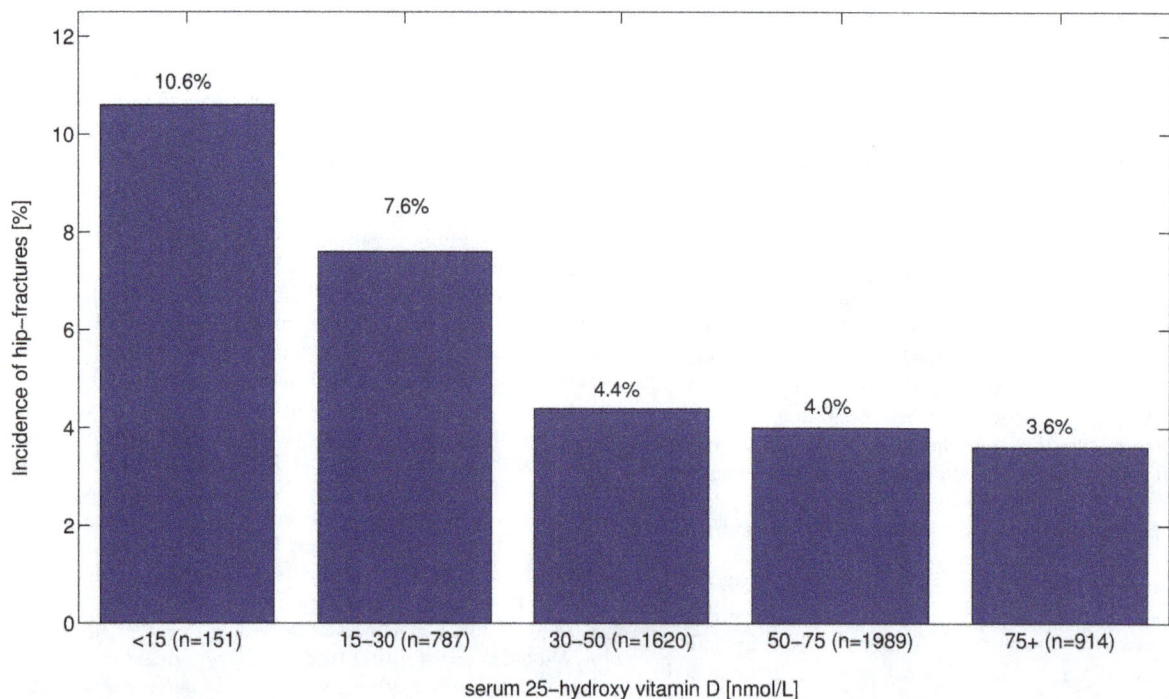

Figure 1. Hip fracture incidence (%) during a follow-up of 5.4 years (SD1.5) among AGES participants (N = 5461) according to serum baseline categories of 25(OH)D. Unadjusted values.

additional mechanisms, independent of bone density [39]. Specifically, vitamin D supplements may effectively decrease the risk of falling, especially in the institutionally elderly, possibly through actions involving balance and muscle strength [20,40].

It is well known that elderly men have higher mean BMD and lower risk for hip fractures than women [14,27], as confirmed in our study. However, the risk increase associated with low 25(OH)D concentrations was comparable in men and women suggesting that vitamin D status is no less important for lowering fracture risk among elderly men than women.

Concerns have been raised over assays for 25(OH)D giving varying results, casting doubt on the comparability of specific values for vitamin D status [41]. Our study employed a common assay method for 25(OH)D, widely used in clinical settings. Thus we believe that our results are clinically relevant, even though the levels measured by the CLIA method may be systematically lower than those measured by HPLC. Furthermore, systematic errors in absolute serum levels should only affect interpretations of our findings in terms of absolute cut-off values but should not affect the magnitude and strength of the observed association.

The length of follow-up may also be a concern, as single baseline vitamin D values may not represent status many years later [42]. Indeed, the study by Looker [13] showed that vitamin D concentrations predicted major osteoporotic fracture risk only for 10 years of follow up. Importantly, our mean follow-up time was 5.4 years, with mean time to event 3.4 years. Frail individuals may also be selectively advised to take vitamin D supplements, diminishing observed risk. However, results from our 25(OH)D

analysis were not available until at the end of follow up, and thus our subjects could not be informed of their status earlier.

The main strength of our study is the large number of elderly people, displaying a wide variation in serum 25(OH)D values, and sustaining a total of 261 hip fractures. Thus, robust associations could be obtained between vitamin D status and fracture risk. The main limitation to our study, however, is the single baseline measurement of 25(OH)D. Also, as this is an observational study, some residual confounding cannot be excluded. However, as hazard ratios for hip fracture were quite similar in unadjusted and fully adjusted data in both sexes, residual confounding is not likely to substantially affect our main results.

To conclude: Our results lend support to the overarching importance of maintaining serum 25(OH)D above 30 nmol/L for bone health of elderly people while potential benefits of having much higher levels could not be detected.

Acknowledgments

We thank all the participants of the AGES-Reykjavik Study and the clinic staff at the Icelandic Heart Association for their invaluable contribution.

Author Contributions

Conceived and designed the experiments: LS TIH VG GS. Performed the experiments: BOE GE KS SS MFC. Analyzed the data: LS TIH GS. Contributed reagents/materials/analysis tools: KS MFC LJL TBH VG. Wrote the paper: LS TIH GS.

References

1. Dawson-Hughes B (2013) What is the optimal dietary intake of vitamin D for reducing fracture risk? Calcif Tissue Int 92: 184–190.
2. Ross AC, Manson JE, Abrams SA, Aloia JF, Brannon PM, et al. (2011) The 2011 report on dietary reference intakes for calcium and vitamin D from the Institute of Medicine: what the clinicians need to know. J Clin Endocrinol Metab 96: 53–58.
3. Bischoff-Ferrari HA, Giuvannucci E, Willett WC, Dietrich T, Dawson-Hughes B (2006) Estimation of optimal serum concentrations of 25-hydroxyvitamin D for multiple health outcomes. Am J Clin Nutr 84: 18–28.
4. Holick MF (2007) Vitamin D deficiency. N Engl J Med 357: 266–281.
5. Cranney A, Horsley T, O'Donnell S, Weiler H, Puil L, et al. (2007) Effectiveness and safety of vitamin D in relation to bone health. Evid Rep Technol Assess 158:1–235.
6. Chung M, Balk EM, Brendel M, Ip S, Lau J, et al. (2009) Vitamin D and calcium: a systematic review of health outcomes. Evid Rep Technol Assess 183:1–420.
7. Steingrimsdottir L, Gunnarsson O, Indridason OS, Franzson L, Sigurdsson G (2005) Relationship between serum parathyroid hormone levels, vitamin D sufficiency, and calcium intake. JAMA 294: 2336–2341.
8. Avenell A, Gillespie WJ, Gillespie LD, O'Connell D (2009) Vitamin D and vitamin D analogues for preventing fractures associated with involutional and post-menopausal osteoporosis. Cochrane Database Syst Rev 2: CD000227. doi:10.1002/14651858.CD000227.pub3.
9. Gerdhem P, Ringsberg KAM, Obrant KJ, Akesson K (2005) Association between 25-hydroxy vitamin D levels, physical activity, strength and fractures in the prospective population-based OPRA study of elderly women. Osteoporos Int 16: 1425–1431.
10. Looker AC, Mussolino ME (2008) Serum 25-hydroxyvitamin D and hip fracture risk in older US white adults. J Bone Miner Res 23: 143–150.
11. Melhus H, Snellman G, Gedeborg R, Byberg L, Berglund L, et al. (2010) Plasma 25-hydroxyvitamin D levels and fracture risk in a community-based cohort of elderly men in Sweden. J Clin Endocrinol Metab 95: 2637–2645.
12. Robinson-Cohen C, Katz R, Hoofnagle AN, Cauley JA, Furberg CD, et al. (2011) Mineral metabolism markers and the long-term risk of hip fracture: The cardiovascular health study. J Clin Endocrinol Metab 96: 2189–2193.
13. Looker AC (2013) Serum 25-hydroxyvitamin D and risk of major osteoporotic fractures in older U.S adults. J Bone Miner Res 28: 997–1006.
14. Holvik K, Ahmed LA, Forsmo S, Forsmo S, Gjesdal CG, et al. (2013) Low serum levels of 25-hydroxyvitamin D predict hip fracture in the elderly. A NOREPOS study. J Clin Endocrinol Metab 98: 3341-3350. doi:10.1210/jc.2013-1468.
15. Roddam AW, Neale R, Appleby P, Allen NE, Tipper S, et al. (2007) Association between plasma 25-hydroxyvitamin D levels and fracture risk – the EPIC-Oxford study. Am J Epidemiol 166: 1327–1336.
16. Cauley JA, Parimi N, Ensrud KE, Bauer DC, Cawthon PM, et al. (2010) Serum 25-hydroxyvitamin D and the risk of hip and nonspine fractures in older men. J Bone Miner Res 25: 545–553.
17. Barbour KE, Houston DK, Cummings SR, Boudreau R, Prasad T, et al. (2012) Calciotropic hormones and the risk of hip and nonspine fractures in older adults: The Health ABC Study. J Bone Miner Res 27: 1177–1185.
18. Muir SW, Montero-Odasso M (2011) Effect of vitamin D supplementation on muscle strength, gait and balance in older adults: A systematic review and meta-analysis. J Am Geriatr Soc 59: 2291–2300.
19. Schwartz AV, Villa ML, Prill M, Kelsey JA, Galinus JA, et al. (1999) Falls in older Mexican-American women. J Am Geriatr Soc 47: 1371–1378.
20. Kalyani RR, Stein B, Valiyil R, Manno R, Maynard JW, et al. (2010) Vitamin D treatment for the prevention of falls in older adults: systematic review and meta-analysis. J Am Geriatr Soc 58: 1299–1310.
21. Lai JK, Lucas RM, Clements MS, Roddam AW, Banks E (2010) Hip fracture risk in relation to vitamin D supplementation and serum 25-hydroxyvitamin D levels: A systematic review and meta-analysis of randomised controlled trials and observational studies. BMC Public Health 10: 331. doi 10.1186/1471-2458-10-331.
22. The DIPART (vitamin D Individual Patient Analysis of Randomized Trials) Group (2010) Patient level pooled analysis of 68 500 patients from seven major vitamin D fracture trials in US and Europe. BMJ 340:b5463. doi:10.1136/bmj.b5463.
23. Bischoff-Ferrari HA, Willett WC, Orav EJ, Lips P, Meunier PJ, et al. (2012) A pooled analysis of vitamin D dose requirements for fracture prevention. N Engl J Med 367: 40–49.
24. Harris TB, Launer LJ, Eiriksdottir G, Kjartansson O, Jonsson PV, et al. (2007) Age, Gene/Environment Susceptibility-Reykjavik Study: multidisciplinary applied phenomics. Am J Epidemiol 165: 1076–1087.
25. Bjornsson G, Bjornsson OJ, Davidsson D, Kristjansson BT, Olafsson O, et al. (1982) Report abc XXIV. Health Survey in the Reykjavik Area. – Women. Stages I-III, 1968–1969, 1971–1972 and 1976–1978. Participants, Invitation, Response etc. The Icelandic Heart Association, Reykjavik.
26. Eysteinsdottir T, Thorsdottir I, Gunnarsdottir I, Steingrimsdottir L (2012) Assessing validity of a short food-frequency questionnaire on present dietary intake of elderly Icelanders. Nutr J 11:12. doi:10.1186/1475-2891-11-12
27. Sigurdsson G, Aspelund T, Chang M, Jonsdottir B, Sigurdsson S, et al. (2006) Increasing sex difference in bone strength in old age: The Age, Gene/Environment Susceptibility-Reykjavik study (AGES-REYKJAVIK). Bone 39: 644–651.
28. Siggeirsdottir K, Aspelund T, Sigurdsson G, Mogensen B, Chang M, et al. (2007) Inaccuracy in self-report of fractures may underestimate association with health outcomes when compared with medical record based fracture registry. Eur J Epidemiol 22: 631–639.

29. Grimnes G, Joakimsen R, Figenschau Y, Torjesen PA, Almås B, et al. (2012) The effect of high-dose vitamin D on bone mineral density and bone turnover markers in postmenopausal women with low bone mass-a randomized controlled 1-year trial. Osteoporos Int 23: 201–211.

30. Johnell O (2006) Review: Vitamin D plus calcium, but not vitamin D alone, prevents osteoporotic fractures in older people. Evid Based Med 11: 13. doi:10.1136/ebm.11.1.13

31. Bouillon R, Van Schoor NM, Gielen E, Boonen S, Mathieu C, et al. (2013) Optimal vitamin D status: a critical analysis on the basis of evidence-based medicine. J Clin Endocrinol Metab 98:E1283-304. doi: 10.1210/jc.2013-1195.

32. Jackson RD, LaCroix AZ, Gass M, Wallace RB, Robbins J, et al. (2006) Women's Health Initiative Investigators. Calcium plus vitamin D supplementation and the risk of fractures. N Engl J Med 354: 669–683.

33. Sanders KM, Stuart AL, Williamson EJ, Simpson JA, Kotowicz MA, et al. (2010) Annual high-dose oral vitamin D and falls and fractures in older women: a randomized controlled trial. JAMA. 303: 1815–1822.

34. Boonen S, Lips P, Bouillon R, Bischoff-Ferrari HA, Vanderschueren D, et al. (2007) Need for additional calcium to reduce the risk of hip fracture with vitamin d supplementation: evidence from a comparative metaanalysis of randomized controlled trials. J Clin Endocrinol Metab 92: 1415–1423.

35. Rianon NJ, Lang TF, Siggeirsdottir K, Sigurdsson G, Eiriksdottir G, et al. (2014) Fracture risk assessment in older adults using a combination of selected quantitative computed tomography bone measures. A sub-analysis of the Age, Gene/Environment Susceptibility-Reykjavik Study. J Clin Densitom 17: 25–31.

36. Black DM, Bouxsein ML, Marshall LM, Cummings SR, Lang TF, et al. (2008) Osteoporotic Fractures in Men (MrOS) Research Group. Proximal femoral structure and the prediction of hip fracture in men: a large prospective study using QCT. J Bone Miner Res 23: 1326–1333.

37. Cummings SR, Black DM, Nevitt MC, Browner W, Cauley J, et al. (1993) Bone density at various sites for prediction of hip fractures. The Study of Osteoporotic Fractures Research Group. Lancet 341: 72–75.

38. Marshall D, Johnell O, Wedel H (1996) Meta-analysis of how well measures of bone mineral density predict occurrence of osteoporotic fractures. BMJ 312: 1254–1259.

39. Rabenda V, Bruyère O, Reginster JY (2011) Relationship between bone mineral density changes and risk of fractures among patients receiving calcium with or without vitamin D supplementation: a meta-regression. Osteoporos Int 22: 893–901.

40. Cameron ID, Gillespie LD, Robertson MC, Murray GR, Hill KD, et al. (2012) Interventions for preventing falls in older people in care facilities and hospitals. Cochrane Database Syst Rev doi: 10.1002/14651858.CD005465.pub3.

41. Snellman G, Melhus H, Gedeborg R, Byberg L, Berglund L, et al. (2010) Determining vitamin D status: a comparison between commercially available assays. PLoS One doi: 10.1371/journal.pone.0011555.

42. Jorde R, Sneve M, Hutchinson M, Emaus N, Figenschau Y, et al. (2010) Tracking of serum 25-hydroxyvitamin D levels during 14 years in a population-based study and during 12 months in an intervention study. Am J Epidemiol 171: 903–908.

12

Numerical Simulation of Callus Healing for Optimization of Fracture Fixation Stiffness

Malte Steiner[1]*, Lutz Claes[1], Anita Ignatius[1], Ulrich Simon[2], Tim Wehner[1]

1 Institute of Orthopaedic Research and Biomechanics, Center of Musculoskeletal Research Ulm, University Hospital Ulm, Ulm, Germany, **2** Scientific Computing Centre Ulm, University of Ulm, Ulm, Germany

Abstract

The stiffness of fracture fixation devices together with musculoskeletal loading defines the mechanical environment within a long bone fracture, and can be quantified by the interfragmentary movement. *In vivo* results suggested that this can have acceleratory or inhibitory influences, depending on direction and magnitude of motion, indicating that some complications in fracture treatment could be avoided by optimizing the fixation stiffness. However, general statements are difficult to make due to the limited number of experimental findings. The aim of this study was therefore to numerically investigate healing outcomes under various combinations of shear and axial fixation stiffness, and to detect the optimal configuration. A calibrated and established numerical model was used to predict fracture healing for numerous combinations of axial and shear fixation stiffness under physiological, superimposed, axial compressive and translational shear loading in sheep. Characteristic maps of healing outcome versus fixation stiffness (axial and shear) were created. The results suggest that delayed healing of 3 mm transversal fracture gaps will occur for highly flexible or very rigid axial fixation, which was corroborated by *in vivo* findings. The optimal fixation stiffness for ovine long bone fractures was predicted to be 1000–2500 N/mm in the axial and >300 N/mm in the shear direction. In summary, an optimized, moderate axial stiffness together with certain shear stiffness enhances fracture healing processes. The negative influence of one improper stiffness can be compensated by adjustment of the stiffness in the other direction.

Editor: João Costa-Rodrigues, Faculdade de Medicina Dentária, Universidade do Porto, Portugal

Funding: This study was intramurally funded by the Center of Musculoskeletal Research Ulm, University of Ulm, Germany. The funders had no role in study design, data collection and analysis, decision to publish, or preparation of the manuscript.

Competing Interests: The authors have declared that no competing interests exist.

* Email: malte.steiner@uni-ulm.de

Introduction

Fractures typically heal successfully, however five to ten per cent of all fractures show complications such as healing delays or non-unions [1,2,3]. These complications are of great clinical relevance due to the large incidence of fractures, which stand as one of the most frequent injuries to the musculoskeletal system [4,5]. Apart from numerous biological factors [6,7], local mechanical conditions within a diaphyseal, long bone fracture zone determine the healing course and success decisively [8,9,10]. A measure for the mechanical conditions within the fracture site is the interfragmentary movement (IFM), which under physiological loading [11] in fractured human tibiae is highly complex and consists of axial motion, bending, and torsional and translational shear [12,13].

To stabilize long bone fractures against these loading influences, surgeons use either external fixation, plate fixation, or intramedullary nailing [14]. Each of these different fixation methods show different predominant IFM directions. External and plate fixation lead to predominant axial compressive IFM through bending because of the relatively low bending stiffness of the devices [15]. Intramedullary nails can create remarkable shear movements in the fracture gap caused by the play of the nail within the medullary canal [16].

Based on animal experiments in sheep, it was found that both magnitude and direction of IFM perform important roles; while small and moderate axial compressive IFM are widely accepted to

stimulate healing [17,18,19,20,21], translational shear can delay or inhibit healing processes [22,23,24], as do large motion magnitudes in general [25].

This indicates that some of the occuring healing complications might be the result of inhibitive mechanical conditions arising from improper fixation stiffness. Thus, finding an optimal fixation stiffness was aspired by means of sheep experiments [21]. Nevertheless, due to the very limited numbers of *in vivo* experiments and investigated fixation device samples, a general statement of the correlation between fixation stability and healing outcome is hard to achieve from *in vivo* data.

Numerical fracture healing simulation, however, has the abilities to freely define the fixation stiffness independent of the design of the fixation devices used, to define and control the acting loading situation, and to simulate large numbers of arbitrarily defined fixation scenarios. Given a proper corroboration by available and suitable *in vivo* results, *in silico* simulations have large potential to provide insights into the mechanical influence on the healing outcome.

Hence, the aim of the present study was to numerically simulate healing outcomes for sheep diaphyseal fractures under physiological loading, being treated by fixations with various combinations of different axial and translational shear fixation stiffness. Thereby, optimal as well as detrimental configurations of fixation stiffness should be identified.

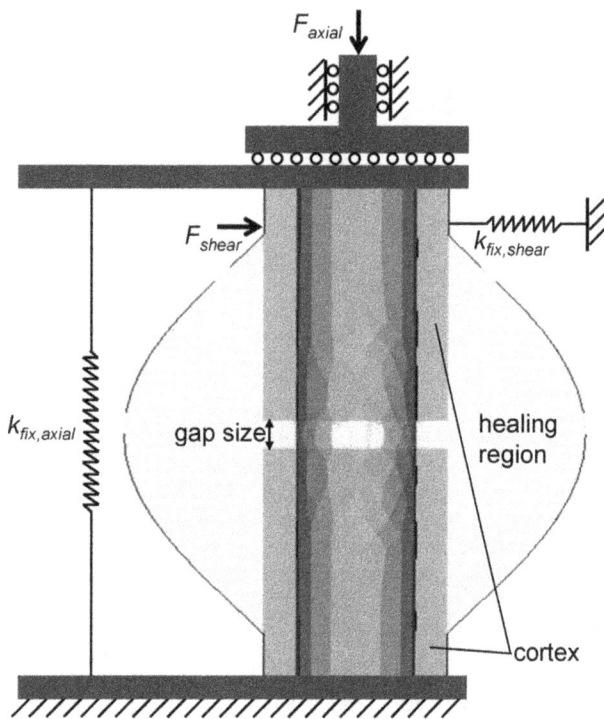

Figure 1. Boundary conditions of the superimposed loading case.

Methods

Numerical fracture healing model

For the present computational study, a three-dimensional finite element model of an idealized mid-diaphyseal, transversal, osteotomy geometry in the ovine tibia (endosteal diameter: 13 mm, periosteal diameter: 20 mm, gap sizes: 1 mm, 3 mm) and its healing region was created and meshed in ANSYS (v14.0, ANSYS Inc., Canonsburg, PA, USA) using tetrahedral elements. Material properties were obtained in a previous study [26] (cf. Table 1) and were assumed as linear elastic and isotropic. Due to large variations in the literature, average loading magnitudes were calculated based on data from three different *in vivo* studies [27,28,29] to represent physiological loading conditions in the mid-diaphyseal sheep tibia. Thus, assuming a mean bodyweight of 63 kg [21], an axial compressive load of 840 N and a translational shear load of 200 N, was applied. To represent the use of intramedullary nailing for fracture fixation, the intramedullary (endosteal) healing region was not modeled. Implemented boundary conditions for loading and fixation behavior are shown

in Figure 1. Elements within the healing region initially consist of connective tissue that develops into cartilage or bone during the healing process, depending on the local mechanical conditions. This is controlled by a previously published numerical fracture healing simulation algorithm that was described in detail elsewhere [30,31]. Briefly, the algorithm applies a set of 20 linguistic fuzzy logic rules (Fuzzy Logic Toolbox in MATLAB (v7.11, R2010b), The MathWorks, Inc., Natick, MA, USA) that controls how tissue composition and vascularization for each finite element changes depending on local mechanical and biological stimuli in an iterative process, representing the healing progress. The rules are based on the mechanoregulatory model proposed by Claes and Heigele [32] and represent intramembranous ossification, chondrogenesis, endochondral ossification, revascularization and tissue destruction. The outputs of this model are the courses of IFM and tissue distribution over the healing time. Additionally, the bending stiffness was calculated for each iteration step by a cantilever bending simulation. The respective bending stiffness $k_{Bend} = EI$ is defined as

$$EI = \frac{F_{bend} \cdot L^3}{3 \cdot u_{bend}}, \qquad (1)$$

where L is the overall length of the bone model, u_{bend} is the applied displacement, and F_{bend} is the corresponding reaction bending force. In a previous study [26] the healing algorithm was further calibrated to properly predict fracture healing processes under various loading conditions (particularly under axial compression, torsional and translational shear loading) in sheep. In contrast to previous studies, where a certain initial IFM was allowed by the fixation, in the present work the stiffness of the initial callus material had a remarkable influence. Therefore the existing model was expanded by adding a maturation of the initial connective tissue over the healing time (i.e. a sigmoidal increase from 0.1 MPa, representing fracture hematoma, to 1.4 MPa, representing mature connective tissue, within 8 weeks). Preceding simulations showed that this had no notable influence on predicting our previous calibration load cases [26] properly.

Characteristic maps of bending stiffness correlated to fixation stability

To create characteristic maps of healing outcome resulting from fixation stability, healing processes were simulated for a total of 96 different combinations of axial ($k_{fix,axial} = 1$, 50, 500, 1000, 1500, 2000, 2500, 3000, 3500, 5000, 7500, 10000 N/mm) and translational shear ($k_{fix,shear} = 1$, 100, 200, 300, 400, 500, 600, 1000 N/mm) fixation stiffness for two gap sizes: most in vivo studies in sheep apply gaps of 2–3 mm, therefore a gap size of 3 mm was chosen, additionally, a small gap size of 1 mm was investigated. For each combination, the bending stiffness was

Table 1. Material properties of the involved tissues, according to Steiner et al. [26].

	Young's Modulus,	Poisson's Ratio,
	E_{tiss} in MPa	ν_{tiss}
Cortical bone	15750	0.325
Woven bone	538	0.33
Fibrocartilage	28	0.3
Connective tissue	1.4	0.33

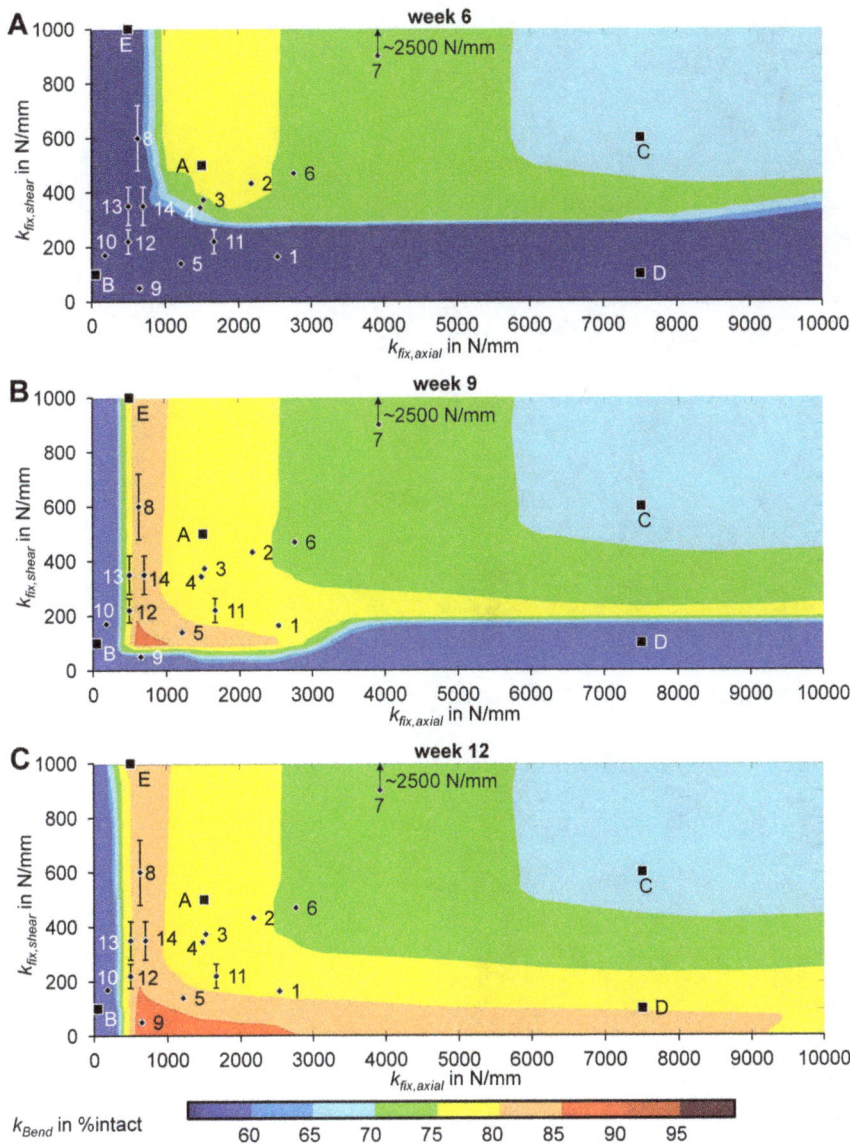

Figure 2. 3 mm osteotomy: characteristic maps of bending stiffness depending on the fracture fixation stiffness in axial ($k_{fix,axial}$) and shear ($k_{fix,shear}$) direction after A 6 weeks of healing B 9 weeks of healing C 12 weeks of healing. Bending stiffness (k_{Bend}) is given as the percentage of the intact (contralateral) bone bending stiffness. Numbered data points refer to experimental data in Table 3, error bars indicate estimated values (20% error) for unknown shear stiffness of the devices. Letters indicate positions of the exemplary simulation results in Figure 5.

reported relatively to the bending stiffness of the respective intact tibial bone (i.e. contralateral side, $EI = 100$ Nmm^2) at several healing time points (i.e. 6, 9, and 12 weeks). We used a surface-fitting tool implemented in MATLAB (v7.11, R2010b, The MathWorks, Inc.) to create the continuous characteristic maps from the single data points.

Extracortical callus volume as predictor of the healing progress

As another indicator for the healing progress, the extracortical bony callus volume was calculated as a percentage of the numerically predefined healing region, where callus formation can take place. This is reported at different healing time points for several exemplary simulations in order to describe the progress of callus development and correlate it to their respective healing success. A further parameter for the callus size is the callus index,

which is defined as the ratio between callus and cortex diameters ($CI = diam_{callus} / diam_{cortex}$).

Corroboration on literature data of different fixation stiffness

For comparison of the created characteristic maps with experimental data, the literature regarding studies which investigated the influence of mechanics on fracture healing in sheep was reviewed. Experimental conditions of the reviewed studies needed to strongly agree with the present simulation parameters. Thus, *in vivo* cases with osteotomies in ovine long bone diaphyses with appropriate gap sizes were chosen. Studies which did not properly characterize the stiffness of the fixation device could not be included. Additionally, only fixations with steady, linear stiffness behavior could be included, and therefore study results where a non-linear fixation stiffness was used (e.g. very rigid fixation allows

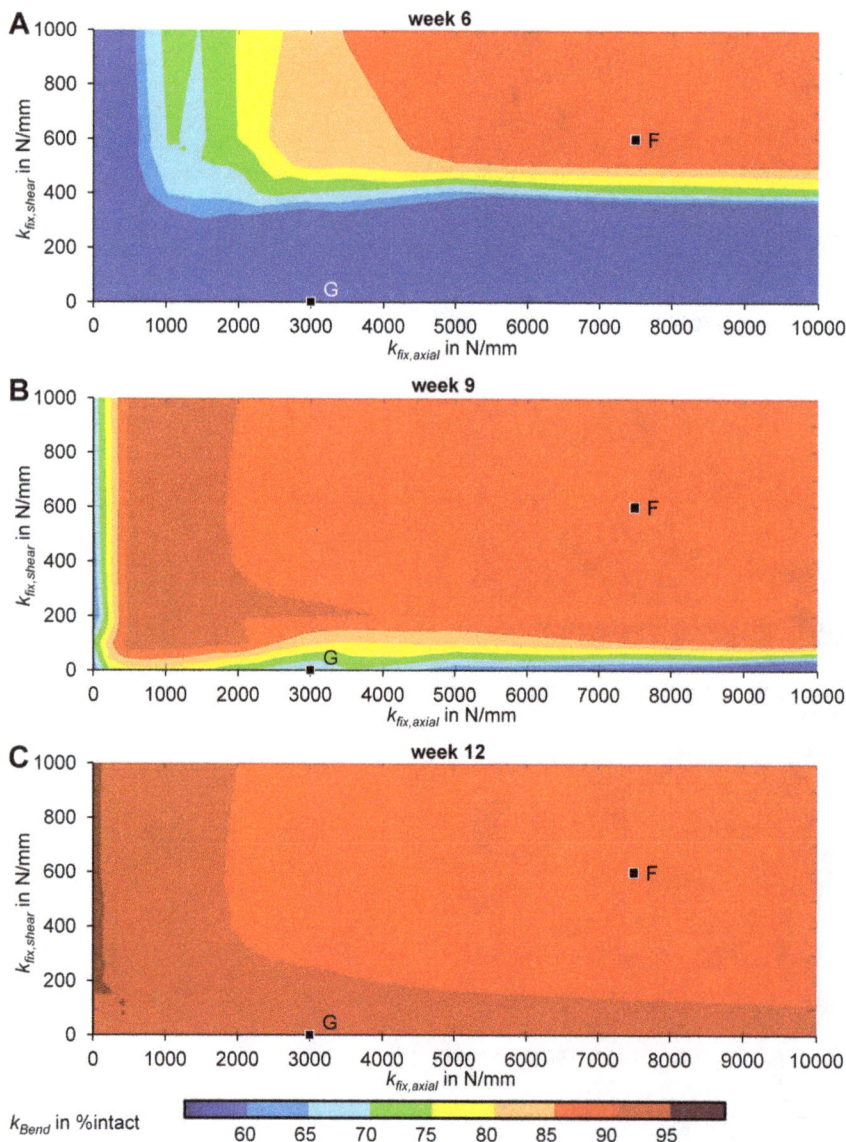

Figure 3. 1 mm osteotomy: characteristic maps of bending stiffness depending on the fracture fixation stiffness in axial ($k_{fix,axial}$) and shear ($k_{fix,shear}$) direction after A 6 weeks of healing B 9 weeks of healing C 12 weeks of healing. Bending stiffness (k_{Bend}) is given as the percentage of the intact (contralateral) bone bending stiffness. Letters indicate positions of the exemplary simulation results in Figure 6.

a certain amount of initial IFM by very low fixation stiffness, cf. Claes et al. [10]) were not taken into account. Furthermore, IFM should only result from the stiffness behavior of the bone-implant construct passively under physiological loading; active IFM applied by actuators could not be included in this study.

Results

Characteristic maps of bending stiffness correlated to fixation stability

The bending stiffness depends on the fixation stiffness in both the shear and axial loading directions as shown in Figure 2 at three healing time points for the physiological loading of an ovine, diaphyseal fracture with 3 mm gap size. At week 6 (Figure 2A), cases with 1000 N/mm–2500 N/mm axial stiffness combined with stiffness greater than 300 N/mm in shear direction are bridged with a resulting bending stiffness greater than 75% of the

respective intact bone. Cases with axial stiffness larger than 3000 N/mm also show bridging but develop a bending stiffness smaller than 75%. A large proportion of cases still show no bridging (i.e. black area). At week 9 (Figure 2B), cases with axial stiffness of 500 N/mm–1000 N/mm show bridging with large callus development, leading to high bending stiffness, greater than 80%, even for more flexible shear stiffness (>100 N/mm). No healing is observed for overly flexible fixation in both stiffness directions. At week 12 (Figure 2C), only cases which are overly flexible in the axial direction continue to show non-unions. Cases with small shear rigidity developed large calluses, which lead to bending stiffness greater than 80%.

Bending stiffness for the same fixation stabilities but for a small gap size of 1 mm show less impact of the fixation stability as compared to a medium gap size of 3 mm. At week 6 (Figure 3A), a large proportion of cases with large stiffness in both directions (i.e. >400 N/mm in shear; and >2500 N/mm in axial direction)

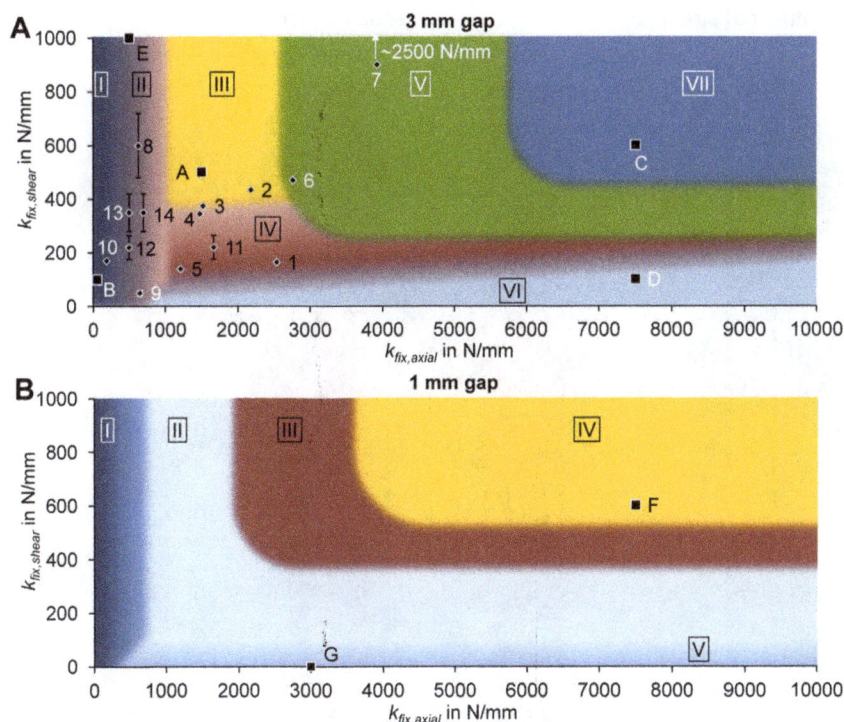

Figure 4. Qualitative characteristic maps of healing outcome depending on the fracture fixation stiffness in axial ($k_{fix,axial}$) and shear ($k_{fix,shear}$) direction for A 3 mm fracture gap; B 1 mm fracture gap. Roman numerals refer to areas of different healing outcomes as explained in detail in Table 3. Letters indicate positions of the exemplary simulation results in Figures 5 and 6.

already show healing with large bending stiffness greater than 80%. At week 9 (Figure 3B), only cases with very flexible stiffness in both directions still show non-unions. However, these are healed at 12 weeks (Figure 3C) and demonstrate very large resulting bending stiffness (>90%).

Qualitatively, the characteristic map for the 3 mm fracture gap can be classified into seven different regions according to Figure 4A and Table 2. Hence, the optimal range (region III, light grey) is 1000 N/mm–2500 N/mm axial stiffness, combined with stiffness greater than 300 N/mm in shear direction (cf. Figure 5, case A). Overly flexible fixation in either direction (approximately < 200 N/mm in axial and <100 N/mm in shear direction) results in delayed healing due to instability and high tissue strains (cf. Figure 5, case B). Impeding influences of low shear stiffness can be compensated by adjusting the axial stiffness; vice versa, this compensatory effect is limited (i.e. increased shear stiffness does not improve the negative effect of low axial stiffness). Furthermore, very high axial stiffness (approximately >3000 N/mm) of the fixation device also results in delayed healing (cf. Figure 5, case C). This effect can, in turn, be partly compensated by decreasing the shear stiffness to approximately 200 N/mm. Furthermore, cases with predominant shear movements (i.e. large axial rigidity, low shear stiffness, cf. Figure 5, case D) show delayed healing when compared against cases with predominant axial movements (cf. Figure 5, case E).

The findings for the 3 mm fracture gap were qualitatively classified into five different categories according to Figure 4B and Table 2. Thus, the best healing results are obtained for very high fixation rigidity (cf. Figure 6, case F), due to a direct gap ossification healing mechanism. For more flexible fixations, healing is delayed compared to the 3 mm gap results. However,

those delayed healing cases do not result in non-unions (cf. Figure 6, case G).

Extracortical callus volume as predictor of the healing progress

As another measure of the healing outcome, the relative extracortical callus volume was investigated for exemplary cases A–E with a gap size of 3 mm. This reveals that the optimal stiffness configuration (cf. Figure 5, case A) leads to only moderate callus formation of 20–30% (CI = ~1.6). Overly flexible configurations lead to extracortical, bony callus formation of less than 50%, which does not result in bony bridging (Figure 5, case B). Likewise, for overly rigid configurations no extracortical bony callus is developed (>4000 N/mm axial stiffness combined with > 400 N/mm shear stiffness leads to <10% extracortical bony callus). In a majority of these cases, bony bridging occurs early in the healing process, but only intercortically with minimal extracortical bone formation (cf. Figure 5, case C).

The largest CI is shown in case B at week 3, which however results in non-union after 9 weeks, whereas case A shows optimal healing (within 5–6 weeks) although it has developed only a moderate CI of 1.6 after 6 weeks. Furthermore, the CI is not directly correlated to the actual callus size, since it only accounts for the largest callus diameter, but not for the total callus volume. This is visible when comparing cases D and E in Figure 5, which both show a large CI of 2.5, and 2.2 after 9 weeks, respectively but a callus volume which differs by a factor of 2.

Corroboration on literature data of different fixation stiffness

Review of the literature on fracture healing experiments in sheep revealed only a limited number of studies which could be

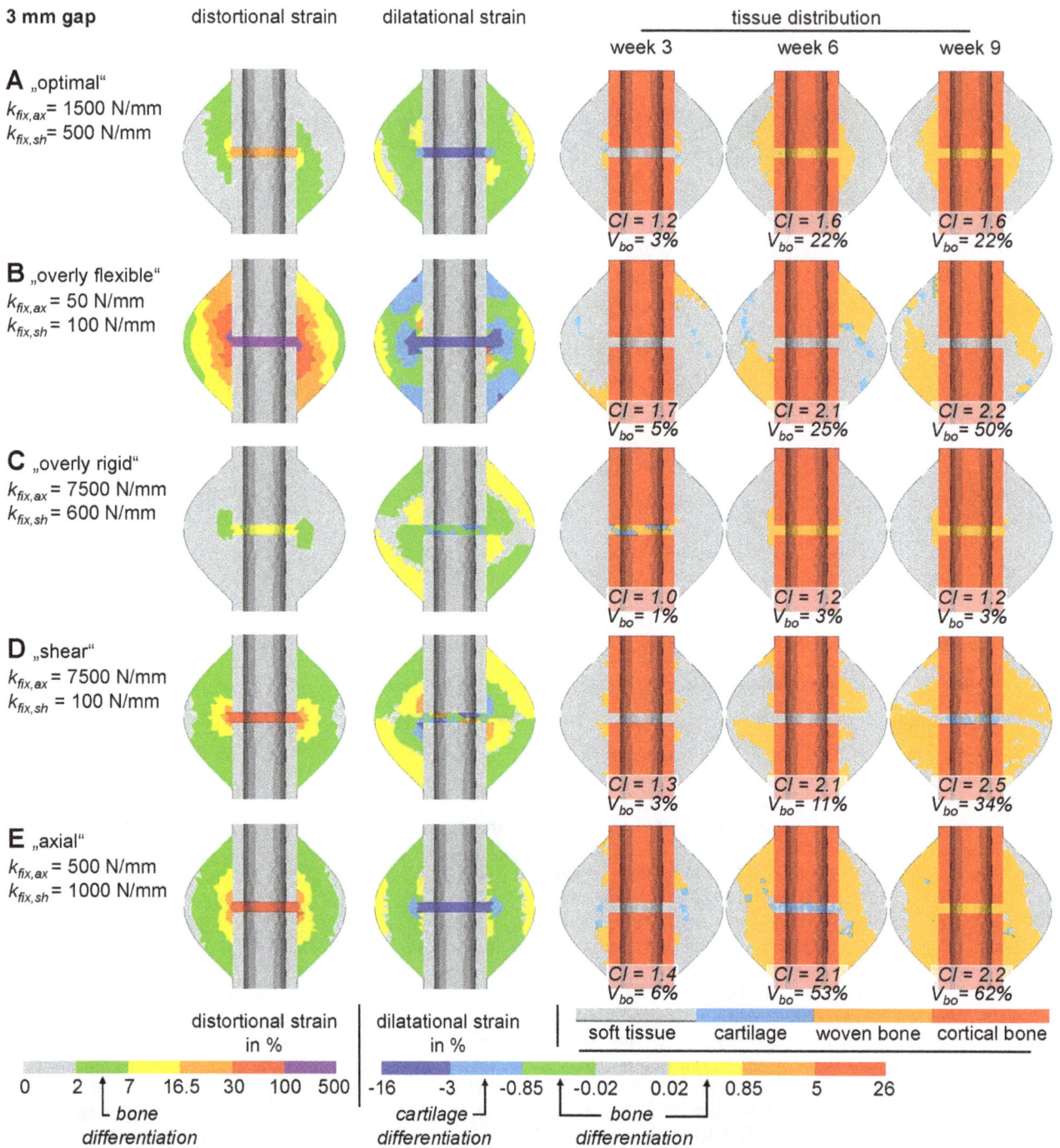

Figure 5. Five different exemplary simulations for a 3 mm gap size. For each case the initial distortional and dilatational strain field is shown, which determine the tissue differentiation following the hypothetic rules of Claes and Heigele [32]. Respective tissue stimulating strain ranges are indicated at the color bars. Additionally, the tissue distribution, as well as the percentage of extracortical bony callus volume (V_{bo}), and the callus index (CI) at 3, 6, and 9 weeks of healing are displayed for **A** optimal fracture fixation; **B** overly flexible fixation leading to non-union; **C** overly rigid fixation leading to inhibition of callus development with unstable bending stiffness; **D** a predominant shear load case; **E** a predominant axial load case. Letters are according to diagrams in Figures 2 and 4.

applied to corroborate the obtained computational results, as listed in Table 3. Only experiments which applied 2–3 mm osteotomies could be included and were assigned to the simulations of 3 mm gap size. Moreover, only few studies reported values for the stiffness of their fixation devices in both, axial as well as shear direction. Thus, also cases were included where only the axial stiffness was reported. For these, ranges of shear stiffness (20% -

error bars in Figures 2 and 4) were estimated based on comparable fixation devices. This data acts as orientation to classify existing fixation methods within the characteristic map presented, and to evaluate the validity of the numerical predictions. Due to the variety of different criteria of measuring healing outcomes in the included studies, a direct quantitative comparison between them and to the present results could not be realized. Qualitatively, the

Table 2. Comments on the qualitative characteristic maps in Figure 4.

	3 mm gap	1 mm gap
I	**Non-union** due to overly flexible fixation	**Delayed healing** with large callus formation and high bending stiffness (>95%) after 12 weeks
II	**Slightly delayed healing** with large callus formation and high bending stiffness (>80%) after 9 weeks	**Slightly delayed healing** with large callus formation and high bending stiffness (>90%) after 9 weeks
III	**Optimal healing** with fast formation of moderate callus volume showing a high bending stiffness (>75%) after 6 weeks	**Quick healing** with moderate callus formation showing sufficient bending stiffness (>85%) after 6 weeks
IV	**Slightly delayed healing** with moderate callus formation showing sufficient bending stiffness (>75%) after 9 weeks	**Optimal healing** - fast formation of moderate callus volume showing a high bending stiffness (>90%) after 6 weeks
V	**Suboptimal healing** - overly rigid fixation stiffness shows rapid but small callus formation resulting in insufficient bending stiffness (kB<75%) at 6 weeks, which does not increase further	**Delayed healing** with large callus formation and high bending stiffness (>90%) after 12 weeks
VI	**Delayed healing** with large callus formation and high bending stiffness (>85%) after 12 weeks	–
VII	**Unfavorable healing** - overly rigid fixation stiffness shows rapid but very small callus formation resulting in unstable bending stiffness (kB<70%) at 6 weeks, which does not increase further	–

predictions are generally in good accordance to experimental results. The best healing outcomes are predicted for cases 2, 3, and 4, which were also experimentally classified [21] as "good" or "excellent healing" (i.e. torsional moment at failure after 9 weeks between 66.3% and 83% of contra-lateral intact tibia, cf. Table 3). Desirable healing outcomes are also predicted for case 8, as confirmed by the respective experiments [33,34]. Slightly delayed but still acceptable healing times are predicted for cases 1, 5, 12, 13, and 14, which does not conflict with the *in vivo* findings [21,34,35]. However, when compared to case 13, the simulations predicted an advanced healing for case 14, which is in contrast to the experiment where a greater healing delay was observed for case 14 [34]. Delayed healing is simulated for cases 6 and 9. For case 6, this is in acceptable agreement with the *in vivo* findings [21] whereas for case 9 experimental results show continuation of non-unions after 6 months [25] while the simulation suggests healing at around 10 weeks. The worst healing is predicted for cases 7 and 10. This was experimentally verified for case 7 [33], whereas the simulation for case 10 predicts worse healing than experimentally detected [36]. In general, but especially for cases 3, 4, 5 and 11, our model tends to predict slightly faster healing than experimentally measured [21,37].

Discussion

Besides systemic, biological factors, the mechanical conditions within a fracture gap influence the bone healing process decisively. The present study focuses on these mechanical effects. Thus, characteristic maps were created which show the bending stiffness of an osteotomized sheep tibia as a function of superimposed translational shear and axial compressive fixation stiffness at several healing time points under physiological loading conditions. To evaluate the validity of the obtained simulation results, numerous outcomes of appropriate experiments were compared to the generated characteristic maps.

The findings presented go beyond the *in vivo* experimental conclusions of Epari et al. [21], who found that enhanced healing outcomes can be achieved especially through optimization of the axial stiffness to moderate values and limitation of the translational shear flexibility. Our results confirm these findings, and further-more show that both loading directions are able to accelerate as well as delay healing. Positive or negative influences of one directional stiffness can be diminished by adjusting the stiffness of the other direction appropriately. Our results suggest that positive healing effects due to appropriate axial stiffness can only be impaired to a limited extent by disadvantageous shear stiffness. Vice versa, negative impacts of too low of a shear stiffness can clearly be compensated by favorable axial stiffness. Due to the small magnitudes of loading in shear direction and superimposed influences of axial loading, these results are not in contrast to our previous findings [24], which stated that, under equal mechanical conditions, isolated shear movements are more detrimental for fracture healing processes than isolated axial compressive move-ments. Because of the limited number of appropriate *in vivo* studies, our findings could only be corroborated for 3 mm gap situations, nonetheless we also investigated a small gap size of 1 mm. We found that small gaps result in desirable healing almost independently of the stiffness configuration. We assume that this is the effect of direct gap ossification, as was found in other experiments applying minimal IFM on small defects in sheep [18,38]. However, for more flexible fixations, healing is delayed compared to the 3 mm gap results, which is due to the larger strains that arise from the small gap size being exposed to the same loading conditions as the larger 3 mm gap. Regarding the effects of different fixation devices, the present characteristic maps suggest ranges of fixation stiffness in axial and shear direction with the best healing outcome, which are most closely reached by external fixators. Tibial nails or internal plates in their current designs are found to be less stimulatory due to their large rigidity in axial direction [39,40]. To overcome these negative influences for

Table 3. Literature data of numerous experiments, investigating the healing outcome under different fixation devices on osteotomies in long bone diaphyses of sheep.

#	Fixation device	Healing outcome	Axial stiffness in N/mm	Shear stiffness in N/mm
1	Medially mounted monolateral external fixator [21]	Torsional moment at failure after 9 weeks: 61.5% of contra-lateral intact tibia	2540	164
2	Anteromedially mounted monolateral external fixator [21]	Torsional moment at failure after 9 weeks: 83% of contra-lateral intact tibia	2177	433
3	Rigid monolateral external fixator [21]	Torsional moment at failure after 9 weeks: 68.2% of contra-lateral intact tibia	1523	374
4	Semirigid monolateral external fixator [21]	Torsional moment at failure after 9 weeks: 66.3% of contra-lateral intact tibia	1479	344
5	Unreamed tibial nail [21]	Torsional moment at failure after 9 weeks: 52.8% of contra-lateral intact tibia	1213	139
6	Angle-stable tibial nail [21]	Torsional moment at failure after 9 weeks: 64.1% of contra-lateral intact tibia	2762	469
7	Locked plating [33]	Torsional strength after 9 weeks: ~42% of contra-lateral intact tibia	3922*	2500*
8	Far cortical locked plating [33]	Torsional strength after 9 weeks: ~67% of contra-lateral intact tibia	628**	600**
9	Mechanically critical external fixator [25]	Torsional moment at failure after 9 weeks: 14% of contra-lateral intact tibia	650	50***
10	Unilateral external fixator [36]	Bending stiffness after 6 weeks: 60% of contra-lateral intact tibia	183	170
11	Rigid unilateral external fixator/ actuator [37] (2 mm gap)	Bending stiffness after 6 weeks: 24% of contra-lateral intact tibia	1666	220***
12	Rigid unilateral external fixator/actuator [35] (2.6 mm gap)	Bending stiffness after 8 weeks: 60–69% of contra-lateral intact tibia	498	220***
13	Monolateral external fixator [34], 35 mm pin offset	Week 6: advanced healing, week 12: bony bridging	500	350***
14	Monolateral external fixator [34], 25 mm pin offset	Week 6: less advanced healing, week 12: bony bridging	700	350***

*shear and axial stiffness numerically calculated (FE-model) – shear stiffness exceeds characteristic map and is marked by an arrow.
**axial stiffness prior to bony contact of the pins, shear stiffness estimated with 20% error.
***shear stiffness assumed based on comparable devices −20% error estimated.

internal plates, a far cortical locking method was developed, which shifts the axial stiffness to that of external fixators leading to more favorable healing success in sheep experiments [33,41]. Another approach was the development of dynamic locking screws, which also increased axial motion especially at the near-plate cortex [42,43]. For intramedullary nails this problem was faced by decreasing their axial stiffness to achieve accelerated healing without changing the torsional or translational shear rigidity of the nails [40]. However, intramedullary nails are widely used and show good clinical outcomes in general [44]. As explanation, we assume that sufficient stimulatory axial IFM is created by the relatively low bending rigidity of intramedullary nails [21,45].

The characteristic maps presented indicate areas where mechanical stimulation is insufficient for callus formation for the 3 mm gap. According to Perren et al. [46], this effect can be regarded as primary bone healing under very stable conditions.

Our simulations predict the development of very small woven bone callus around the gap (Figure 5, case C), which provides no sufficient stabilization of the fracture and might lead to re-fractures. This is expressed by the low bending stiffness arising from the small callus area moment of inertia and the low material stiffness of the new developed woven bone tissue (cf. Table 1). These findings are confirmed by clinical studies which report re-fractures after the removal of very rigid osteosynthesis devices, especially of internal plates in the forearm [47], femur [48], clavicle, and tibia [49], even though they had been classified as "successfully healed" before removal. Therefore, these very rigid cases lead to unfavorable healing outcomes under physiological conditions.

An examination on the ability of the callus size (CI or callus volume) to serve as an indicator for the success of fracture healing revealed that no dependable prognosis of the healing outcome can

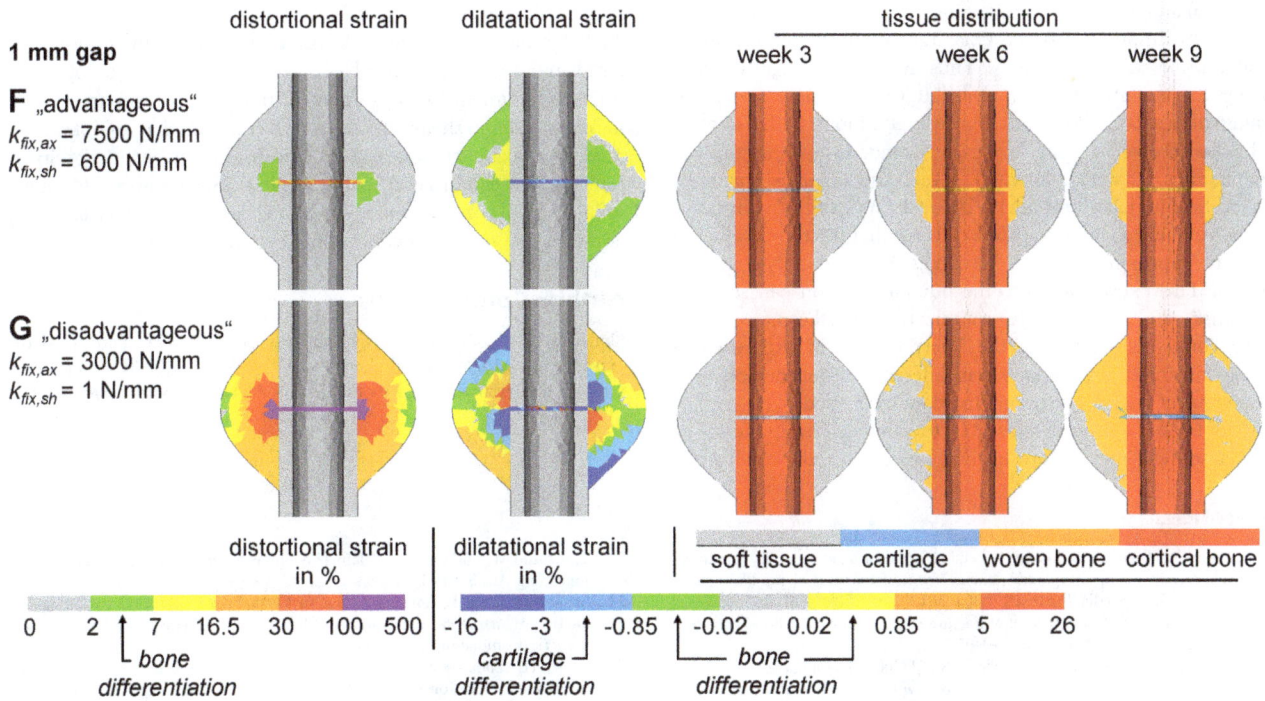

Figure 6. Exemplary simulations for a 1 mm gap size. For each case the initial distortional and dilatational strain field is shown, which determine the tissue differentiation following the hypothetic rules of Claes and Heigele [32]. Respective tissue stimulating strain ranges are indicated at the color bars. Additionally, the tissue distribution at 3, 6, and 9 weeks of healing are displayed for **F** advantageous fixation; **G** disadvantageous (overly flexible) fixation. Letters are according to diagrams in Figures 3 and 4.

be made solely based on the callus size at early healing time points. This is according to Marsh [50], who stated that stiffness measurement is more appropriate than the CI to predict functional outcome of fracture healing in patients. Furthermore, neither the CI nor the callus volume account for the shape of the callus, which can be symmetrical under axial dominated IFM or asymmetrical under shear dominated IFM. The latter show smaller total callus volume, which still has the ability to bridge in the far periphery, resulting in delayed healing compared to axially dominated cases with symmetrical callus development (cf. case D versus case E in Figure 5).

The results of this study show that the optimal healing outcome is reached with a moderate callus volume. For very small calluses, we predict unstable healing due to insufficient mechanical stimulation, whereas large calluses can result in healing, delayed healing or even non-unions despite the large callus volume. The latter can be characterized as hypertrophic non-unions, where large calluses are developed which will not result in bony bridging due to large persisting IFM.

There are two major drawbacks which influence the clinical relevance of the present study: (1) it is a numerical study which is accompanied with several modeling assumptions and limitations. First, we excluded endosteal healing regions; this was reasonable since it represents the situation for intramedullary nailing, and pre-investigations indicated that it has no remarkable effect on the simulated healing results. Furthermore, revascularization after fracture is mainly derived rather from surrounding soft tissue and periosteum than from the bone marrow [51,52,53]. Second, we used a linear description for our callus model which includes linear elastic and isotropic material properties as well as a linear behavior of the fixation device. Third, we applied a simplified, superimposed, and averaged loading scenario, consisting of axial

compressive and translational shear loading. This represents the physiological conditions at the fracture site in sheep only to a limited extent since additionally axial distraction, bending, and torsional shear occurs [27,28,29] and forces for other activities than normal walking (i.e. running, jumping, and short impact forces) are not known and could not be considered. From a mechanical point of view, it is reasonable to focus on axial compression and translational shear, which represent the predominant loading directions within a fracture site since bending mainly produces axial compression within the fracture gap and stiff fixation devices such as intramedullary nails produce shear loading due to play within the medullary canal [16]. Despite these model limitations, our study uses the advantages of numerical simulation to deliver unprecedented, continuous data maps of fixation stiffness and their resulting healing outcomes, by extending results from previous *in vivo* experiments, which themselves provide only punctual information due to their limited number. Furthermore, the corroboration of the numerical simulations depends on the availability of adequate *in vivo* data, which is still limited. Although for numerous cases the respective shear stiffness could only be estimated and was assigned with 20%-error bars, the underlying algorithm was calibrated on various loading conditions in sheep [26] and the characteristic maps of the present study were corroborated by several suitable *in vivo* data points. Thereby, the applied model reaches a relatively high validity to properly predict fracture healing processes in sheep.

(2) This study simulated the fracture healing processes in sheep. Apart from differences between sheep and humans in the loading situation [11,12,13] and the fracture geometry, our results are not directly transferable to the human situation because, clinically, large variations of different fracture types and circumstances occur. However, our results can approximately be extrapolated to

the clinical situation by comparing our results for idealized sheep fractures to simple, transverse tibia fractures in patients without additional injuries and diseases. Thus, Marsh [50] reports rapid healing in patients to occur after 10 weeks, whereas delayed healing takes around 20 weeks. This was also found by Claes et al. [54], who observed healing for simple, closed, Type A fractures in patients after 10 weeks; for more severe and complex fractures, delayed healing takes around 15–20 weeks. With this quantitative data, we assume as an extrapolation factor that fracture healing in sheep is approximately 1.7–1.8 times faster than in human patients. This extrapolation to the human situation can serve as orientation for fracture care optimization. Furthermore, these results could be helpful for the interpretation of experimental findings on fracture healing, when different fixation devices (e.g. intramedullary nails vs. external fixation) were used.

In summary, this study was able to simulate the influence of fixation stiffness on fracture healing processes and revealed the

optimal fixation stiffness configuration for rapid fracture healing. The presented findings provide numerous insights into desirable or disadvantageous mechanical conditions which help to optimize fracture treatment by adjustment of the fracture fixation stability in both axial and shear directions. We conclude that an optimized, moderate axial stiffness together with certain shear rigidity is essential for enhanced fracture healing. Furthermore, inhibiting influences of one loading direction can be compensated by adjusting the other directional stiffness appropriately.

Author Contributions

Conceived and designed the experiments: MS LC TW. Performed the experiments: MS. Analyzed the data: MS US TW LC AI. Contributed reagents/materials/analysis tools: MS LC AI US. Wrote the paper: MS.

References

1. Bhandari M, Tornetta P, Sprague S, Najibi S, Petrisor T, et al. (2003) Predictors of reoperation following operative management of fractures of the tibial shaft. Journal of Orthopaedic Trauma 17: 353–361.
2. Einhorn TA (1995) Enhancement of fracture healing. Journal of Bone and Joint Surgery-American Volume 77A: 940–956.
3. Karladani AH, Granhed H, Karrholm J, Styf J (2001) The influence of fracture etiology and type on fracture healing: a review of 104 consecutive tibial shaft fractures. Archives of Orthopaedic and Trauma Surgery 121: 325–328.
4. Brinker MR, O'Connor DP (2004) The incidence of fractures and dislocations referred for orthopaedic services in a capitated population. Journal of Bone and Joint Surgery-American Volume 86A: 290–297.
5. Praemer A, Furner S, Rice DP (1992) Musculoskeletal conditions in the United States. Rosemont, IL: American Academy of Orthopaedic Surgeons Park Ridge.
6. Claes L, Recknagel S, Ignatius A (2012) Fracture healing under healthy and inflammatory conditions. Nature Reviews Rheumatology 8: 133–143.
7. Einhorn TA (1998) The cell and molecular biology of fracture healing. Clinical Orthopaedics and Related Research: S7–S21.
8. Pauwels F (1960) [A new theory on the influence of mechanical stimuli on the differentiation of supporting tissue]. Z Anat Entwicklungsgesch 121: 478–515.
9. Carter DR, Blenman PR, Beaupre GS (1988) Correlations between mechanical stress history and tissue differentiation in initial fracture healing. J Orthop Res 6: 736–748.
10. Claes L, Augat P, Suger G, Wilke HJ (1997) Influence of size and stability of the osteotomy gap on the success of fracture healing. J Orthop Res 15: 577–584.
11. Wehner T, Claes L, Simon U (2009) Internal loads in the human tibia during gait. Clin Biomech 24: 299–302.
12. Gardner TN, Evans M, Hardy J, Kenwright J (1997) Dynamic interfragmentary motion in fractures during routine patient activity. Clinical Orthopaedics and Related Research: 216–225.
13. Duda GN, Sollmann M, Sporrer S, Hoffmann JE, Kassi JP, et al. (2002) Interfragmentary motion in tibial osteotomies stabilized with ring fixators. Clinical Orthopaedics and Related Research: 163–172.
14. Bhandari M, Guyatt GH, Swiontkowski MF, Tornetta P 3rd, Hanson B, et al. (2001) Surgeons' preferences for the operative treatment of fractures of the tibial shaft. An international survey. J Bone Joint Surg Am 83-A: 1746–1752.
15. Bottlang M, Feist F (2011) Biomechanics of far cortical locking. J Orthop Trauma 25 Suppl 1: S21–28.
16. Wehner T, Penzkofer R, Augat P, Claes L, Simon U (2011) Improvement of the shear fixation stability of intramedullary nailing. Clinical Biomechanics 26: 147–151.
17. Kenwright J, Richardson J, Cunningham J, White S, Goodship A, et al. (1991) Axial movement and tibial fractures. A controlled randomised trial of treatment. Journal of Bone & Joint Surgery, British Volume 73-B: 654–659.
18. Claes LE, Wilke HJ, Augat P, Rubenacker S, Margevicius KJ (1995) Effect of dynamization on gap healing of diaphyseal fractures under external fixation. Clin Biomech (Bristol, Avon) 10: 227–234.
19. Claes LE, Heigele CA, Neidlinger-Wilke C, Kaspar D, Seidl W, et al. (1998) Effects of mechanical factors on the fracture healing process. Clin Orthop Relat Res: S132–147.
20. Larsson S, Kim W, Caja VL, Egger EL, Inoue N, et al. (2001) Effect of early axial dynamization on tibial bone healing - A study in dogs. Clinical Orthopaedics and Related Research: 240–251.
21. Epari DR, Kassi JP, Schell H, Duda GN (2007) Timely fracture-healing requires optimization of axial fixation stability. J Bone Joint Surg Am 89: 1575–1585.
22. Augat P, Burger J, Schorlemmer S, Henke T, Peraus M, et al. (2003) Shear movement at the fracture site delays healing in a diaphyseal fracture model. J Orthop Res 21: 1011–1017.

23. Yamagishi M, Yoshimura Y (1955) The biomechanics of fracture healing. J Bone Joint Surg Am 37: 1035–1068.
24. Steiner M, Claes L, Ignatius A, Simon U, Wehner T (2014) Disadvantages of interfragmentary shear on fracture healing – mechanical insights through numerical simulation. J Orthop Res In press.
25. Schell H, Thompson MS, Bail HJ, Hoffmann JE, Schill A, et al. (2008) Mechanical induction of critically delayed bone healing in sheep: radiological and biomechanical results. J Biomech 41: 3066–3072.
26. Steiner M, Claes L, Ignatius A, Niemeyer F, Simon U, et al. (2013) Prediction of fracture healing under axial loading, shear loading and bending is possible using distortional and dilatational strains as determining mechanical stimuli. Journal of the Royal Society Interface 10: 20130389.
27. Heller MO, Duda GN, Ehrig RM, Schell H, Seebeck P, et al. (2005) Muskuloskeletale Belastungen im Schafshinterlauf: Mechanische Rahmenbedingungen der Heilung. Mat-wiss u Werkstofftech 2005, 36, No 12 36: 775–780.
28. Duda GN, Eckert-Hubner K, Sokiranski R, Kreutner A, Miller R, et al. (1998) Analysis of interfragmentary movement as a function of musculoskeletal loading conditions in sheep. J Biomech 31: 201–210.
29. Grasa J, Gomez-Benito MJ, Gonzalez-Torres LA, Asiain D, Quero F, et al. (2010) Monitoring in vivo load transmission through an external fixator. Ann Biomed Eng 38: 605–612.
30. Simon U, Augat P, Utz M, Claes L (2011) A numerical model of the fracture healing process that describes tissue development and revascularisation. Comput Methods Biomech Biomed Engin 14: 79–93.
31. Wehner T, Claes L, Niemeyer F, Nolte D, Simon U (2010) Influence of the fixation stability on the healing time-a numerical study of a patient-specific fracture healing process. Clin Biomech 25: 606–612.
32. Claes LE, Heigele CA (1999) Magnitudes of local stress and strain along bony surfaces predict the course and type of fracture healing. J Biomech 32: 255–266.
33. Bottlang M, Lesser M, Koerber J, Doornink J, von Rechenberg B, et al. (2010) Far cortical locking can improve healing of fractures stabilized with locking plates. J Bone Joint Surg Am 92: 1652–1660.
34. Goodship AE, Watkins PE, Rigby HS, Kenwright J (1993) The role of fixator frame stiffness in the control of fracture healing. An experimental study. J Biomech 26: 1027–1035.
35. Bishop NE, van Rhijn M, Tami I, Corveleijn R, Schneider E, et al. (2006) Shear does not necessarily inhibit bone healing. Clin Orthop Relat Res 443: 307–314.
36. Wolf S, Janousek A, Pfeil J, Veith W, Haas F, et al. (1998) The effects of external mechanical stimulation on the healing of diaphyseal osteotomies fixed by flexible external fixation. Clin Biomech (Bristol, Avon) 13: 359–364.
37. Hente R, Fuchtmeier B, Schlegel U, Ernstberger A, Perren SM (2004) The influence of cyclic compression and distraction on the healing of experimental tibial fractures. J Orthop Res 22: 709–715.
38. Claes L, Mutschler W (1981) Quantitative investigations on newly-built bone in defects - its time-dependent changes of morphological and biomechanical properties Archives of Orthopaedic and Trauma Surgery 98: 257–261.
39. Lujan TJ, Henderson CE, Madey SM, Fitzpatrick DC, Marsh JL, et al. (2010) Locked Plating of Distal Femur Fractures Leads to Inconsistent and Asymmetric Callus Formation. Journal of Orthopaedic Trauma 24: 156–162 110.1097/BOT.1090b1013e3181be6720.
40. Dailey HL, Daly CJ, Galbraith JG, Cronin M, Harty JA (2012) A novel intramedullary nail for micromotion stimulation of tibial fractures. Clinical Biomechanics 27: 182–188.
41. Bottlang M, Doornink J, Lujan TJ, Fitzpatrick DC, Marsh L, et al. (2010) Effects of Construct Stiffness on Healing of Fractures Stabilized with Locking Plates. Journal of Bone and Joint Surgery-American Volume 92A: 12–22.
42. Dobele S, Horn C, Eichhorn S, Buchholtz A, Lenich A, et al. (2010) The dynamic locking screw (DLS) can increase interfragmentary motion on the near

cortex of locked plating constructs by reducing the axial stiffness. Langenbecks Archives of Surgery 395: 421–428.

43. Plecko M, Lagerpusch N, Andermatt D, Frigg R, Koch R, et al. (2013) The dynamisation of locking plate osteosynthesis by means of dynamic locking screws (DLS)–An experimental study in sheep. Injury 44: 1346–1357.

44. Bhandari M, Guyatt GH, Swiontkowski MF, Schemitsch EH (2001) Treatment of open fractures of the shaft of the tibia - A systematic overview and meta-analysis. Journal of Bone and Joint Surgery-British Volume 83B: 62–68.

45. Penzkofer R, Maier M, Nolte A, von Oldenburg G, Püschel K, et al. (2009) Influence of intramedullary nail diameter and locking mode on the stability of tibial shaft fracture fixation. Archives of Orthopaedic and Trauma Surgery 129: 525–531.

46. Perren SM, Huggler A, Russenberger M, Allgower M, Mathys R, et al. (1969) The reaction of cortical bone to compression. Acta Orthop Scand Suppl 125: 19–29.

47. Beaupre GS, Csongradi JJ (1996) Refracture risk after plate removal in the forearm. Journal of Orthopaedic Trauma 10: 87–92.

48. Davison BL (2003) Refracture following plate removal in supracondylar-intercondylar femur fractures. Orthopedics 26: 157–159.

49. Ochs BG, Gonser CE, Baron HC, Stockle U, Badke A, et al. (2012) Refracture of long bones after implant removal. Unfallchirurg 115: 323–329.

50. Marsh D (1998) Concepts of fracture union, delayed union, and nonunion. Clinical Orthopaedics and Related Research: S22–S30.

51. Rhinelander FW (1974) Tibial Blood Supply in Relation to Fracture Healing. Clinical Orthopaedics and Related Research 105: 34–81.

52. Strachan R, McCarthy I, Fleming R, Hughes S (1990) The role of the tibial nutrient artery. Microsphere estimation of blood flow in the osteotomised canine tibia. Journal of Bone & Joint Surgery, British Volume 72-B: 391–394.

53. Triffitt PD, Cieslak CA, Gregg PJ (1993) A quantitative study of the routes of blood flow to the tibial diaphysis after an osteotomy. Journal of Orthopaedic Research 11: 49–57.

54. Claes L, Grass R, Schmickal T, Kisse B, Eggers C, et al. (2002) Monitoring and healing analysis of 100 tibial shaft fractures. Langenbecks Arch Surg 387: 146–152.

13

BMP-Non-Responsive Sca1$^+$CD73$^+$CD44$^+$ Mouse Bone Marrow Derived Osteoprogenitor Cells Respond to Combination of VEGF and BMP-6 to Display Enhanced Osteoblastic Differentiation and Ectopic Bone Formation

Vedavathi Madhu, Ching-Ju Li, Abhijit S. Dighe, Gary Balian, Quanjun Cui*

Orthopaedic Research Laboratories, Department of Orthopaedic Surgery, University of Virginia, Charlottesville, Virginia, United States of America

Abstract

Clinical trials on fracture repair have challenged the effectiveness of bone morphogenetic proteins (BMPs) but suggest that delivery of mesenchymal stem cells (MSCs) might be beneficial. It has also been reported that BMPs could not increase mineralization in several MSCs populations, which adds ambiguity to the use of BMPs. However, an exogenous supply of MSCs combined with vascular endothelial growth factor (VEGF) and BMPs is reported to synergistically enhance fracture repair in animal models. To elucidate the mechanism of this synergy, we investigated the osteoblastic differentiation of cloned mouse bone marrow derived MSCs (D1 cells) *in vitro* in response to human recombinant proteins of VEGF, BMPs (-2, -4, -6, -9) and the combination of VEGF with BMP-6 (most potent BMP). We further investigated ectopic bone formation induced by MSCs pre-conditioned with VEGF, BMP-6 or both. No significant increase in mineralization, phosphorylation of Smads 1/5/8 and expression of the ALP, COL1A1 and osterix genes was observed upon addition of VEGF or BMPs alone to the cells in culture. The lack of CD105, Alk1 and Alk6 expression in D1 cells correlated with poor response to BMPs indicating that a greater care in the selection of MSCs is necessary. Interestingly, the combination of VEGF and BMP-6 significantly increased the expression of ALP, COL1A1 and osterix genes and D1 cells pre-conditioned with VEGF and BMP-6 induced greater bone formation *in vivo* than the non-conditioned control cells or the cells pre-conditioned with either VEGF or BMP-6 alone. This enhanced bone formation by MSCs correlated with higher CADM1 expression and OPG/RANKL ratio in the implants. Thus, combined action of VEGF and BMP on MSCs enhances osteoblastic differentiation of MSCs and increases their bone forming ability, which cannot be achieved through use of BMPs alone. This strategy can be effectively used for bone repair.

Editor: Xing-Ming Shi, Georgia Regents University, United States of America

Funding: This work was supported by grants from the Orthopaedic Research and Education Foundation (OREF) http://www.oref.org/site/PageServer, the Musculoskeletal Transplant Foundation (MTF) https://www.mtf.org/ and the Orthopaedic Trauma Association (OTA) http://ota.org/ to QC. The funders had no role in study design, data collection and analysis, decision to publish, or preparation of the manuscript.

Competing Interests: The authors have declared that no competing interests exist.

* Email: QC4Q@hscmail.mcc.virginia.edu

Introduction

Injuries to the postnatal skeleton are repaired through natural healing which is a complex, well-orchestrated process that recapitulates the pathway of embryonic development. It involves a variety of cell types and signaling molecules. Deficiencies in mesenchymal stem cells (MSCs) [1–2], angiogenesis induced by vascular endothelial growth factor (VEGF) [3–4] and bone morphogenetic proteins (BMPs) signaling [5–7] are associated with fractures that do not heal. It is estimated that of the 7.9 million fractures sustained each year in the United States, 5% to 20% result in delayed or impaired healing [8].

Clinical trials conducted using BMP-2 and BMP-7 to enhance bone repair showed that the method is not cost effective [9–11]. A recent review of 11 randomized controlled trials and 4 economical evaluations of BMPs for fracture repair concluded that only one study showed a difference in fracture healing between the BMP treated and control groups, but there was some suggestion that no

second intervention was needed in the groups treated with BMP [10]. Several investigators have reported that BMPs fail to enhance mineralization and ALP expression in MSCs *in vitro* [12–21]; however the reasons that underlie the non-responsiveness of these cells are not understood. The limited success of clinical trials that used BMP-2 or BMP-7 could be due to suboptimal response of the osteoprogenitor cells as these stem cells play a pivotal role in BMP-induced bone repair [22]. The clinical trials using MSCs have shown promising results for fracture repair [23–24] which can be further enhanced through combined use of MSCs and BMPs if BMP-responsiveness of MSCs is better understood.

Combined delivery of MSCs, VEGF and BMPs (BMP-2, -4 and -7) has been immensely successful in enhancing fracture repair and bone formation in various animal models. We have systematically reviewed these studies recently [25]. These studies have shown that delivery of any single factor or combination of any two factors was less effective in inducing osteogenesis in comparison to that induced by MSCs, VEGF and BMP together. Synergistic enhancement of bone formation was BMP-type specific as VEGF and MSCs showed more influence on osteogenesis with BMP-4 than that with BMP-2 whereas there was no synergy with BMP-7 [26–28].

Since BMP-6 is reported to be more potent than BMP-2, -4 and -7 [29–30] and BMP-6 is resistant to inhibition by noggin while other BMPs are susceptible to noggin [31] which is predominantly expressed in non-union fractures [6–7], BMP-6 would be an ideal candidate to enhance fracture repair with VEGF and MSCs. We have demonstrated earlier that cloned mouse bone marrow derived mesenchymal stem cells (mBMMSCs) (D1 cells) co-expressing human VEGF and BMP-6 genes or VEGF and lim mineralization protein 1 (LMP1) genes induce significantly greater osteogenesis in vivo in comparison with that induced by D1 cells alone or by D1 cells expressing only one of those genes [32–33]. LMP-1 is a known downstream signal transducer of BMP-6 signaling pathway. To confirm these findings using primary cells, we transduced rat BMMSCs with adenoviral vector co-expressing VEGF and BMP-6 genes and showed that non-transduced rat BMMSCs failed to induce ectopic bone formation while trans-duced BMMSCs induced ectopic bone formation successfully [34]. We have also shown recently that simultaneous activation of intracellular VEGF and BMP-6 pathways enhances osteogenic differentiation of human adipose derived stem cells (hADSCs) [35]. However, the exact mechanism of enhanced bone formation by transiently transfected D1 cells expressing VEGF and BMP-6 [32] or VEGF and LMP-1 [33] was not completely understood. It remained elusive as to what role was played by exogenously added D1 cells and what was contribution of VEGF and BMP-6 secreted by the cells in enhancing bone formation. To gain more detailed insight into this paradigm, we sought to determine role of exogenously added MSCs in this study. We examined if cross-talk between VEGF and BMP-6 signaling pathways enhances osteogenic differentiation of D1 cells in vitro using human recombinant proteins of VEGF and BMP-6. We also characterized D1 cells for expression of MSCs-specific surface markers, expression of VEGF and BMP receptors and investigated bone formation elicited by D1 cells in vivo after they were pre-conditioned with VEGF and BMP-6 in this study.

Methods

Ethics statement

8–10 weeks old Balb/c mice (Taconic, NY, USA) were housed in the SPF Vivarium at the University of Virginia, which is fully accredited by the American Association for Accreditation of Laboratory Animal Care. This study was carried out in strict accordance with the recommendations in the Guide for the Care and Use of Laboratory Animals of the National Institutes of Health under Public Health Assurance number A3245-01. The protocol was approved by the University of Virginia Institutional Animal Care and Use Committee (protocol number 3701). All surgeries were performed under general anesthesia, and post-operative analgesia was given to all animals to minimize suffering.

Cells, media, growth factors and culture conditions

We used D1 cells that were isolated in our laboratory from a BALB/c mouse bone marrow [36]. The D1 cells are also available from American Type Culture Collection (ATCC) under the product number CRL-12424. The D1 cells (passage 5) were grown in Dulbecco's Modified Eagle's Medium (Gibco BRL, Gaithers-burg, MD., USA) containing 10% fetal bovine serum (Hyclone Laboratories, Logan, VT., USA), 50 μg/ml sodium ascorbate,

100 IU/ml penicillin G, and 100 μg/ml streptomycin in a humidified atmosphere of 5% carbon dioxide at 37°C. The medium was designated as basal medium (BM) and to induce osteogenesis, 10 mM β-glycerophosphate was added to BM to prepare osteogenic medium (OM). For all the experiments related to osteogenesis, the D1 cells were seeded at a density of 0.5×10^4 cells/cm² in a 24-well plate. Human recombinant proteins BMP-2, -4, -6; VEGF (Prospec, Israel) and BMP-9 (Assay Designs/Enzo Life Sciences, USA) were added to OM at the specified concentrations. Culture medium was replaced twice a week. The mineralization was determined using OM supplemented with 1, 10 and 100 ng of VEGF or individual BMPs and OM supplemented with a combination of 10 ng of VEGF and 10 ng of BMP-6. To determine mRNA expression of runx2 and osterix in presence of BMPs, the cells were grown in BM, OM and OM supplemented with 10 ng of BMP proteins. The Smads 1/5/8 phosphorylation was quantified using cells grown in BM, OM, OM containing 10 ng VEGF or 10 ng individual BMPs or combination of 10 ng VEGF and 10 ng BMP-6. The influence of cross-talk between VEGF and BMP-6 pathways on expression of osteogenic genes was investigated in cells grown in BM, OM and OM supplemented with 10 ng VEGF or BMP-6 or both. To investigate if pre-conditioning of the cells improves their bone formation ability, cells were grown in OM, OM supplemented with 10 ng VEGF or BMP-6 or both for 7 days and then implanted in sub-cutaneous tissues of Balb/c mice.

The staining of cytoplasm and the nuclei

The D1 cells were seeded at a density of 1×10^3 cells/cm² in a 24-well plate and maintained in BM for 4 days. At day 5, the cells were stained using the methods described earlier [35].

Alizarin red and Sudan IV staining

Mineralization was quantified using alizarin red staining as described earlier [35]. To determine if the D1 cells are capable of differentiation along an adipogenic lineage, the cells were cultured in BM containing 10^{-7} M dexamethasone for 14 days to induce adipogenesis. The differentiated cells were stained with Sudan IV, a stain for fat, counterstained with hematoxylin, and visualized by light microscopy (20X).

RNA extraction, preparation of cDNA, conventional PCR and real time PCR

The methods used for RNA extraction, cDNA and quantification of expression of osteogenic markers using real time PCR were described earlier [35] and the primer sequences used are described in Table 1 RNA extraction from the harvested implant was performed using a TissueLyser as described earlier [37].

A measure of the mRNA for BMP-receptors (ActR-I/Alk2, BMPR-IA/Alk3, BMPR-IB/Alk6), TGF-receptors (Alk1, TβR-I/Alk5), VEGF receptors (membrane VEGFR1/mFlt-1, soluble VEGFR1/sFlt-1, VEGFR2/Flk1,) was determined using a cDNA template and gene specific primers by conventional PCR. The amplified DNA products from the PCR reactions were resolved in a 1% agarose gel and stained with ethidium bromide. The primers used are described in Table 2.

Fluorescence Activated Cell Sorting

The D1 cells were grown in BM and harvested after 5 days. A homogeneous suspension of cells in PBS was prepared, washed and then incubated with anti-mouse CD16/CD32 monoclonal antibody Clone 2.4G2 (BD Biosciences, MD, USA) to block the Fc receptors. The D1 cells (1×10^6 cells) were stained using specific

Table 1. List of primers used in real time PCR.

Name	Sequence
18S Forward	5'-CGGCGACGACCCATTCGAAC-3'
18 S Reverse	5'-GAATCGAACCCTGATTCCCCGTC-3'
Alkaline Phosphatase Forward	5'-ACGAGATGCCACCAGAGG-3'
Alkaline Phosphatase Reverse	5'-ACGAGATGCCACCAGAGG-3'
Runx2 Forward	5'-TTATCAAGGGAATAGAGGG-3'
Runx2 Reverse	5'-AGGACAGAGGGAAACAAC-3'
Osterix Forward	5'-ACCAGGTCCAGGCAACAC-3'
Osterix Reverse	5'-GCAAAGTCAGATGGGTAAGT-3'
Dlx5 Forward	5'-GATCCCTATGACAGGAGTGGGAC-3'
Dlx5 Reverse	5'-GGACTCGAGATCTAATAAAGCGTC-3'
COL1A1 Forward	5'-CGCCATCAAGGTCTACTGC-3'
COL1A1 Reverse	5'-GAATCCATCGGTCATGCTCT-3'
OPG Forward	5'-GCTGAGTGTTTTGGTGGACAGTT-3'
OPG Reverse	5'-GCTGGAAGGTTTGCTCTTGTG-3'
RANKL Forward	5'-TGCAGCATCGCTCTGTTCC-3'
RANKL Reverse	5'-CCCACAATGTGTTGCAGTTCC-3'
CADM1 Forward	5'-ATTCTGGGCCGCTATTTTG-3'
CADM1 Reverse	5'-TGTCCTCCTTCTGCATTGATT-3'

monoclonal antibodies for 30 minutes. The list of antibodies is described in Table 3. The cells were washed three times with a solution of 1% BSA in PBS and analyzed using a FACS caliber flow cytometer (BD Biosciences, MD, USA); the data was analyzed using FloJo software (TreeStar, OR, USA).

Western blotting

The D1 cells were grown in BM or OM or with OM supplemented with VEGF or one of the BMP proteins or a combination of VEGF and BMP-6 for 24 hours and then lysed with SDS sample buffer without bromophenol blue (125 mM Tris-HCl pH 6.8, 150 mM β-mercaptoethanol, 1% SDS and 20%

Table 2. List of primers used in PCR.

Name	Sequence
Alk1 Forward	5'-GTGTGGCGGTCAAGATTTTC-3'
Alk1 Reverse	5'-GGTTAGGGATGGTGGGTG-3'
Alk2 Forward	5'-CTGGACCAGAGGAACAAAGG-3'
Alk2 Reverse	5'-GGCGGGGTCTTACACGTCA-3'
Alk3 Forward	5'-TTATTCTGCTGCTTGTGGTCTGTG-3'
Alk3 Reverse	5'-CTTTACATCCTGGGATTCAAC-3'
Alk5 Forward	5'-GCGAAGGCATTACAGTGTTCT-3'
Alk5 Reverse	5'-TCTGAAATGAAAGGGCGATCTAGTGATGG-3'
Alk6 Forward	5'-GAAGATCAAGTGAATGCTGCACAG-3'
Alk6 Reverse	5'-GAACCAGCTGGCTTCCTC-3'
VEGFR2 Forward	5'-AGAACACCAAAAGAGAGAGGAACG-3'
VEGFR2 Reverse	5'-GCACACAGGCAGAAACCAGTAG-3'
mFlt1 Forward	5'-GTCACAGATGTGCCGAATGG-3'
mFlt1 Reverse	5'-TGAGCGTGATCAGCTCCAGG-3'
sFlt1 Forward	5'-GTCACAGATGTGCCGAATGG-3'
sFlt1 Reverse	5'-TGACTTTGTGTGGTACAATC-3'
β-actin Forward	5'-GCTGTATTCCCCTCCATCCTG-3'
β-actin Reverse	5'- CACGGTTGGCCTTAGGGTTCAG-3'

Table 3. List of antibodies used for fluorescence activated cell sorting.

Name	Clone	Label	Source
Anti Sca-1	D7	Phycoerythrin (PE)	eBiosciences
Anti CD105		Fluorescein (FITC)	R and D System
Anti CD90	30-H12	PE	eBiosciences
Anti CD73	TY/11.8	Alexa Fluor 647	Biolegend
Anti CD45	A20	FITC	eBiosciences
Anti CD34	RAM 34	FITC	eBiosciences
Anti CD44	IM7	PE	eBiosciences
Anti CD146	ME-9F1	PE	Biolegend
Anti CD133	13A4	Peridinin-chlorophyll-protein complex (PerCP)	eBiosciences
Anti Nestin	25	Alexa Fluor 647	BD Biosciences

glycerol) in the presence of 1X protease inhibitor cocktail (Santa Cruz Biotechnology) and 1 mM PMSF (Santa Cruz Biotechnology). The lysates were immediately placed on ice. The protein concentration was determined using a Bradford protein assay kit (Biorad) and equal amounts of total cell proteins were resolved on 8–12% SDS-polyacrylamide gels, electro-transferred to nitrocellulose membranes (Thermo Scientific), membranes were blocked with 5% non-fat dry milk in TBST (50 mM Tris, pH 7.6, 150 mM NaCl, 0.05% tween 20) for 1 hour at room temperature, washed and incubated overnight at 4°C in 5% BSA in TBST containing anti-phospho-Smad1/5/8 (1:1000) or anti-GAPDH antibodies (1:1000) (Cell Signaling, USA). The membranes were then incubated with HRP-conjugated secondary antibody (1:2000 in 5% non-fat dry milk in TBST) (Cell Singling, USA) for 1 hour at room temperature followed by chemiluminescent substrate for HRP antibody (Thermo Scientific) and enhancer solution (Thermo Scientific) mixed in a 1:1 ratio. The membranes were incubated in the dark with CL-Xposure films (Pierce) and the films were developed to visualize the bands. To measure the density of bands quantitatively, electronic images were generated by placing the X-ray films in a GS-800 calibrated densitometer (Biorad, USA); images were quantified using ImageJ software.

Mice and osteogenesis induced by the D1 cells activated with VEGF or BMP-6 or the combination of VEGF and BMP-6

The D1 cells were grown in OM or OM supplemented with VEGF or BMP-6 or both for 1 week. After one week, D1 cells were harvested, suspended in PBS and were mixed (1:1 volume ratio) with Matrigel (BD Biosciences, NJ, USA) at 4°C and kept chilled in a syringe until injected in the mice. The mice were anesthetized using intra-peritoneal injection of ketamine (80 mg/kg) and xylazine (10 mg/kg). D1 cells (passage 4, 1×10^6 cells/0.3 mL) in Matrigel suspension were injected on the dorsum of experimental mice. The detailed procedure is described earlier [37]. The mice from each group were sacrificed at week 2 and week 4 and at each time point harvested implants (n = 8) were used for radiography and H and E staining.

Radiographs

The details of the methods are described earlier [37]. At 2 and 4 weeks the implants were surgically removed from the subcutaneous tissue and placed on an x-ray film, radiographs were taken; the films were subsequently developed and placed into a GS-800

Calibrated Densitometer (Bio-rad, CA, USA) to convert the radiograph films into digital images. Density measurements of radiographs were performed with the ImageJ software.

Histology & Microscopy

For histological analysis, implants retrieved at week 2 and week 4 were decalcified using 0.25 M EDTA and fixed in 10% neutral buffered formalin, then dehydrated and embedded in paraffin. Six micrometer sections were stained with hematoxylin and eosin and evaluated by light microscopy.

Statistical analysis

All *in vitro* experiments were repeated three times and bone formation in the sub-cutaneous tissue was repeated two times. Data from one individual set are represented in the manuscript. Statistical analysis of the averages of optical densities measured at 405 nm for the Alizarin Red staining assay, average of densities from radiographs, band densities in the western blot analysis, and the relative gene expression from real time PCR was performed. To determine whether the differences between the means of different groups were statistically significant, one-way ANOVA was used, followed by the LSD test using SPSS 18.0 software. The OM group was treated as the control. Statistical significance level was set at $p < 0.05$.

Results

In vitro mineralization of mesenchymal stem cells

Human recombinant proteins of VEGF or BMP-6 did not enhance mineralization of D1 cells at concentrations of 1 or 10 or 100 ng at day 7, 14 and 21 (Fig. 1). We therefore tested if other BMPs, BMP-2, -4 or -9 could enhance the mineralization. A similar trend was observed for all BMPs (Fig. 1). A combination of 10 ng VEGF and 10 ng BMP-6 also failed to enhance mineralization at day 7, 14 and 21.

Expression of runx2 and osterix genes and activation of Smads 1/5/8

Since VEGF, BMP-6 and other BMPs did not enhance mineralization, we determined if addition of these proteins would influence osteogenesis through modulation of the osteogenic transcription factors runx2 and osterix because both transcription factors are master regulators of osteogenesis. Surprisingly, transcription factor gene expression remained unchanged in

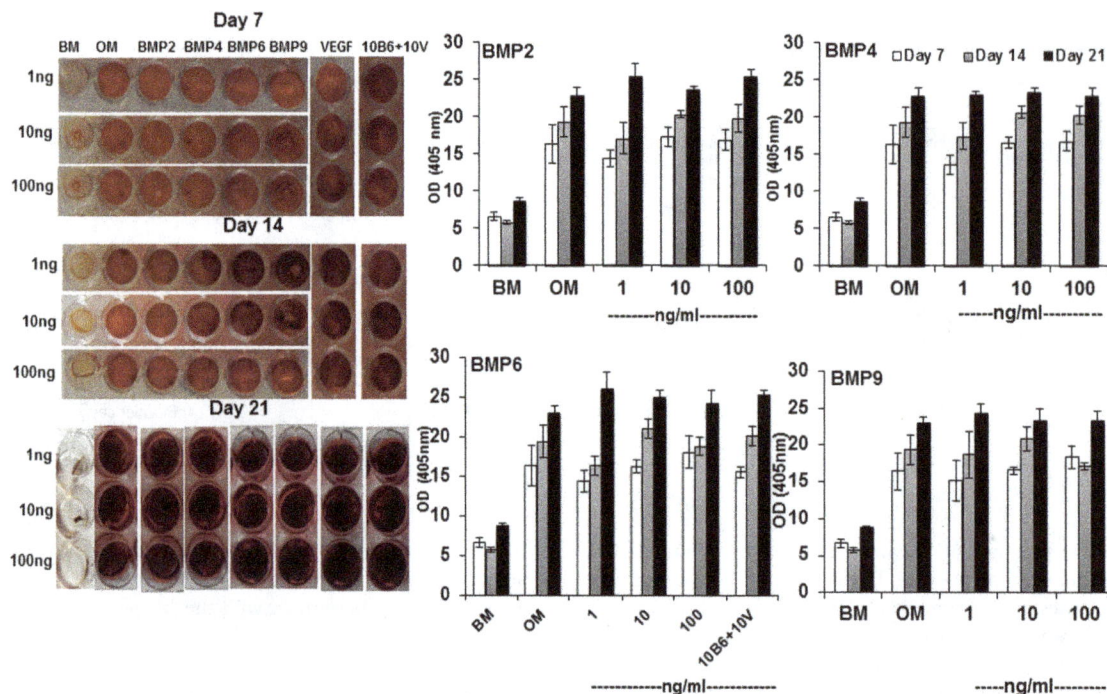

Figure 1. BMPs do not enhance mineralization. The mineralization of D1 cells was measured quantitatively using alizarin red staining. The cells were stained at day 7, 14 and 21 using alizarin red (left panel). The dye was extracted and intensity of color was quantified at 405 nm using a spectrophotometer (right panel).

response to the VEGF or BMP-6 or other BMPs (Fig. 2). Furthermore, Smads 1/5/8, which are downstream modulators of the BMP-signaling pathway, did not show increased phosphorylation upon treatment of D1 cells with VEGF or BMP-6 alone. Smad 1/5/8 phosphorylation increased when the cells were treated with the combination of VEGF and BMP-6 in comparison with all other groups. However, this increase was not statistically significant.

Expression of mesenchymal stem cell surface markers and VEGF and BMP receptor genes

To determine if lack of BMP-responsiveness of D1 cells correlates with expression of receptors, we determined expression of the receptor genes and found D1 cells expression of Alk2, Alk3 but a lack of expression of Alk1 and Alk6 (Fig. 3). It is known that BMP-2 and -4 bind to Alk3 as well as to Alk6; BMP-6 binds strongly to Alk2 and weakly to Alk6, and BMP-9 binds to Alk1 and Alk2. Therefore the D1 cells showed expression of at least one receptor for each of the BMPs that we tested i.e. BMP-2, -4, -6 and -9. In addition, D1 cells expressed the TGF-β binding receptor Alk5 (Fig. 3). The main receptor for VEGF165 is VEGFR2 (Flk-1) which was expressed in D1 cells but the cells did not express either the membrane form or the soluble form of VEGFR1 (Flt-1) (Fig. 3) that binds to VEGF thereby modulating the amount of VEGF available for VEGFR2. BMP-6 enhanced gene expression for VEGFR2 significantly. Cell surface analysis of the D1 cells showed a surface expression profile of CD105−CD90−CD73+CD45−CD34- (Fig. 3) which is not a classical CD105+CD90+CD73+CD45−CD34− mesenchymal stem cell characteristic. However, the D1 cells expressed Sca-1 (~80%), CD44 (~80%) and nestin (~30%) receptors that are known to be expressed by mesenchymal stem cells.

D1 cells are capable of differentiation into adipogenic and osteogenic lineages in vitro

The D1 cells have large nuclei that occupy most of the cytoplasmic space (Fig. 4). In the presence of dexamethasone, D1 cells in culture differentiate into an adipogenic lineage and exhibit lipid vesicles. Similarly, in the presence of osteogenic medium, the D1 cells differentiate into the osteogenic lineage in vitro and display mineralization.

Cross-talk between intracellular VEGF and BMP-6 pathways enhances expression of the ALP, COL1A1 and osterix genes

Despite our observation that VEGF, BMP-6 and combination of VEGF plus BMP-6 did not enhance mineralization of D1 cells significantly, we considered that the combination of VEGF and BMP-6 might enhance expression of osteogenic markers ALP and COL1A1 genes. When the combination of 10 ng VEGF and 10 ng BMP-6 was added to the OM, ALP and COL1A1 gene expression at day 7 was increased significantly (Fig. 5) with a corresponding significant increase in osterix gene expression.

Preconditioning of the D1 cells with the combination of VEGF and BMP-6 enhances osteogenesis in vivo

Since the combination of 10 ng VEGF and 10 ng BMP-6 enhanced expressions of ALP, COL1A1 and osterix genes at week 1, we wanted to test if preconditioning of the D1 cells with the combination of VEGF and BMP-6 for 1 week could promote osteogenesis in vivo. The preconditioning with VEGF or BMP-6 or both did not enhance osteogenesis in comparison with OM group at week 2 (Fig. 6). At week 4, however, the D1 cells preconditioned with VEGF and BMP-6 induced significantly greater osteogenesis in comparison with that induced by other

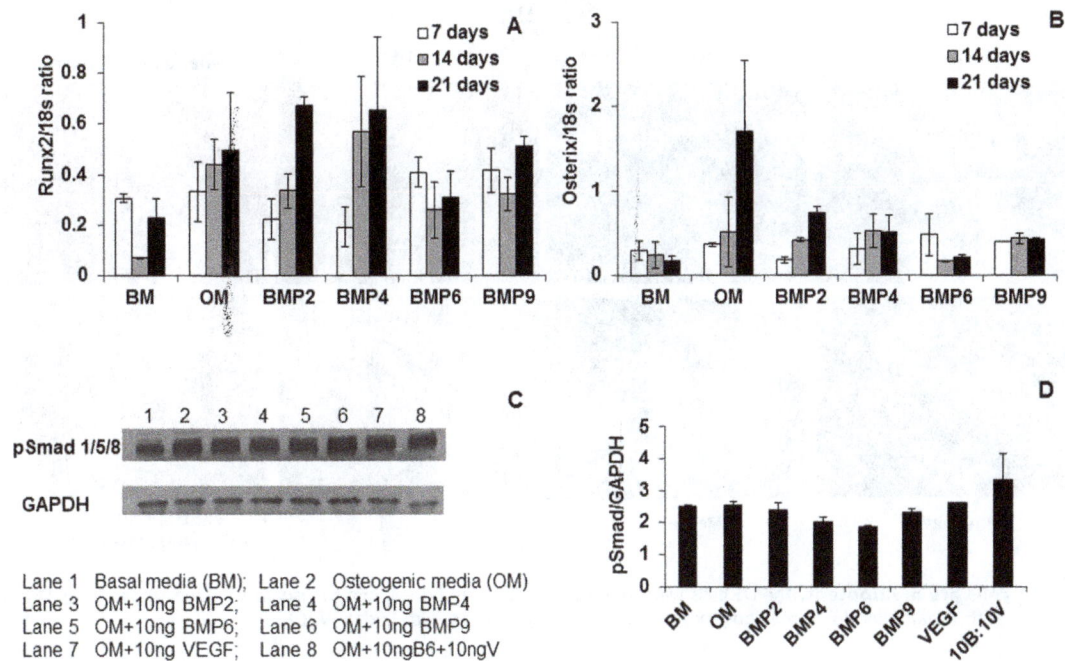

Lane 1   Basal media (BM);   Lane 2   Osteogenic media (OM)
Lane 3   OM+10ng BMP2;   Lane 4   OM+10ng BMP4
Lane 5   OM+10ng BMP6;   Lane 6   OM+10ng BMP9
Lane 7   OM+10ng VEGF;   Lane 8   OM+10ngB6+10ngV

Figure 2. BMPs do not enhance Smad 1/5/8 phosphorylation and expression of runx2 and osterix genes. mRNA levels of runx2 (A) and osterix (B) were quantified using real time PCR. Smad phosphorylation was determined by western blots (C) and band intensity was quantified using ImageJ software (D).

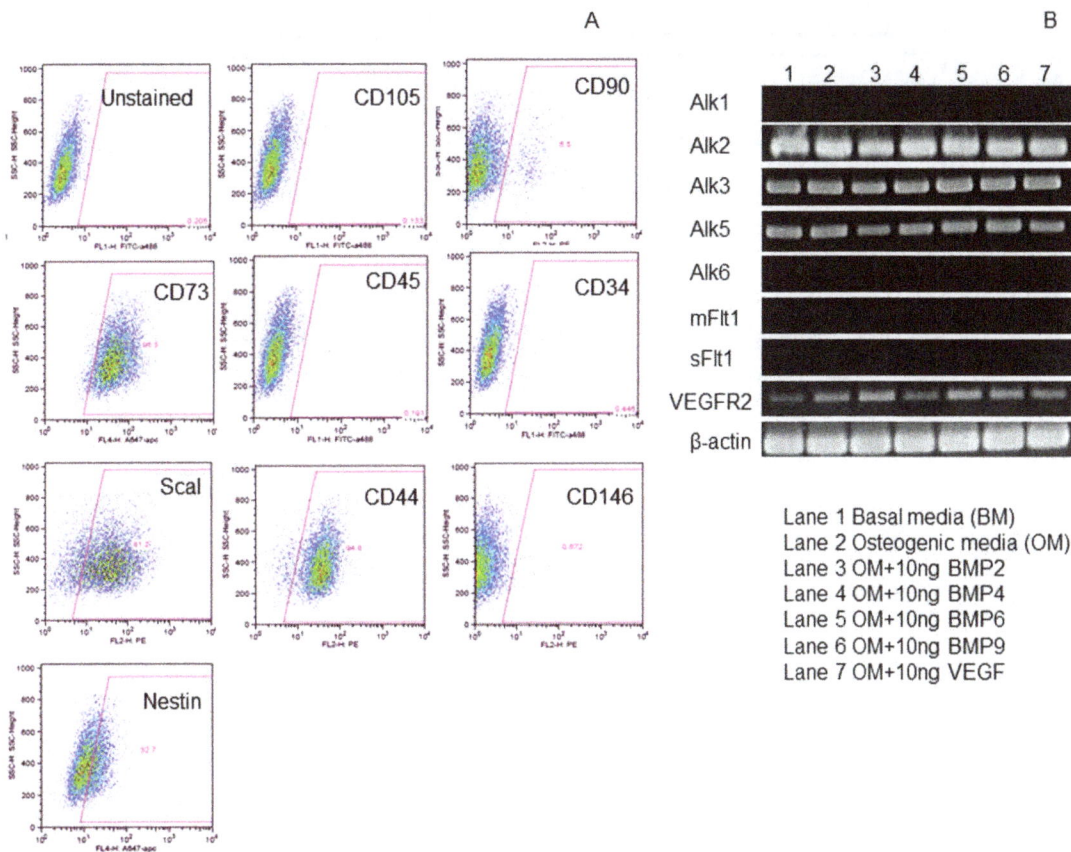

Lane 1 Basal media (BM)
Lane 2 Osteogenic media (OM)
Lane 3 OM+10ng BMP2
Lane 4 OM+10ng BMP4
Lane 5 OM+10ng BMP6
Lane 6 OM+10ng BMP9
Lane 7 OM+10ng VEGF

Figure 3. The D1 cells do not express CD105, Alk1 and Alk6 receptors. Using labeled monoclonal antibodies expression of stem cell markers (A) was determined by flow cytometry. Expression of VEGF and BMP receptors was determined by PCR followed by agarose gel electrophoresis (B).

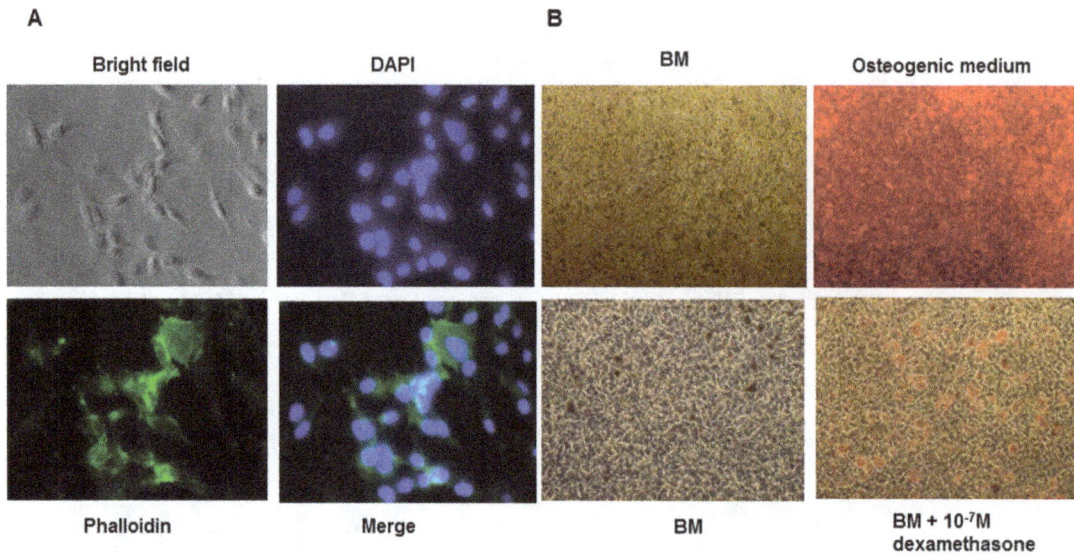

Figure 4. The D1 cells are multipotent. The D1 cells were stained with DAPI and phalloidin to visualize cell morphology (A). Osteogenesis was assayed by staining with Alizarin Red (B) and adipogenesis was assayed by staining with Sudan IV (C).

groups. The enhanced osteogenesis at week 4 correlated with higher ratio of mRNA levels of osteoprotegrin (OPG) to receptor activator of nuclear factor-kappaB ligand (RANKL) genes (Fig. 6) and higher expression of CADM1 (Fig. 7) in implants of D1 cells

pre-conditioned with the combination of VEGF and BMP-6. We did not find any correlation between enhanced bone formation at week 4 and expression of ALP, COL1A1 genes or expression of genes of transcription factors osterix and Dlx5 in the implants at

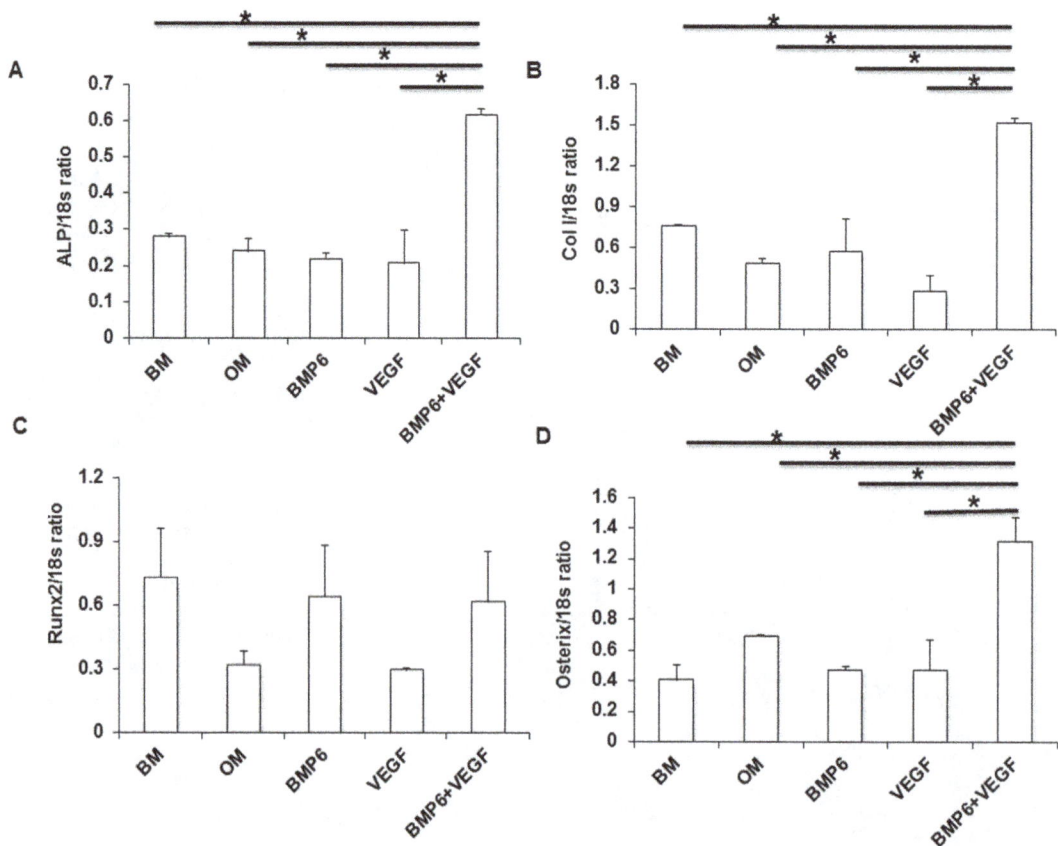

Figure 5. Combination of VEGF and BMP-6 enhances expression of osteogenic genes. Expression of ALP (A), COL1A1 (B), runx2 (C) and osterix (D) genes were determined by real time PCR at day 7. * denotes $p < 0.05$.

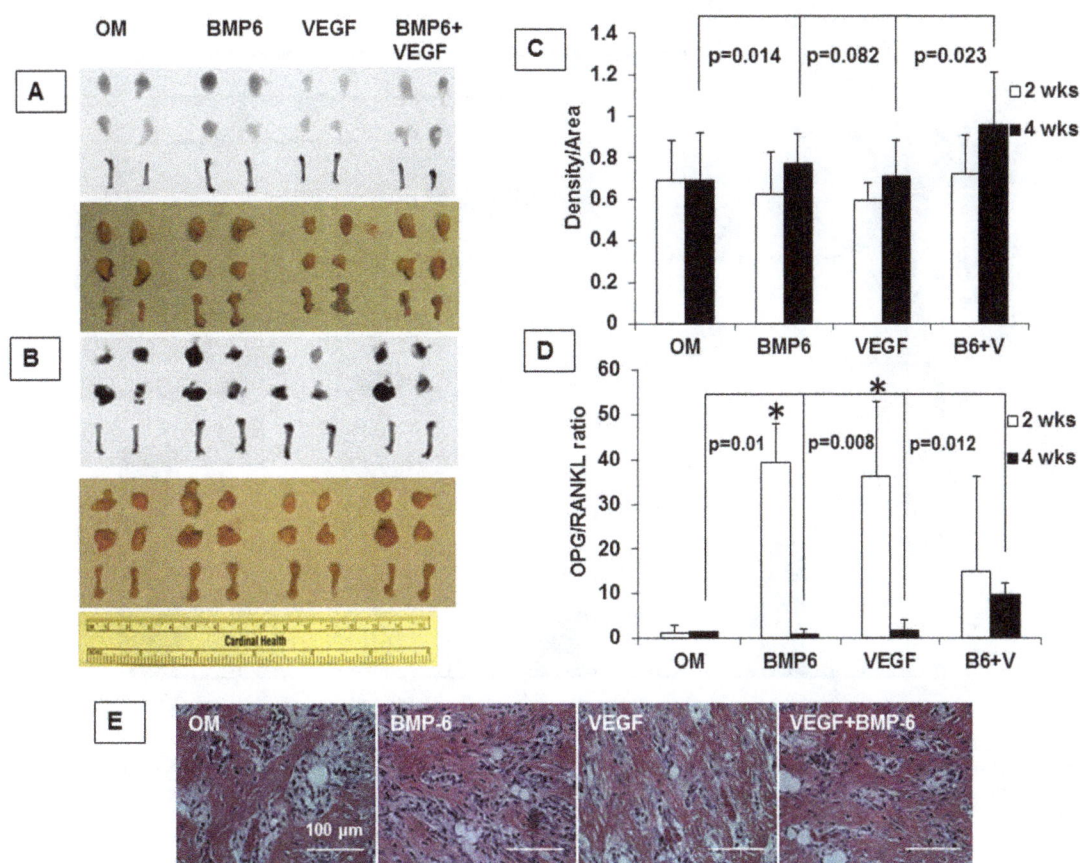

Figure 6. Preconditioning of BMP-non-responsive D1 cells with VEGF and BMP-6 enhances their ability to induce ectopic bone formation. The bone density of harvested implants was measured by radiography and Image J software (A-C). Representative images are shown in the figure. H and E staining revealed typical histology of bone (E). Real time PCR showed modulation of RANKL/OPG ratio (D). * denotes p<0.05 compared with OM group at weeks 2.

week 4 (Fig. 8). However, expression of ALP gene in the implants correlated with expression of osterix and Dlx5 genes while COL1A1 expression correlated with Dlx5 expression.

Discussion

The purpose of this study was to gain insight into synergistic interaction between MSCs, VEGF and BMP in enhancing fracture repair. Various growth factors (BMPs, GDF-5, TGF-β, VEGF, angiopoetins, FGF, PDGF) and cell types (platelets, endothelial cells, macrophages, MSCs, chondrocytes, osteoclasts, osteoblasts) are known to be involved during fracture repair [25]. However, involvement of MSCs, VEGF and BMP is crucial as deficiencies in these factors can lead to fractures non-unions [1–7]. Interactions between these growth factors and cells during fracture repair are complex and are not completely understood. In the last decade several investigators have shown that exogenous addition MSCs, VEGF and BMP synergistically enhances bone formation but the exact mechanism remains elusive. It is difficult to explain this synergy through VEGF induced increased angiogenesis since our previous studies on synergistic aspect [32–33] revealed that increase in angiogenesis did not always correlate with increase in osteogenesis. While complete inhibition of angiogenesis is known to inhibit bone formation [3–4] the number of vessels and VEGF expression levels are reported to be similar in non-union fractures and fractures that heal [38–39]. Taken together, these facts suggest that synergistic enhancement of bone formation by MSCs, VEGF

and BMP involves additional mechanisms than increase in angiogenesis which are not understood. Our data reveals these additional mechanisms as −1. Cross-talk between intracellular signaling pathways of VEGF and BMP-6 enhances osteoblastic differentiation of MSCs (Fig. 5) and 2. Paracrine factors produced by MSCs preconditioned with the combination of VEGF and BMP-6 modulate osteoclastogenesis through modulation of RANKL/OPG ratio (Fig. 6) and enhance osteogenic potential of MSCs as revealed by CADM1 expression (Fig. 7). CADM1 has been recently identified as a marker of higher bone forming capacity of MSCs [40]. The findings of this study shed light on possible mechanism for our earlier findings that D1 cells transiently (≤1 week) expressing VEGF and BMP-6 genes [32] or VEGF and LMP-1 genes [33] induced significantly greater bone formation at week 3 than that induced by D1 cells alone or D1 cells expressing any single gene. It appears from our present study (Fig. 6) and our previous findings [32–33] that transient VEGF and BMP-6 (or LMP-1) activation of D1 cells for about a week is sufficient to warrant superior bone formation. A recent study nicely demonstrated using conditional knock-out mice that intracellular levels of VEGF and VEGF signaling in MSCs control fate of differentiation of MSCs into osteogenic versus adipogenic lineage and this function of VEGF is quite distinct than that of secreted VEGF functions [41].

Synergistic enhancement of bone formation using MSCs, VEGF and BMP is reported to be cell-type specific as VEGF

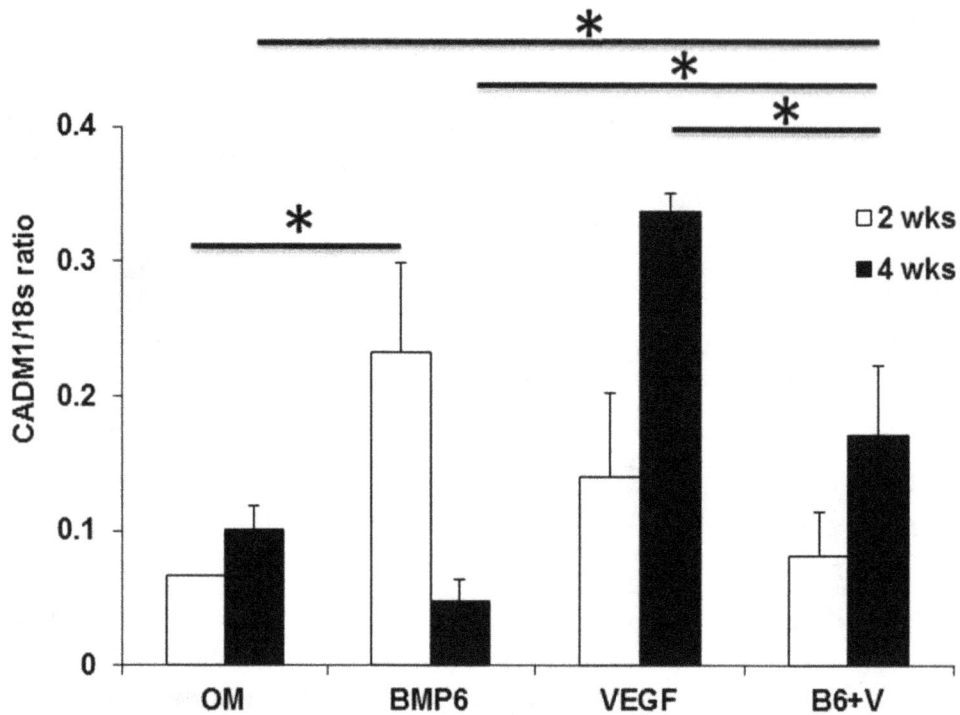

Figure 7. Enhanced expression of CADM1 in implants of D1 cells preconditioned with VEGF and BMP-6. RNA was isolated from the harvested implants and converted into cDNA. Using this cDNA as a template, mRNA expression of CADM1 was quantitatively determined in real time PCR. * denotes $p < 0.05$.

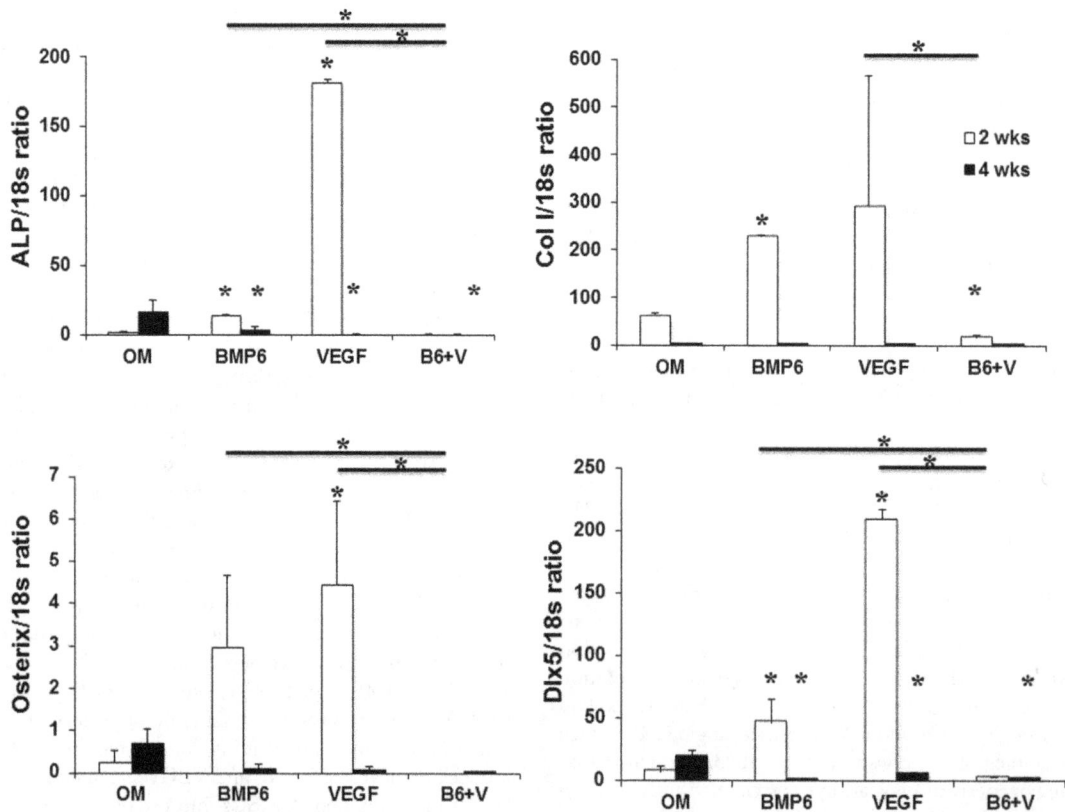

Figure 8. Expression of ALP and COL1 genes and genes for transcription factors osterix and Dlx5 in the implants of D1 cells. mRNA expression was quantified using gene specific primers and real time PCR. cDNA prepared from RNA isolated from the harvested implants was used as the template. * denotes $p < 0.05$ compared with OM group of the respective time point, unless indicated otherwise by the horizontal lines.

and BMP-4 co-expressing C2C12 cells made more bone in comparison with that made by NIH3T3 cells [42]. The D1 cells did not exhibit increased mineralization in response to BMPs (Fig. 1). This data is in agreement with reported findings that BMPs do not enhance mineralization of MSCs *in vitro* [12-21]. We also found that BMP-6 alone did not enhance expression of runx2, osterix, ALP, COL1A1 genes (Fig. 5) and phosphorylation of Smads 1/5/8 (Fig. 2) in D1 cells.

We investigated why D1 cells did not respond to BMPs. Although the D1 cells expressed the main receptors for BMPs, they did not express Alk1 and Alk6 (Fig. 3). Alk6 is not required for ALP expression and mineralization in MSCs [15], but we do not know if Alk6 is required for up regulation of runx2 and osterix genes and phosphorylation of Smads 1/5/8 in MSCs in response to BMP-6. Although the D1 cells were capable of differentiation into adipogenic and osteogenic lineages *in vitro* (Fig. 4) they did not express CD105 and CD90 receptors (Fig. 3) making it difficult to distinguish them as MSCs. Non-responsiveness of D1 cells to BMPs can be attributed to the lack of surface expression of CD105 because CD105 is the co-receptor for BMP-signaling [43].

Interestingly, we discovered that BMP-nonresponsive phenotype of D1 cells *in vitro* could be partially overcome with preconditioning using a combination of VEGF and BMP-6 (Fig. 5). Most importantly, ability of BMP-non-responsive D1 cells to induce bone formation *in vivo* was significantly enhanced if the cells were pre-conditioned with VEGF and BMP-6 through paracrine modulation of RANKL/OPG ratio (Fig. 6) and expression of CADM1 (Fig. 7). This strategy can be effectively used for enhancement of fracture repair.

Conclusion

The data presented in this report demonstrates that: 1. osteoprogenitor cells that do not express CD105, Alk1 and Alk6

receptors do not respond well to BMPs *in vitro*, 2. These cells respond to a combination of VEGF and BMP-6 *in vitro*, moreover, VEGF signaling is required for a major response of MSCs to BMPs and, 3. Preconditioning of these cells with the combination of VEGF and BMP-6 enhances their ability to induce ectopic bone formation through paracrine modulation of the RANKL/OPG ratio and expression of CADM1. Overall, the data suggests that signaling interplay between the VEGF and the BMPs that are produced during fracture repair together with the endogenous or exogenously added MSCs is critical for bone repair. Therefore, greater care should be exercised while selecting MSCs for tissue engineering purposes since MSCs that do not express essential receptors might be less responsive to BMPs. Use of either MSCs alone, or VEGF or BMPs alone might not be suitable for bone repair but the combined use of MSCs, VEGF and BMP-6 is likely to be a useful approach for the development of therapies that would enhance fracture repair.

Acknowledgments

We thank Dr. Chunxi Yang, Department of Orthopaedic Surgery, Shanghai Tenth People's Hospital (Tenth People's Hospital of Tongji University), Shanghai 200072, China, for his help in statistical analysis of the data. We also thank Ms. Pinar Smith, School of Medicine, University of Virginia, Charlottesville, VA 22908, USA, for her technical assistance.

Author Contributions

Conceived and designed the experiments: ASD QC. Performed the experiments: VM CL ASD. Analyzed the data: VM ASD QC. Contributed reagents/materials/analysis tools: GB. Wrote the paper: ASD GB QC.

References

1. Bajada S, Marshall MJ, Wright KT, Richardson JB, Johnson WE (2009) Decreased osteogenesis, increased cell senescence and elevated Dickkopf-1 secretion in human fracture non union stromal cells. Bone 45: 726–735.
2. Mathieu M, Rigutto S, Ingels A, Spruyt D, Stricwant N, et al. (2013) Decreased pool of mesenchymal stem cells is associated with altered chemokines serum levels in atrophic nonunion fractures. Bone 53: 391–398.
3. Street J, Bao M, deGuzman L, Bunting S, Peale FV Jr, et al. (2002) Vascular endothelial growth factor stimulates bone repair by promoting angiogenesis and bone turnover. Proc Natl Acad Sci U S A 99: 9656–9661.
4. Hausman MR, Schaffler MB, Majeska RJ (2001) Prevention of fracture healing in rats by an inhibitor of angiogenesis. Bone 29: 560–564.
5. Niikura T, Hak DJ, Reddi AH (2006) Global gene profiling reveals a downregulation of BMP gene expression in experimental atrophic nonunions compared to standard healing fractures. J Orthop Res 24: 1463–1471.
6. Fajardo M, Liu CJ, Egol K (2009) Levels of Expression for BMP-7 and Several BMP Antagonists May Play an Integral Role in a Fracture Nonunion: A Pilot Study. Clin Orthop Relat Res 467: 3071–3078.
7. Kloen P, Lauzier D, Hamdy RC (2012) Co-expression of BMPs and BMP-inhibitors in human fractures and non-unions. Bone 51: 59–68.
8. Aspenberg P, Genant HK, Johansson T, Nino AJ, See K, et al. (2010) Teriparatide for acceleration of fracture repair in humans: a prospective, randomized, double-blind study of 102 postmenopausal women with distal radial fractures. J Bone Miner Res 25: 404–414.
9. Delimar D, Smoljanovic T, Bojanic I (2012) Could the use of bone morphogenetic proteins in fracture healing do more harm than good to our patients? Int Orthop 36: 683.
10. Nauth A, Ristiniemi J, McKee MD, Schemitsch EH (2009) Bone morphogenetic proteins in open fractures: past, present, and future. Injury 40: 27–31.
11. Garrison KR, Shemilt I, Donell S, Ryder JJ, Mugford M, et al. (2010) Bone morphogenetic protein (BMP) for fracture healing in adults. Cochrane Database Syst Rev 6: 1–158.
12. Chou YF, Zuk PA, Chang TL, Benhaim P, Wu BM (2011) Adipose-derived stem cells and BMP2: Part 1. BMP2-treated adipose-derived stem cells do not improve repair of segmental femoral defects. Connect Tissue Res 52: 109–118.

13. Zuk P, Chou YF, Mussano F, Benhaim P, Wu BM (2011) Adipose-derived stem cells and BMP2: Part 2. BMP2 may not influence the osteogenic fate of human adipose-derived stem cells. Connect Tissue Res 52: 119–132.
14. Mizuno D, Agata H, Furue H, Kimura A, Narita Y, et al. (2010) Limited but heterogeneous osteogenic response of human bone marrow mesenchymal stem cells to bone morphogenetic protein-2 and serum. Growth Factors 28: 34–43.
15. Osyczka AM, Diefenderfer DL, Bhargave G, Leboy PS (2004) Different effects of BMP-2 on marrow stromal cells from human and rat bone. Cells Tissues Organs 176: 109–119.
16. Diefenderfer DL, Osyczka AM, Reilly GC, Leboy PS (2003) BMP responsiveness in human mesenchymal stem cells. Connect Tissue Res 44: 305–311.
17. Diefenderfer DL, Osyczka AM, Garino JP, Leboy PS (2003) Regulation of BMP-induced transcription in cultured human bone marrow stromal cells. J Bone Joint Surg Am 85: 19–28.
18. Puleo DA (1997) Dependence of mesenchymal cell responses on duration of exposure to bone morphogenetic protein-2 in vitro. J Cell Physiol 173: 93–101.
19. Hanada K, Dennis JE, Caplan AI (1997) Stimulatory effects of basic fibroblast growth factor and bone morphogenetic protein-2 on osteogenic differentiation of rat bone marrow-derived mesenchymal stem cells. J Bone Miner Res 12: 1606–1614.
20. Jørgensen NR, Henriksen Z, Sørensen OH, Civitelli R (2004) Dexamethasone, BMP-2, and 1, 25-dihydroxyvitamin D enhance a more differentiated osteoblast phenotype: validation of an in vitro model for human bone marrow-derived primary osteoblasts. Steroids 69: 219–226.
21. Kyllönen L, Haimi S, Säkkinen J, Kuokkanen H, Mannerström B, et al. (2013) Exogenously added BMP-6, BMP-7 and VEGF may not enhance the osteogenic differentiation of human adipose stem cells. Growth Factors 31: 141–153.
22. Takagi K, Urist MR (1982) The role of bone marrow in bone morphogenetic protein-induced repair of femoral massive diaphyseal defects. Clin Orthop Relat Res 171: 224–231.
23. Waese EY, Kandel RA, Stanford WL (2008) Application of stem cells in bone repair. Skeletal Radiol 37: 601–608.
24. Steinert AF, Rackwitz L, Gilbert F, Nöth U, Tuan RS (2012) Concise review: the clinical application of mesenchymal stem cells for musculoskeletal regeneration: current status and perspectives. Stem Cells Transl Med 1: 237–247.

25. Cui Q, Dighe AS, Irvine JN (2013) Combined angiogenic and osteogenic factor delivery for bone regenerative engineering. Curr Pharm Des 19: 3374–3383.

26. Peng H, Wright V, Usas A, Gearhart B, Shen HC, et al. (2002) Synergistic enhancement of bone formation and healing by stem cell-expressed VEGF and bone morphogenetic protein-4. J Clin Invest 110: 751–719.

27. Peng H, Usas A, Olshanski A, Ho AM, Gearhart B, et al. (2005) VEGF improves, whereas sFlt1 inhibits, BMP2-induced bone formation and bone healing through modulation of angiogenesis. J Bone Miner Res 20: 2017–2027.

28. Roldan JC, Detsch R, Schaefer S, Chang E, Kelantan M, et al. (2010) Bone formation and degradation of a highly porous biphasic calcium phosphate ceramic in presence of BMP-7, VEGF and mesenchymal stem cells in an ectopic mouse model. J Craniomaxillofac Surg 38: 423–430.

29. Li JZ, Li H, Sasaki T, Holman D, Beres B, et al. (2003) Osteogenic potential of five different recombinant human bone morphogenetic protein adenoviral vectors in the rat. Gene Ther 10: 1735–1743.

30. Kang Q, Sun MH, Cheng H, Peng Y, Montag AG, et al. (2004) Characterization of the distinct orthotopic bone-forming activity of 14 BMPs using recombinant adenovirus-mediated gene delivery. Gene Ther 11: 1312–1320.

31. Song K, Krause C, Shi S, Patterson M, Suto R, et al. (2010) Identification of a key residue mediating bone morphogenetic protein (BMP)-6 resistance to noggin inhibition allows for engineered BMPs with superior agonist activity. J Biol Chem 285: 12169–12180.

32. Cui F, Wang X, Liu X, Dighe AS, Balian G, et al. (2010) VEGF and BMP-6 enhance bone formation mediated by cloned mouse osteoprogenitor cells. Growth Factors 28: 306–317.

33. Wang X, Cui F, Madhu V, Dighe AS, Balian G, et al. (2011) Combined VEGF and LMP-1 delivery enhances osteoprogenitor cell differentiation and ectopic bone formation. Growth Factors 29: 36–48.

34. Seamon J, Wang X, Cui F, Keller T, Dighe AS, et al. (2013) Adenoviral Delivery of the VEGF and BMP-6 Genes to Rat Mesenchymal Stem Cells Potentiates Osteogenesis. Bone Marrow Res 2013: 737580.

35. Zhang Y, Madhu V, Dighe AS, Irvine JN Jr, Cui Q (2012) Osteogenic response of human adipose-derived stem cells to BMP-6, VEGF, and combined VEGF plus BMP-6 in vitro. Growth Factors 30: 333–343.

36. Diduch DR, Coe MR, Joyner C, Owen ME, Balian G (1993) Two cell lines from bone marrow that differ in terms of collagen synthesis, osteogenic characteristics, and matrix mineralization. J Bone Joint Surg Am 75: 92–105.

37. Dighe AS, Yang S, Madhu V, Balian G, Cui Q (2012) Interferon gamma and T cells inhibit osteogenesis induced by allogeneic mesenchymal stromal cells. J Orthop Res 31: 227–234.

38. Reed AA, Joyner CJ, Brownlow HC, Simpson AH (2002) Human atrophic fracture non-unions are not avascular. J Orthop Res 20: 593–599.

39. Sarahrudi K, Thomas A, Braunsteiner T, Wolf H, Vécsei V, et al. (2009) VEGF serum concentrations in patients with long bone fractures: a comparison between impaired and normal fracture healing. J Orthop Res 27: 1293–1297.

40. Mentink A, Hulsman M, Groen N, Licht R, Dechering KJ, et al. (2013) Predicting the therapeutic efficacy of MSC in bone tissue engineering using the molecular marker CADM1. Biomaterials 34: 4592–601.

41. Liu Y, Berendsen AD, Jia S, Lotinun S, Baron R, et al. (2012) Intracellular VEGF regulates the balance between osteoblast and adipocyte differentiation. J Clin Invest 122: 3101–3113.

42. Li G, Corsi-Payne K, Zheng B, Usas A, Peng H, et al. (2009) The dose of growth factors influences the synergistic effect of vascular endothelial growth factor on bone morphogenetic protein 4-induced ectopic bone formation. Tissue Eng Part A 15: 2123–2133.

43. Barbara NP, Wrana JL, Letarte M (1999) Endoglin is an accessory protein that interacts with the signaling receptor complex of multiple members of the transforming growth factor-beta superfamily. J Biol Chem 274: 584–594.

14

Clinical Efficacy and Safety of Pamidronate Therapy on Bone Mass Density in Early Post-Renal Transplant Period: A Meta-Analysis of Randomized Controlled Trials

Zijie Wang[¶], Zhijian Han[¶], Jun Tao[¶], Pei Lu, Xuzhong Liu, Jun Wang, Bian Wu, Zhengkai Huang, Changjun Yin, Ruoyun Tan*, Min Gu*

Department of urology, the first affiliated hospital of Nanjing Medical University, Nanjing, China

Abstract

Introduction: The overall effect of pamidronate on bone mass density (BMD) in the early renal transplant period varies considerably among studies. The effects of pamidronate on graft function have not been determined.

Materials and Methods: A comprehensive search was conducted in PubMed, the Cochrane Central Register of Controlled Trials (CENTRAL) and Embase independently by two authors. Randomized controlled trials of pamidronate evaluating bone loss in the first year of renal transplantation were included. Methods reported in the "Cochrane Handbook for Systematic Reviews of Interventions 5.0.2" were used to evaluate changes of lumbar spine and femoral neck BMD, and serum creatinine, calcium and intact parathyroid hormone (iPTH) levels. Fixed or random effect models were used as appropriate.

Results: Six randomized trials evaluating 281 patients were identified. One hundred forty-four were treated with pamidronate and 137 were control patients. Administration of pamidronate was associated with significant reduction of bone loss in the lumbar spine, compared to the control group (standardized mean difference (SMD) = 24.62 [16.25, 32.99]). There was no difference between the pamidronate treated and control femoral neck BMD (SMD = 3.53 [−1.84, 8.90]). A significant increase in the serum creatinine level of the intervention group was seen, compared to the control group. The serum calcium and iPTH of the pamidronate and control groups were not different after 1 year (serum creatinine: SMD = −3.101 [−5.33, −0.89]; serum calcium: SMD = 2.18 [−0.8, 5.16]; serum iPTH: SMD = 0.06 [−0.19, 0.31]). Heterogeneity was low for serum calcium and iPTH and high for serum creatinine.

Conclusions: This meta-analysis demonstrated the beneficial clinical efficacy of pamidronate on BMD with no association with any alteration in graft function during the first year of renal transplantation. Significant heterogeneity precludes the conclusion of the relationship between serum creatinine and pamidronate.

Editor: Sudha Agarwal, Ohio State University, United States of America

Funding: This project is sponsored by the grants from the National Natural Science Foundation of China(81100532), the Science and Education Health Project of Jiangsu Province for important talent (RC2011055), "333 high level talents project" in Jiangsu province (2011 and 2013), Jiangsu province six talents peak from Department of human resources, social security office of Jiangsu Province of China (2010WSN-56 and 2011-WS-033), General program of Department of Health of Jiangsu Province of China(H2009907), and the Priority Academic Program Development of Jiangsu Higher Education Institutions (JX10231801). The funders had no role in study design, data collection and analysis, decision to publish, or preparation of the manuscript.

Competing Interests: The authors have declared that no competing interests exist.

* Email: njmuwzj@qq.com (RT); njmuwzj1990@hotmail.com (MG)

¶ These authors are first authors on this work.

Introduction

Kidney transplantation is an established treatment option for end-stage renal disease (ESRD) [1]. Bone mass density (BMD) loss induced by pre-transplantation bone disease, drug treatments for immunosuppression, secondary hyperparathyroidism and adynamic bone disease are major risk factors for complications such as infection and transplant rejection [2]. Smerud [3] reported that 0.5% of total femur and 1.9% of ultradistal radius BMD was lost during the first 12 months after a successful kidney transplant.

Pamidronate, a bisphosphonate (BP), is effective in preventing and treating post-transplant renal osteodystrophy. Pamidronate

significantly reduces the rate of bone reabsorption and turnover and increases BMD. It maintains or improves the structural and material properties of bone and reduces the risk of fractures [4,5]. Studies comparing pamidronate with traditional medicines, such as vitamin D and calcium, demonstrated pamidronate's effectiveness in protecting against early post-transplant bone loss [6,7]. However, overall efficacy of pamidronate on bone loss during the early period of transplantation varies considerably across studies [6–9]. The safety of pamidronate on graft function in post-transplant recipients is not completely clear, although Lee S [10] has reported that pamidronate could attenuate post-renal transplant bone loss without leading to renal dysfunction. There are no previous meta-analyses of this topic.

Methods

Literature Search

A comprehensive search was conducted in PubMed, the Cochrane Central Register of Controlled Trials (CENTRAL) and Embase (updated on December 15th 2013) by two independent authors (Wang and Han). The Mesh search heading terms included "renal transplantation" or "kidney transplantation" combined with "pamidronate". The reference lists of all studies included in the meta-analysis and abstracts of the Annual Meeting of the American Society of Nephrology, the International Transplant Society and the European Dialysis and Transplantation Association were also reviewed.

Study Selection

The inclusion criteria were: (1) a randomized controlled trial (RCT) which investigated the use of pamidronate in renal transplant recipients with a control group receiving no treatment or placebo, alone or in combination with calcium and/or vitamin D in both groups; (2) a homogenous group of *de novo* adult renal transplant recipients; (3) at least one outcome of interest for our study. Two authors independently assessed the inclusion criteria and selected trials for final analysis. Disagreements were resolved after discussion.

Study Quality

The quality of the eligible trials was assessed using the Jadad guidelines. Three specific domains, including random allocation, double-blinding and description of withdrawals and dropouts, were considered as the quality items [11]. A score of 0 to 5 was assigned to each study, 0 being the lowest and 5 being the best quality.

Data Extraction

Changes in the BMD of the lumbar spine and femoral neck, and serum creatinine, calcium and intact parathyroid hormone (iPTH) levels from all eligible studies were extracted. Data extracted from previously published studies included study design, the size of the intervention and control groups, mean age of both groups, intervention protocol, dosage of pamidronate, immunosuppressive drug protocol, duration of the trial, and BMD at baseline and after follow-up. The standard deviation (SD) of the BMD of the lumbar spine and femoral neck of two studies and the mean and SD value of serum creatinine, calcium and iPTH of all eligible trials were estimated using a statistical method based on the Cochrane handbook [12]. Attempts were made to obtain missing data from the first or corresponding author of such studies.

Statistical Analysis

BMD of the lumbar spine and femoral neck, and changes of serum creatinine, calcium and iPTH levels, were calculated separately from baseline to last follow-up in both groups. Data were analyzed using the methods of the "Cochrane Handbook for Systematic Reviews of Interventions 5.0.2". I^2 was calculated to estimate heterogeneity among trials. I^2 was calculated as 100%* (Q-df)/Q, where Q was the Cochran's heterogeneity statistic and df was the number of degrees of freedom. A fixed-effect model set at low statistical inconsistency ($I^2 < 25\%$) was used. If I^2 was greater than 25%, a random-effects model was used [12,13]. The average differences of each included trial were expressed as the standardized mean difference (SMD) and 95% confidence interval

(CI). Forest plots were used to present overall results. STATA (release 12.0, College Station, TX) was used to complete all meta-analyses.

Results

Literature Search

Using the key words mentioned above, 21 citations were identified. Ten of these were selected for full-text review and 11 citations were excluded as they did not meet the inclusion criteria based on their titles or abstracts. Three of the 10 were excluded after full-text review, because they were case reports, did not have a full text, or were follow-up publications. One additional trial was excluded after attempting to contact the author due to the incompleteness of the available BMD values. Six RCTs with 281 participants were included in our meta-analysis [7–9,14,15] (Figure 1).

Included trials

The characteristics and quality of the trails included are shown in Table 1. All trials administered intravenous pamidronate to the intervention group and oral calcium to both groups. In addition, oral cholecalciferol (800 IU/d) was supplied in one study for 12 months in both groups [8]. Another study added with Vitamin D_3 [14]. Participants in two other studies received calcitriol in both the pamidronate group and the control group.

Pamidronate was administered at doses ranging from 30 mg to 90 mg per intravenous injection. Two studies administered 0.5 mg/kg and 1.0 mg/kg pamidronate, respectively. Coco M [15] reported the lowest pamidronate treatment dose (60 mg) and Omidvar B [9] the highest.

BMD was determined using dual energy X-ray absorptiometry (DEXA) in six trials. Lumbar spine BMD change was reported in five studies and BMD changes of the femoral neck were reported in four studies [15]. Serum creatinine, calcium and iPTH levels were reported in four trials. All eligible studies performed administration of pamidronate and placebo agents preemptively as no osteoporosis was present in enrolled patients.

The quality of trials involved was assessed by two independent authors using Jadad guidelines [11] for estimating the risk of bias. One study [8] received a score of 4 for double-blinding without detailed explanations. Other reports [6,7,9,14,15] were not scored above 3 due to the lack of double-blinding.

Quantitative Data Analysis

We selected the later data point if BMD was evaluated at both 6 months and 12 months. Changes of BMD in the lumbar spine, femoral neck and serum creatinine, calcium, and iPTH levels were analyzed in our meta-analysis.

The pamidronate treated group had significantly less decline in lumbar spine BMD than the control group (Figure 2) (SMD = 24.62 [16.25, 32.99], p for effect <0.001, p for heterogeneity < 0.001, $I^2 = 98.4\%$). Five studies with 188 patients were evaluated. A random effects model was used to evaluate the femoral neck (Figure 2). The pamidronate treated group and control group had similar declines in femoral neck BMD (SMD = 3.53 [−1.84, 8.90], p for effect = 0.198, p for heterogeneity <0.001, $I^2 = 97.6\%$). Four studies with 129 patients were evaluated.

A significant increase in the serum creatinine (Figure 3) was found in the intervention group, and control group (SMD = − 3.101 [−5.33, −0.89], p for effect = 0.006, p for heterogeneity < 0.001, $I^2 = 97.1\%$). Four studies with 221 patients were evaluated. There was no difference in the serum calcium (Figure 3) levels of the two groups (SMD = 2.18 [−0.8, 5.16], p for effect = 0.151, p

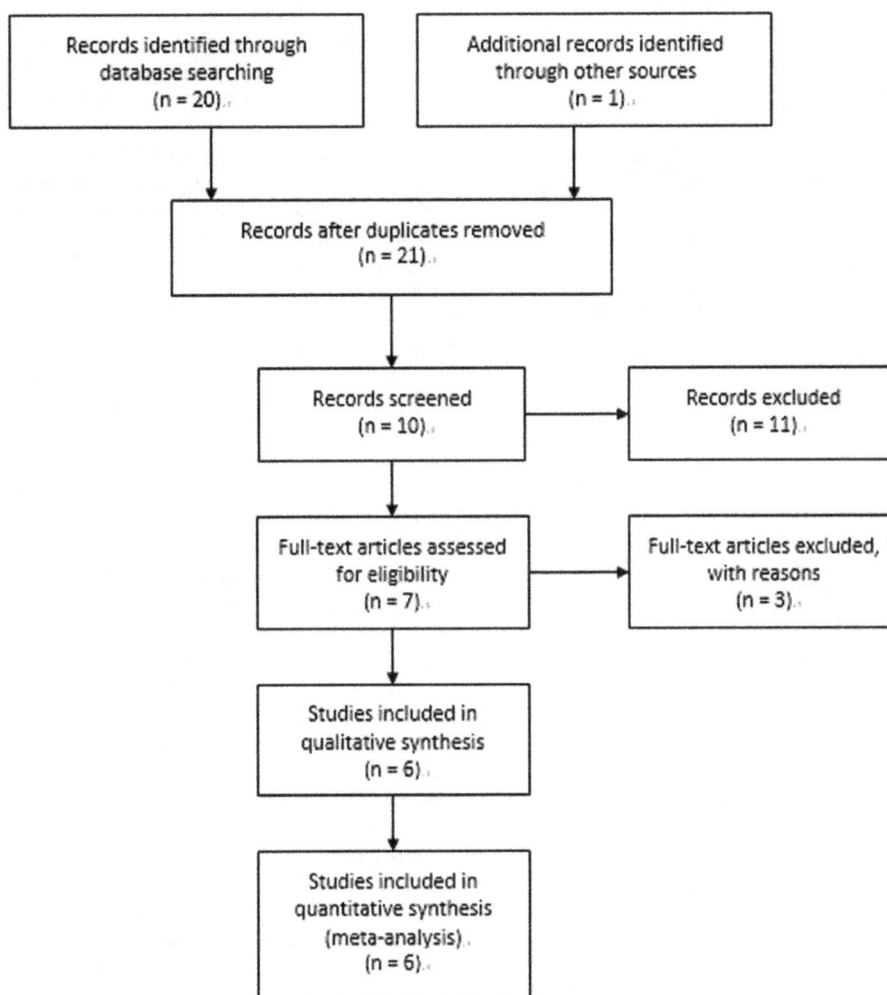

Figure 1. Flow diagram. Flow chart of trial selection.

for heterogeneity <0.001, $I^2 = 98.3\%$). Five studies with 246 patients were evaluated. I^2 from the I-squared test was 0.00% for iPTH, so a fixed effect model was used. The pamidronate and control groups had similar serum iPTH levels (Figure 3) at 1 year (SMD $= 0.06$ [-0.19, 0.31], p for effect $= 0.646$, p for heterogeneity $= 0.836$, $I^2 = 0.00\%$). Five studies with 246 patients were evaluated.

Sensitivity analysis was performed. BMD of the lumbar spine and femoral neck and serum calcium findings were not altered by omitting any single trial. Significant heterogeneity was identified in the serum creatinine analysis. No study characteristic was related to the lack of homogeneity in the relationship between serum creatinine and pamidronate.

Bone fractures and adverse effects

Coco M [15] reported three new vertebral fractures at 12 months, one in the pamidronate group and two in the control group. Torregrosa [8] reported one peripheral fracture at 6 months in the pamidronate group. No other new fractures were reported in the other four studies.

Walsh [6] reported 5 episodes of transient hypocalcemia (8.6%) in pamidronate group which could be considered as pamidronate-related adverse events. No withdrawal of pamidronate administration was reported during experiment due to adverse effects.

Graft function and immunosuppression

There was no acute rejection reported due to the administration of pamidronate in any of the trials included. Torregrosa JV [8] observed seven rejections, four in the pamidronate group and three in control group, during follow-up. This constituted 18% of the renal transplant cases. There was no difference in the incidence of acute rejection of the two groups.

Two-drug or three-drug immunosuppressive regimens, including steroids and calcineurin inhibitors such as cyclosporine and FK506 (tacrolimus), were used in five trials. No induction phase was reported in the trial reported by Nam [7]. There was no significant difference in the doses of immunosuppressive drugs administered to the two groups.

Discussion

Nitrogen-containing BPs such as Alendronate and Pamidronate are taken up preferentially by the skeleton and suppress bone resorption. They are widely used in the treatment of Paget's disease of bone, metastatic and osteolytic bone disease, hypercalcemia of malignancy, and glucocorticoid-induced osteoporosis [4,16]. Recipients of kidney transplantation may experience rapid bone loss during the first 12–18 months and may continue to undergo persistent bone loss for many years, which could lead to

Table 1. Description of the 6 trials included in the meta-analysis.

Author/year/area	Sample size (PAMI/CON)	PAM group age (mean ±SD)	CON group age (mean ±SD)	Intervention	PAM administration (months after transplantation)	Control	Follow-up (months)	Immunosuppression	BMD measurements (months)	Quality score
Nam JH/2000/South Korea(4)	35(15/20)	44	44	PAM + calcium	30 mg i.v. (0, 1, 2, 3, 4, 5, 6 months)	Calcium	6	Not mentioned	0, 6	1
Torregrosa JV/2011/ Spain(7)	29(19/10)	53.99±13.79	56.53±15.48	PAM + calcium + cholecalciferol	30 mg i.v. (7 d, 10 d, 3 months)	Placebo + calcium + cholecalciferol	12	Steroids + cyclosporine + MMF	0, 6, 12	4
Fan SL/2000/UK(8)	25(13/12)	53	50	PAM + calcium + Vit D	0.5 mg/kg i.v. (0, 1 month)	Placebo + calcium + Vit D	12	Steroids + AZA + cyclosporine	0, 3, 12	2
Coco M/2003/US(9)	59(31/28)	43.8±2.3	44.3±2.3	PAM + calcium + calcitriol	60 mg i.v. (0); 30 mg i.v. (1, 2, 3, 6 months)	Calcium + calcitriol	12	Steroids + cyclosporine/ FK506	0, 6, 12	3
Omidvar B/2011/Iran(10)	40(20/20)	38.3	37.2	PAM+ calcium + calcitriol	90 mg i.v. (0, 1, 2, 3 months)	Alendronate + calcium + calcitriol	6	Steroids + cyclosporine + MMF	0, 6	2
Walsh SB/2009/UK(4)	93(46/47)	46.1±12.77	46.1±12.93	PAM + calcium + Vit D + cholecalciferol	1 mg/kg i.v. at 0, 1, 4, 8, 12 months	Calcium + Vit D + cholecalciferol	12	Steroids + cyclosporine	0, 3, 6, 12, 24	3

Abbreviation: PAM: pamidronate; CON: control; BMD: bone mineral density; SD: standard Deviation; Vit D: vitamin D; AZA: azathioprine; MMF: mycophenolate mofetil; FK506: tacrolimus.

post-transplant osteoporosis [17,18].Practice guidelines for kidney transplantation recommend vitamin D and calcium supplements in the absence of contraindications and BPs for the prevention of bone loss in the early post-transplant period [19,20]. All six studies performed pamidroante administration after kidney transplantation preemptively, which could be considered as prophylaxis for post-transplant rapid bone loss and osteoporosis. Outcomes of our meta-analysis are consistent with the mechanism of action of BPs mentioned above and the recommendation of these guidelines.

Our meta-analysis confirmed that pamidronate reduced bone loss of the lumbar spine and not the femoral neck. Bone cells have heterogeneous responses to pamidronate according to whether the bone is cancellous or cortical. Cortical osteoclasts seem to be unaffected by the use of BPs [21], possibly accounting for the different BMD outcomes in the lumbar spine and femoral neck. Boyce [22] reported that human parathyroid hormone (1–34) [hPTH (1–34)] plus risedronate was superior to hPTH (1–34) plus 1, 25(OH)$_2$ D$_3$ in preventing osteoporosis of the cortical envelope. The action of iPTH and pamidronate requires a long time to become apparent. Thus, longer follow-up may be needed to demonstrate the protective efficacy of pamidronate on the femoral neck.

Administration of pamidronate was not associated with renal toxicity during the first year of kidney transplantation since there was no significant difference in the relationship between serum calcium, iPTH and the administration of pamidronate. In contrast, some other BPs including alendronate, have been shown to have some detrimental effect on renal function [23–25].However, a slight increase in serum creatinine level with a high degree of heterogeneity was seen. No study characteristic was found to be related to the lack of homogeneity in the relationship between serum creatinine and pamidronate. Different treatment criteria, different dosages used and different durations of treatment in 4 of the trials may have contributed to this heterogeneity. In addition to the poor quality of included articles, the pooled data of serum creatinie must be interpreted with caution and the relationship between serum creatine and pamidronate remained to be determined.

The optimal drug to prevent BMD should provide predictable effects, be easy to administer with no adverse events, and have no withdrawal effects at the end of infusion [26]. Pamidronate is well-tolerated, long-lasting and needs minimal additional monitoring during treatment. In contrast, alendronate is associated with gastrointestinal complications after sudden withdrawal of the medication. None of the 6 trials reported serious adverse events from pamidronate. Pamidronate administration is sometimes associated with fever and flu-like symptoms at the start of treatment, the so-called "post-dose" symptoms. These effects are transient and occur predominantly after the first intravenous administration of pamidronate, probably due to the release of pro-inflammatory cytokines [16,27,28]. Moreover, jaw osteonecrosis and atypical femoral fractures were also reported in few trials with administration of pamidronate in the general population, which remained to be observed in transplant recipients[29,30].Torregrosa [8] used low doses of pamidronate (30 mg i.v., on days 7 and 10, and 3 months after transplant) to reduce bone turnover, a simple regimen to administer regimen.

Some new bone turnover markers, including iPTH, osteocalcin (OC), procollagen type I N propeptide (PINP), serum C-terminal cross-linking telopeptide of type I collagen (sCTX) and bone-specific alkaline phosphatase (BSAP) have been used to monitor bone remodeling and bone reabsorption. Torregrosa [8] analyzed the performance of PINP and CTX in administration of pamidronate. The bone remodeling markers of PINP and CTX

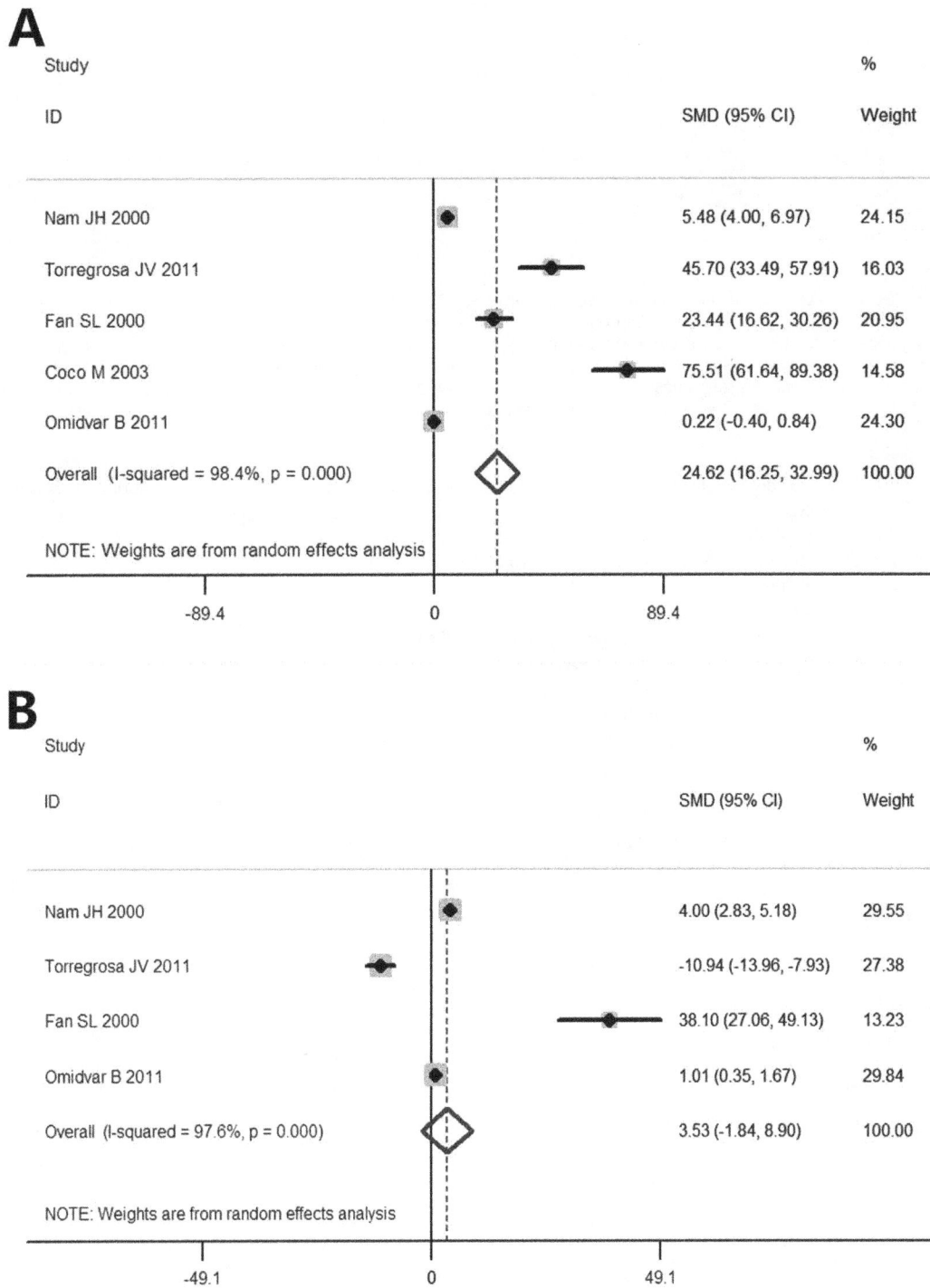

Figure 2. Forest plot of lumbar spine and femoral neck BMD change. (A). The administration of pamidronate was associated with significant benefit to the intervention group, compared to the control group. (SMD = 24.62 [16.25, 32.99], p for effect <0.001, p for heterogeneity <0.001, I^2 =98.4%). Five studies with 188 patients were analyzed. (B). No significant difference was found in the BMD of the intervention and control groups (SMD =3.53 [−1.84, 8.90], p for effect =0.198, p for heterogeneity <0.001, I^2 =97.6%). Four studies with 129 patients were analyzed. BMD: bone mineral density; SMD: standardized mean difference.

fall initially during the first 3 months in pamidronate group and control group, and distinct outcomes, recovering starting in control group and continuous slight decrease in pamidronate group, was found during 12 months, although differences between two groups were not significant. The experience with all these, except for iPTH, is limited. We did not observe any significant differences in the iPTH levels of the pamidronate and control groups. Biomarkers specific to bone turnover and remodeling [31], such as CTX in urine and serum, PINP and OC, might be more

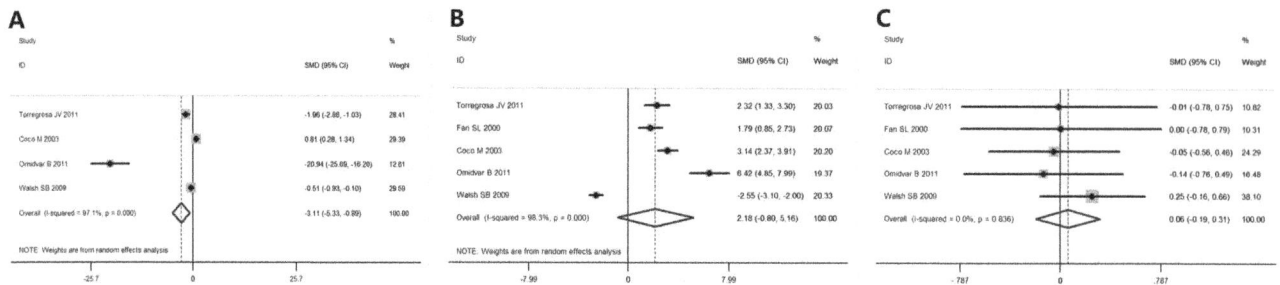

Figure 3. Forest plot of the change in serum creatinine, calcium and iPTH. (A). There was a significant increase in the serum creatinine of the intervention group (SMD = −3.101 [−5.33, −0.89], p for effect = 0.006, p for heterogeneity <0.001, I^2 = 97.1%). Four studies with 221 patients were analyzed.(B). No significant difference was detected in the serum calcium of the intervention and control groups (serum calcium: SMD = 2.18 [−0.8, 5.16], p for effect = 0.151, p for heterogeneity <0.001, I^2 = 98.3%). Five studies with 246 patients were analyzed. (C). There was no difference in the serum iPTH of the intervention and control groups at 1-year follow-up (SMD = 0.06 [−0.19, 0.31], p for effect = 0.646, p for heterogeneity = 0.836, I^2 = 0.00%). Five studies with 246 patients were analyzed. iPTH: intact parathyroid hormone. SMD: standardized mean difference.

sensitive indicators of bone metabolism. Their efficacy remains to be validated in clinical studies.

Our meta-analysis had some limitations. Roschger [32] showed that cancellous and cortical bone are both strengthened by the BPs alendronate and pamidronate. This was confirmed by a four-year study of bone loss with pamidronate [33]. In contrast, we did not see a positive outcome in the femoral neck. This may be due to the relatively short, one-year follow-up time. Longer studies are needed to better examine this treatment effect. The small number and low quality of some ariticles introduced a high risk of bias. A large number of multicenter randomized controlled trials with long term follow-up would better evaluate the actions of pamidronate.

In conclusion, our meta-analysis suggests that pamidronate, which is simple to administer and well tolerated without any serious adverse effects, is beneficial to bone loss and is not correlated with renal toxicity in the first year after renal transplantation. Further clinical studies are needed to confirm

our conclusions. The best way to monitor these patients' bone turnover is yet to be determined.

Acknowledgments

We acknowledge Deng Xiaheng and Liu Kang for their professional advice and support.

Author Contributions

Conceived and designed the experiments: RT MG. Performed the experiments: ZW Z. Han. Analyzed the data: ZW Z. Han JT. Contributed reagents/materials/analysis tools: PL XL JW. Wrote the paper: ZW. Checked and polished the article: BW Z. Huang CY.

References

1. Epstein S, Stuss M (2011) Transplantation osteoporosis. Endokrynol Pol 62: 472–485.
2. Okamoto M, Suzuki T, Fujiki M, Nobori S, Ushigome H, et al. (2010) The consequences for live kidney donors with preexisting glucose intolerance without diabetic complication: analysis at a single Japanese center. Transplantation 89: 1391–1395.
3. Smerud KT, Dolgos S, Olsen IC, Asberg A, Sagedal S, et al. (2012) A 1-year randomized, double-blind, placebo-controlled study of intravenous ibandronate on bone loss following renal transplantation. Am J Transplant 12: 3316–3325.
4. Papapoulos SE (2008) Bisphosphonates: how do they work? Best Pract Res Clin Endocrinol Metab 22: 831–847.
5. Mitterbauer C, Schwarz C, Haas M, Oberbauer R (2006) Effects of bisphosphonates on bone loss in the first year after renal transplantation–a meta-analysis of randomized controlled trials. Nephrol Dial Transplant 21: 2275–2281.
6. Walsh SB, Altmann P, Pattison J, Wilkie M, Yaqoob MM, et al. (2009) Effect of pamidronate on bone loss after kidney transplantation: a randomized trial. Am J Kidney Dis 53: 856–865.
7. Nam JH, Moon JI, Chung SS, Kim SI, Park KI, et al. (2000) Pamidronate and calcitriol trial for the prevention of early bone loss after renal transplantation. Transplant Proc 32: 1876.
8. Torregrosa JV, Fuster D, Monegal A, Gentil MA, Bravo J, et al. (2011) Efficacy of low doses of pamidronate in osteopenic patients administered in the early post-renal transplant. Osteoporos Int 22: 281–287.
9. Omidvar B, Ghorbani A, Shahbazian H, Beladi Mousavi SS, Shariat Nabavi SJ, et al. (2011) Comparison of alendronate and pamidronate on bone loss in kidney transplant patients for the first 6 months of transplantation. Iran J Kidney Dis 5: 420–424.
10. Lee S, Glicklich D, Coco M (2004) Pamidronate used to attenuate post-renal transplant bone loss is not associated with renal dysfunction. Nephrol Dial Transplant 19: 2870–2873.

11. Jadad AR, Moore RA, Carroll D, Jenkinson C, Reynolds DJ, et al. (1996) Assessing the quality of reports of randomized clinical trials: is blinding necessary? Control Clin Trials 17: 1–12.
12. Higgins JPT GS, Cochrane Collaboration. (2008) Cochrane handbook for systematic reviews of interventions. Chichester, England; Hoboken, NJ: WileyBlackwell.
13. Biondi-Zoccai G, Lotrionte M, Landoni G, Modena MG (2011) The rough guide to systematic reviews and meta-analyses. HSR Proc Intensive Care Cardiovasc Anesth 3: 161–173.
14. Fan SL, Almond MK, Ball E, Evans K, Cunningham J (2000) Pamidronate therapy as prevention of bone loss following renal transplantation. Kidney Int 57: 684–690.
15. Coco M, Glicklich D, Faugere MC, Burris L, Bognar I, et al. (2003) Prevention of bone loss in renal transplant recipients: a prospective, randomized trial of intravenous pamidronate. J Am Soc Nephrol 14: 2669–2676.
16. Russell RG (2011) Bisphosphonates: the first 40 years. Bone 49: 2–19.
17. Julian BA, Laskow DA, Dubovsky J, Dubovsky EV, Curtis JJ, et al. (1991) Rapid loss of vertebral mineral density after renal transplantation. N Engl J Med 325: 544–550.
18. Durieux S, Mercadal L, Orcel P, Dao H, Rioux C, et al. (2002) Bone mineral density and fracture prevalence in long-term kidney graft recipients. Transplantation 74: 496–500.
19. National Kidney F (2002) K/DOQI clinical practice guidelines for chronic kidney disease: evaluation, classification, and stratification. Am J Kidney Dis 39: S1–266.
20. Transplantation EEGoR (2002) European best practice guidelines for renal transplantation. Section IV: Long-term management of the transplant recipient. Nephrol Dial Transplant 17 Suppl 4: 1–67.
21. Chappard D, Petitjean M, Alexandre C, Vico L, Minaire P, et al. (1991) Cortical osteoclasts are less sensitive to etidronate than trabecular osteoclasts. J Bone Miner Res 6: 673–680.

Clinical Efficacy and Safety of Pamidronate Therapy on Bone Mass Density in Early...

135

22. Boyce RW, Paddock CL, Franks AF, Jankowsky ML, Eriksen EF (1996) Effects of intermittent hPTH(1-34) alone and in combination with 1,25(OH)(2)D(3) or risedronate on endosteal bone remodeling in canine cancellous and cortical bone. J Bone Miner Res 11: 600–613.

23. Body JJ, Diel I, Bell R (2004) Profiling the safety and tolerability of bisphosphonates. Semin Oncol 31: 73–78.

24. Cremers S, Papapoulos S (2011) Pharmacology of bisphosphonates. Bone 49: 42–49.

25. Guy JA, Shea M, Peter CP, Morrissey R, Hayes WC (1993) Continuous alendronate treatment throughout growth, maturation, and aging in the rat results in increases in bone mass and mechanical properties. Calcif Tissue Int 53: 283–288.

26. Pasin L, Greco T, Feltracco P, Vittorio A, Neto CN, et al. (2013) Dexmedetomidine as a sedative agent in critically ill patients: a meta-analysis of randomized controlled trials. PLoS One 8: e82913.

27. Sanders JM, Ghosh S, Chan JM, Meints G, Wang H, et al. (2004) Quantitative structure-activity relationships for gammadelta T cell activation by bisphospho-nates. J Med Chem 47: 375–384.

28. Thompson K, Rogers MJ (2004) Statins prevent bisphosphonate-induced gamma, delta-T-cell proliferation and activation in vitro. J Bone Miner Res 19: 278–288.

29. Migliorati CA (2003) Bisphosphanates and oral cavity avascular bone necrosis. J Clin Oncol 21: 4253–4254.

30. Meier RP, Perneger TV, Stern R, Rizzoli R, Peter RE (2012) Increasing occurrence of atypical femoral fractures associated with bisphosphonate use. Arch Intern Med 172: 930–936.

31. Biver E (2012) Use of bone turnover markers in clinical practice. Curr Opin Endocrinol Diabetes Obes 19: 468–473.

32. Roschger P, Rinnerthaler S, Yates J, Rodan GA, Fratzl P, et al. (2001) Alendronate increases degree and uniformity of mineralization in cancellous bone and decreases the porosity in cortical bone of osteoporotic women. Bone 29: 185–191.

33. Fan SL, Kumar S, Cunningham J (2003) Long-term effects on bone mineral density of pamidronate given at the time of renal transplantation. Kidney Int 63: 2275–2279.

15

Novel Intramedullary-Fixation Technique for Long Bone Fragility Fractures Using Bioresorbable Materials

Takanobu Nishizuka[1]*, Toshikazu Kurahashi[1], Tatsuya Hara[1], Hitoshi Hirata[1], Toshihiro Kasuga[2]

1 Department of Hand Surgery, Nagoya University Graduate School of Medicine, Nagoya, Japan, **2** Department of Frontier Materials, Nagoya Institute of Technology, Nagoya, Japan

Abstract

Almost all of the currently available fracture fixation devices for metaphyseal fragility fractures are made of hard metals, which carry a high risk of implant-related complications such as implant cutout in severely osteoporotic patients. We developed a novel fracture fixation technique (intramedullary-fixation with biodegradable materials; IM-BM) for severely weakened long bones using three different non-metallic biomaterials, a poly(L-lactide) (PLLA) woven tube, a nonwoven polyhydroxyalkanoates (PHA) fiber mat, and an injectable calcium phosphate cement (CPC). The purpose of this work was to evaluate the feasibility of IM-BM with mechanical testing as well as with an animal experiment. To perform mechanical testing, we fixed two longitudinal acrylic pipes with four different methods, and used them for a three-point bending test (N = 5). The three-point bending test revealed that the average fracture energy for the IM-BM group (PLLA + CPC + PHA) was 3 times greater than that of PLLA + CPC group, and 60 to 200 times greater than that of CPC + PHA group and CPC group. Using an osteoporotic rabbit distal femur incomplete fracture model, sixteen rabbits were randomly allocated into four experimental groups (IM-BM group, PLLA + CPC group, CPC group, Kirschner wire (K-wire) group). No rabbit in the IM-BM group suffered fracture displacement even under full weight bearing. In contrast, two rabbits in the PLLA + CPC group, three rabbits in the CPC group, and three rabbits in the K-wire group suffered fracture displacement within the first postoperative week. The present work demonstrated that IM-BM was strong enough to reinforce and stabilize incomplete fractures with both mechanical testing and an animal experiment even in the distal thigh, where bone is exposed to the highest bending and torsional stresses in the body. IM-BM can be one treatment option for those with severe osteoporosis.

Editor: Jie Zheng, University of Akron, United States of America

Funding: This work was supported by Japan Science and Technology Agency (AS2414028P, http://www.jst.go.jp/tt/EN/univ-ip/a-step.html#supportContent). The funders had no role in study design, data collection and analysis, decision to publish, or preparation of the manuscript.

Competing Interests: The authors have declared that no competing interests exist.

* Email: nishizuka1@mail.goo.ne.jp

Introduction

Metallic implants such as locked plating or intramedullary nailing can instantaneously strengthen weakened long bone metaphyses; however, they sometimes cause complications such as cutout because the strength of the bone is much less than that of the metallic implants in severely osteoporotic patients [1]. We therefore developed a new technique, intramedullary-fixation with biodegradable materials (IM-BM), to instantaneously strengthen severely weakened long bone metaphyses, imitating vertebroplasty. Vertebroplasty [2] can immediately make the collapsed vertebrae stronger using calcium phosphate cement (CPC) [3]; however, there is no such procedure with CPC for long bone metaphyses due to the limited torsional and bending strength associated with CPC [3,4]. We therefore combined a poly(L-lactide) (PLLA) woven tube with CPC based on a concept of reinforced concrete in order to strengthen severely weakened long bone.

Reinforced concrete is one of the most widely used modern building materials to strengthen the framework. Typical concrete has high resistance to compressive stresses (about 28 MPa); however, any appreciable tension (*e.g.*, due to bending) will break the microscopic rigid lattice, resulting in cracking and concrete separation. Reinforced concrete is a composite material made by inserting steel bars in concrete, and resists not only compression but also bending and torsional stresses.

We also combined a nonwoven polyhydroxyalkanoates (PHA) fiber mat to prevent cement leakage from the fracture site. PHA are biodegradable materials and show excellent extendibility.

The purpose of this work was to evaluate the feasibility of IM-BM in both mechanical testing and animal experiment models. The present work demonstrated that IM-BM was strong enough to reinforce and stabilize incomplete fractures with both mechanical testing and an animal experiment even in the distal thigh, where bone is exposed to the highest bending and torsional stresses in the body.

Materials and Methods

Ethics statement

The Institutional Committee for Animal Care of Nagoya University approved the experimental protocol (reference number: 25166).

Intramedullary-fixation with Biodegradable Materials (IM-BM)

The procedure for IM-BM begins with reaming the intramedullary cavity and inserting a PLLA woven tube into the cavity, followed by injection of CPC paste both inside and outside the tube using a syringe. However, massive CPC paste leakage occurs from the fracture site, and it appears likely to inhibit bone union. Therefore, we use a nonwoven PHA fiber mat to prevent CPC leakage. The 3-hydroxybutyrate (3HB) and 4-hydroxybutyrate (4HB) copolymers (poly [P](3HB-co-4HB)) used in the PHA fiber mat in this work demonstrate both strength and flexibility (Figure 1). The nonwoven PHA fiber mat can prevent CPC leakage. Therefore, when we injected the CPC paste inside and outside the PLLA woven tube, the nonwoven PHA fiber mat was expanded until it fit the cavity (Figures 2 and 3).

Preparation of PLLA Woven Tube

Nipro Co., Ltd. (Tokyo, Japan) produced the PLLA woven tube used in this study. First, a plain-stitch fabric was knitted using PLLA monofilaments (0.2 mm in diameter). Then, three sheets of fabric were stacked, and formed into a cylindrical shape by painting with dichloromethane (Wako Junyaku Kogyo Co., Ltd., Osaka, Japan), with a resulting external and internal diameter of 10 and 7 mm, respectively. Finally, they were cut and shortened to 65 mm in length for mechanical testing. Smaller size PLLA woven tubes for the animal experiment, with external and internal diameters of 5 and 4 mm, respectively, were also prepared. They were cut and shortened to 38 mm in length. Our previous experiment indicated that the mean modulus of elasticity in bending for these tubes was 46.7 MPa.

Preparation of a Nonwoven PHA Fiber Mat

PHA represent a complex class of biopolymers consisting of various hydroxyalkanoic acids. Microorganisms synthesize PHA as storage compounds for energy [5]. PHA exhibit biodegradable, biocompatible, thermoplastic and elastomeric properties once extracted from the cells [6]. Attempts have been made for many years to develop PHA applications in medical devices [7]. Polymerization of 4HB with other hydroxyl acids such as 3HB can produce elastomeric compositions at moderate 4HB contents (15%–35%), and relatively hard rigid polyesters at lower 4HB contents [7]. 3HB and 4HB copolymer (P(3HB-co-4HB)) at 18% 4HB content (G5 JAPAN Co., Ltd., Osaka, Japan) was used in our work as a tool to prevent CPC leakage.

Electrospinning is a process that can generate a polymer fiber mat with high flexibility and porosity [8,9]. A porous material with continuous pore structure is expected to be useful for implants used in the regeneration of damaged tissue, because the pore would allow penetration of nutriments and/or ingrowth of tissues, blood vessels, and cells [10]. The nonwoven fiber mat consisting of a biodegradable polymer may be one of the best biomaterial candidates, because the interlocking fibers easily form large connective pores [11]. A nonwoven PHA fiber mat with 3HB and 4HB copolymers was prepared using an electrospinning method. First, 2 g of PHA powder consisting of P(3HB-co-4HB) copolymers containing 18% 4HB (G5 JAPAN Co.) were dissolved in chloroform at 6 wt% to prepare the solution for electrospinning. The samples were then spun on the electrospinning unit (NEU, Kato Tech Co., Kyoto, Japan). The solution for electrospinning was loaded into a glass syringe and pushed out at a flow rate of 30 μl/min through a metallic needle (22 gauge) that was connected to a +10 kV electrical field at room temperature and approximately 55% relative humidity. The fibers were collected on an aluminum drum rotating at 2000 mm/min, traversing at 100 mm/min, and positioned 80 mm from the tip of the needle. The nonwoven PHA fiber mat, consisting of microfibers with diameters of approximately 10 μm (Figure 4), was produced with a final thickness of 100 μm after spinning for 120 min. The resulting nonwoven PHA fiber mat showed excellent expandability (Figure 1); it did not fracture easily even when the CPC paste was injected to expand it (Figure 3).

CPC Preparation

The CPC used in the present work was Biopex-R® (advanced type) (BPRad, HOYA Co., Ltd., Tokyo, Japan). The CPC powder consisted of α-tricalcium phosphate (α-Ca$_3$(PO$_4$)$_2$; α-TCP), tetracalcium phosphate (Ca$_4$(PO$_4$)$_2$O; TECP), dicalcium phosphate dihydrate (CaHPO$_4$·2H$_2$O), hydroxyapatite (Ca$_{10}$(PO$_4$)$_6$(OH)$_2$; HAp) and magnesium phosphate (Mg$_3$(PO$_4$)$_2$). The malaxation liquid was composed of sodium chondroitin sulfate, disodium succinate ((CH$_2$COONa)$_2$), sodium hydrogensulfite (NaHSO$_3$) and water (H$_2$O). The CPC powder was mixed with the malaxation liquid, turning it into a paste, which hardened over time via hydration to form a hydroxyapatite structure [12]. Twelve grams of powder and 4 ml of malaxation liquid were used in the present mechanical testing and animal experiment. BPRad takes only 1 day to reach maximum compressive strength after kneading of the powder and malaxation liquid mixture.

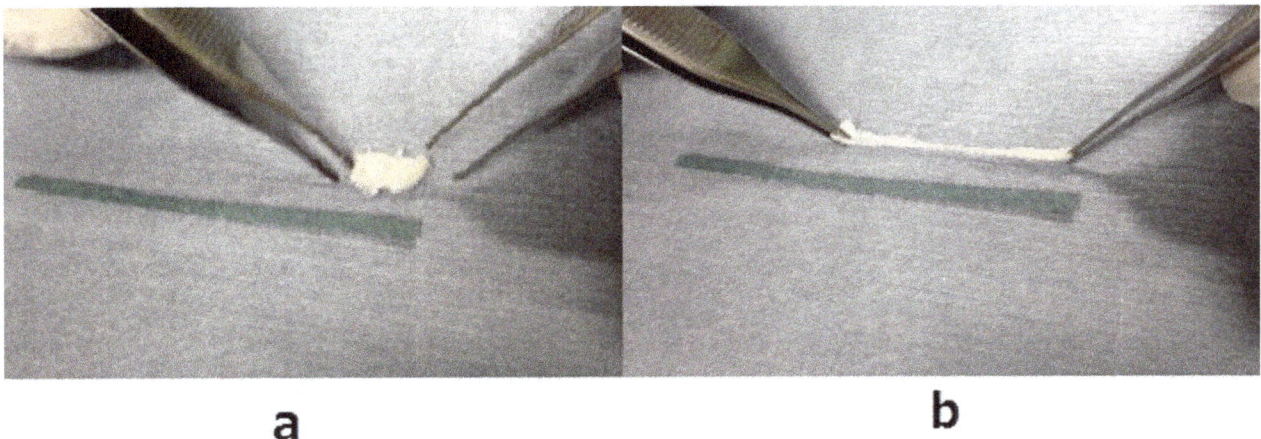

a   b

Figure 1. Expandability of PHA fiber mat. Before elongation (a) and after elongation (b).

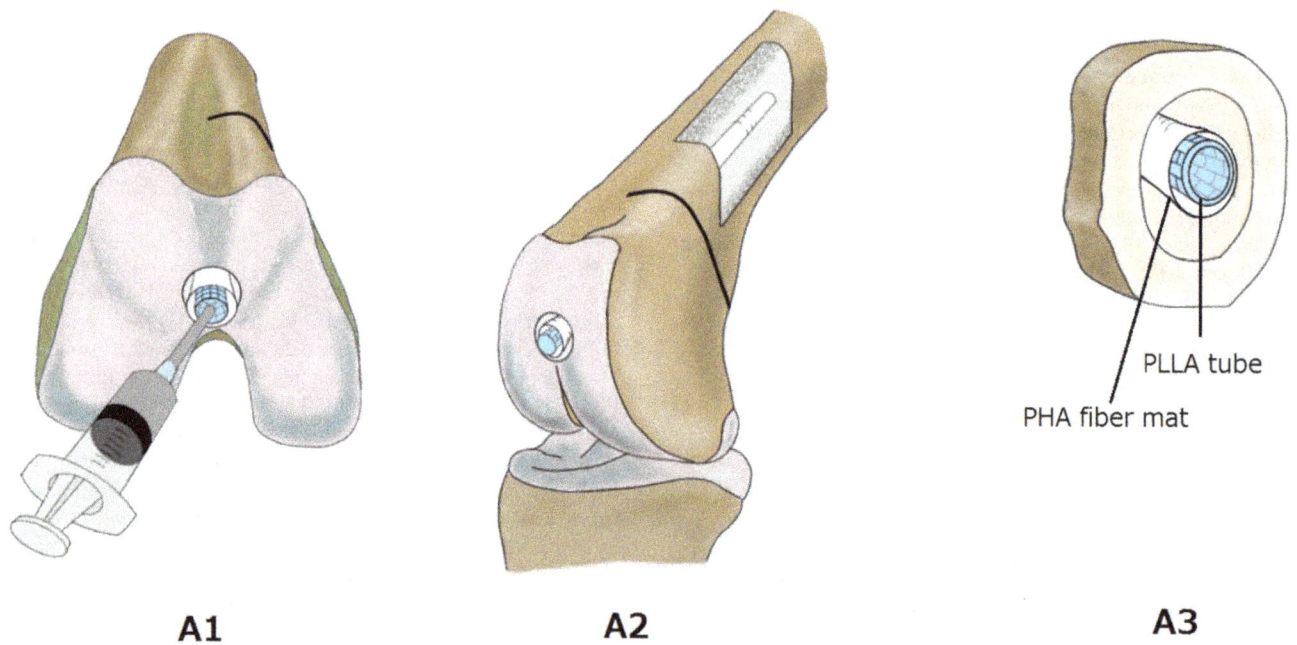

Figure 2. IM-BM procedures. View of the distal femur (A1, A2) and schema of bone cross section (A3) before CPC injection. PLLA: PLLA woven tube; PHA: PHA fiber mat; CPC: calcium phosphate cement.

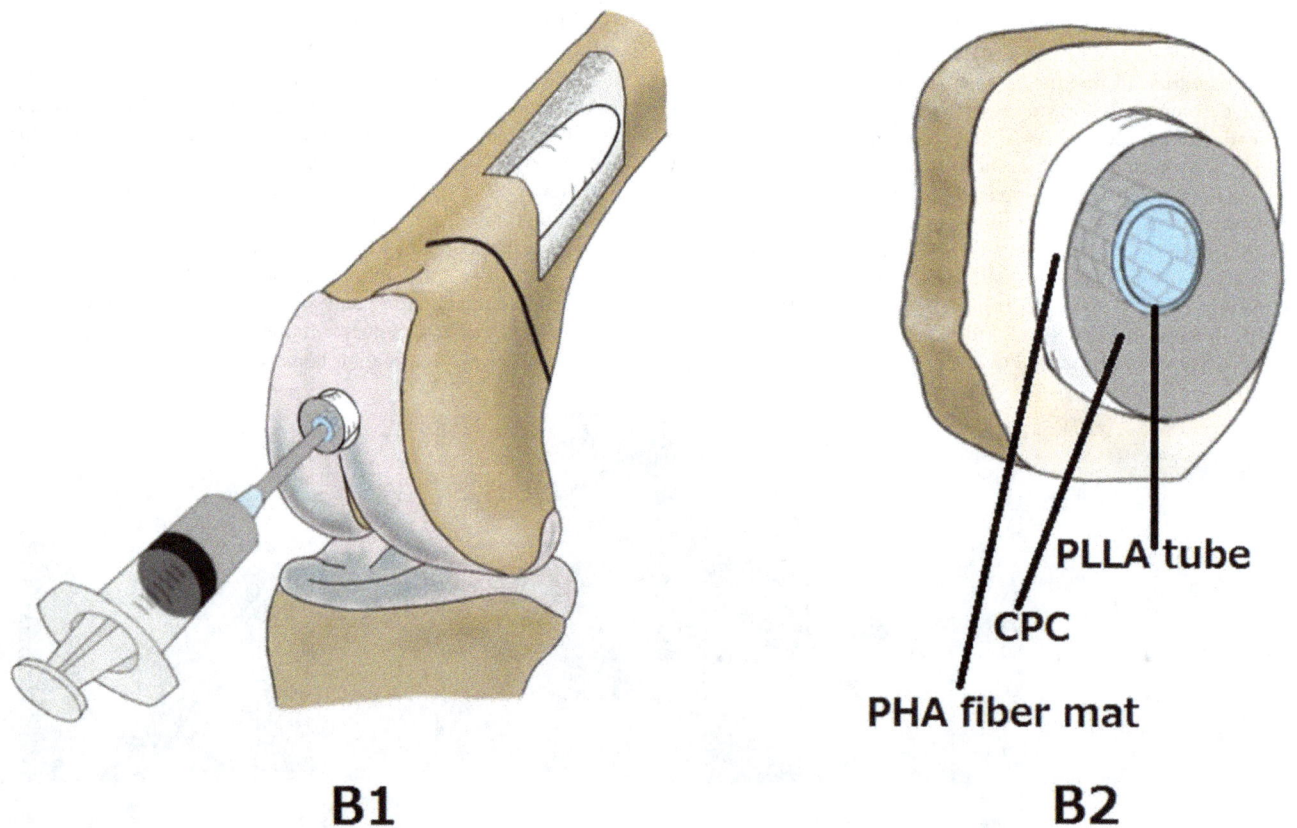

Figure 3. IM-BM procedures. View of the distal femur (B1) and bone cross section schema (B2) after CPC injection. PLLA: PLLA woven tube; PHA: PHA fiber mat; CPC: calcium phosphate cement.

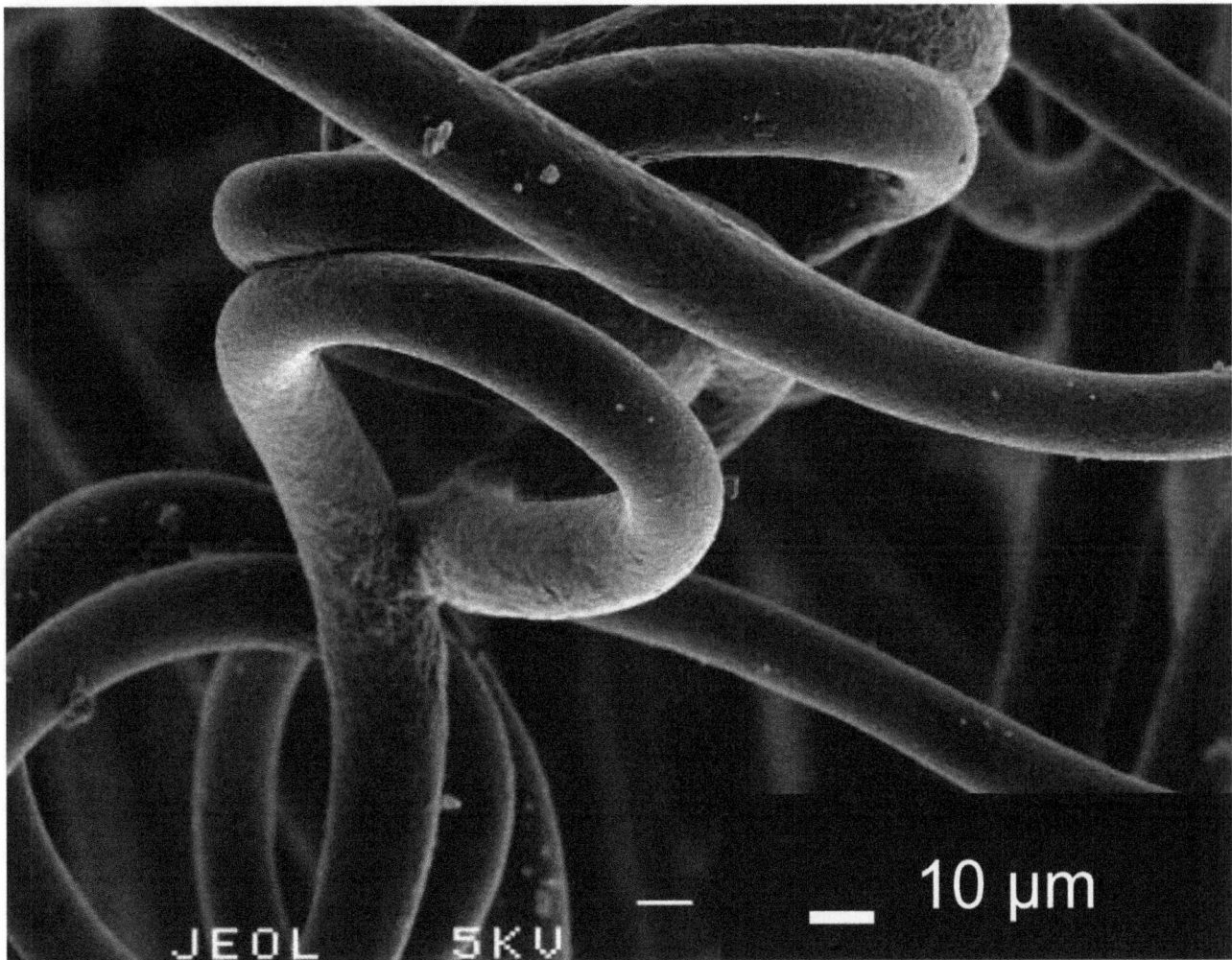

Figure 4. Scanning Electron Microscopy (SEM) photograph of a nonwoven PHA fiber mat. A nonwoven PHA fiber mat, consisting of microfibers with diameters of approximately 10 μm.

Mechanical Testing

Five profile specimens were tested for each sample composition. As shown in Figure 5, we fixed two longitudinal acrylic pipes with four different methods. For group 1, the PLLA woven tube was wrapped by the nonwoven PHA fiber mat, and it was inserted into two acrylic pipes placed longitudinally. The outer diameter of the pipe was 16 mm, and the length of each pipe was 35 mm. The powder and the liquid in the incubator (NTT-2200, EYELA, Tokyo, Japan) were warmed to 30°C before the injection. Just after kneading, the CPC paste was injected inside and outside the PLLA woven tube using a syringe. After the injection, the specimens were submerged in simulated body fluid (Na$^+$ 142.0, K$^+$ 5.0, Mg^{2+} 1.5, Ca^{2+} 2.5, Cl$^-$ 148.8, HCO$_3^-$ 4.2, PO$_4^{2-}$ 1.0, and SO$_4^{2-}$ 0.5 mM and buffered at pH 7.40 with trishydroxymethyl-aminomethane) [13] maintained at 37°C. The CPC started to harden gradually. After 10 min, a three-point bending test was performed using 858 Mini Bionix II (MTS, Eden Prairie, MN) following the Japanese Industrial Standard (JIS) K 7074. The cross-head speed was 0.5 mm/min, and the support span was 60 mm. For group 2, the PLLA woven tube was inserted into two acrylic pipes placed longitudinally. Then, the CPC paste was injected inside and outside the PLLA woven tube. For group 3, the cylindrical shape of the nonwoven PHA fiber mat was inserted into

acrylic pipes. Then, the CPC paste was injected into the nonwoven PHA fiber mat. Only the CPC paste was injected into acrylic pipes for group 4.

The maximum flexural strength was determined using the following equation:

$$\delta_{fmax} = 8F_{max}L/\pi d^3,$$

where δ_{fmax} is the maximum flexural strength (MPa), F_{max} is the maximum load (N), L is the support span (mm), and d is the diameter of the specimen (mm).

The modulus of elasticity in bending was determined using the following equation:

$$E_f = \left(4L^3/3\ \pi d^4\right) \times (\Delta F/\Delta S),$$

where E_f is the modulus of elasticity in bending (MPa), L is the support span (mm), d is the diameter of the specimen (mm), ΔF is the variation of the load (N), and ΔS is the variation of the central deflection (mm).

Fracture energy (J/m^2) was determined using integral calculus from the beginning to the yield point at the stress–strain curve. A

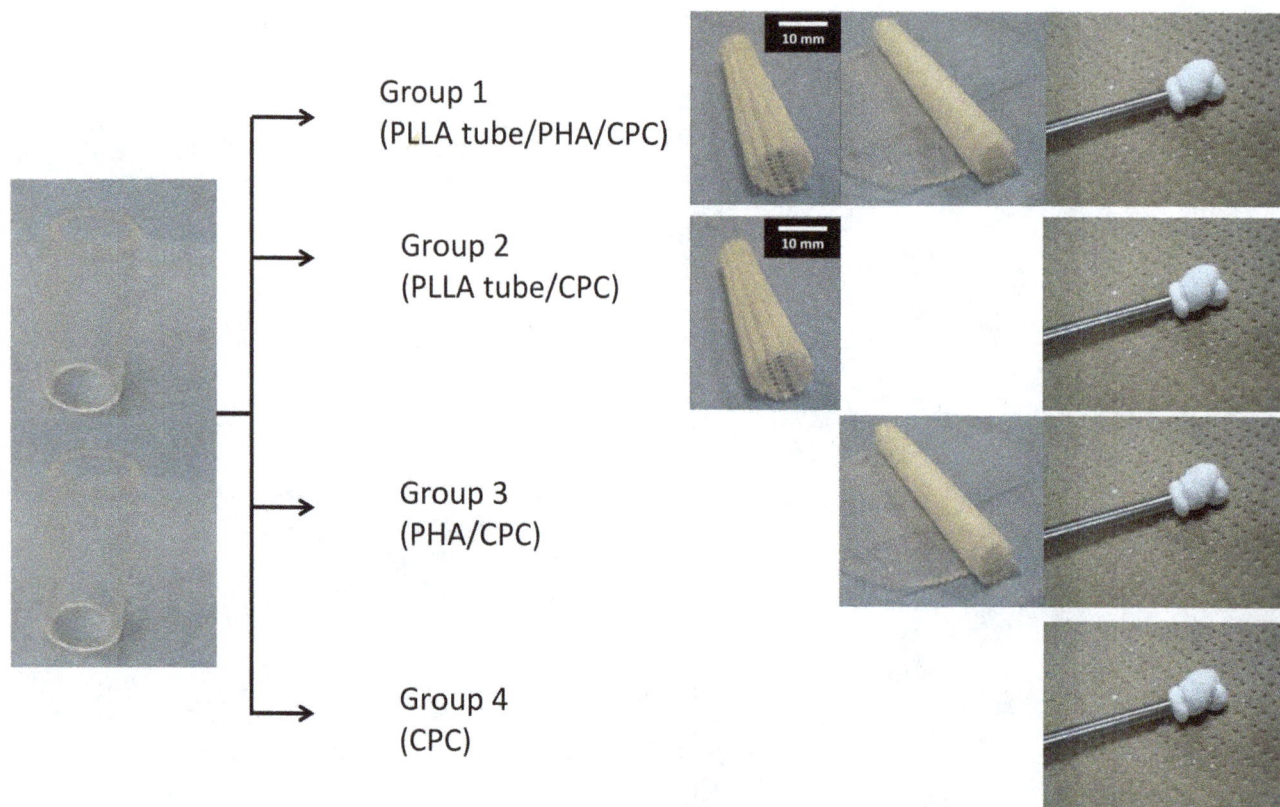

Figure 5. Method of mechanical testing. Two acrylic pipes placed longitudinally were fixed in four groups by the different method. Pictures of group 1 show a PLLA woven tube, a nonwoven PHA fiber mat, and CPC paste sequentially from the left.

mean value and standard deviation were calculated concerning the δ_{fmax}, the modulus of elasticity in bending, and the fracture energy.

All statistical analyses were conducted using SPSS version 19.0 (SPSS, Tokyo, Japan). Data from multiple groups were compared using a one-way analysis of variance (ANOVA). We performed multiple comparisons of the three treatment groups using the Bonferroni test when significant differences were detected. Significance levels of all the tests were established at $p < 0.05$.

Experimental Animal Model of Osteoporosis and Surgical Procedure

Sixteen skeletally mature, 8-month-old (3.0–3.5 kg body weight), female New Zealand white rabbits were used. Experimental rabbit osteoporosis models were made by performing bilateral ovariectomy followed by intramuscular injection with methylprednisolone sodium succinate (Solu-Medrol; Pfizer, Tokyo, Japan) at a dosage of 1 mg/kg/day for four consecutive weeks, as previously described by Castaneda et al. [14] The sixteen rabbits were then randomly allocated into four experimental groups. The first was an IM-BM group (PLLA woven tube + CPC + nonwoven PHA fiber mat). The second was a PLLA + CPC group. The third was a CPC group. The fourth was a Kirschner wire (K-wire) group.

All the PLLA woven tubes and the nonwoven PHA fiber mat used in our animal experiments were sterilized with ethylene oxide gas (20% by weight; CO_2 80% by weight) with 50% H_2O at 45°C for 5 h. The rabbits were anesthetized with an intramuscular injection of ketamine hydrochloride (75 mg/kg body weight) and xylazine (10 mg/kg body weight) 8 weeks after the ovariectomy.

The surgical site was shaved and prepared with a solution of Betadine (povidone-iodine). A lateral parapatellar incision was made, and the patella was medially dislocated. A half-round fracture was produced 10 mm proximal to the distal end of the femur with an electrical cutter to reproduce an insufficiency fracture. In the K-wire group, two 1.5-mm K-wires were inserted intramedullary from the intercondylar area 5 mm proximal from the edge of the intercondylar notch until penetrating the proximal bone cortex. Finally, the fascia and the skin wounds were closed. In the IM-BM group, PLLA + CPC group, and the CPC group, a drill hole was produced in the intercondylar area 5 mm proximal from the edge of the intercondylar notch using 1.5-mm K-wire. Next, an intramedullary cavity was reamed from 3 mm to 7 mm by the drill reamer, and the cavity was curetted.

In the IM-BM group, the PLLA tube wrapped with nonwoven PHA fiber mat was inserted into the cavity (Figure 2-A1, A2, A3). Next, CPC paste was injected into the lumen of the PLLA tube just after kneading the powder and malaxation liquid, which was preheated to 30°C in the incubator (Figure 3-B1, B2). The paste began to harden about 10 min after kneading. In the PLLA + CPC group, CPC paste was injected after insertion of the PLLA woven tube. In the CPC group, only CPC paste was injected. A small amount of CPC paste leaked from the fracture site in the PLLA + CPC group and the CPC group. In the IM-BM group, the PLLA + CPC group, and the CPC group, the fascia and the skin wounds were closed within 15 min after kneading of the CPC paste, and the rabbits began to bear weight a few hours after the operation.

Postoperative lesions were evaluated with the use of soft X-ray (SOFTEX, Yokohama, Japan) at weeks 1, 4, 8, 12, and 20. Lateral radiographs were made with an exposure of 45 kV, 10 mA, and 15 s. The soft X-ray data at postoperative week 1 from multiple groups were compared using a one-way ANOVA. When significant differences were detected in ANOVA, we performed multiple comparisons of the four treatment groups using the Bonferroni test. A significance level for the test was established at $p < 0.05$.

With pentobarbital overdose, two of the four rabbits in the IM-BM group were sacrificed at week 20, and the other two in the IM-BM group were sacrificed at week 52. A 15 mm segment of the metaphyseal portion of the femur was removed for histological examination. The specimens were fixed with 0.2% glutaraldehyde for 24 h and then in 10% phosphate-buffered formalin for 48 h. The specimens were subsequently dehydrated in ethanol and embedded in methyl methacrylate (MMA). The embedded blocks were trimmed with a cutter and ground with abrasive paper. Thereafter, the sections were further ground to a final thickness of approximately 10 μm. Finally, the specimens were stained with hematoxylin and eosin, and examined under the microscope.

Results

Mechanical Testing

Table 1 shows the mean maximum flexural strength values for each group at 10 min immediately following the CPC injection. The group 1 values (PLLA + CPC + PHA; 2.71±0.66 MPa) were significantly higher ($p < 0.001$) than the values of group 3 (CPC + PHA; 0.79±0.23 MPa) and group 4 (CPC only; 0.52±0.24 MPa). Although there is no statistically significant difference, the values of group 1were higher than the values of group 2 (PLLA + CPC; 2.37±0.13 MPa) ($p = 0.15$). Table 1 also shows the average fracture energy at 10 min following the CPC injection. The group 1 values (PLLA + CPC + PHA; 1210±334 J/m^2) were significantly higher ($p < 0.001$) than the group 2 values (PLLA + CPC; 434±63 J/m^2), the group 3 values (CPC + PHA; 19.4±6.4 J/m^2) and the group 4 values (CPC only; 5.5±5.7 J/m^2). Figure 6 shows the representative stress–strain curves for group 1 (PLLA + CPC + PHA) and group 4 (CPC only). In group 1, the curve can be categorized into four zones (zone 1: steep slope zone, zone 2: gentle slope zone, zone 3: almost flat slope zone, and zone 4: negative slope zone). In zones 1 and 2, the stress kept increasing and the curve did not drop until the end of zone 3. In contrast, in groups 3 and 4, the curve immediately reached the yield point. Once the curve reached the yield point, the curve dropped abruptly due to the fragmentation of the materials. The average moduli of elasticity in bending in group 1 were 179±89 MPa in zone 1 and 18.2±8.7 MPa in zone 2. The average moduli of elasticity in bending in groups 2, 3, and 4 were 144±31 MPa, 183±64 MPa and 223±69 MPa, respectively.

Animal Experiments

Soft X-ray photographs revealed that there were no fracture displacements (0/4) over the entire postoperative period in the IM-BM group (Figure 7a), whereas two of four rabbits in PLLA + CPC group, three of four rabbits in the CPC group (Figure 7f), and three (including one cutout) of four rabbits in the K-wire group (Figure 7d) had fracture displacements at postoperative week 1. Although statistical analysis did not indicate a significant difference, IM-BM group had fewer fracture displacements than other groups (PLLA + CPC, CPC, K-wire) ($p = 0.35, 0.143, 0.143$, respectively: all Bonferroni multiple comparison test), as shown in Table 2. Figure 7b shows that all rabbits in the IM-BM group achieved bony union in 8 weeks. There were no postoperative infections or clinical signs of implant reaction in the IM-BM group. On the other hand, all rabbits in the PLLA + CPC group showed CPC leakage from the fracture site (Figure 7e), and three of four rabbits in the CPC group had wound dehiscence within the first postoperative week.

Histologic examination at week 20 in the IM-BM group indicated that the PLLA tube was not degraded yet (Figure 8a). Histologic examination at week 52 in the IM-BM group showed that the PLLA tube seemed to have degraded gradually (Figure 8b). A multinucleated giant cell and neovascularization were observed in the PHA fiber mat layer (Figure 8c).

Discussion

The incidence of fragility fractures has been increasing in developed countries. Since Galibert et al. in 1987 introduced percutaneous poly (methyl methacrylate) (PMMA)-assisted vertebroplasty [15], many authors have reported treatment outcomes for vertebroplasty or balloon kyphoplasty. PMMA has excellent compressive, bending, and tensile strength [16]. However, PMMA monomer toxicity produces a risk of hypotension [17], and can damage surrounding cells due to heat evolution during the hardening process. In addition to these problems, PMMA is not osteoconductive and does not enhance bone remodeling.

Alternatively, CPC (Biopex) is one of the most commonly used injectable bone cement pastes and is highly biocompatible, with excellent osteoconductivity [12]. The cement is absorbed progressively from the outer surface and replaced by bone tissue through the normal remodeling process [12]. Moreover, it can set without heat evolution. However, CPC is brittle and has generally low mechanical strength [3,4], except for compressive strength. Thus far, CPC has been mainly limited to vertebroplasty and balloon kyphoplasty, which require a high compressive strength.

We inserted a PLLA woven tube into the intramedullary cavity with injection of CPC paste in order to overcome the abovementioned problems. We wrapped the PLLA tube with nonwoven PHA fiber mat to prevent both CPC leakage from the fracture site

Table 1. The mean maximum flexural strength values and the mean fracture energy for each group.

	Group 1 (PLLA tube/PHA/CPC)	Group 2 (PLLA tube/CPC)	Group 3 (PHA/CPC)	Group 4 (CPC)
Maximum flexural strength (MPa)	*2.71±0.66	2.37±0.13	0.79±0.23	0.52±0.2
Fracture energy (J/m^2)	*1210±334	434±63	19.4±6.4	5.5±5.7

*Significant difference (p<0.001) in the maximum flexural strength between group 1(*) and group 3/group 4 (Bonferroni test).
*Significant difference (p<0.001) in the fracture energy between group 1(*) and group 2/group 3/group 4 (Bonferroni test).
PLLA: poly(ʟ-lactide); PHA: polyhydroxyalkanoates; CPC: calcium phosphate cement.

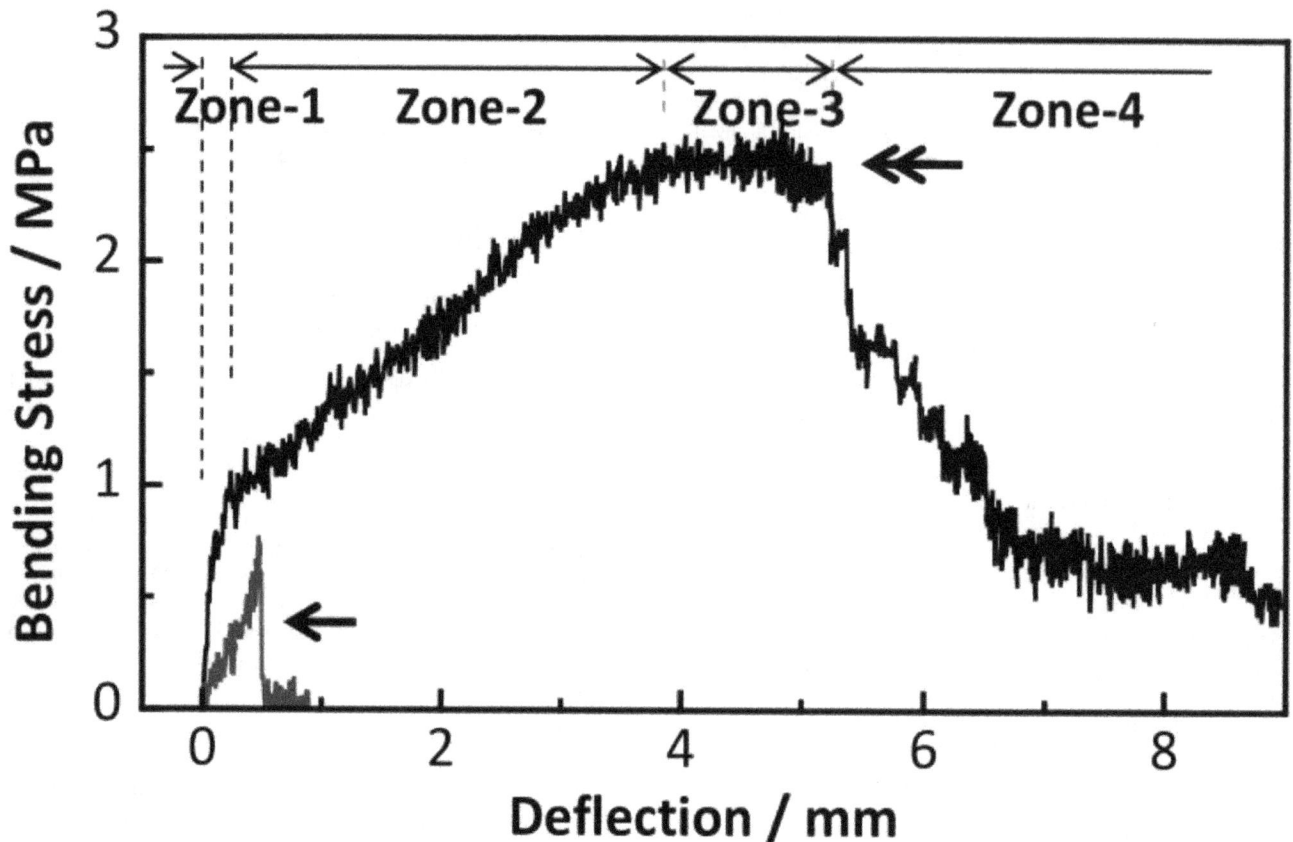

Figure 6. Result of mechanical testing. A representative stress–strain curve 10 min after the CPC injection in group 1 (double arrow) and group 4 (arrow).

and embolism. The PHA used in the present work was comprised of the copolymers 3HB and 18% 4HB. We also attempted to use a nonwoven poly(lactic-co-glycolic acid) (PLGA) fiber mat as a leakage prevention material in a preliminary trial with acrylic tubes. However, the PLGA mat did not extend far enough into the cavity and easily ruptured during injection of CPC paste. In contrast, the present animal experiment demonstrated that a nonwoven PHA fiber mat wrapped around a PLLA tube can efficiently prevent cement leakage from the fracture site and allow almost complete filling of the reamed cavity with CPC, as observed by postoperative soft X-ray analysis as well as histologic examination (Figures 7a and 8a).

This animal experiment also demonstrated that IM-BM markedly improved mechanical strength when compared with CPC only. Rabbits in the IM-BM group had no fracture displacement, whereas three of four rabbits in the CPC group had fracture displacements within 1 week after the surgery. Furthermore, the IM-BM also revealed the better results than

other two groups (PLLA + CPC, K-wire). Two of four rabbits in the PLLA + CPC group and three of four rabbits in the K-wire group suffered fracture displacement, and one of four rabbits in the K-wire group suffered cutout at postoperative week 1. Histologic examination at week 52 in the IM-BM group showed partial degradation of the PLLA tube in the CPC. It has been previously reported that it takes 1.5–5 years for the degradation of PLLA to be complete, as shown in Table 3 [7]. The absorption of the nonwoven PHA fiber mat is preferable, because it enables the CPC to make contact with the bone gradually. However, partial absorption of the nonwoven PHA fiber mat was unclear at weeks 20 and 52. A multinucleated giant cell and neovascularization were observed in the PHA fiber mat layer. This suggests that the PHA used in our study have good biocompatibility. We are now conducting a long-term study to evaluate the degradation behavior of PHA.

Mechanical testing has clearly shown that the combination of the PLLA woven tube with CPC and PHA fiber mat improved the

Table 2. Fracture displacement rate in four groups at postoperative week 1.

	IM-BM group	PLLA + CPC group	CPC group	K-wire group
Fracture displacement rate	0/4	2/4	3/4	3/4

IM-BM group had fewer fracture displacements than the PLLA + CPC, the CPC, and the K-wire groups although statistical analysis did not indicate a significant difference ($p = 0.35, 0.143, 0.143$, respectively: all Bonferroni multiple comparison test).
IM-BM: intramedullary-fixation with biodegradable materials; CPC: calcium phosphate cement; K-wire: Kirschner wire.

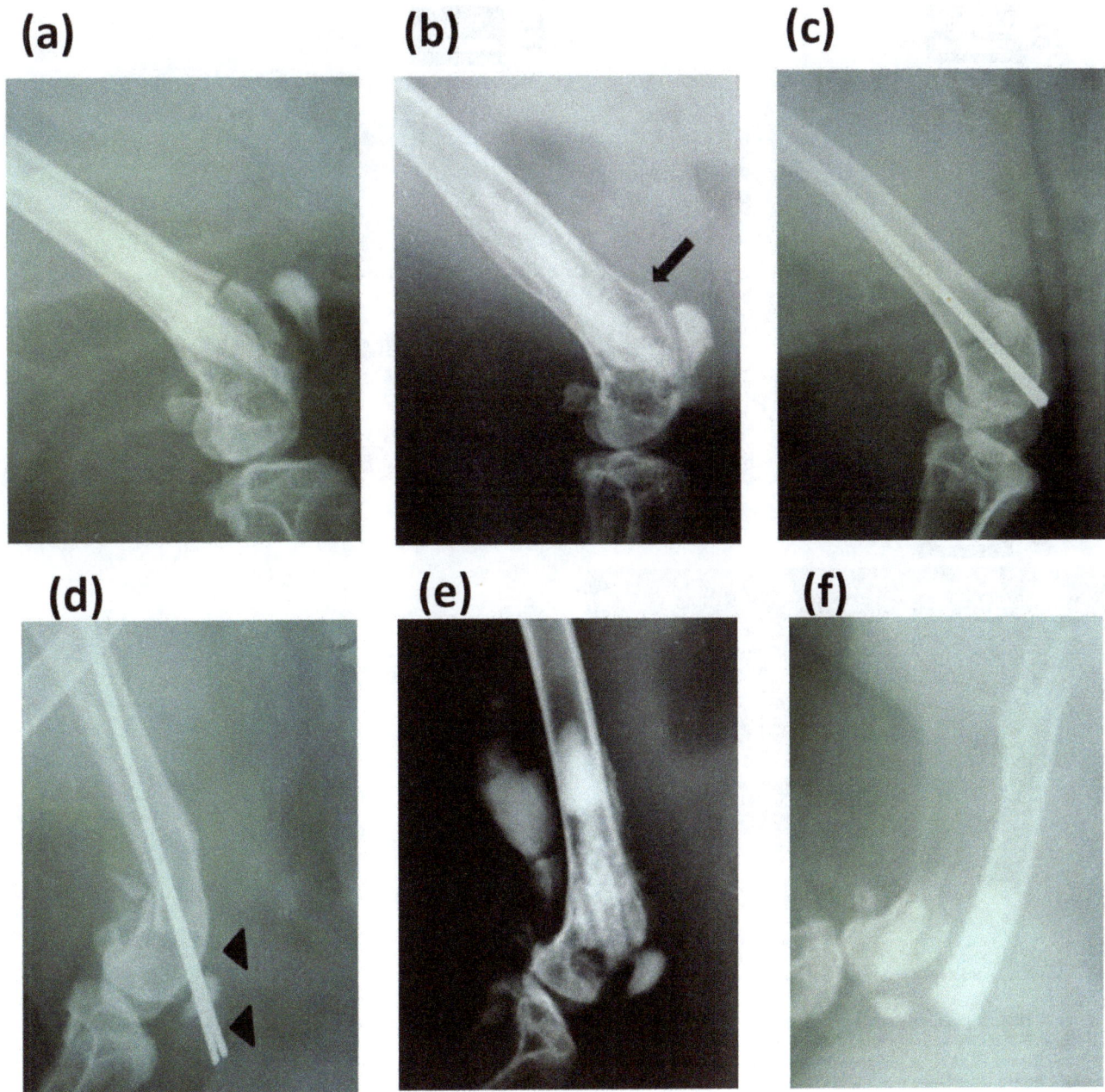

Figure 7. Representative postoperative radiographs. Representative postoperative radiographs in the IM-BM group (PLLA + CPC + PHA) at week 0 (a) and week 8 (b). (b) The fracture site obtained complete bony union (arrow). Representative postoperative radiographs in the Kirschner wire group at week 0 (c) and week 1 (d). (d) Cutout happened at the fracture site (arrowhead). Representative postoperative radiograph in the PLLA + CPC group at week 0 (e). (e) It showed CPC leakage from the fracture site. Representative postoperative radiograph in the CPC group at week 1 (f). (f) It showed fracture displacement.

apparent mechanical properties, including a significant increase in fracture energy and flexural strength. All the stress–strain curves for group 1 (PLLA + CPC + PHA) showed slope changes at the end of zone 1 (Figure 6). The change may be due to fracture of bonding at the interface between the CPC and the PHA fiber mat. Thus, cracks in the CPC followed the fracture of bonding. The slope in zone 2 was smaller than that in zone 1. It is thought that the PLLA woven tube mainly supported the load with the CPC, because the PHA fiber mat prevented the CPC from breaking into pieces. In zone 3, the slope became flat. The PLLA woven tube was believed to be considerably deformed. In zone 4, the slope

became negative. The CPC was not able to support the load any further because it was broken into pieces.

It should be emphasized that the average fracture energy for the IM-BM group (PLLA + CPC + PHA) was 60 to 200 times greater than that of CPC + PHA group and CPC group in our mechanical testing. Considering the result that the mean fracture energy of PLLA + CPC + PHA group (1210 ± 334 J/m^2) was 3 times higher ($p < 0.001$) than that of the PLLA + CPC group (434 ± 63 J/m^2), the enhanced fracture energy of PLLA + PHA + CPC implant was mainly due to the PLLA tube, but PHA fiber mat also improved the fracture energy significantly.

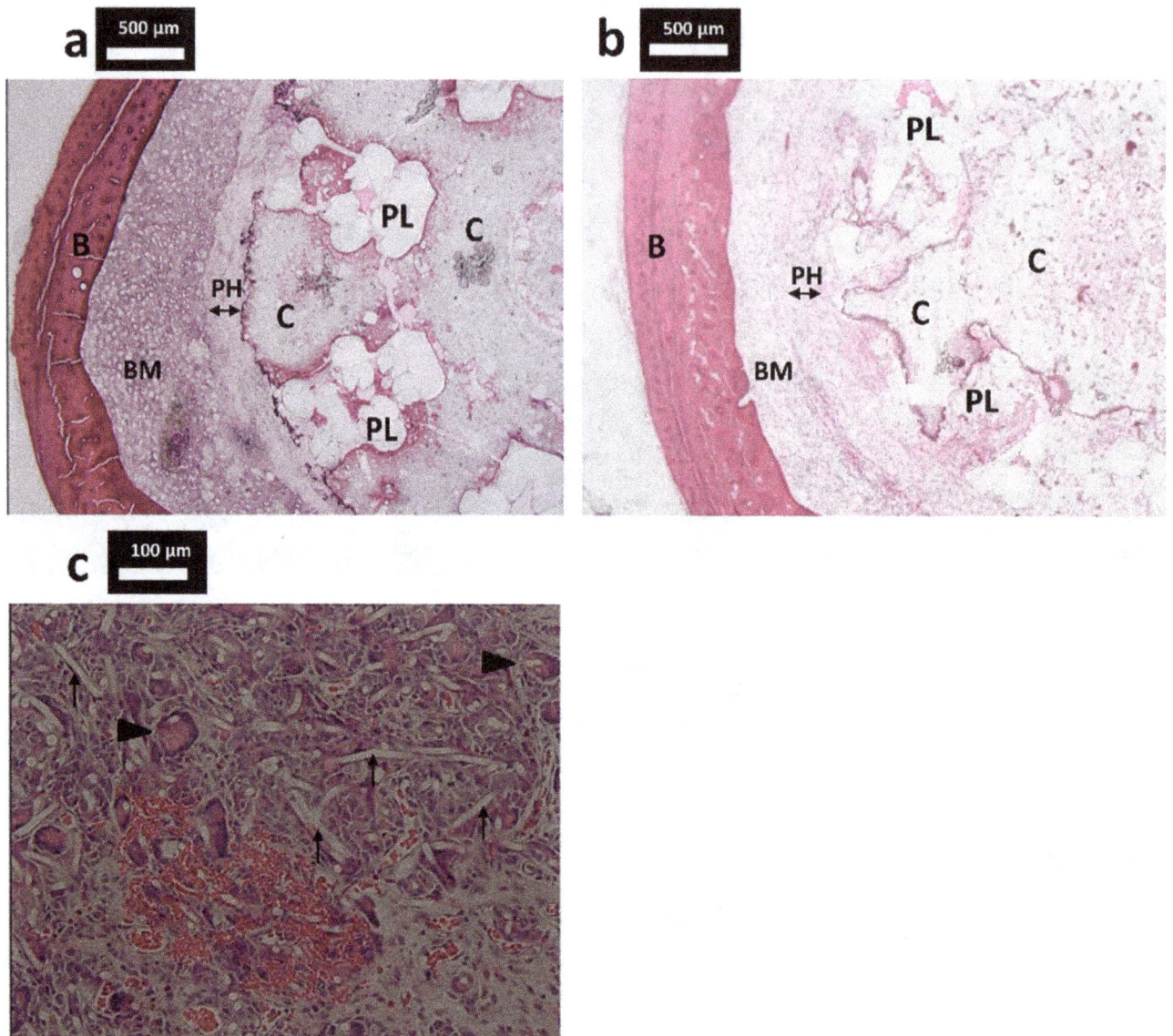

Figure 8. Histologic cross sections of specimens from the IM-BM group. Histologic cross sections of specimens from the IM-BM group (PLLA + CPC + PHA) stained with hematoxylin and eosin. (a) A PHA fiber mat layer surrounded the CPC, and the PLLA tube was not degraded at week 20. (b) At week 52, the PLLA tube seemed to have degraded gradually. (c) Multinucleated giant cell (arrowhead) and neovascularization were observed in the PHA fiber mat layer at week 52. PHA fiber (arrow). PL: PLLA woven tube; PH: PHA fiber mat C: CPC; B: bone cortex; BM: bone marrow.

Table 3. Properties of biodegradable thermoplastic polyesters. (Wu Q. 2009 [7]).

	Tm (°C)	Tg (°C)	Tensile strength (MPa)	Tensile modulus (GPa)	Elongation at break (%)	Absorption rate
PGA	225	35	70	6900	<3	6 weeks
PLLA	175	65	28–50	1200–2700	6	1.5–5 years
PDLLA	Amorphous	50–55	29–35	1900–2400	6	3 months
P(3HB)	180	1	36	2500	3	2 years
P(3HB-co-4HB) (4HB 16%)	152	−8	26	Not measured	444	Unknown

PGA: poly glycolic acid; PLLA: poly(L-lactide); PDLLA: poly(D L–lactide); P(3HB): poly(3-hydroxybutyrate); P(3HB-co-4HB) (4HB 16%): poly(3-hydroxybutyrate-co-16% 4-hydroxybutyrate); Tm: melting temperature; Tg: glass transition temperature.

The maximum flexural strength of K-wire fixation in our previous mechanical study using two 1.6-mm K-wires was almost same as that of PLLA + PHA + CPC group in our current study (3.0 MPa in K-wire group vs 2.71 MPa in PLLA + PHA + CPC group). However, we think that IM-BM was strong enough to reinforce and stabilize incomplete fractures even in the distal thigh where bone is exposed to the highest bending and torsional stresses. In fact, a benefit of the IM-BM implant is that it is not harder than necessary and the risk of cutout is low, whereas metallic implants sometimes cause cutout in severely osteoporotic patients. The current study indicates that IM-BM can also be applied to insufficiency fractures in other areas in the body such as rib and proximal humerus.

Conclusions

In conclusion, the present work demonstrated that IM-BM was strong enough to reinforce and stabilize incomplete fractures with both mechanical testing and an animal experiment even in the distal thigh, where bone is exposed to the highest bending and torsional stresses in the body. The combination of three biomaterials with different physical and biological properties can be one treatment option for those with severe osteoporosis.

Acknowledgments

We thank Dr. Seiichi Kato of the Pathology Department at Nagoya University Hospital for advice on histology.

Author Contributions

Conceived and designed the experiments: TN HH T.Kasuga. Performed the experiments: TN T.Kurahashi TH. Analyzed the data: TN. Contributed reagents/materials/analysis tools: T.Kasuga. Contributed to the writing of the manuscript: TN HH T.Kasuga.

References

1. Owsley K, Gorczyca JT (2008) Fracture displacement and screw cutout after open reduction and locked plate fixation of proximal humeral fractures [corrected]. J Bone Joint Surg 90: 233–240.
2. Nakano M, Hirano N, Matsuura K, Watanabe H, Kitagawa H, Ishihara H, et al. (2002) Percutaneous transpedicular vertebroplasty with calcium phosphate cement in the treatment of osteoporotic vertebral compression and burst fractures. J Neurosurg 97: 287–293.
3. Ambard AJ, Mueninghoff L (2006) Calcium phosphate cement: review of mechanical and biological properties. J Prosthodont 15: 321–328.
4. Ishikawa K, Asaoka K (1995) Estimation of ideal mechanical strength and critical porosity of calcium phosphate cement. J Biomed Mater Res 29: 1537–1543.
5. Valappil SP, Misra SK, Boccaccini AR, Roy I (2006) Biomedical applications of polyhydroxyalkanoates, an overview of animal testing and in vivo responses. Expert Rev Med Devices 3: 853–868.
6. Steinbüchel A, Hustede E, Liebergesell M, Pieper U, Timm A (1992) Molecular basis for biosynthesis and accumulation of polyhydroxyalkanoic acids in bacteria. FEMS Microbiol Rev 9: 217–230.
7. Wu Q, Wang Y, Chen GQ (2009) Medical application of microbial biopolyesters polyhydroxyalkanoates. Artif Cells Blood Substit Immobil Biotechnol 37: 1–12.
8. Sill TJ, von Recum HA (2008) Electrospinning: applications in drug delivery and tissue engineering. Biomaterials 29: 1989–2006.
9. Li WJ, Laurencin CT, Caterson EJ, Tuan RS, Ko FK (2002) Electrospun nanofibrous structure: a novel scaffold for tissue engineering. J Biomed Mater Res 60: 613–621.
10. Mizutani Y, Hattori M, Okuyama M, Kasuga T, Nogami M (2005) Preparation of porous poly(L-lactic acid) composite containing hydroxyapatite whiskers. Chemistry Letters 34: 1110–1111.
11. Bhattarai SR, Bhattarai N, Yi HK, Hwang PH, Cha DI (2004) Novel biodegradable electrospun membrane: scaffold for tissue engineering. Biomaterials 52: 2595–2602.
12. Kurashina K, Kurita H, Kotani A, Takeuchi H, Hirano M (1997) In vivo study of a calcium phosphate cement consisting of alpha-tricalcium phosphate/dicalcium phosphate dibasic/tetracalcium phosphate monoxide. Biomaterials 18: 147–151.
13. Kokubo T, Kushitani H, Sakka S, Kitsugi T, Yamamuro T (1990) Solutions able to reproduce in vivo surface-structure changes in bioactive glass-ceramic A-W. J Biomed Mater Res 24: 721–734.
14. Castañeda S, Calvo E, Largo R, González-González R (2008) Characterization of a new experimental model of osteoporosis in rabbits. J Bone Miner Metab 26: 53–59.
15. Galibert P, Deramond H, Rosat P, Le Gars D (1987) Preliminary note on the treatment of vertebral angioma by percutaneous acrylic vertebroplasty. Neurochirurgie 33: 166–168.
16. Yamamuro T, Nakamura T, Iida H, Kawanabe K, Matsuda Y, et al. (1998) Development of bioactive bone cement and its clinical applications. Biomaterials 19: 1479–1482.
17. Phillips H, Cole PV, Lettin AW (1971) Cardiovascular effects of implanted acrylic bone cement. Br Med J 3: 460–461.

16

Interaction of Age and Mechanical Stability on Bone Defect Healing: An Early Transcriptional Analysis of Fracture Hematoma in Rat

Andrea Ode[1,2], **Georg N. Duda**[1,2,3]*, **Sven Geissler**[1,2], **Stephan Pauly**[1,3], **Jan-Erik Ode**[1], **Carsten Perka**[1,2,3], **Patrick Strube**[1,3]

1 Julius Wolff Institute, Charité - Universitätsmedizin, Berlin, Germany, 2 Berlin-Brandenburg Center for Regenerative Therapies, Berlin, Germany, 3 Klinik für Orthopädie, Centrum für Muskuloskeletale Chirurgie, Charité - Universitätsmedizin, Berlin, Germany

Abstract

Among other stressors, age and mechanical constraints significantly influence regeneration cascades in bone healing. Here, our aim was to identify genes and, through their functional annotation, related biological processes that are influenced by an interaction between the effects of mechanical fixation stability and age. Therefore, at day three post-osteotomy, chip-based whole-genome gene expression analyses of fracture hematoma tissue were performed for four groups of Sprague-Dawley rats with a 1.5-mm osteotomy gap in the femora with varying age (12 vs. 52 weeks - biologically challenging) and external fixator stiffness (mechanically challenging). From 31099 analysed genes, 1103 genes were differentially expressed between the six possible combinations of the four groups and from those 144 genes were identified as statistically significantly influenced by the interaction between age and fixation stability. Functional annotation of these differentially expressed genes revealed an association with *extracellular space, cell migration* or *vasculature development*. The chip-based whole-genome gene expression data was validated by q-RT-PCR at days three and seven post-osteotomy for MMP-9 and MMP-13, members of the mechanosensitive matrix metalloproteinase family and key players in cell migration and angiogenesis. Furthermore, we observed an interaction of age and mechanical stimuli *in vitro* on cell migration of mesenchymal stromal cells. These cells are a subpopulation of the fracture hematoma and are known to be key players in bone regeneration. In summary, these data correspond to and might explain our previously described biomechanical healing outcome after six weeks in response to fixation stiffness variation. In conclusion, our data highlight the importance of analysing the influence of risk factors of fracture healing (e.g. advanced age, suboptimal fixator stability) in combination rather than alone.

Editor: Dimitrios Zeugolis, National University of Ireland, Galway (NUI Galway), Ireland

Funding: This study was supported partly by the Federal Ministry of Education and Research (BMBF, Grant 0315848A) excellence cluster, Berlin-Brandenburg Center for Regenerative Therapies, and partly by the German Research Foundation (DFG SFB 760). The funders had no role in study design, data collection and analysis, decision to publish, or preparation of the manuscript.

Competing Interests: The authors have declared that no competing interests exist.

* Email: Georg.Duda@charite.de

Introduction

Due to the ageing of the population the high incidents of delayed or mal-unions after fracture trauma develops to a growing concern. The classical boundary conditions that influence healing (mechanics, surgery, accompanying traumata) are overlapped by the age-related changes in regenerative capacity.

Fracture consolidation is significantly influenced by many biological and mechanical factors. An important biological risk factor is the age of the patient. Animal experiments in rats and clinical studies in humans show a delayed course of bone healing with increasing age[1–3]. Possible reasons for this could be a diminished number of mesenchymal progenitor cells, their reduced migration potential and higher susceptibility towards senescence, and reduced local or systemic blood flow in older individuals [4,5]. Inadequate fracture stability - determined by fixation stability - is the principle mechanical factor that leads to a non-union [6,7]. An optimal mechanical stimulus enables successful fracture healing, whereas too little or too much disables

it. Especially the early phase of bone healing seems to be sensitive to mechanical loading conditions [8]. In clinical cases biological and mechanical boundary conditions both jointly interact with each other and influence regeneration. The negative influence of mechanical instability on the biological factor of vascularity, endochondral ossification and maturation is an important example for this [9,10]. Vascularity is not only disturbed by the trauma itself and/or by surgical disruption but also by (initial) instability at the fracture site[6][11]. A failure of angiogenesis is critical, since angiogenesis is not only responsible for the oxygen supply, but also a prerequisite for the resorption of necrotic tissue and recruitment of different cell types including mesenchymal progenitor cells, which is necessary for a mechanically stable repair of the bone defect [12]. However, it remains unclear whether one stressor to regeneration - mechanical stability or age - dominates or how they interact.

In recent animal studies we provided evidence that the healing outcome of bone regeneration depends not only on mechanical stability or age alone, but more importantly, on the overlap of both stressors [1,9]. Our data revealed a statistically significant interaction between the effects of mechanical stability and age on radiological outcome at two and six weeks and on biomechanical callus competence at six weeks post-operative. For example, in young rats, the biomechanical parameters torsional stiffness and maximum torque at failure were improved when bone defects were rigidly fixated, whereas the opposite was true for old rats [1]. However, on a more microscopically level, results were not as explicit. Micro-computed tomography could not reveal an interaction between the effects of mechanical stability and age on callus size, geometry, microstructure, and mineralization. Similar results were observed for histological analysis of vascularity and bone remodelling. Rather, we found a complex mixture of differences in the investigated parameters between the groups. For example, fixator stability influences callus size and geometry, whereas age influences callus strut thickness and perforation within these struts [9].

Gene expression in the early fracture hematoma is also known to be influenced by either age or fixation stability. For example, Meyer et al. found significantly lower levels of mRNA levels for Indian hedgehog and bone morphogenetic protein 2 (BMP2) in the fracture callus of old rats compared to young ones [13]. Comparative analysis of stabilized and non-stabilized fractures in small animals revealed differences in molecular signals controlling chondrogenesis [14]. In large animals, mRNA expression levels of members of the BMP-, tumor necrosis factor (TNF)- and matrix metalloproteinase (MMP) families as well as genes involved in bone matrix generation were lower in the critical fixation compared to the rigid fixation group at several time points [10]. However, little is known about the interaction between the effects of mechanical stability and age on gene expression. This is especially important during the early phase of bone healing, which has been shown to be mechanically sensitive and therefore crucial for the healing outcome [8].

In the present study we performed a chip-based whole-genome gene expression analysis of fracture hematoma tissue from young and old rats that underwent rigid and semi-rigid bone defect fixation. Our aim was to identify genes and, through their functional annotation, related biological processes that are influenced by an interaction between the effects of mechanical stability and age. In conclusion, we identified a number of genes and their functional annotation revealed an association with cell migration and blood vessel formation, which is so far unknown.

Materials and Methods

Animals and groups

All animal experiments were carried out according to the policies established by the Animal Welfare Act, the NIH Guide for Care and Use of Laboratory Animals, and the National Animal Welfare Guidelines and were approved by the local legal representative (LAGeSo Berlin, G0190/05).

Operations and postoperative care were performed according to a previously published protocol and employed a standardized biomechanically validated external fixation device [15]. Preoperatively the animal husbandry was performed in large cages (ground area 1800 cm², height 19 cm, ground covered with soft-wood granule animal bedding) with a maximum of 6 animals per cage. After operation we changed to single animal husbandry in a smaller cage (ground area 810 cm², height 19 cm, soft-wood granule bedding). Housing facility was specific pathogen free with a 12/12 h light/dark rhythm and a room temperature of 24°C. Animals had free access to water and food (pressed diet pellets for

rodents). Preoperatively, as well as before surgical intervention for harvesting the fracture hematoma rectal temperature was measured to detect possible infections (temperature >38 °C). Postoperatively the animals were visited daily and if necessary analgesia was given. The experimental model has been previously described [1] and is briefly summarized here. For gene-chip and q-RT-PCR (day 3) analysis thirty-six and for q-RT-PCR analysis (day 7) twenty female Sprague–Dawley (Sprague-Dawley SD (Aged for old groups) Outbred rats, Harlan Laboratories, Indianapolis, USA) rats were divided into four groups with nine (day 3) respectively five (day 7) animals each group. Groups were defined by variation of fixator stabilities (rigid vs. semi-rigid) and age (12 vs. 52 weeks): young rigid (YR), young semi-rigid (YSR), old rigid (OR), and old semi-rigid (OSR). Weights of the old animals ranged at 313.4 ± 17.4 g whereas that of the young ones was 251.9 ± 15.3 g ($p < 0.001$ in t-test). Animals were not restricted in weight bearing. In cases of adverse events (infection, major bleeding, pin loosening, implant failure or complications related to anaesthesia) the animal was sacrificed as described and a new animal was included/operated to gain the planned group sizes. Regarding this, two animals of the YSR group died for unknown reasons during primary surgery in general anaesthesia, and two aged rats (one OR, one OSR) presented with pin loosening prior to harvesting at day 7.

Surgical procedure

Using an anterolateral approach, the left femur was osteotomized at the midshaft, distracted to a gap of 1.5 mm and externally fixated employing a previously described fixation system [1]. The distance between fixator and bone (offset) was set to 7.5 mm in the rigid configuration (leading to a torsional 8.13 Nmm/° and axial 25.21 N/mm fixator stiffness) and 15 mm in the semi-rigid configuration (torsional 6.62 Nmm/°, axial 10.39 N/mm stiffness) (Figure 1). Before sacrifice and under general anaesthesia (see anaesthesia protocol published before [16]) the wound was reopened, inter-fragmentary fracture hematoma was harvested with a sterile forceps, directly transferred into a sterile container and frozen immediately in liquid nitrogen. For the gene-chip-analysis follow-up was three days, for q-RT-PCR analysis follow-up was three (RNA of the gene chip animals was used) and seven days. Animal sacrifice was performed in deep general anaesthesia by intracardial injection of 5 ml potassium chloride (7.45%, B.Braun Melsungen AG, Melsungen, Germany) [16].

RNA Isolation, cDNA Synthesis, and Quantitative Reverse Transcription-Polymerase Chain Reaction

At day three and seven post-OP, total RNA was isolated from fracture hematoma by using Trizol (following the instructions of the manufacturer) starting with an initial stepwise mechanical destruction of the tissue with syringe cannulas of three different diameters until liquid was homogeneous without visible tissue particles. Next, RNA was reversely transcribed to cDNA using iScript cDNA Synthesis kit (Bio-Rad, Munich, Germany) according to the manufacturer's instructions. RNA quality was evaluated by visualizing the 18S/28S rRNA on a 1.5% agarose gel. Quantification of MMP-2, MMP-9, MMP-13, and TIMP-2 were assessed by quantitative reverse transcription-polymerase chain reaction (q-RT-PCR) using the iQ SYBR Green Supermix and the iQ 5 Multicolor Realtime PCR Detection System and software (Bio-Rad, Munich, Germany) using the delta-Ct-method. The transcript expression was normalized versus the housekeeping gene β-actin (ACTB), elongation factor 1-alpha 1 (EEF1A), and glyceraldehyde-3-phosphate dehydrogenase (GAPDH). The primers used in the real-time PCR assay were commercially purchased

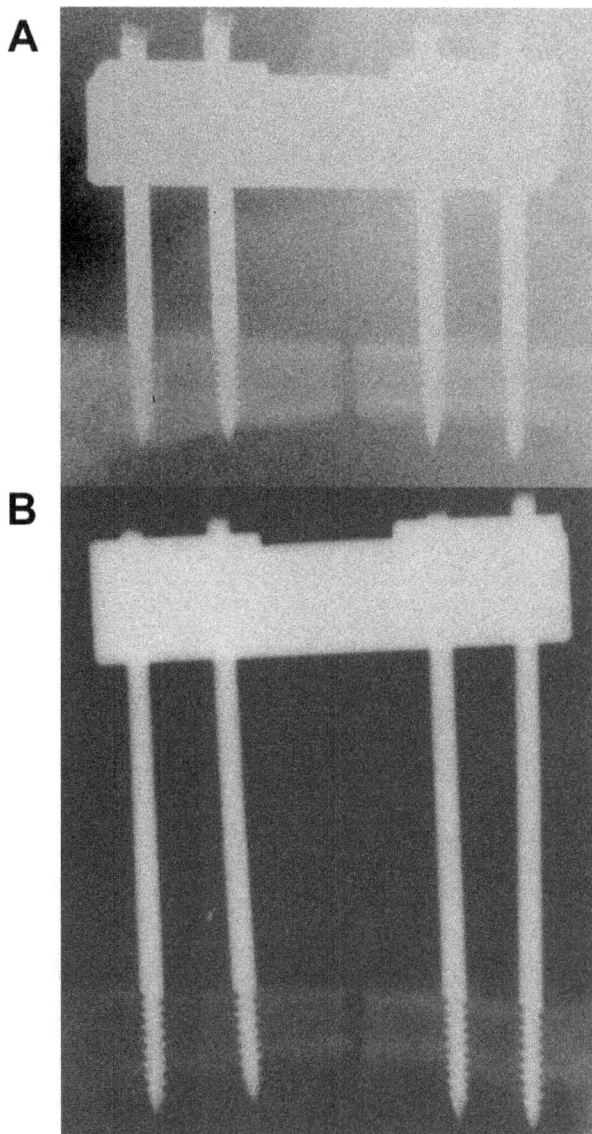

Figure 1. Radiographs of the two fixator configurations varying in the distance between bone and fixator crossbar (offset). (A) Rigid configuration with a 7.5 mm offset. (B) Semi-rigid configuration with a 15 mm offset. Osteotomy gap was set to 1.5 mm.

(Invitrogen, Karlsruhe, Germany; Table 1). Amplification efficiency (E) was assessed to be between 1.9 and 2. At day 7, transcripts from five animals were analyzed. At day 3, analysis was performed with three pools of total RNA from three animals per pool. Each experiment was conducted in triplicates.

Affymetrix gene chip hybridization

The amplification and labeling of the RNA samples, isolated at day three post-OP, were carried out according to the manufacturer's instructions (Affymetrix, Santa Clara, CA). Briefly, total RNA was quantified by UV-spectroscopy and its quality was checked by analysis on a LabChip (BioAnalyzer, AGILENT Technologies, Santa Clara, CA). Between one to three micrograms from each sample were synthesized into double-stranded cDNA using SuperScript transcriptase II (Life Technologies, Inc., Carlsbad, CA) and with an oligo(dT)24 primer containing a T7

RNA polymerase promoter (TIBMOL Biol, Berlin, Germany). After RNAse H – mediated (Roche, Germany) second strand cDNA synthesis, the product was purified and served as template in the subsequent in vitro transcription (IVT) reaction. Labeled complementary RNA (cRNA) was prepared from double-stranded cDNA by in vitro transcription using the GeneChip RNA transcript labeling kit (Affymetrix, Santa Clara, CA). After cleanup (Qiagen, Hilden, Germany), the biotin-labeled cRNA was fragmented by alkaline treatment [40 mmol/L Trisacetate (pH 8.2), 100 mmol//L potassium acetate, and 50 mmol//L magnesium acetate] at 94°C for 35 minutes. 15 µg of each cRNA sample was hybridized for 16 hours at 45°C to an Affymetrix Rat GeneChip Array 230 2.0. Chips were washed and stained with streptavidin-phycoerythrin using a fluidics station according to the protocols recommended by the manufacturer. Finally, probe arrays were scanned at 1.56-µm resolution using the Affymetrix GeneChip System confocal scanner 3000. Raw data were submitted to Affymetrix Expression Console software (v.1.3) to generate probe set summarization (CHP) files from feature intensity (CEL) files using PLIER algorithm. Analysis of differentially expressed genes was performed with Affymetrix Transcriptome Analysis Console (TAC) Software and PASW Statistics 18 (SPSS Inc., Chicago, USA). To conduct functional categorizing, all differentially expressed genes were submitted to the Database for Annotation, Visualization and Integrated Discovery (DAVID) V6.7 (http://david.abcc.ncifcrf.gov/) [17]. P-values were determined using EASE, followed by a Benjamini-Hochberg correction for multiple comparisons. Summary and visualization of Gene Ontology (GO) terms was performed with REVIGO (http://revigo.irb.hr/) [18]. For each condition group (YSR, YR, OSR, OR) three Affymetrix gene chip hybridizations were performed with separate pools of total RNA. Each pool comprised of total RNA from three animals. Thus, the analysis is based on total RNA from nine animals per condition group.

MSC isolation, culture and mechanical stimulation

MSCs were isolated from bone marrow of 12 months old Sprague–Dawley rats selected by plastic adherence (Dobson et al., 1999). Dulbecco's modified Eagle's medium (DMEM) (Gibco, NY, USA) supplemented with 10% fetal calf serum (FCS) (Biochrom AG, Berlin, Germany) and 10 U/ml penicillin plus 100 µg/ml streptomycin was used as expansion medium for MSCs. Only cells from passages 2–4 were used for experiments. The bioreactor system used has been described previously [15]. Briefly, MSCs were trypsinized, and 2×106 cells in 350 µl of bioreactor medium (culture medium containing 2.4% Trasylol [Bayer, Leverkusen, Germany]) were mixed with 300 µl of fibrinogen/bioreactor medium (1:2) mixture and 50 µl of thrombin S/bioreactor medium (1:2) mixture (Tissucol; Baxter, Munich, Germany). This MSC/fibrinogen/thrombin mixture was placed between two spongiosa bone chips and allowed to solidify for 30 minutes at 37°C. The sandwich construct was placed into the bioreactor, and 25 ml of bioreactor medium was added. A strain of approximately 20% at a frequency of 1 Hz was applied in accordance with in vivo measurements of interfragmentary movement [19]. Mechanical loading was carried out for 72 hours. Afterwards, cells within the fibrin construct were isolated by 225 U trypsin/1 ml PBS.

Transwell Migration Assay

Random migration (i.e. equal concentrations of bioactive molecules in both compartments) was measured by a modified Boyden chamber assay (Falk et al., 1980) using polycarbonate filters (8 µm pore size; Nunc, Wiesbaden, Germany) coated with or without Collagen I (100 µg/ml; Pure Col, Inamed Biomaterials,

Table 1. Primer sequences.

Protein	Gene	Primer Sequence (forward/reverse)
matrix metalloproteinase 9	Mmp-9	5' GTCTGGATAAGTTGGGGCTA 3'
		5' GCCTTGTCTTGGTAGTGAAA 3'
matrix metalloproteinase 13	Mmp-13	5' CAGTCTCTCTATGGTCCAGG 3'
		5' TGGTCAAAAACAGTTCAGGC 3'
actin cytoplasmic 1 (β-actin)	Actb	5' TGTCACCAACTGGGACGATA 3'
		5' GGGGTGTTGAAGGTCTCAAA 3'
glyceraldehyde-3-phosphate dehydrogenase	Gapdh	5' ATGGGAAGCTGGTCATCAAC 3'
		5' GTGGTTCACACCCATCACAA 3'
elongation factor 1-alpha 1	Eef1a	5' CCCTGTGGAAGTTTGAGACC 3'
		5' CTGCCCGTTCTTGGAGATAC 3'

Fremont, U.S.), which is the most abundant extracellular protein of bones (Rossert and de Crombrugghe, 2002). MSCs (4×10^4) were seeded onto the filters and incubated for 5 h at 37°C. Equal cell seeding was validated by an MTS test. Non-migrated cells were removed from the upper side of the filter by scraping, and remaining migrated cells were stained with 10μg/ml Hoechst-33342 (Invitrogen, Karlsruhe, Germany). The average numbers of migrated cells from five microscopic fields (1 mm×0.8 mm) per filter (0.47 cm²) were analysed using the NIH ImageJ software package (http://rsb.info.nih.gov/nih-image/). MSCs were isolated form three (old MSCs) and five (young MSCs) different animals followed by separate migration assays, which were performed in duplicates, i.e. two wells per group, the mean value being used for statistical analysis.

Statistical analyses

The statistical analysis of q-RT-PCR data was performed using statistics software PASW Statistics 18 (SPSS Inc., Chicago, USA). If not stated otherwise, the influence of age and mechanical stability and their interaction on gene expression and migration were tested with a 2-tailed, 2-way Analysis of Variance (ANOVA) and posthoc Bonferroni correction. The parameters time (gene expression) and coating (migration) were set as covariates. The assumption of normality was tested using the Shapiro-Wilk normality test. For graphical presentation, results are presented in boxplots. The dark line in the middle of the boxes is the median. The box represents the interquartile range (IQR = Q3-Q1). The whiskers indicate 1.5xIQR. Outliers are circles between 1.5xIQR and 3xIQR of the quartiles. Extreme values are stars more than 3xIQR away from quartiles. For statistical analysis of chip-based

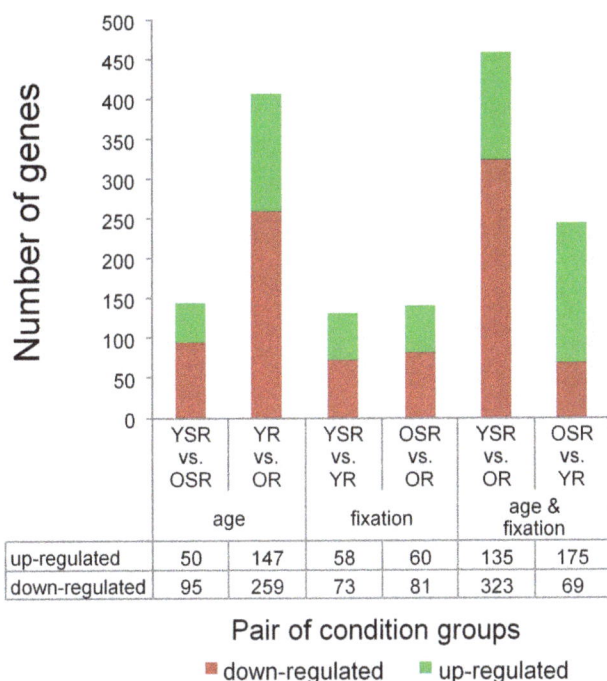

	age		fixation		age & fixation	
	YSR vs. OSR	YR vs. OR	YSR vs. YR	OSR vs. OR	YSR vs. OR	OSR vs. YR
up-regulated	50	147	58	60	135	175
down-regulated	95	259	73	81	323	69

Figure 2. Number of differentially expressed genes for each pair of condition groups. With Affymetrix Transcriptome Analysis Console (TAC) a traditional unpaired One-Way Analysis of Variance (ANOVA) for each pair of condition groups was performed (Linear Fold Change <−2 or > 2; ANOVA p-value (condition pair) <0.05).

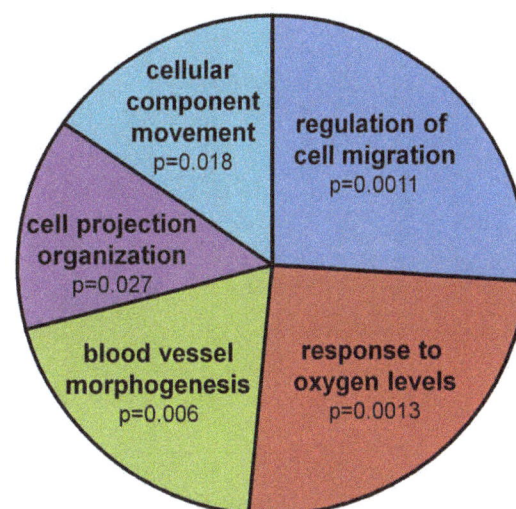

Figure 3. Functional annotation of 144 genes that are affected by a statistically significant interaction between age and fixation stability. Pie Chart view of REVIGO results: The single GO terms (Table S8 in File S3) are joined into clusters of related terms, visualized as sectors with different colours. Size of the sectors is adjusted (log10p-value) to reflect the p-values.

Table 2. Gene list of cluster *Regulation of cell migration*.

Affymetrix ID	Gene Name	Linear Fold Change						p-value
		(YSR vs. YR)	(OSR vs. OR)	(YSR vs. OSR)	(YR vs. OR)	(YSR vs. OR)	(OSR vs. YR)	(2-way ANOVA)
1393403_AT	angiopoietin-like 3	-2.9	2.2	-1.5	4.1	1.4	-1.9	1.87E-02
1369814_AT	chemokine (C-C motif) ligand 20	1.2	-2.6	4.3	1.4	1.7	-3.5	2.35E-02
1370634_X_AT	chemokine (C-X-C motif) ligand 3	-3.0	-1.7	1.2	2.1	-1.4	-3.6	3.50E-02
1388459_AT	collagen, type XVIII, alpha 1	1.1	-1.8	-1.1	-2.2	-2.0	1.2	2.04E-02
1369113_AT	gremlin 1, cysteine knot superfamily, homolog (Xenopus laevis)	-1.2	-2.9	-3.2	-8.1	-9.3	2.8	4.81E-02
1369166_AT	matrix metallopeptidase 9	1.0	-5.0	-2.0	-10.4	-10.1	2.1	3.97E-03
1398275_AT	matrix metallopeptidase 9	2.0	-4.8	-1.8	-17.7	-8.7	3.7	4.67E-03
1370642_S_AT	platelet derived growth factor receptor, beta polypeptide	-1.0	-1.8	-1.1	-2.0	-2.1	1.1	2.35E-02
1393456_AT	podoplanin	-1.2	2.0	1.2	2.8	2.3	-1.4	3.90E-02
1391369_AT	serum response factor (c-fos serum response element-binding transcription factor)	-1.0	2.0	1.1	2.1	2.1	-1.1	1.22E-04
1382685_AT	slit homolog 2 (Drosophila)	1.2	-1.9	-1.1	-2.6	-2.2	1.4	4.26E-02
1392382_AT	transforming growth factor, beta 2	-1.4	1.5	-2.7	-1.2	-1.8	1.9	4.80E-02
1371240_AT	tropomyosin 1, alpha	-1.3	6.9	-1.2	7.4	5.7	-1.1	3.90E-02

Bold: Linear Fold Change <-2 or >2.

Table 3. Gene list of cluster *Response to oxygen levels.*

Affymetrix ID	Gene Name	Linear Fold Change						p-value
		(YSR vs. YR)	(OSR vs. OR)	(YSR vs. OSR)	(YR vs. OR)	(YSR vs. OR)	(OSR vs. YR)	
1393902_AT	aldo-keto reductase family 1, member C1 (dihydrodiol dehydrogenase 1; 20-alpha (3-alpha)-hydroxysteroid dehydrogenase)	1.9	-3.2	1.9	-3.2	-1.7	1.0	8.82E-03
1398333_AT	endothelial PAS domain protein 1	-1.1	-3.0	-1.1	-3.0	-3.3	1.0	4.07E-02
1370604_AT	leptin receptor	1.0	-3.8	1.0	-3.8	-3.8	1.0	1.24E-02
1388204_AT	matrix metallopeptidase 13	-1.1	-4.2	-1.5	-6.0	-6.4	1.4	4.47E-02
1369166_AT	matrix metallopeptidase 9	1.0	-5.0	-2.0	-10.4	-10.1	2.1	3.97E-03
1398275_AT	matrix metallopeptidase 9	2.0	-4.8	-1.8	-17.7	-8.7	3.7	4.67E-03
1387410_AT	nuclear receptor subfamily 4, group A, member 2	1.6	-1.8	1.4	-2.1	-1.3	1.2	1.30E-03
1370642_S_AT	platelet derived growth factor receptor, beta polypeptide	-1.0	-1.8	-1.1	-2.0	-2.1	1.1	2.35E-02
1393456_AT	podoplanin	-1.2	2.0	1.2	2.8	2.3	-1.4	3.90E-02
1368170_AT	solute carrier family 6 (neurotransmitter transporter, GABA), member 1	1.0	2.8	-2.8	1.0	1.0	2.8	3.70E-05
1392382_AT	transforming growth factor, beta 2	-1.4	1.5	-2.7	-1.2	-1.8	1.9	4.80E-02

Bold: Linear Fold Change < -2 or > 2.

whole-genome gene expression data see section 2.4 Affymetrix gene chip hybridization. The level of significance for all statistical tests was defined $p < 0.05$.

Results

The data discussed in this publication have been deposited in NCBI's Gene Expression Omnibus [20] and are accessible through GEO Series accession number GSE53256 (http://www.ncbi.nlm.nih.gov/geo/query/acc.cgi?acc = GSE53256).

In total, 31099 genes were analysed with Affymetrix Transcriptome Analysis Console (TAC). TAC computes and summarizes a traditional unpaired One-Way (single factor) Analysis of Variance (ANOVA) for each pair of condition groups and for all six condition groups. In our study, 1103 genes were differentially expressed between the six possible combinations (Linear Fold Change < -2 or > 2; ANOVA p-value (condition pair) < 0.05). To illustrate the differences between the six possible combinations the numbers of up- and down-regulated genes for each pair of condition groups are displayed in Figure 2 and listed in Table S1–S6 in File S1. Since TAC cannot examine the combined effect of age and fixation stability on gene expression, a two-way ANOVA was conducted with PASW Statistics 18. However, complete analysis of 31099 genes would be computationally intensive. Therefore, 521 genes were pre-selected for analysis under the following conditions: (1) ANOVA p-value (All conditions) < 0.05 and (2) Linear Fold Change < -2 or > 2 in at least one of the six condition pairs. Statistical analysis of these 521 genes revealed a statistically significant interaction between age and fixation stability on gene expression of 144 genes (2-way ANOVA $p < 0.05$). A complete list of these genes, the pre-selection criteria, Linear Fold Change in all six condition pairs and the results of 2-way ANOVA analysis can be found in Table S7 in File S2.

To identify biological processes related to these differently expressed genes, functional categorizing was conducted using DAVID v6.7. Functional annotation of these differentially expressed genes resulted in a list of Gene Ontology terms related to biological processes (Table S8 in File S3). Single GO terms were then joined into five clusters of related terms using REVIGO; the two dominant clusters, based on p-values, being *Regulation of cell migration* and *Response to oxygen levels* (Figure 3 and Table S9–S11 in File S4). The respective genes that were functionally categorized to these clusters by the functional annotation tool DAVID v6.7 are listed in Table 2 and 3.

Interestingly, among the genes listed in Table 2 and 3 with a noticeable Linear Fold Change in gene expression are members of the family of matrix metalloproteinases (MMPs): MMP-9 and MMP-13. To validate the results of Affymetrix chip-based whole-genome gene expression analyses, the expression level of MMP-9 and -13 were analysed via qRT-PCR at day 3 and also day 7. There was also a statistically significant interaction between the effects of fixation and age on gene expression of MMP-9 ($p = 0.009$) and MMP-13 ($p = 0.016$). MMP-9 and -13 expression is also influenced by time (MMP-9, $p = 0.001$; MMP-13, $p = 0.007$). Thus results are presented separately for day 3 and day 7 (Figure 4). Post-hoc inter-group comparison revealed that MMP-9 expression is significantly higher in YSR than in OSR ($p = 0.019$) at day 7; for MMP-13 a trend was observed between YSR and OSR ($p = 0.057$).

Functional annotation clustering of the 144 genes that were influenced by a significant interaction between age and fixation stability revealed the cluster *Regulation of cell migration* having the most significant p-value. To validate whether this biological process is influenced by a significant interaction between age and

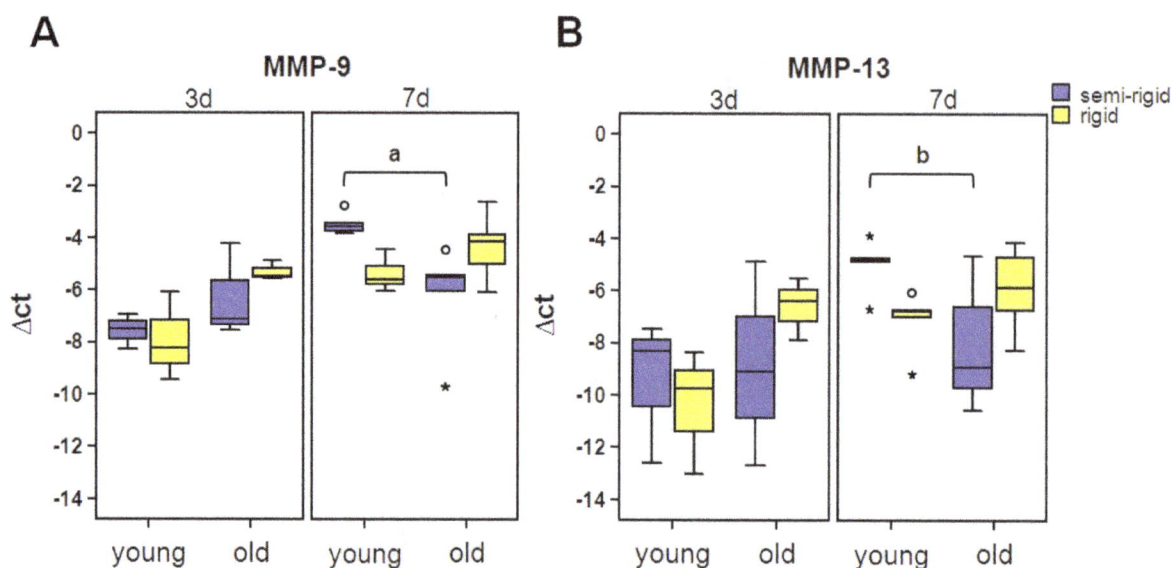

Figure 4. Gene expression of MMP-9 and -13 were significantly affected by the interaction of fixation and age. The expression of mRNA of YR, YSR, OR and OSR was evaluated by quantitative qRT-PCR, normalized for the housekeeping genes (HKG) *Actb*, *Gapdh*, and *Eef1a* and quantified using the delta-Ct-method: Δct = ct (geo mean HKG) - ct (gene of interest). (day 3, n = 3 RNA pools á 3 animals; day 7, n = 5; a, *p* = 0.019; b, *p* = 0.057; °, outlier; *, extreme value)

mechanical stability, we investigated this parameter in a simplified *in vitro* model. In order to do so, we mimicked the early phase fracture gap conditions by embedding mesenchymal stromal cells (MSCs) in fibrin, the major extracellular matrix of the hematoma, and by stimulating these cells with cyclic-compressive loading. MSCs were chosen as cell source, because they are known to be mechanosensitive and key players in bone regeneration, and they are present in the fracture hematoma by day three post-fracture [21–23], the same day we harvested the hematoma tissue for gene expression analyses. The MSCs were isolated from young (10–12 weeks; data published in [24]) and old (12 months) rats (yMSCs and oMSCs, respectively) in accordance with the *in vivo* experiments. To apply two different mechanical loading regimes to MSCs, similar to the ones *in vivo* (semi-rigid and rigid fixation allowing more or less interfragmentary movement, respectively), the cells underwent cyclic compression in a bioreactor (loaded) and were compared to nonloaded controls. Although the loading regimes *in vivo* (more or less movement) and *in vitro* (cyclic or no compression) did not perfectly match, the migratory behaviour of MSCs was found to be influenced by the interaction between age and mechanical stimulation (p = 0.007). Coating of the migration filter with collagen I had no influence on the results compared to no coating (p = 0.942). Thus results are displayed together (Figure 5). Inter-group comparison revealed that migration of nonloaded yMSCs is significantly higher compared to loaded yMSCs (p<0.001), nonloaded oMSCs (p = 0.005) and loaded oMSCs (p = 0.003). No statistical significance was observed between the latter three groups. A summary of the work flow in this study is given in Figure 6.

Discussion

This study is a follow-up of two previous ones [1,9]. Our aim in this study was to compare gene expression in fracture hematoma tissue of young and old rats that underwent either rigid or semi-rigid fixation. By using Affymetrix chip-based whole-genome gene expression analyses our aim was to identify genes and related

biological processes that are influenced by an interaction between the effects of mechanical stability and age. By this we wanted to gain insights into the early hematoma's biological processes that led to the previously reported biomechanical long-term outcomes in bone defect healing, which were influenced by age and varying fixator configurations, i.e. fixation stiffness. In total, we had four experimental groups: young semi-rigid (YSR), young rigid (YR), old semi-rigid (OSR) and old rigid (OR).

The majority of fractures heal by secondary, or indirect, fracture healing involving callus formation [22]. This process is both spatially and temporally regulated [25]. By using a model of experimental fracture healing in the rat the healing cascade has been elucidated [21]. Compared to human fractures, the rat fracture healing cascade proceeds at about twice the speed [23]: Initially, bone fracture is accompanied by disruption of bone marrow, bone matrix, blood vessels, and surrounding soft tissue. Within the first 24 hours, bleeding of these tissues and releasing of bone marrow into the fracture gap give rise to the initial hematoma [26]. Degranulating platelets and inflammatory cells release cytokines and growth factors that induce migration of MSCs from bone marrow and acute inflammatory cells and further aggregation of platelets. From day two to six, in the area between the cortices, soft callus begins to form via endochondral ossification, where MSCs begin to proliferate by day three [21–23].

In our study fracture hematoma tissue was harvested at three days post-osteotomy. From 31099 analysed genes, 1103 genes were differentially expressed between the six possible combinations and from those 1103 genes 521 genes were selected to be analysed with a two-way ANOVA. In total, 144 genes were identified as statistically significantly influenced by the interaction between age and fixation stability. Functional annotation of these genes revealed an involvement in cell migration. Thus far, there is no data published that report on the interaction of age and mechanical stimulation on cell migration *in vivo*.

We have two possible explanations for the observations in our study: either (1) the cell type composition in the fracture

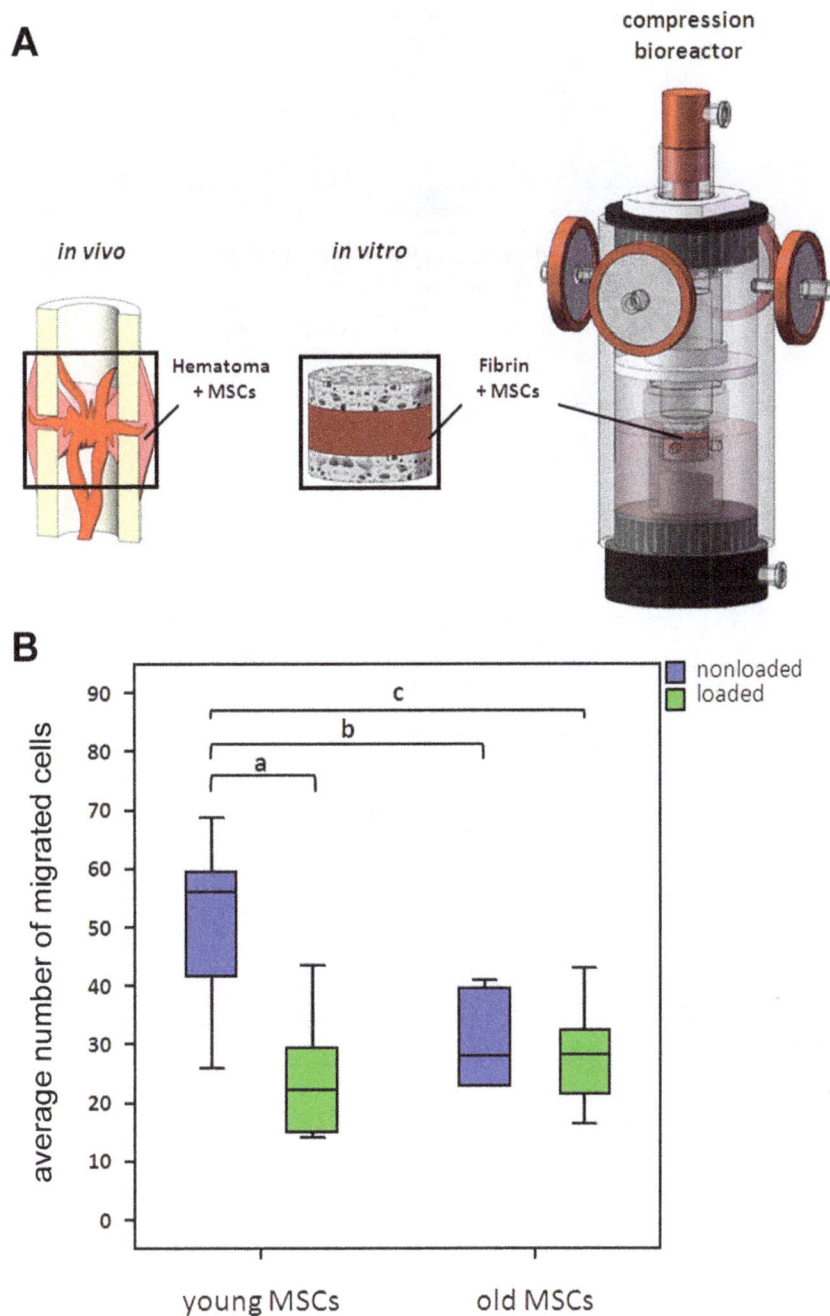

Figure 5. Migration of mechanically stimulated young and old MSCs. (A) Experimental set-up to investigate the effect of mechanical loading of MSC/fibrin constructs. MSCs were embedded in fibrin, placed between two cancellous bone chips and mechanically stimulated. (B) MSC migration was investigated in a modified Boyden-Chamber assay. The average number of migrated cells from five microscopic fields per filter was analysed using NIH ImageJ software. (young MSCs, n = 10; old MSCs, n = 6, a, p<0.001; b, p = 0.005; c, p = 0.003).

hematoma of young and old animals varies so that different cells respond differently to mechanical stimulation or (2) the cell type composition is similar, but the ability of these cells to sense and adapt to mechanical stimulation has changed during aging. We recently reported that migration of young MSCs, key players in bone regeneration and present in the fracture hematoma, is reduced *in vitro* if the cells underwent mechanical stimulation compared to non-stimulated controls [24]. Therefore, we now compared migration of young and old MSCs in response to cyclic-compressive loading. Interestingly, a statistically significant inter-

action between the effects of mechanical stimulation and age on MSC migration could also be observed in this setting. These results point towards a reduced ability of MSCs to sense and/or adapt to mechanical stimulus with advanced age. Based on several studies, it was proposed that fracture hematoma and bone tissue of old individuals is less responsive to mechanical stimulation than that of young ones. For example, an obvious growth of the loaded tibia was reported in young but not in old animals [27]. And a higher mechanical loading threshold was needed for initiation of bone growth during remodelling in old compared to young rats

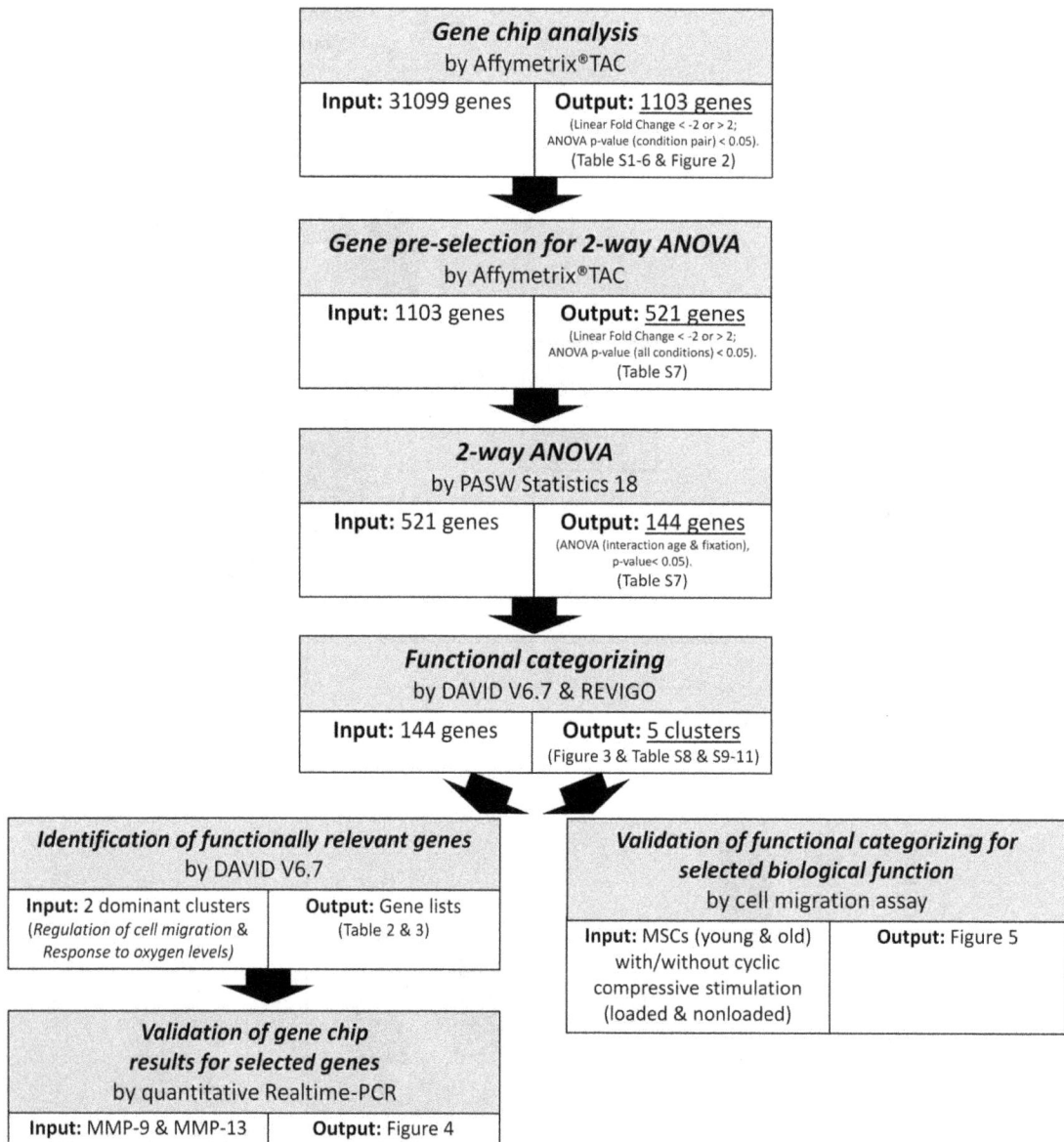

Figure 6. Summary and overview of the work flow in this study.

[28]. We recently reported that mechanical loading *in vitro* stimulates the paracrine pro-angiogenic capacity of MSCs and human fracture hematoma [29,30]. Interestingly, in the latter study, the angiogenic regulator *vascular endothelial growth factor* (VEGF) was up-regulated in hematoma of young but not old patients in response to mechanical loading.

The chip-based whole-genome gene expression analysis revealed that members of the family of matrix metalloproteinases (MMPs), MMP-9 and -13, were strongly influenced by an interaction of the effects of age and mechanical stability. Therefore, these results were further validated by q-RT-PCR with similar outcome. MMPs degrade most components of the extracellular matrix (ECM), such as aggrecan, collagens, elastin, or vitronectin, as well as many non-ECM molecules. Thereby, MMPs allow cell migration, participate in cleavage or release of biologically active molecules and regulate cellular behaviour such as cell attachment, growth, differentiation, and apoptosis [31,32]. During successful enchondral ossification, MMP-9 and -13 play an

important role in the fracture callus [33]. They coordinate not only cartilage matrix degradation, but also the recruitment and differentiation of endothelial cells, osteoclasts, chondroclasts and osteoprogenitors. Lack of MMP-9 in mice results in non-unions and delayed unions of their fractures caused by persistent cartilage at the injury site [34]. MMP-13-null mice showed profound defects in growth plate cartilage [35]. Several studies provided evidence for the regulation of MMP mRNA by mechanical loading *in vitro*. For example, mRNA level of MMP-9 increased as early as 3-6 h after the application of cyclic tensile load on cultured chondrocytes isolated from young rabbits [36]. MMP-13 mRNA up-regulation has been described after stretching of murine osteoblasts [37]. This is the first study that describes the simultaneous influence of age and mechanical stimuli on their expression. However, it is known that MMP function is spatially and temporally regulated at transcriptional, post-transcriptional, and post-translational levels via MMP controlled activation, inhibition and cell surface localization. Therefore, it is now crucial to validate these results also on protein level.

In summary, our results indicate that cellular migration is differently affected by fixator stability in young and old rats three days post-osteotomy possibly leading to the previously reported biomechanical long-term outcomes in bone defect healing. In conclusion, our data highlight the importance of analysing the influence of risk factors of fracture healing (e.g. advanced age, suboptimal fixator stability) in combination rather than alone.

Supporting Information

File S1 Table S1–S6. Up- and down-regulated genes for each pair of condition groups identified by Affymetrix Transcriptome Analysis Console (TAC)

File S2 Table S7. Genes that are influenced by the interaction between age and fixation stability identified by 2-way ANOVA.

References

1. Strube P, Sentuerk U, Riha T, Kaspar K, Mueller M, et al. (2008) Influence of age and mechanical stability on bone defect healing: Age reverses mechanical effects. Bone 42: 758–764. doi:10.1016/j.bone.2007.12.223.
2. Meyer RA, Tsahakis PJ, Martin DF, Banks DM, Harrow ME, et al. (2001) Age and ovariectomy impair both the normalization of mechanical properties and the accretion of mineral by the fracture callus in rats. J Orthop Res 19: 428–435. doi:10.1016/S0736-0266(00)90034-2.
3. Skak SørV, Jensen TT (1988) Femoral shaft fracture in 265 children: Log-normal correlation with age of speed of healing. Acta Orthop Scand 59: 704–707.
4. Kasper G, Mao L, Geissler S, Draycheva A, Trippens J, et al. (2009) Insights into Mesenchymal Stem Cell Aging: Involvement of Antioxidant Defense and Actin Cytoskeleton. STEM CELLS 27: 1288–1297. doi:10.1002/stem.49.
5. Bloomfield SA, Hogan HA, Delp MD (2002) Decreases in bone blood flow and bone material properties in aging Fischer-344 rats. Clin Orthop Relat Res: 248–257.
6. Panagiotis M (2005) Classification of non-union. Injury 36: S30–S37. doi:10.1016/j.injury.2005.10.008.
7. Hayda RA, Brighton CT, Esterhai JL (1998) Pathophysiology of delayed healing. Clin Orthop Relat Res: S31–40.
8. Klein P, Schell H, Streitparth F, Heller M, Kassi J, et al. (2003) The initial phase of fracture healing is specifically sensitive to mechanical conditions. Journal of Orthopaedic Research 21: 662–669. doi:10.1016/S0736-0266(02)00259-0.
9. Mehta M, Strube P, Peters A, Perka C, Hutmacher D, et al. (2010) Influences of age and mechanical stability on volume, microstructure, and mineralization of the fracture callus during bone healing: Is osteoclast activity the key to age-related impaired healing? Bone 47: 219–228. doi:10.1016/j.bone.2010.05.029.
10. Lienau J, Schmidt-Bleek K, Peters A, Weber H, Bail HJ, et al. (2010) Insight into the Molecular Pathophysiology of Delayed Bone Healing in a Sheep Model. Tissue Engineering Part A 16: 191–199. doi:10.1089/ten.tea.2009.0187.
11. Claes L, Blakytny R, Göckelmann M, Schoen M, Ignatius A, et al. (2009) Early dynamization by reduced fixation stiffness does not improve fracture healing in a rat femoral osteotomy model. Journal of Orthopaedic Research 27: 22–27. doi:10.1002/jor.20712.
12. Carano RA, Filvaroff EH (2003) Angiogenesis and bone repair. Drug Discov Today 8: 980–989. doi:10.1016/S1359-6446(03)02866-6.
13. Meyer RA Jr, Meyer MH, Tenholder M, Wondracek S, Wasserman R, et al. (2003) Gene expression in older rats with delayed union of femoral fractures. J Bone Joint Surg Am 85-A: 1243–1254.
14. Le AX, Miclau T, Hu D, Helms JA (2001) Molecular aspects of healing in stabilized and non-stabilized fractures. Journal of Orthopaedic Research 19: 78–84. doi:10.1016/S0736-0266(00)00006-1.
15. Strube P, Mehta M, Putzier M, Matziolis G, Perka C, et al. (2008) A new device to control mechanical environment in bone defect healing in rats. Journal of Biomechanics 41: 2696–2702. doi:10.1016/j.jbiomech.2008.06.009.
16. Kaspar K, Schell H, Toben D, Matziolis G, Bail HJ (2007) An easily reproducible and biomechanically standardized model to investigate bone healing in rats, using external fixation/Ein leicht reproduzierbares und biomechanisch standardisiertes Modell zur Untersuchung der Knochenheilung in der Ratte unter Verwendung eines Fixateur Externe. bmte 52: 383–390. doi:10.1515/BMT.2007.063.
17. Huang DW, Sherman BT, Lempicki RA (2008) Systematic and integrative analysis of large gene lists using DAVID bioinformatics resources. Nat Protocols 4: 44–57. doi:10.1038/nprot.2008.211.

File S3 Table S8. Functional annotation of differentially expressed genes using DAVID v6.7.

File S4 Table S9–S11. Single GO terms were joined into five clusters of related terms using REVIGO.

Acknowledgments

The authors would like to thank Dr. Ute Ungethuem from the Laboratory of Functional Genome Research Charité Core Facility for performing Affymetrix hybridization. We are grateful to Dr. Nicola Ott, Martin Textor, Liliya Schumann, Annett Kurtz, Marcel Gaetjen, Delia Koennig, and Claudia Schaar for excellent technical support.

Author Contributions

Conceived and designed the experiments: AO GND SG SP JEO CP PS. Performed the experiments: AO SG JEO PS. Analyzed the data: AO GND SG SP JEO CP PS. Wrote the paper: AO GND JEO PS.

18. Supek F, Bošnjak M, Škunca N, Šmuc T (2011) REVIGO Summarizes and Visualizes Long Lists of Gene Ontology Terms. PLoS ONE 6: e21800. doi:10.1371/journal.pone.0021800.
19. Claes LE, Heigele CA, Neidlinger-Wilke C, Kaspar D, Seidl W, et al. (1998) Effects of mechanical factors on the fracture healing process. Clin Orthop Relat Res: S132–147.
20. Edgar R, Domrachev M, Lash AE (2002) Gene Expression Omnibus: NCBI gene expression and hybridization array data repository. Nucl Acids Res 30: 207–210. doi:10.1093/nar/30.1.207.
21. Einhorn TA (1998) The cell and molecular biology of fracture healing. Clin Orthop Relat Res: S7–21.
22. Dimitriou R, Tsiridis E, Giannoudis PV (2005) Current concepts of molecular aspects of bone healing. Injury 36: 1392–1404. doi:10.1016/j.injury.2005.07.019.
23. Phillips AM (2005) Overview of the fracture healing cascade. Injury 36: S5–S7. doi:10.1016/j.injury.2005.07.027.
24. Ode A, Kopf J, Kurtz A, Schmidt-Bleek K, Schrade P, et al. (2011) CD73 and CD29 concurrently mediate the mechanically induced decrease of migratory capacity of mesenchymal stromal cells. Eur Cell Mater 22: 26–42.
25. Gerstenfeld LC, Cullinane DM, Barnes GL, Graves DT, Einhorn TA (2003) Fracture healing as a post-natal developmental process: Molecular, spatial, and temporal aspects of its regulation. Journal of Cellular Biochemistry 88: 873–884. doi:10.1002/jcb.10435.
26. Barnes GL, Kostenuik PJ, Gerstenfeld LC, Einhorn TA (1999) Growth Factor Regulation of Fracture Repair. Journal of Bone and Mineral Research 14: 1805–1815. doi:10.1359/jbmr.1999.14.11.1805.
27. Rubin CT, Bain SD, McLeod KJ (1992) Suppression of the osteogenic response in the aging skeleton. Calcif Tissue Int 50: 306–313.
28. Turner CH, Takano Y, Owan I (1995) Aging changes mechanical loading thresholds for bone formation in rats. Journal of Bone and Mineral Research 10: 1544–1549. doi:10.1002/jbmr.5650101016.
29. Groothuis A, Duda GN, Wilson CJ, Thompson MS, Hunter MR, et al. (2010) Mechanical stimulation of the pro-angiogenic capacity of human fracture haematoma: Involvement of VEGF mechano-regulation. Bone 47: 438–444. doi:10.1016/j.bone.2010.05.026.
30. Kasper G, Dankert N, Tuischer J, Hoeft M, Gaber T, et al. (2007) Mesenchymal Stem Cells Regulate Angiogenesis According to Their Mechanical Environment. STEM CELLS 25: 903–910. doi:10.1634/stemcells.2006-0432.
31. Ortega N, Behonick D, Stickens D, Werb Z (2003) How Proteases Regulate Bone Morphogenesis. Annals of the New York Academy of Sciences 995: 109–116. doi:10.1111/j.1749-6632.2003.tb03214.x.
32. Sternlicht MD, Werb Z (2001) How matrix metalloproteinases regulate cell behavior. Annu Rev Cell Dev Biol 17: 463–516. doi:10.1146/annurev.cellbio.17.1.463.
33. Uusitalo H, Hiltunen A, Söderström M, Aro HT, Vuorio E (2000) Expression of Cathepsins B, H, K, L, and S and Matrix Metalloproteinases 9 and 13 During Chondrocyte Hypertrophy and Endochondral Ossification in Mouse Fracture Callus. Calcified Tissue International 67: 382–390. doi:10.1007/s002230001152.
34. Colnot C, Thompson Z, Miclau T, Werb Z, Helms JA (2003) Altered fracture repair in the absence of MMP9. Development 130: 4123–4133.
35. Stickens D, Behonick DJ, Ortega N, Heyer B, Hartenstein B, et al. (2004) Altered endochondral bone development in matrix metalloproteinase 13-deficient mice. Development 131: 5883–5895. doi:10.1242/dev.01461.

17

Novel Mutations in *FKBP10* and *PLOD2* Cause Rare Bruck Syndrome in Chinese Patients

Peiran Zhou, Yi Liu, Fang Lv, Min Nie, Yan Jiang, Ou Wang, Weibo Xia, Xiaoping Xing, Mei Li*

Department of Endocrinology, Key Laboratory of Endocrinology of Ministry of Health, Peking Union Medical College Hospital, Peking Union Medical College, Chinese Academy of Medical Sciences, Beijing, China

Abstract

Bruck syndrome (BS) is an extremely rare form of osteogenesis imperfecta characterized by congenital joint contracture, multiple fractures and short stature. We described the phenotypes of BS in two Chinese patients for the first time. The novel compound heterozygous mutations c.764_772dupACGTCCTCC (p.255_257dupHisValLeu) in exon 5 and c.1405G>T (p.Gly469X) in exon 9 of *FKBP10* were identified in one proband. The novel compound heterozygous mutations c.1624delT (p.Tyr542Thrfs*18) in exon 14 and c.1880T>C (p.Val627Ala) in exon 17 of *PLOD2* were identified in another probrand. Intravenous zoledronate was a potent agent for these patients, confirmed the efficacy of bisphosphonates on this disease. In conclusion, the novel causative mutations identified in the patients expand the genotypic spectrum of BS.

Editor: Andreas R. Janecke, Innsbruck Medical University, Austria

Funding: This study was supported by the National Natural Science Foundation of China (81100623) and National Key Program of Clinical Science. The funders had no role in study design, data collection and analysis, decision to publish, or preparation of the manuscript.

Competing Interests: The authors have declared that no competing interests exist.

* Email: limeilzh@sina.com

Introduction

Osteogenesis imperfecta (OI) is a remarkably heterogeneous monogenic disease characterized by bone fragility and low bone mass, more than 90% of which are caused by dominant mutations in encoding genes of type I procollagen chains proα1 (*COL1A1*, MIM 120150) or proα2 (*COL1A2*, MIM 120160) [1,2]. Bruck syndrome (BS, MIM 259450 and 609220) is an extremely rare autosomal recessive form of OI, which is defined by congenital large joint contracture, bone fragility, multiple bone fractures starting in infancy or early childhood [2–4]. According to the latest genetic research, mutations of genes encoding new proteins involved in post translational modifications and folding of type I collagen have been identified to give rise to autosomal recessive forms of OI, including *CRTAP, LEPRE1, PPIB, SERPINF1, BMP1, WNT1, TMEM38B. FKBP10* (MIM 607063) and *PLOD2* (MIM 601865), encoding FKBP65 and lysyl hydroxylase 2 (LH2), are also reported as targeted genes of the recessive forms of OI [1,5].

FKBP65 is a rough endoplasmic reticulum resident protein which belongs to the family of prolyl *cis–trans* isomerases. FKBP65 acts as an important collagen chaperone-like protein participating in folding of type I procollagen [6]. LH2 is the key enzyme responsible for hydroxylation of lysine residues outside the major triple helix of type I collagen, crucial to formation of mature intermolecular cross-links in bone and cartilage [5,7]. BS is caused by mutations of *FKBP10* or *PLOD2* [6–11]. According to different causative genes, BS is delineated into phenotypically indistinguishable type 1 (BS1) and type 2 (BS2), which are caused by mutations of *FKBP10* and *PLOD2*, respectively [7,9,11].

Genetic and phenotypic heterogeneity of BS has not been completely recognized. Up to now, only 48 individuals with *FKBP10* mutations and 10 individuals with *PLOD2* mutations have been reported all over the world, however, no information of BS is reported in Chinese.

Therefore, we identified the mutations of causative genes, described the clinical phenotype and evaluated the effects of bisphosphonates (BPs) for the first time in two new patients with BS.

Materials and Methods

Affected Family and Control

Two Chinese patients from different non-consanguineous families were diagnosed as BS in the department of endocrinology, Peking Union Medical College Hospital (PUMCH) from 2012 to 2013.

Family 1

The proband was a 9-year-old boy, who was born through full-term normal delivery. The birth weight was 3500 g (the 50th centile) with unknown body length and head circumference. The boy had congenital symmetrical flexion deformity of knees. Bilateral thumb-in-palm deformities were presented at birth and then were corrected by an orthopedic surgery at the age of five years. When he was 1.5, 6.0, 8.5 and 8.8 years old, multiple bone fractures occurred at right femur for one time and at left femur for three times following trivial trauma. Although the fractures healed uneventfully under conservative treatment, he was still unable to stand and walk because of the severe contractures of knees and curvature deformities of femora. Intellect and other milestones of development were normal. The family history was non-contributory. Physical examination showed that he had short stature with deformities of knees. His height was 2.3 SD less than the average. He had no blue sclerae, hearing loss, dentinogenesis imperfecta or clubfoot. Bilateral knee arthrogryposis with pterygia and small joint laxity were shown in Figure 1A–C. The X-ray films revealed severe generalized osteoporosis with presence of wormian bone in cranium, flattening of vertebral bodies with scoliosis, thoracic cage collapse, deformity of pelvis, bowing femora with old healed fractures, slender long bone with thin cortices, metaphyseal enlargement of distal femur, narrowed joint space of knees (Figure 2A–E). We gave the patient alendronate (ALN) (Fosamax, Merck Sharp & Dohme Pharmaceutical Co., LTD) 70 mg weekly for 3 months. Because of adverse effects of gastrointestinal tract, he turned to accept infusion of zoledronic acid (ZOL) (Aclasta, Novartis Pharma Stein AG) at dose of 5 mg yearly. 500 mg calcium plus 200 IU vitamin D_3 was supplemented daily.

Family 2

The proband was a 22-year-old man. He was the only child of a non-consanguineous couple. He was born at full-term with footling presentation and suffered from a right femoral fracture during difficult delivery. Since then, nearly twenty times of fractures occurred at his bilateral ribs, right humerus and femora. Notably, the patient presented left pes equinovarus and mild limitation of joint movement of knees and right elbow. Camptodactyly was found at right thumb, fourth to fifth finger, left third to fourth fingers and fourth toes (Figure 1D–H). He had apparent kyphoscoliosis (Figure 1I). His stature was 3.6SD shorter than the average. He could not walk independently because of contractures of knees and discrepancy of lower limb length. He

had normal sclerae, hearing, dentition and intelligence. His parents were healthy without family history of OI. The X-ray films also revealed severe generalized osteoporosis with wormian bone in cranium, multiple vertebral compression fractures with rotation kyphoscoliosis, collapsed right thoracic cage, deformity of pelvis, slender long bone with thin cortices (Figure 2F–J). He took 70 mg ALN weekly for 16 months. Since bone mineral density (BMD) gain was not obvious, he accepted infusion of 5 mg ZOL yearly. Supplementation of 500 mg calcium and 200 IU vitamin D_3 was given daily.

100 unaffected, unrelated, ethnically matched, healthy subjects were recruited from the outpatients in the department of endocrinology, PUMCH. This study was approved by the Ethic Committee of PUMCH. Signed informed consents were obtained from all subjects included in this study or from their parents.

Mutation Analysis

Genomic DNA of the probands, their parents and ethnically matched control was extracted from peripheral leukocytes with a QIAamp DNA Mini Kit (50) (Qiagen, Germany). All exons of *FKBP10* and *PLOD2*, exon–intron junctions were amplified by polymerase chain reaction (PCR) in 23 reactions. Primers were designed using the software Oligo 7.0 (Table S1). Taq DNA polymerase (Biomed, China) and its standard buffer were used in all reactions under the following conditions: initial denaturation at 95°C for 2 min, followed by 35 cycles at 95°C for 30 s, 53–63°C for 30 s, and 72°C for 45/90 s. Direct sequencing reactions of PCR products were performed using BigDye Terminators Cycle Sequencing Ready Reaction Kit, version 3.1 (Applied Biosystems), and analyzed with an ABI 3130 automatic sequencer (Applied Biosystems) using standard methods. The results of sequencing were compared with the reference nucleotide sequence of

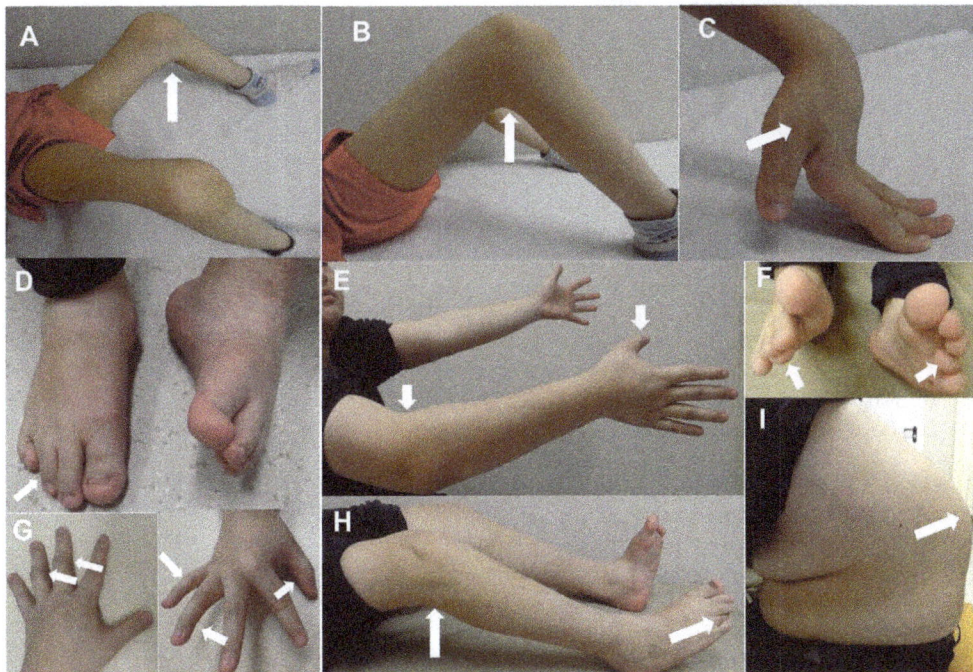

Figure 1. Clinical phenotypes in probands with Bruck syndrome. For proband 1, (A)–(B) severe flexion deformity of knees (white arrows); (C) small joint laxity of hand and scar of orthopedic surgery for correcting thumb-in-palm deformity (white arrow). For proband 2, (D) left pes equinovarus and invisible right fourth toe because of camptodactyly (white arrow); (E) congenital joint contracture of right elbow and camptodactyly of right thumb (white arrow); (F) camptodactyly of fourth toes (white arrows); (G) mild camptodactyly of left 3–4th fingers and right thumb, 4–5 fingers (white arrows); (H) limited movement of knees and invisible right fourth toe from this view (white arrows); (I) severe ithyokyphosis.

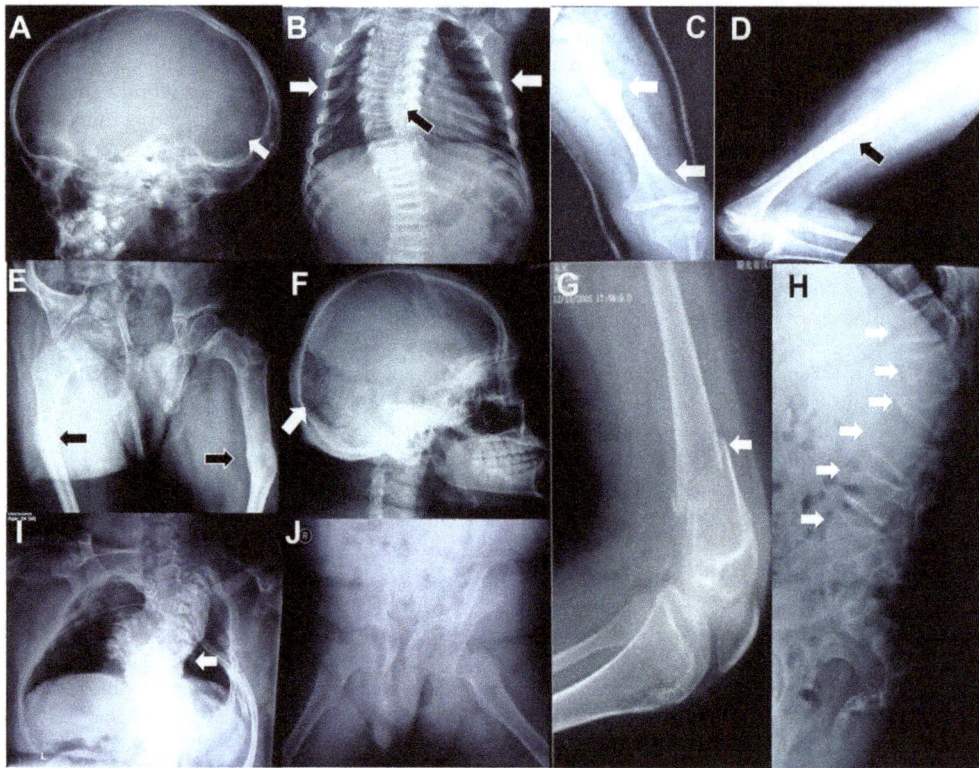

Figure 2. Radiological findings in the two probands with Bruck syndrome. For proband 1, (A) occipital wormian bone (white arrow); (B) scoliosis (black arrow) and thoracic cage collapse (white arrows); (C)–(D) slender femur with thin cortices (black arrow), metaphyseal enlargement of distal femur (white arrow) and old fracture (white arrow); (E) old fractures and bending of femora (black arrows), severe deformity of pelvis and osteoporosis. For proband 2, (F) occipital wormian bone (white arrow); (G) embedded fracture of right distal femur (white arrow); (H) multiple vertebral compression fractures (white arrows) and ithyokyphosis; (I) rotation kyphoscoliosis (white arrow), indistinct ribs and thoracic cage collapse; (J) severe deformity of pelvis and osteoporosis.

FKBP10 (NM_021939.3) and *PLOD2* (NM_182943.2). Genetic mutations identified in our patients were submitted to the OI database (https://oi.gene.le.ac.uk).

Assessment of Effect and Safety of Bisphosphonates

New fracture was determined by medical history and X-ray films of bone. BMD at lumbar spine 2–4 (L2–L4), femoral neck (FN) and total hip (TH) was measured at baseline and after 6 and 12 months of treatment by dual-energy x-ray absorptiometry (DXA, Lunar Prodigy Advance, GE Healthcare, USA) according to the manufacturer's protocol. The BMD Z scores were calculated according to BMD of the age matched boys in Beijing, China [12,13]. BMD of the first proband's parents was also measured.

Serum levels of calcium, phosphate, alanine aminotransferase (ALT) and creatinine were detected by automatic analyzer. Serum levels of β-isomerized carboxy-telopeptide of type I collagen (β-CTX, bone resorption marker), total alkaline phosphatase (TALP, bone formation marker), 25 hydroxy vitamin D (25(OH)D, marker of vitamin D nutritional status) and intact parathyroid hormone (PTH) were measured by automated electrochemiluminescence system (E170; Roche Diagnostics, Switzerland). All biochemical tests were performed in the clinical central laboratory of PUMCH.

All adverse events were recorded in detail during the follow-up. Safety of the treatment was assessed by the records of adverse effects, physical examination and assessment of hematologic biochemical markers of liver and kidney functions.

Results

Mutations Identified in *FKBP10* and *PLOD2*

For the first proband, DNA sequence analysis indicated compound heterozygous mutations in *FKBP10* gene: 9 base pairs duplication (c.764_772dup ACGTCCTCC) in exon 5 resulting in three amino acids duplication (p.255_257dupHisValLeu) and c.1405G>T transition in exon 9 leading to the substitution of glycine at position 469 by premature termination codon (p.Gly469X) (Figure 3A). This duplication occurred in the second peptidyl-prolyl cis-trans isomerase (PPIase) domain of FKBP65 (Figure 4A), among a region of highly conserved residues (Figure 4B). The nonsense mutation occurred in the fourth PPIase domain of FKBP65 (Figure 4A), generating a premature truncation of the protein. The parents were heterozygous carriers for one of the compound mutations, respectively.

For the second proband, compound heterozygous mutations in *PLOD2* gene were identified in DNA sequence analysis: one base pairs deletion (c.1624delT) in exon 14 resulting in frame shift (p.Tyr542Thrfs*18) and c.1880T>C transition in exon 17 leading to the substitution of valine at position 627 by alanine (p.Val627Ala) (Figure 3B). His parents were heterozygous carriers for one of the compound mutations, respectively.

The four kinds of novel mutations were absent in the 100 unrelated control subjects and were not classed as polymorphisms in all public databases.

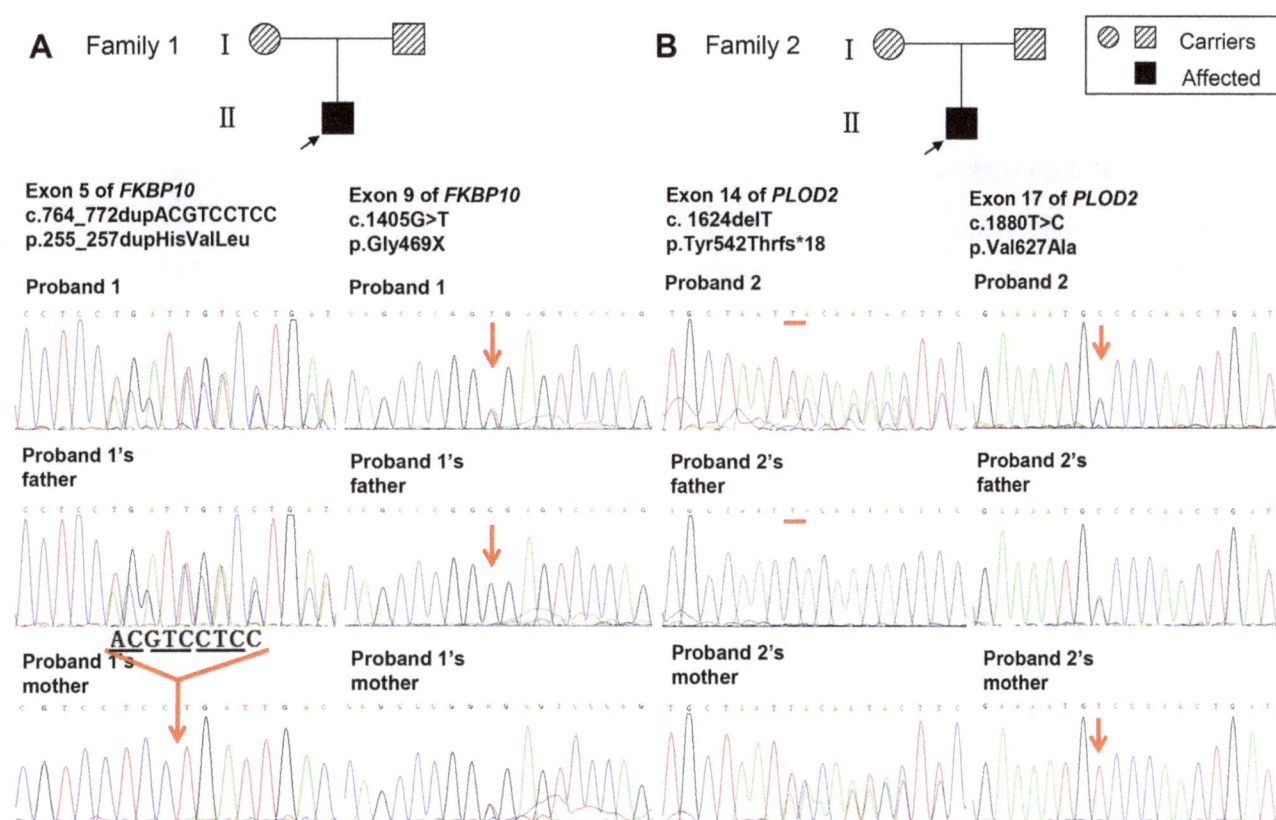

Figure 3. Pedigree of the two families displaying Bruck syndrome and mutation analysis. Probands are indicated by the arrows. Black symbols indicate individuals with Bruck syndrome; shadow symbols represent carriers. (A) In proband 1, novel compound heterozygous mutations of *FKBP10* were identified as: c.764_772dupACGTCCTCC (p.255_257dupHisValLeu) in exon 5 and c.1405G>T (p.Gly469X) in exon 9. (B) In proband 2, novel compound heterozygous mutations of *PLOD2* were identified as: c. 1624delT (p.Tyr542Thrfs*18) in exon 14 and c.1880T>C (p.Val627Ala) in exon 17. The probands' parents were both asymptomatic heterozygous carriers for the compound mutations, respectively.

Effect and Safety of Bisphosphonates

At baseline, the first proband had increased level of β-CTX and normal levels of calcium, phosphate, PTH and TALP (Table 1). BMD and Z scores at L2–L4, FN and TH were extremely low (Table 1). After 9 months treatment of BPs, serum β-CTX level was decreased from 1.3 ng/mL to 1.0 ng/mL and serum TALP level was decreased from 353 U/L to 194 U/L (Table 1). BMD at L2–L4, FN and TH was significantly increased by 125.5%, 31.4%, 49.3% compared to baseline, respectively (Figure S1A). The Z scores of BMD at all above sites were increased from −4.1, −3.9 and −2.9 of baseline to −2.5, −3.1 and −1.2, respectively (Figure S1B). However, two times of new fractures at different positions of left femur recurred after 2 weeks and 10 months of ZOL treatment. The laboratory results and BMD of his patients were all normal. His father's BMD Z scores at L2–L4, FN and TH were −0.6, 0.0 and −0.7, respectively. His mother's BMD Z scores at above sites were −1.1, 0.0 and −0.1, respectively.

At baseline, the second proband had mildly increased TALP and ALT levels, normal β-CTX level (Table 2). The DXA films of spine showed the severe kyphoscoliosis with dim shapes of ribs (Figure S2C). BMD at proximal femur was low. BMD at lumber spine was normal. However, severe deformity of lumbar spine would lead to bias of measurement. After 23 months treatment of BPs, serum β-CTX level was decreased from 0.4 ng/mL to 0.3 ng/mL and serum TALP level was decreased from 124 U/L to 113 U/L. BMD at L2–L4, FN and TH was significantly increased by 11.6%, 21.2%, 3.9% compared to baseline,

respectively (Figure S2A). The Z scores of BMD at all above sites were increased from 0.2, −1.2 and −0.8 of baseline to 1.7, 0.7 and −0.4, respectively (Figure S2B). No new fracture occurred during period of BPs treatment.

The ability of daily activities of the two probands was significantly improved after BPs treatment. Both of the patients had mild fever and muscle soreness in the second day after infusion of ZOL, with the highest body temperature of 37.3 and 37.8 centigrade respectively. The adverse effects were in remission after 2 to 3 days spontaneously without special management. No osteonecrosis of jaw or other adverse effects were observed.

Discussion

BS is an exceedingly rare form of OI, which presents the concurrence of bone fragility and congenital joint contractures in an individual. In 1897, Bruck reported a man with bone fragility and joint contractures, which was the first description of this syndrome [14]. We reported two new patients with this rare disease for the first time in Chinese. They presented with recurrent fractures, multiple congenital arthrogryposis, postnatal short stature and progressive scoliosis, but without blue sclerae, dentinogenesis imperfecta or hearing loss. The causative mutations were identified as novel compound heterozygous mutations in *FKBP10* and *PLOD2*, respectively, and their parents are asymptomatic heterozygous carriers for one of the compound mutations.

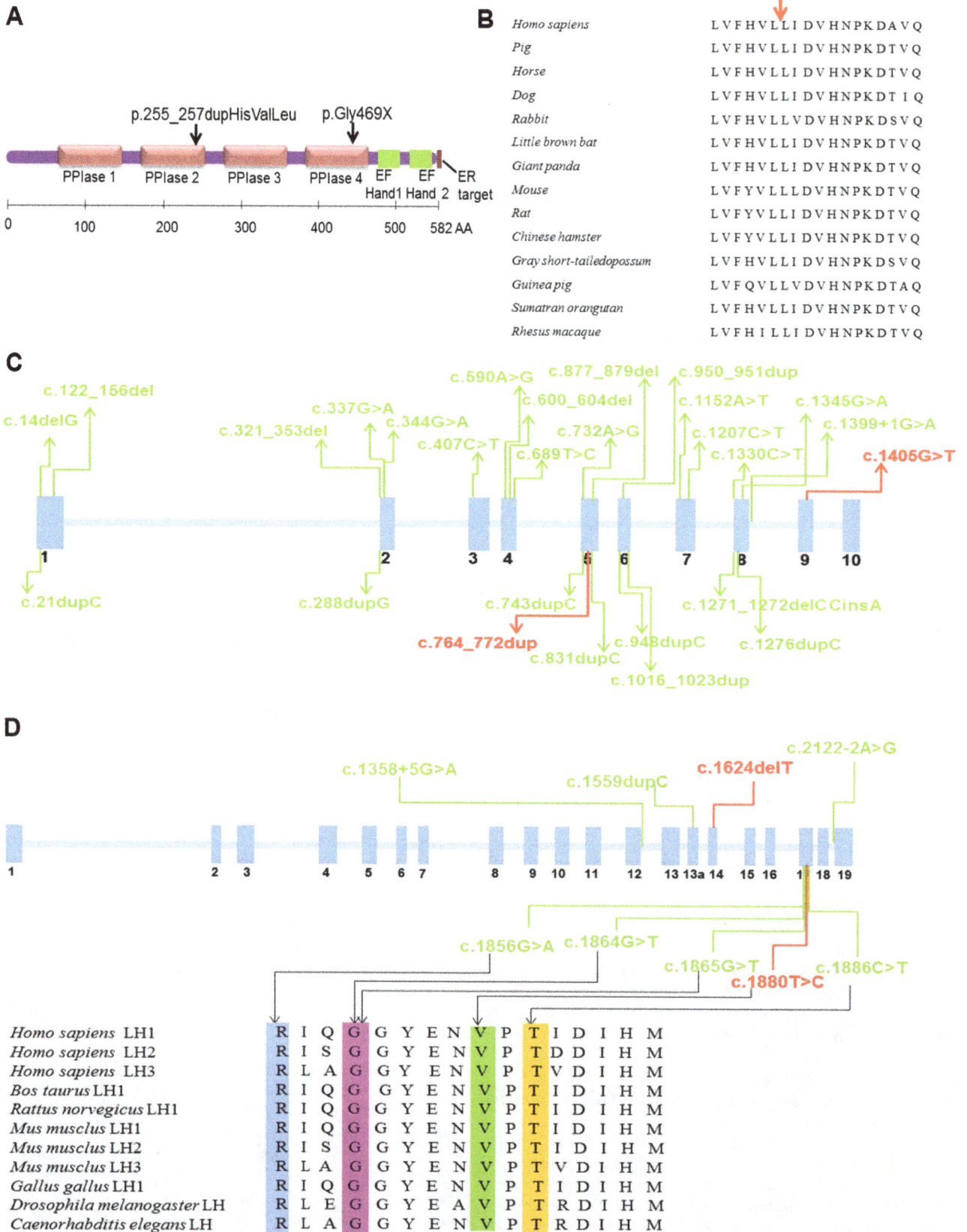

Figure 4. Mutation information of *FKBP10* and *PLOD2*. (A) Representation of FKBP65 with the location of mutations in proband 1 (black arrows). (B) The whole stretch sequence around Leu258 is highly conserved in FKBP65 among 14 different species. Red arrow indicates position of p.255_257dupHisValLeu mutation. (C) Blue boxes indicate all exons of *FKBP10*. Mutations were identified in *FKBP10* in patients with Bruck syndrome and osteogenesis imperfecta. The two kinds of mutations in our study are shown in red. (D) Blue boxes indicate all exons of *PLOD2*. Mutations were

identified in *PLOD2* in patients with Bruck syndrome and osteogenesis imperfecta. The two kinds of mutations in this study are shown in red. Mutation in exon 17 of proband 2 will lead to change of amino acid in lysyl hydroxylase at highly conserved among 11 different species.

FKBP10 and *PLOD2* locate at 17q2 and 3q24, respectively. They are reported to be causative loci for moderate to severe isolated recessive OI, as well as BS [7,15,16]. 25 kinds of mutations have been identified over whole exons of *FKBP10* gene, which mainly focus on exon 5 (32.26%) and exon 6 (24.73%) (Figure 4C) (https://oi.gene.le.ac.uk). Duplication mutations (54.84%) in *FKBP10* resulting in frame shift of the amino acid sequence are the majority cause of recessive OI with or without joint contractures (https://oi.gene.le.ac.uk). Only 7 kinds of mutations in *PLOD2* have been identified which mainly focus on exon 17 (60%) (Figure 4D)(https://oi.gene.le.ac.uk). Substitution mutations (80%) in *PLOD2* are the majority causes of recessive OI with or without joint contractures. Deletion mutation in exon 14 of *PLOD2* in our patients is identified for the first time (https://oi.gene.le.ac.uk). In our patients, compound heterozygous mutations of c.764_772dupACGTCCTCC in exon 5 and c.1405G>T in exon 9 of *FKBP10*, and c.1624delT in exon 14 and c.1880T>C in exon 17 of *PLOD2* are all novel mutations of causative gene of BS.

FKBP65 has four PPIase domains that catalyze the interconversion of cis/trans isomers of peptidyl-prolyl bonds in proteins containing proline [17]. Since approximately one-sixth of the collagen sequence consists of proline residues, this conversion is the rate-limiting step in the folding process of nascent proteins [18]. FKBP65 prevents premature cross-links between procollagen chains and assists proper registration, folding into the collagen triple helix, and subsequent trafficking [19,20]. Moreover, FKBP65 could modulate type I collagen cross-linking indirectly and is crucial for the stability or activity of LH2 [15,19,21]. Inactivating mutations of *FKBP10* could lead to loss function of

FKBP65, marked diminution of lysyl hydroxylation, instable secreted type I procollagen similar to mutations in *SERPINH1* [22–24]. The compound variants of *FKBP10* in our patient affect the second and fourth PPIase domain, which will reduce folding and cross-linking of type I procollagen.

Fibrillar collagen molecules in tissues are connected through lysyl- and hydroxylysyl-derived cross-links. The involved lysyl residues locate in the amino-terminal and carboxyl-terminal telopeptides and two sites in the triple-helical domain. LH2 is highly expressed in bone and is mainly responsible for hydroxylation of the triple-helical cross-linking lysyl residues. In this study, mutation c. 1624delT in exon 14 of *PLOD2* results in frame shift. Mutation c.1880T>C of *PLOD2* causes the substitution of valine by alanine at position 627, which is close to previously identified variants of p.Arg619His(c.1856G>A), p.Gly622Cys(c.1864G>T), p.Gly622Val(c.1865G>T) and p.Thr629Ile(c.1886C>T) in patients with BS (Figure 4D) [5,7,25]. This region is proposed to be an important functional domain of LH2 enzyme and is highly conserved throughout the species [25]. Moreover, the missense mutation may lead to damage of protein predicted by SIFT online software (http://sift.jcvi.org/). Impaired function of LH2 will lead to abnormal hydroxylation of the triple-helical cross-linking lysyl residues, and then will affect the installment and secretion of the collagen fibers from osteoblasts.

The phenotypes of Chinese patients are generally similar to clinical spectrum in other ethnical patients with BS (Table 2). Mutations of either *FKBP10* or *PLOD2* gene lead to congenital joint contractures of knees, elbows and other joints. Talipes and camptodactyly seem to be the more common sign of patients with *PLOD2* mutations. However, since there are few patients recorded

Table 1. Clinical characteristics of the two patients with BS.

Characteristics	Proband 1		Proband 2		Reference values
	Baseline	9M visit	Baseline	23M visit	
Age (years)	9	10	22	24	
Height (cm)	120	120	150	150	
Weight (kg)	19.5	20.0	79	79	
Serum calcium (mmol/L)	2.39	2.34	2.40	2.36	2.13–2.70
Serum phosphate (mmol/L)	1.68	1.86	1.05	0.95	0.81–1.45
Serum TALP (U/L)	353	194	124	113	30–120 (adult)
					42–390 (child)
Serum β-CTX (ng/mL)	1.3	1.0	0.4	0.3	0.26–0.512
Serum creatinine (μmol/L)	24	25	46	55	59–104 (adult)
					18–62 (child)
Serum ALT (U/L)	10	10	77	64	5–40
Serum intact PTH (pg/mL)	18.7		37.5		12–65
Serum 25(OH)D (ng/mL)	25.4		12.7		
L2–L4 BMD (mg/cm²)(Z score)	216 (−4.1)	487 (−2.5)	1186 (0.2)	1324 (1.7)	
FN BMD (mg/cm²) (Z score)	338 (−3.9)	444 (−3.1)	877 (−1.2)	1063 (0.7)	
TH BMD (mg/cm²) (Z score)	469 (−2.9)	700 (−1.2)	906 (−0.8)	941 (−0.4)	

BS, Bruck syndrome; TALP, total alkaline phosphatase; β-CTX, β-isomerized carboxy-telopeptide of type I collagen; ALT, alanine aminotransferase; PTH, parathyroid hormone; 25(OH)D, 25 hydroxy vitamin D; L2–L4, lumbar spine 2–4; FN, femoral neck; TH, total hip.

Table 2. Clinical, radiological and genetic information of patients with BS.

Patients	Proband 1 in Chinese	Proband 2 in Chinese	Patients with *FKBP10* mutations [4,7,9,15,16,23,26–29]	Patients with *PLOD2* mutations [5,7,25]
Causitive mutations	*FKBP10* c.764_772dupACGTCCTCC, c.1405G>T	*PLOD2* c.1624delT, c.1880T>C	Mostly duplication mutations	Mostly substitutionmutations
Race	Han	Han	Variable	Variable
Sex	Male	Male	Both	Both
Positive family history	-	-	+/-	+/−
Consanguineous pedigree	-	-	Most	Most
Postnatal short stature	+	+	+	+
First fracture age	18 months	At birth	Early infancy	Early infancy
Times of fracture	6	nearly 20	Variable	Variable
Congenital joint contractures	Knees	Knees, right elbow	Mostly knees, elbows and ankles; wrists and hips also reported	Mostly knees and elbows; wrists and ankles also reported
Camptodactyly	thumbs	4th toes, right thumb and 4–5 fingers, left 3–4 fingers	8/38 cases	2/6 cases
Clubfoot	-	left	15/38 cases	5/6 cases
Scoliosis/kyphoscoliosis	+	+	Most	Most
Blue sclerae	-	-	- (almost all)	- (almost all)
Dentinogenesis imperfecta	-	-	-	-
Wormian bones	+	+	Most	Most
Mobility	Difficulty in walking with limping			

BS, Bruck syndrome; N.A, not available.

with BS, the genotype-phenotype correlation still needs to be investigated in more patients. The overlapped phenotype induced by *FKBP10* and *PLOD2* mutations possibly attribute to the common mechanisms affecting collagen cross-link formation through diminution of telopeptide lysyl hydroxylation. However, age of initial fracture, times of fracture and limitation of joints movement are variable among patients with BS. In order to elucidate the detail mechanism of BS caused by *FKBP10* and *PLOD2* mutations, we should further analyze the molecular stability and post-translational modification of type I procollagen through culturing fibroblasts or osteoblasts of the patients with BS using Western blot analysis or immunocytochemical analysis of proteins. The C18 reverse-phase HPLC is helpful to complete quantitative analysis of the cross-link of type I collagen [15].

Effective treatment for BS is still deficient. BPs are widely used to treat osteoporosis through potent inhibition of osteoclasts [30]. Since increasing osteoclast activity contributes to pathogenesis of OI [31], pamidronate, risedronate, ALN or ZOL are demonstrated to reduce fracture incidence and improve musculoskeletal function of patients with OI [32–36]. We chose ZOL to treat this rare disease because of its convenience and no gastrointestinal adverse effect. Significant increases in areal BMD and its Z scores at lumbar spine and proximal hip in patients with BS were observed after treatment of ZOL. The bone resorption biomarker level was decreased and the ability of daily activities of the patients was improved after treatment of BPs. ZOL was generally well tolerated to BPs. However, the efficacy and safety of BPs on BS still needs to be further confirmed in large sampled clinical study.

Conclusions

BS is an extremely rare, autosomal recessively inherited, moderate or severe type of OI, which is characterized by congenital joint contracture, multiple fractures and postnatal short stature. Novel compound heterozygous mutations c.764_772dupACGTCCTCC (p.255_257dupHisValLeu) and c.1405G>T (p.Gly469X) in *FKBP10*, c.1624delT (p.Tyr542Thrfs*18) and c.1880T>C (p.Val627Ala) in *PLOD2* are the new genetic mechanisms of BS. Moreover, intravenous zoledronic acid is probably an effective treatment option for patients with BS.

Supporting Information

Figure S1 Effects of bisphosphonates on proband 1 with Bruck syndrome. (A)–(B) BMD and Z score at all sites were significantly increased after 9 months of bisphosphonates treatment. (C) Bone morphology was improved in spine and right femur after 9 months of treatment, which was showed in images of DXA. BMD, bone mineral density; DXA, dual-energy x-ray absorptiometry; L2–L4, lumbar spine 2–4; FN, femoral neck; TH, total hip; ALN, alendronate; ZOL, zoledronate acid.

Figure S2 Effects of bisphosphonates on proband 2 with Bruck syndrome. (A)–(B) BMD and Z score were increased at L2–L4 after bisphosphonates treatment. BMD and Z score at proximal femur was decreased after 16 months of ALN treatment but was significantly increased after 7 months of ZOL treatment. (C) In images of DXA, color of lumbar spine became darker after 23 months of treatment. No significant change in image of proximal femur was observed after treatment. BMD, bone mineral density; DXA, dual-energy x-ray absorptiometry; L2–L4, lumbar spine 2–4; FN, femoral neck; TH, total hip; ALN, alendronate; ZOL, zoledronate acid.

Table S1 List of primers for PCR-amplification of all exons and exon–intron junctions of *FKBP10* and *PLOD2*.

Acknowledgments

We thank all patients with BS and their families for their participation in this research and thank all unaffected, unrelated individuals for providing control DNA samples.

Author Contributions

Conceived and designed the experiments: ML. Performed the experiments: PRZ YL FL. Analyzed the data: PRZ. Contributed reagents/materials/analysis tools: ML MN YJ OW WBX XPX. Wrote the paper: PRZ ML.

References

1. Rohrbach M, Giunta C (2012) Recessive osteogenesis imperfecta: clinical, radiological, and molecular findings. Am J Med Genet C Semin Med Genet 160C: 175–189.
2. Byers PH, Pyott SM (2012) Recessively inherited forms of osteogenesis imperfecta. Annu Rev Genet 46: 475–497.
3. Viljoen D, Versfeld G, Beighton P (1989) Osteogenesis imperfecta with congenital joint contractures (Bruck syndrome). Clin Genet 36: 122–126.
4. Caparrós-Martin JA, Valencia M, Pulido V, Martínez-Glez V, Rueda-Arenas I, et al. (2013) Clinical and molecular analysis in families with autosomal recessive osteogenesis imperfecta identifies mutations in five genes and suggests genotype-phenotype correlations. Am J Med Genet A 161: 1354–1369.
5. Ha-Vinh R, Alanay Y, Bank RA, Campos-Xavier AB, Zankl A, et al. (2004) Phenotypic and molecular characterization of Bruck syndrome (osteogenesis imperfecta with contractures of the large joints) caused by a recessive mutation in PLOD2. Am J Med Genet A 131: 115–120.
6. Alanay Y, Avaygan H, Camacho N, Utine GE, Boduroglu K, et al. (2010) Mutations in the gene encoding the RER protein FKBP65 cause autosomal-recessive osteogenesis imperfecta. Am J Hum Genet 86: 551–559.
7. Puig-Hervás MT, Temtamy S, Aglan M, Valencia M, Martínez-Glez V, et al. (2012) Mutations in PLOD2 cause autosomal-recessive connective tissue disorders within the Bruck syndrome—osteogenesis imperfecta phenotypic spectrum. Hum Mutat 33: 1444–1449.
8. Marini JC, Blissett AR (2013) New genes in bone development: what's new in osteogenesis imperfecta. J Clin Endocrinol Metab 98: 3095–3103.
9. Shaheen R, Al-Owain M, Sakati N, Alzayed ZS, Alkuraya FS (2010) FKBP10 and Bruck syndrome: phenotypic heterogeneity or call for reclassification? Am J Hum Genet 87: 306–307.
10. Bank RA, Robins SP, Wijmenga C, Breslau-Siderius LJ, Bardoel AF, et al. (1999) Defective collagen crosslinking in bone, but not in ligament or cartilage, in Bruck syndrome: indications for a bone-specific telopeptide lysyl hydroxylase on chromosome 17. Proc Natl Acad Sci U S A 96: 1054–1058.
11. Yapicioğlu H, Ozcan K, Arikan O, Satar M, Narli N, et al. (2009) Bruck syndrome: osteogenesis imperfecta and arthrogryposis multiplex congenita. Ann Trop Paediatr 29: 159–162.
12. Genant HK, Grampp S, Glüer CC, Faulkner KG, Jergas M, et al. (1994) Universal standardization for dual x-ray absorptiometry: patient and phantom cross-calibration results. J Bone Miner Res 9: 1503–1514.
13. Zhang LW, Liu JC, Zhai FY, Cao RX, Duan JL (2003) Normal reference values for bone mineral density in children and adolescents aged 6–18 years, Beijing, China. Chin J Osteoporosis 9: 134–136.
14. Viljoen D, Versfeld G, Beighton P (1989) Osteogenesis imperfecta with congenital joint contractures (Bruck syndrome). Clin Genet 36: 122–126.
15. Schwarze U, Cundy T, Pyott SM, Christiansen HE, Hegde MR, et al. (2013) Mutations in FKBP10, which result in Bruck syndrome and recessive forms of osteogenesis imperfecta, inhibit the hydroxylation of telopeptide lysines in bone collagen. Hum Mol Genet 22: 1–17.
16. Shaheen R, Al-Owain M, Faqeih E, Al-Hashmi N, Awaji A, et al. (2011) Mutations in FKBP10 cause both Bruck syndrome and isolated osteogenesis imperfecta in humans. Am J Med Genet A 155A: 1448–1452.
17. Göthel SF, Marahiel MA (1999) Peptidyl-prolylcis-trans isomerases, a super-family of ubiquitous folding catalysts. Cell Mol Life Sci 55: 423–436.
18. Murphy LA, Ramirez EA, Trinh VT, Herman AM, Anderson VC, et al. (2011) Endoplasmic reticulum stress or mutation of an EF-hand Ca²⁺-binding domain directs the FKBP65 rotamase to an ERAD-based proteolysis. Cell Stress Chaperones 16: 607–619.
19. Barnes AM, Cabral WA, Weis M, Makareeva E, Mertz EL, et al. (2012) Absence of FKBP10 in recessive type XI osteogenesis imperfecta leads to diminished collagen cross-linking and reduced collagen deposition in extracellular matrix. Hum Mutat 33: 1589–1598.
20. Ishikawa Y, Vranka J, Wirz J, Nagata K, Bächinger HP (2008) The rough endoplasmic reticulum-resident FK506-binding protein FKBP65 is a molecular chaperone that interacts with collagens. J Biol Chem 283: 31584–31590.
21. Barnes AM, Duncan G, Weis M, Paton W, Cabral WA, et al. (2013) Kuskokwim syndrome, a recessive congenital contracture disorder, extends the phenotype of FKBP10 mutations. Hum Mutat 34: 1279–1288.
22. Christiansen HE, Schwarze U, Pyott SM, AlSwaid A, Al Balwi M, et al. (2010) Homozygosity for a missense mutation in SERPINH1, which encodes the collagen chaperone protein HSP47, results in severe recessive osteogenesis imperfecta. Am J Hum Genet 86: 389–398.
23. Kelley BP, Malfait F, Bonafe L, Baldridge D, Homan E, et al. (2011) Mutations in FKBP10 cause recessive osteogenesis imperfecta and Bruck syndrome. J Bone Miner Res 26: 666–672.
24. Venturi G, Monti E, Dalle Carbonare L, Corradi M, Gandini A, et al. (2012) A novel splicing mutation in FKBP10 causing osteogenesis imperfecta with a possible mineralization defect. Bone 50: 343–349.
25. van der Slot AJ, Zuurmond AM, Bardoel AF, Wijmenga C, Pruijs HE, et al. (2003) Identification of *PLOD2* as telopeptide lysyl hydroxylase, an important enzyme in fibrosis. J Biol Chem 278: 40967–40972.
26. Setijowati ED, van Dijk FS, Cobben JM, van Rijn RR, Sistermans EA, et al. (2012) A novel homozygous 5 bp deletion in FKBP10 causes clinically Bruck syndrome in an Indonesian patient. Eur J Med Genet 55: 17–21.
27. Yapicioğlu H, Ozcan K, Arikan O, Satar M, Narli N, et al. (2009) Bruck syndrome: osteogenesis imperfecta and arthrogryposis multiplex congenita. Ann Trop Paediatr 29: 159–162.
28. Mokete L, Robertson A, Viljoen D, Beighton P (2005) Bruck syndrome: congenital joint contractures with bone fragility. J Orthop Sci 10: 641–646.
29. McPherson E, Clemens M (1997) Bruck syndrome (osteogenesis imperfecta with congenital joint contractures): review and report on the first North American case. Am J Med Genet 70: 28–31.
30. Olmos JM, Zarrabeitia MT, Hernández JL, Sañudo C, González-Macías J, et al. (2012) Common allelic variants of the farnesyl diphosphate synthase gene influence the response of osteoporotic women to bisphosphonates. Pharmaco-genomics J 12: 227–232.
31. Brenner RE, Vetter U, Bollen AM, Mörike M, Eyre DR (1994) Bone resorption assessed by immunoassay of urinary cross-linked collagen peptides in patients with osteogenesis imperfecta. J Bone Miner Res 9: 993–997.
32. Andiran N, Alikasifoglu A, Alanay Y, Yordam N (2008) Cyclic pamidronate treatment in Bruck syndrome: proposal of a new modality of treatment. Pediatr Int 50: 836–838.
33. Bishop N, Adami S, Ahmed SF, Antón J, Arundel P, et al. (2013) Risedronate in children with osteogenesis imperfecta: a randomised, double-blind, placebo-controlled trial. Lancet 382: 1424–1432.
34. Barros ER, Saraiva GL, de Oliveira TP, Lazaretti-Castro M (2012) Safety and efficacy of a 1-year treatment with zoledronic acid compared with pamidronate in children with osteogenesis imperfecta. J Pediatr Endocrinol Metab 25: 485–491.
35. Pavón de Paz I, Iglesias Bolaños P, Durán Martínez M, Olivar Roldán J, Guijarro De Armas G, et al. (2010) Effects of zoledronic acid in adults with osteogenesis imperfecta. Endocrinol Nutr 57: 245–250.
36. Sousa T, Bompadre V, White KK (2014) Musculoskeletal functional outcomes in children with osteogenesis imperfecta: associations with disease severity and pamidronate therapy. J Pediatr Orthop 34: 118–122.

18

Osteoblast-Specific *Krm2* Overexpression and *Lrp5* Deficiency Have Different Effects on Fracture Healing in Mice

Astrid Liedert[1]*, Viktoria Röntgen[1], Thorsten Schinke[2], Peggy Benisch[3], Regina Ebert[3], Franz Jakob[3], Ludger Klein-Hitpass[4], Jochen K. Lennerz[5], Michael Amling[2], Anita Ignatius[1]

1 Institute of Orthopaedic Research and Biomechanics, Center of Musculoskeletal Research, University of Ulm, Ulm, Germany, 2 Department of Osteology and Biomechanics, University Medical Center Hamburg-Eppendorf, Hamburg, Germany, 3 Orthopaedic Center for Musculoskeletal Research, University of Würzburg, Würzburg, Germany, 4 Institute of Cell Biology, University of Duisburg-Essen, Duisburg, Germany, 5 Institute of Pathology, University of Ulm, Ulm, Germany

Abstract

The canonical Wnt/β-catenin pathway plays a key role in the regulation of bone remodeling in mice and humans. Two transmembrane proteins that are involved in decreasing the activity of this pathway by binding to extracellular antagonists, such as Dickkopf 1 (Dkk1), are the low-density lipoprotein receptor related protein 5 *(Lrp5)* and Kremen 2 *(Krm2)*. *Lrp 5* deficiency *(Lrp5$^{-/-}$)* as well as osteoblast-specific overexpression of Krm2 in mice *(Col1a1-Krm2)* result in severe osteoporosis occurring at young age. In this study, we analyzed the influence of Lrp5 deficiency and osteoblast-specific overexpression of Krm2 on fracture healing in mice using flexible and semi-rigid fracture fixation. We demonstrated that fracture healing was highly impaired in both mouse genotypes, but that impairment was more severe in *Col1a1-Krm2* than in *Lrp5$^{-/-}$* mice and particularly evident in mice in which the more flexible fixation was used. Bone formation was more reduced in *Col1a1-Krm2* than in *Lrp5$^{-/-}$* mice, whereas osteoclast number was similarly increased in both genotypes in comparison with wild-type mice. Using microarray analysis we identified reduced expression of genes mainly involved in osteogenesis that seemed to be responsible for the observed stronger impairment of healing in *Col1a1-Krm2* mice. In line with these findings, we detected decreased expression of sphingomyelin phosphodiesterase 3 (Smpd3) and less active β-catenin in the calli of *Col1a1-Krm2* mice. Since Krm2 seems to play a significant role in regulating bone formation during fracture healing, antagonizing KRM2 might be a therapeutic option to improve fracture healing under compromised conditions, such as osteoporosis.

Editor: Jan Peter Tuckermann, University of Ulm, Germany

Funding: This study was funded by the German Research Foundation (DFG) (Research Unit FOR793, IG18/7-2 and SCHI 504/5-2). The funder had no role in study design, data collection and analysis, decision to publish, or preparation of the manuscript.

Competing Interests: The authors have declared that no competing interests exist.

* Email: astrid.liedert@uni-ulm.de

Introduction

The canonical Wnt/β-catenin pathway has been intensively investigated over the past decade because of its key role in the regulation of skeletal development and bone mass maintenance [1]. The remarkable finding that loss-of-function mutations in the Wnt coreceptor low-density lipoprotein receptor related protein 5 (LRP5) gene cause the osteoporosis-pseudoglioma syndrome (OPPG), a rare autosomal recessive disorder of severe juvenile osteoporosis and congenital blindness, and that gain-of-function mutations in this gene result in a high bone mass phenotype, provided first evidence for the considerable influence of Lrp5 signaling on bone remodeling [2,3]. In addition, studies using transgenic mouse models are currently reflecting the high impact of Wnt signaling on bone mass regulation [4–6]. Thus, targeted disruption of Lrp5 in mice results in a low bone mass phenotype due to decreased osteoblast proliferation and function [7]. The osteoporotic phenotype and persistent eye vascularization recapitulates the human OPPG syndrome. Although most of the transgenic animal models that affect bone mass specifically target

canonical Wnt signaling, there is increasing evidence that noncanonical Wnt signaling pathways, the Wnt-planar cell polarity (Wnt-PCP) and the Wnt-calcium (Ca2+) pathway, play a significant role in bone mass homeostasis. Thus, it has been demonstrated that there may be a crosstalk between these pathways and that some Wnts are able to activate more than one of these pathways in a receptor-dependent manner. [1,5].

There is evidence that canonical Wnt signaling needs to be downregulated in mature osteoblasts to enable bone matrix mineralization [8]. Therefore, extracellular antagonists, including Dickkopf 1 (Dkk1), a member of a small family of secreted proteins, are upregulated during osteoblast differentiation [6,8]. Dkk1 binds to both coreceptors, Lrp5/6 and with high affinity to the transmembrane proteins Kremen 1 or 2 (Krm1, Krm2), thereby forming a ternary complex that undergoes rapid endocytosis and removal of the Lrp coreceptors from the cell membrane, resulting in an inhibition of Wnt/β-catenin signaling [9]. Deleting both, Krm1 and additionally Krm2 expression in mice leads to an increase of bone volume, which was comparable to that observed in haploinsufficient Dkk1 (+/−) mice [10].

Osteoblast-specific overexpression of Krm2 in transgenic mice (*Col1a1-Krm2*) results in severe osteoporosis that is associated with an impaired osteoblast maturation and bone formation as well as increased bone resorption [6]. Consequently, these data demonstrate that Krm2, at least in mice, is an important regulator of bone remodeling by inhibiting bone formation while increasing bone resorption.

Various studies have already shown the crucial role of Wnt/β-catenin signaling in bone fracture repair [11]. Canonical Wnt signaling has been shown to be important in the early phase of fracture repair to allow differentiation of mesenchymal cells into either chondrocyte or osteoblast lineages [12]. β-Catenin mediated Tcf-dependent transcription is activated during both, chondrogenesis as well as osteogenesis in fracture healing and is downregulated in the later phase of osteogenesis, as osteoblasts mature to osteocytes. Using various transgenic mouse models it has been demonstrated that a precisely stage-specifically regulated canonical Wnt signaling is necessary in order to allow complete fracture healing [13]. Fracture healing was impaired in mice conditionally expressing β-catenin null alleles. These mice had a lack of bone and cartilage and showed immature mesenchymal cells at the fracture site. Fracture healing was also repressed in mice expressing the null allele specifically in osteoblasts. These observations are in line with previous studies demonstrating that activated canonical Wnt signaling can interfere with the differentiation of skeletal precursors into chondrocytes and osteoblasts [14,15]. Canonical Wnt signaling has been shown to maintain mesenchymal stem cells in a less differentiated state during osteogenic differentiation. In contrast, in cells already committed to the osteoblast phenotype, activated β-catenin signaling promotes osteoblastic differentiation and enhances osteogenesis, whereas in osteoblast precursors lacking β-catenin osteoblast differentiation is inhibited and they develop into chondrocytes [16,17].

It has been shown that suppression of Wnt pathway inhibitors [18] and activation of β-catenin signaling can enhance healing, whereas β-catenin pathway inhibitors can delay bone regeneration [19]. Based on all these findings, it is obvious that Wnt/β-catenin signaling activation during a defined time during fracture healing might be an excellent option for the improvement of fracture healing under compromised conditions, such as osteoporosis. However, clarifying the role of signaling molecules regulating this pathway in fracture healing is a prerequisite to expand the small number of anabolic drugs that are currently available and evaluated for bone regeneration.

Apart from molecular factors, the mechanical environment that is determined by the fixation stability has an important influence on the fracture healing outcome [20]. Thus, more rigid fracture stabilization promotes intramembraneous ossification, whereas more flexible fracture fixation increases endochondral bone formation. Previously, we established standardized models for investigating the impact of mechanical factors on bone healing in mice, allowing for the adjustment of flexible and semi-rigid conditions [21].

In the present study we examined the influence of Lrp5 deficiency and osteoblast-specific Krm2 overexpression on fracture healing in mice with flexible and semi-rigid fixation, respectively. Both mouse models are known to be associated with an osteoporotic phenotype due to impaired Wnt signaling. We hypothesized that these mouse models show a genotype-specific delayed healing compared to wild-type mice that is more evident in mice with the more flexible fracture fixation compared to mice with the semi-rigid fracture fixation.

Material and Methods

Animals

The experiments were performed according to international regulations for care and use of laboratory animals, and approved by the local ethical committee (Regierungspräsidium Tübingen, No. 906, Germany). *Col1a1-Krm2* transgenic mice (*C57BL/6* genetic background) were generated as previously described [6]. In brief, the ORF encoding the Dkk receptor Krm2 was placed under the control of an osteoblast-specific *Col1a1* promoter fragment. Schulze et al. performed RT-PCR to confirm the bone-specific expression of the transgene, and using Northern blot analysis with RNA isolated from the femura of the transgenic animals they found that the expression was at lest 20-fold increased compared to the expression in the bone of wildtype animals [6]. *Lrp5*-deficient mice (*Lrp5*$^{-/-}$) mice (*C57BL/6* genetic background) were provided by Jackson Laboratory (005823, Bar Harbor, Maine, USA). Mice were kept in individual cages with a 12 h circadian rhythm and were given ad libitum access to food and water.

Fracture healing study

Female, 26 weeks old mice (n = 78) of each genotype (n = 22–30, 25±3 g body weight) were used for the study. For investigation of fracture healing at day 21 the mice were randomly divided into three groups (*C57BL/6* wildtype, *Lrp5*$^{-/-}$ and *Col1a1-Krm2* mice) with either semi-rigid (n = 7–11/group) or flexible fracture fixation (n = 4–7/group) in order to generate mechanical conditions inducing regular or delayed healing, respectively [21]. Motion and ground reaction forces were monitored during the healing period in order to control proper limb loading [21]. 21 days after surgery the mice were euthanized by carbon dioxide inhalation. The fracture calli of each genotype with either semi-rigid (n = 7–11) or flexible fracture fixation (n = 4–7) were evaluated at day 21 by biomechanical and histological evaluation and by micro-computed tomography (µCT). Additional animals of each genotype with semi-rigidly fixated osteotomy were sacrificed 10 days after surgery for a genome-wide comparative gene expression analysis of the fracture callus (n = 5–6) and for histological and immunohistological (n = 5–6) evaluation.

Surgical procedure

All animals received an analgesic (15 mg/kg, Tramal, Gruenenthal GmbH, Aachen, Germany) subcutaneously during the operation and in the drinking water (25 mg/l) for the first 3 postoperative days. After a subcutaneous injection of atropine sulfate (50 µg/kg, Atropin, Braun, Melsungen, Germany) the mice were anesthetized with 2% isoflurane (Forene, Abbott, Wiesbaden, Germany). For antibiosis the animals received daily subcutaneous injections of clindamycin-2-dihydrogenphosphate (45 mg/kg, Clindamycin, Ratiopharm, Germany) until the 3rd postoperative day. Penetrating the fascia lata between the gluteus superficialis and biceps femoris muscles the femur was exposed. The fixator was fitted in a cranio-lateral position using 4 mini-Schanz screws (Research Implant System, RIS, Davos, Switzerland), placing the 1st and 2nd screw proximal and distal of the trochanter tertius, respectively. In order to provoke regular or delayed bone healing a semi-rigid (axial stiffness 18.1 N/mm) or flexible (axial stiffness 0.82 N/mm) fixator was used [21]. A standardized osteotomy gap of 0.5 mm was created at the mid-shaft of the right femur in the middle between the inner screws by using a 0.45 mm Gigli saw. The muscles were sutured with absorbable (Vicryl, J&J, Norderstedt, Germany), and the skin with nonabsorbable thread (Resolon, Resorba, Nuernberg, Germany). All mice were allowed to move freely immediately post-surgery. Mice were sacrificed 10 or 21 days postoperatively using carbon dioxide inhalation.

Biomechanical testing

In order to determine the mechanical properties of the fracture callus the bending stiffness was analyzed by a non-destructive 3-point bending test after a healing period of 21 days as described before [21]. Briefly, the proximal end of the femur was fixed in an aluminum cylinder with SelfCem (Heraeus Kulzer, Hanau, Germany). The cylinder itself was fixed in a hinge joint, serving as the proximal support for the bending test. The femoral condyles rested on the bending support, the distance between both supports being 20 mm (l). The bending load F was applied on the midshaft and continuously recorded versus sample deflection (d) up to a maximum force of 5 N. Since the callus was not always located in the middle of the supports (l/2), the distances between the load vector and the proximal (a) and distal (b) supports were considered for calculating the bending stiffness $EI = k((a^2b^2)/3 \, l)$ [21].

μCT scanning

At day 21 post fracture the femora were imaged at a resolution of 30 μm, using a μCT Fan Beam Yscope System (Stratec Medizintechnik GmbH, Pforzheim, Germany) operating at a peak voltage of 40 kV and 140 μA. 3D reconstructions were visualized using 3D software (VG Studio Max 1.0; Volume Graphics, Heidelberg, Germany) and total volume (TV), maximum moment of inertia (I_{max}), and bone volume fraction (BV/TV) were measured after segmentation of the former osteotomy gap. Global thresholding was performed to distinguish between mineralized and non-mineralized tissue. The gray value corresponding to 25% of x-ray attenuation of the cortical bone of each specimen was taken as threshold [21].

Histology

The fracture calli harvested 21 days after surgery were processed for undecalcified histology. The bones were fixed in 4% formaldehyde, dehydrated by increasing ethanol concentrations and embedded in methyl methacrylate. 70 μm sections were cut and surface stained with Paragon (Paragon C&C, New York, NY). The newly formed callus was examined qualitatively and quantitatively under light microscopy (Axiophot; Zeiss, Oberkochen, Germany). The relative amounts of bone, cartilage, and soft tissue were determined at the osteotomy gap by the point counting method. Additionally, bony bridging of the fracture gap was evaluated in the histological slides at 4 positions at the fracture gap: anterior and posterior callus each peripherally (periosteal callus) and in between the cortices (intracortical callus). To describe the quality of bony bridging we used a scoring system (4 = complete bony bridging at all 4 locations; 3 = at 3 locations; 2 = at 2 locations; 1 = at 1 location; 0 = no bony bridging).

Additional fracture calli were harvested 10 days after surgery from rigidly fixated groups and processed for decalcified histology. The specimens were fixed in 4% formaldehyde, decalcified in 20% EDTA and embedded in paraffin. Longitudinal sections of 5–7 μm were stained by Giemsa (Merck, Darmstadt, Germany) and the relative amounts of osseous tissue, cartilage, and fibrous tissue were determined as described above.

Immunohistochemistry

Osteoclasts were identified by histochemical staining of tartrat-resistant acid phosphatase (TRAP) (Leucocyte Acid Phosphatase Kit, Sigma Aldrich Chemie GmbH, Steinheim, Germany) and counted in the whole peripheral callus. Additional paraffin sections were used for immunostaining of sphingomyelin phosphodiesterase 3 (Smpd3) by the use of a polyclonal anti-mouse Smpd3 antibody (Santa Cruz Biotechnology Inc., Heidelberg, Germany). To detect the primary antibody, labeled-streptavidin-biotin method (LAB-SA, Histostain-Plus Kit, Life Technologies GmbH, Darmstadt, Germany) was used and 3-amino-9-ethylcarbazole (AEC) was used as chromogen (Zytomed Systems, Berlin, Germany). The monoclonal non-phospho (active) β-catenin antibody (Cell Signaling, Danvers, MA, USA) and the polyclonal anti-collagen type II antibody (Rockland, Gilbertsville, PA, USA) were used together with the Vectastain ABC kit (Vector Laboratories, Burlingham, CA, USA) to detect the stabilized active form of endogenous β-catenin and collagen type II, respectively. Finally, counterstaining with hematoxylin (Waldeck, Münster, Germany) was performed. The sections were qualitatively evaluated under light microscopy.

Whole transcriptome analysis of the fracture callus

Three mice of each wildtype, $Lrp5^{-/-}$ and $Col1a1$-$Krm2$ with semi-rigidly fixated osteotomy were sacrificed 10 days after operation. Whole femur was dissected and immediately shock frozen in liquid nitrogen. Callus region (in the following referred to as callus) between 2nd and 3rd pin hole was homogenized using a knife-rotor homogenizer (T 10 basic ULTRA-TURRAX, IKA-Werke GmbH & Co. KG, Staufen, Germany). Total RNA was isolated with RNeasy Lipid Tissue Mini Kit (Qiagen, Hilden, Germany) according to manufacturer's instructions. Following amplification, labeling and fragmentation according to the Gene Chip 3′IVT Express Kit (Affymetrix, High Wycombe, United Kingdom), 10 μg of cRNA were hybridized on Affymetrix Gene Chips Mouse Genome 430 2.0. Hybridization signals were detected by Affymetrix Gene Chip Scanner 3000 and global normalization was performed by Affymetrix Gene Chip Operating Software 1.4 using the MAS5 algorithm. Normalized data of three calli of wildtype mice were crosswise compared to three calli of $Lrp5^{-/-}$ mice and $Col1a1$-$Krm2$ mice, respectively. Statistical analysis was performed by Partek Genomic Suite (Partek Incorporated, St. Louis, USA) using ANOVA test with multiple testing corrections. The complete data were deposited in NCBI's Gene Expression Omnibus (GEO, http://www.ncbi.nlm.nih.gov/geo/) and are accessible through GEO SuperSeries accession number GSE51686. Differential gene expression in the comparisons $Lrp5^{-/-}$ versus wildtype and $Col1a1$-$Krm2$ versus wildtype was regarded as significantly reliable when gene products (probe sets) fulfilled the following criteria: present calls in all three samples of at least one of the compared groups; change p-value <0.002 for the increased expression and p-value >0.998 for the decreased expression in at least 7 of the 9 cross-comparisons. Categorization of genes into functional groups was done by using Gene Ontology (GO) classification. (http://www.geneontology.org/).

Quantitative real-time PCR

For cDNA synthesis we used 1 μg of total RNA of fracture calli harvested from wildtype mice (n = 6), $Lrp5^{-/-}$ mice (n = 6) and $Col1a1$-$Krm2$ mice (n = 5) including the 3 RNA samples of microarray hybridization. Reverse transcription was performed with Oligo(dT)15 primers (Peqlab Biotechnologie GmbH, Erlangen, Germany) using MMLV reverse transcriptase (Promega GmbH, Mannheim, Germany) according to the manufacturer's instructions. Quantitative real-time PCR (qPCR) was performed using KAPA SYBR FAST Universal 2xqPCR Master Mix (Peqlab Biotechnologie GmbH) and 0.25pmol of sequence specific primers obtained from biomers.net GmbH (Ulm, Germany) (Table 1). Results were calculated with the efficiency-corrected Ct model

Table 1. Quantitative PCR primer sequences.

Gene name	Forward primer (5'-3')	Reverse primer (5'-3')	NCBI Accession No.
Alpl	aacccagacacaagcattcc	gagagcgaagggtcagtcag	NM_007431.2
B2m	gtctttctggtgcttgtctc	agttcagtatgttcggcttc	NM_009735.3
Col1a1	ggcaagaatggagatgatgg	accatccaaaccactgaagc	NM_007742.3
Cyclin D1	ttgactgccgagaagttgtg	ctggcattttggagaggaag	NM_007631.2
Cyclin E1	acagcttggatttgctggac	actgtctttggaggcaatgg	NM_007633.2
Pth1r	accccgagtctaaagagaac	taaatgtaatcgggacaagg	NM_001083936.1
Tnfrsf11b	tgttccggaaacagagaagc	actctcggcattcactttgg	NM_008764.3

[22] with B2m as the house-keeping gene. Groups were compared with non-parametrical Mann-Whitney U test.

Statistics

The statistical methods used for analysis of the microarrays and qPCR were already described in the corresponding paragraphs above. Results are presented as mean and standard deviation (SD). The number of animals included in the different groups (three genotypes with either flexible or more rigid fixation) is indicated in the legends. Biomechanical, μCT, and histochemical data of the groups were compared with non-parametrical Mann-Whitney U test using PASW Statistics 18.0 software (SPSS Inc., Chicago, USA). Level of significance was $p \leq 0.05$.

Results

Alterations in fracture healing do not result from differing limb loading

In order to exclude that alterations in bone healing result from differing mechanical stimuli acting on the regenerating tissue we recorded the ground reaction forces of the operated limb and the activity of the $Lrp5^{-/-}$ and $Col1a1$-$Krm2$ mice. The activity of the animals decreased postoperatively to about 70% of the preoperative value and then tended to increase to preoperative values with regard to wildtype mice (Fig. 1A). On average, the activities of $Lrp5^{-/-}$ and $Col1a1$-$Krm2$ mice did not seem to reach these values. However, there were no significant differences between the three genotypes. The ground reaction forces of the operated limb postoperatively declined by about 20% and remained at this level

during the entire healing period (Fig. 1B). We could not detect any significant differences between the genotypes. It can therefore be suggested that the osteoporotic mice loaded the operated limb properly, ensuring that alterations in bone healing are caused by the genotype and not by differing mechanical conditions in the fracture gap.

Krm2 overexpression in osteoblasts and Lrp5 deficiency impair regular fracture healing

To investigate fracture healing under better mechanical conditions we used a semi-rigid fixator, which has previously been shown to allow fast bone healing by promoting intramembranous with respect to endochondral bone formation [21]. As one important parameter for successful fracture healing we assessed the mechanical competence of both, the healed femurs at day 21 post fracture, the time point of bony bridging of the gap, as well as of the contralateral intact femurs. The stiffness of the intact $Lrp5^{-/-}$ and $Col1a1$-$Krm2$ femurs was significantly decreased compared to the wildtype confirming their osteoporotic phenotype [6,7] (Fig. 2A). The stiffness of the healed femurs was considerably reduced, by 50% in $Lrp5^{-/-}$-deficient mice and by 58% in $Col1a1$-$Krm2$ transgenic mice compared to wildtype controls (Fig. 2A). By comparing the stiffness of the osteotomized to the intact femurs we found that healed bones did not reach the mechanical competence of the intact bones in all mice strains at this time point of evaluation. The relative stiffness was most decreased in $Col1a1$-$Krm2$ mice (Fig. 2A). These data were confirmed by the semiquantitative assessment of bony bridging of the osteotomy gaps. Whereas most of the wildtype mice exhibited

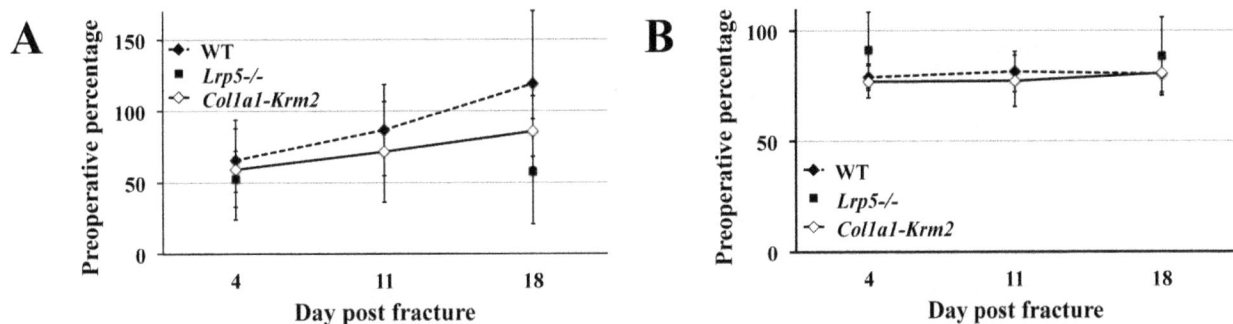

Figure 1. The different genotypes do not affect limb loading during fracture healing. (A) Motion of the mice was measured pre- and postoperatively using an infrared beam detection system. (B) Peak vertical ground reaction forces of the operated limb were recorded during movement of the mice using a force plate. n = 3–7 randomly selected mice per group (wildtype: dashed line (n = 7), $Lrp5^{-/-}$: without line (n = 3), $Col1a1$-$Krm2$: black line (n = 6)). Postoperative values were related to preoperative measurements. Data are expressed as means ± SD.

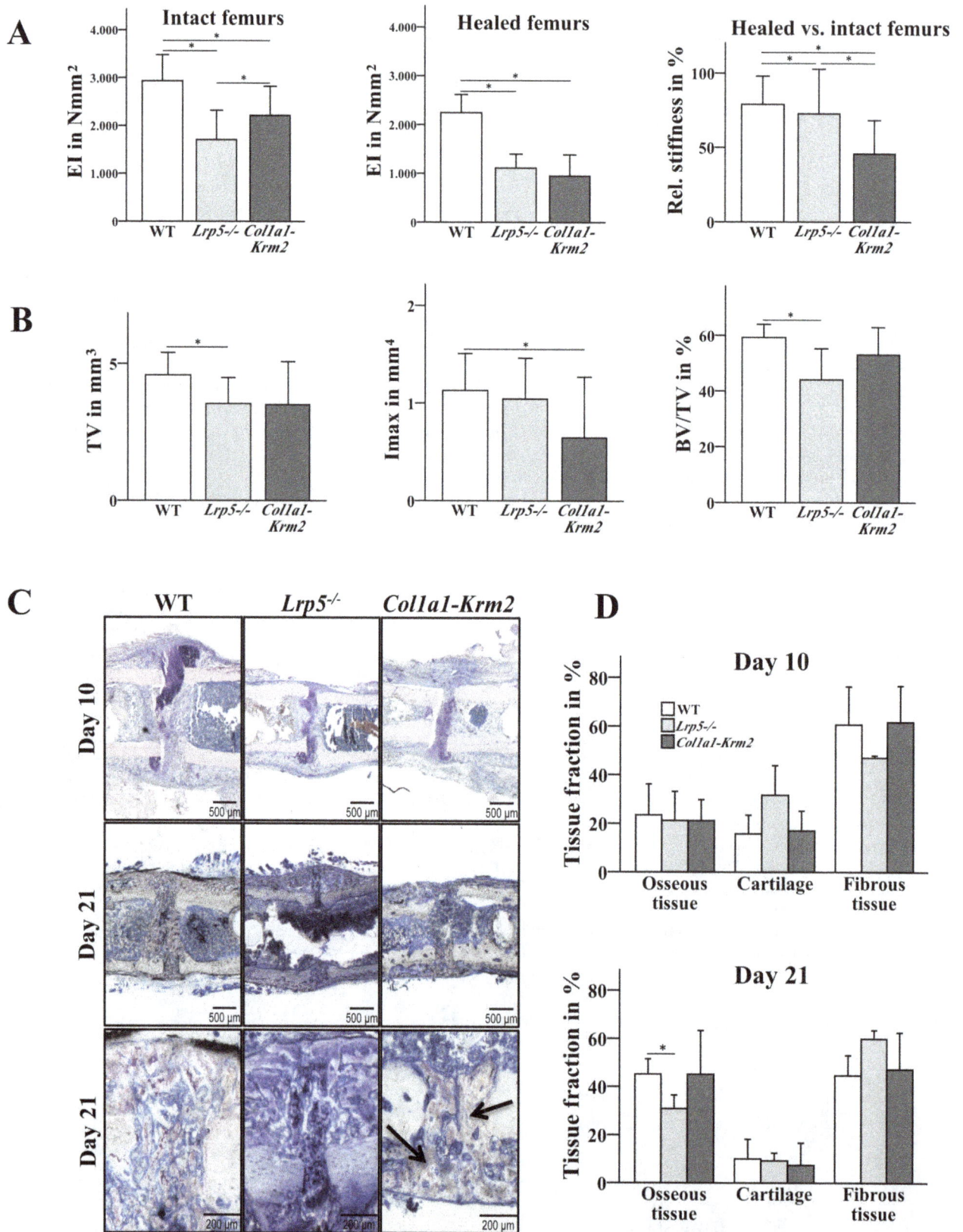

Figure 2. *Krm2* overexpression in osteoblasts and *Lrp5* deficiency impair regular fracture healing. The fractured femurs of wildtype, *Col1a1-Krm2* and *Lrp5*[−/−] mice were stabilized using a semi-rigid fixator in order to provide better mechanical healing conditions as described in the Material and Methods section. (A) In order determine the mechanical competence of the femurs the stiffness of both intact and fractured femurs was measured. Wildtype (n = 8), *Lrp5*[−/−] (n = 9), *Col1a1-Krm2* (n = 7) ± SD * $p<0.05$. (B) μCT analysis was performed to measure callus volume (TV), maximum moment of inertia (Imax) and bone volume fraction (BV/TV). Wildtype (n = 8), *Lrp5*[−/−] (n = 7), *Col1a1-Krm2* (n = 7) ± SD. * $p<0.05$ versus

wildtype. (C) For histological analysis, the paraffin sections of the calli were stained with Giemsa at day 10 post fracture. Sections of methacrylate embedded calli were stained with Paragon at day 21 post fracture. The black arrows indicate crude and less branched bone trabeculae in the callus of *Col1a1-Krm2* mice (D) Histomorphometric evaluation was performed to quantify total osseous tissue, cartilage, and fibrous tissue in the callus at day 10 and 21 post fracture. Wildtype (n = 8), *Lrp5*$^{-/-}$ (n = 5), *Col1a1-Krm2* (n = 5) ± SD. * p<0.05 versus wildtype.

complete bony bridging in the rigidly fixated groups, bridging was less successful in osteoporotic mice with the poorest results in *Col1a1-Krm2* mice (Table 2).

μCT measurements of the fracture calli revealed that the geometrical parameters (total callus volume, maximum moment of inertia) were slightly decreased in the rigidly fixated osteoporotic mouse strains compared to wildtype controls indicating inferior callus formation (Fig. 2B). The relative amount of mineralized tissue in the osteotomy gap (BV/TV) was significantly decreased in *Lrp5*$^{-/-}$ mice but not in *Col1a1-Krm2* mice indicating that the *Col1a1-Krm2* transgenic callus was small but transformed to mineralized tissue (Fig. 2B).

Histologically, we found a lot of cartilage near the osteotomy gap after 10 days, indicating secondary bone formation at this location. Intramembranous bone formation started near the periosteum in some distance to the gap (Fig. 2C). The pattern of tissue distribution was similar in all groups with the more rigid fixation. The histomorphometric data revealed no differences in the relative amount of bone and cartilage after 10 days (Fig. 2D). After 21 days, cartilage and fibrous tissue were decreased in favor of newly formed bone in all mice. Confirming the μCT data, the bone fraction was reduced in *Lrp5*$^{-/-}$ but not in *Col1a1-Krm2* mice. The newly formed bone trabeculae in the callus of the *Col1a1-Krm2* transgenic mice appeared crude and less branched and the osteoblasts covering the bone surfaces displayed an irregular morphology. These morphological abnormalities were not observed in *Lrp5*$^{-/-}$ mice (Fig. 2C).

Fracture healing is more strongly impaired in *Col1a1-Krm2* mice than in *Lrp5*$^{-/-}$ mice

In the used mouse model, flexible fracture fixation provoked the formation of a large callus with inferior mechanical competence indicating delayed bone healing with predominantly endochondral bone formation [21]. The mechanically induced delay of fracture healing was also observed in *Lrp5*$^{-/-}$ and *Col1a1-Krm2* mice. The flexibilization of the fracture fixation reduced the callus stiffness by about 25% in wildtype as well as in *Lrp5*$^{-/-}$ mice with no significant differences between both genotypes, and by 46% in *Col1a1-Krm2* mice (Fig. 3A). The bony bridging of the callus was poor, particularly in the osteoporotic mice (Table 2). μCT analysis revealed that total callus volume and maximum moment of inertia were more than doubled in all flexibly fixated mice compared to the rigidly fixated groups with no significant differences between the genotypes (Fig. 3A). However, the mineralized fraction (BV/TV) of the calli of all genotypes was significantly decreased compared to the rigidly fixated groups indicating inferior bone formation under flexible conditions. Being in line with the mechanical data the reduction of the mineralized tissue fraction was most pronounced in the *Col1a1-Krm2* transgenic mice (Fig. 3B). The histomorphometrical data confirmed the μCT data (Fig. 3C, D). The cartilage fraction in the *Lrp5*$^{-/-}$ calli was reduced compared to *Col1a1-Krm2* and wildtype mice indicating reduced endochondral bone formation. This suggestion was supported by a lower expression of collagen type II in the calli of *Lrp5*$^{-/-}$ mice compared to *Col1a1-Krm2* and wild-type mice (Fig. 3E). Taken together the results revealed that bone healing was most compromised in *Col1a1-Krm2* mice under mechanically unstable conditions.

Identification of differentially expressed genes in fracture calli of *Lrp5*$^{-/-}$ and *Col1a1-Krm2* mice

To identify genes that may be responsible for the observed greater impairment of healing in *Col1a1-Krm2* mice compared to that in *Lrp5*$^{-/-}$ mice, we performed microarray analysis of three independent callus samples from each mouse strain in the semi-rigidly fixated group. We collected the samples 10 days after surgery, because endochondral and intramembraneous bone formation took place and β-catenin-mediated transcription has been shown to be active at this time point [13]. Gene expression profiles of *Lrp5*$^{-/-}$ and *Col1a1-Krm2* mice were each compared to wildtype mice. We obtained 121 differentially expressed gene products in calli of *Lrp5*$^{-/-}$ mice and 829 differentially expressed gene products in *Col1a1-Krm2* mice (Fig. 4A, Table S1). Some of the gene expression changes were identical in both datasets and the overlap comprised 39 gene products with increased expression and 27 gene products with reduced expression (including osteoblast associated genes *Alpl* and *Pthr1*) in both, *Col1a1-Krm2* and *Lrp5*$^{-/-}$ calli. We focused on differentially expressed genes associated with bone/ossification and cartilage, to identify possible candidate genes for the decreased fracture healing potential we observed (Table 3).

We observed a markedly decreased expression of genes involved in chondrocyte and/or osteoblast differentiation as well as endochondral and intramembranous ossification, including *Egfr* [23], *Fgfr2* [24], *Mmp2* [25], *Mmp14* [26] and *Cd276* [27] in calli of *Col1a1-Krm2* mice, but not in Lrp5$^{-/-}$ mice. According to the results of the microarray hybridization, osteoblast marker *Col1a2* was significantly decreased in calli of *Krm2* over-expressing mice compared to wildtype. Another marker for osteoblastogenesis, *Alpl* was decreased in calli of *Col1a1-Krm2* transgenic and *Lrp5*$^{-/-}$ mice, whereas the microarray results did not reveal any reliable differences of other well-established osteoblast differentiation markers, such as *Runx2*, *Col1a1*, *Bglap* or *Spp1*.

We did not observe any alterations in the expression of *Tnfrsf11b*, which encodes for the RANKL antagonist osteoprotegerin that functions as an osteoclastogenesis inhibitor. The gene has been demonstrated to be regulated by canonical Wnt signaling [28] and was shown to be significantly reduced in primary osteoblasts of *Col1a1-Krm2* transgenic mice [6].

Furthermore, our microarray data of *Col1a1-Krm2* calli indicated a significant decrease of *Phex* [29] and *Smpd3* [30] (Table 3), genes described as down-regulated in primary osteoblasts of this mouse strain [6]. The decreased expression of *Smpd3* is in line with the reduced immunohistological staining of Smpd3 protein that we found in *Col1a1-Krm2* transgenic calli (Fig. 5C). In wildtype mice, Smpd3 was mainly present in osteoblasts in the peripheral callus and to a less extend in chondroblasts and precursor cells in the immature tissue in the osteotomy gap. Staining intensity and pattern was similar in *Lrp5*$^{-/-}$ calli. The sphingomyelinase Smpd3 and the product of its enzymatic action on sphingomyelin, ceramide, are inhibitory factors of bone resorption [31].

Increased expression of *Ctse* that encode for cathepsin E, respectively, indicates enhanced osteoclast activity or number in *Col1a1-Krm2* mice in comparison with wildtype mice [32]. Since it has been shown that canonical Wnt signaling affects bone

Table 2. Bony bridging of the fracture callus.

Fixation	Genotypes	Number of Mice with Score					Mean Score
		0	1	2	3	4	
Rigid	WT				2	5	3.7
	Lrp5−/−			3	2		2.5
	Col1a1-Krm2		1	4			1.8
Flexible	WT		2	2			1.5
	Lrp5−/−	1	3				0.7
	Col1a1-Krm2	1	3				0.7

Bony bridging of the fracture callus evaluated at 4 locations in the fracture callus: anterior and posterior callus peripherally (periosteal callus) and in between the cortices (intracortical callus). The quality of bone bridging was described by a scoring system (4 = complete bony bridging at all locations; 3 = at 3 locations; 2 = at 2 locations; 1 = at 1 location; 0 = no bony bridging). The table displays the number of mice with a distinct bridging score within the groups. n = 4–7 mice per group.

resorption, we analyzed osteoclast number in the calli of the three different genotypes. We found a significantly enhanced number of TRAP-positive osteoclasts in the peripheral callus of $Lrp5^{-/-}$ as well as *Col1a1-Krm2* mice (Fig. 5A, B).

Only few genes linked to cartilage were differentially expressed in comparison with wildtype, including Col11a1 that was decreased in $Lrp5^{-/-}$ mice (Table 3). Decrease of *Col11a1* indicates impaired cartilage collagen fibril formation and extracellular matrix formation [33], which may reflect impaired enchondral bone formation.

It was reported that the only genes whose expression was decreased in bone of $Lrp5^{-/-}$ mice were the regulators of cell proliferation *CylcinD1*, *D2* and *E1* [34]. We analyzed two of those genes by qPCR and did not detect differential expression in calli of $Lrp5^{-/-}$ or *Col1a1-Krm2* (Fig. 4B), which might be due to the different origin of the RNA used in our approach.

As β-catenin has been shown to be a key downstream mediator in canonical Wnt/β-catenin signaling (26), we analyzed the occurrence of active β-catenin in the calli of the different genotypes. Unphosphorylated stabilized β-catenin was predominantly present in osteoblastic cells lining the periosteum and newly formed trabeculae as well as in prehypertrophic chondrocytes. Staining intensity was lowest in *Col1a1-Krm2* calli (Fig. 5D). However, $Lrp5^{-/-}$ calli showed also decreased levels of active β-catenin in comparison with its occurrence in the calli of wild-type mice.

Discussion

In the present study, we investigated the influence of *Lrp5* deficiency and osteoblast-specific overexpression of *Krm2* in fracture healing using $Lrp5^{-/-}$ and *Col1a1-Krm2* mice. Our data indicated that fracture healing was highly impaired in both mouse genotypes, but that osteoblast-specific *Krm2* overexpression resulted in an even worse healing phenotype than *Lrp5* deficiency. Moreover, our data revealed that the stronger impairment of healing in *Col1a1-Krm2* was associated with decreased expression of genes mainly involved in osteogenesis.

Although various findings of mouse genetic studies demonstrated the crucial influence of Wnt signaling on bone mass maintenance, the precise biological role of the regulatory molecules in this process has not yet been fully elucidated. Thus, in particular the biological role of *Lrp5* in bone remodeling is controversially discussed [34,35]. Although a positive role has been reported for *Krm2* on *Lrp6*-mediated Wnt signaling, which is presumably facilitated through an interaction with the Wnt signaling agonists of the R-Spondin (Rspo) family [36], the antagonistic effect of Krm2 by binding to the Dkk1 receptors on canonical Wnt signaling has been well described already before [9].

In the present study on bone regeneration in $Lrp5^{-/-}$ and *Col1a1-Krm2* mice, biomechanical testing of the fracture calli of the semi-rigidly fixated groups and comparison of the stiffness of the fractured femur with the stiffness of the respective genotype-specific intact femur revealed a more impaired healing in *Col1a1-Krm2* mice than in $Lrp5^{-/-}$ mice. This fact was supported by analysis of bony bridging of the osteotomy gaps, which was poorest in the *Col1a1-Krm2* group. µCT analysis (bone tissue fraction, maximum of inertia, tissue volume) of the semi-rigidly fixated groups revealed that the calli of the *Col1a1-Krm2* and $Lrp5^{-/-}$ mice comprised a similarly decreased amount of mineralized tissue fraction, but *Col1a1-Krm2* calli seemed to be smaller compared to the calli of wild-type mice. Moreover, histological assessment of the fracture calli showed a stronger impairment of bone

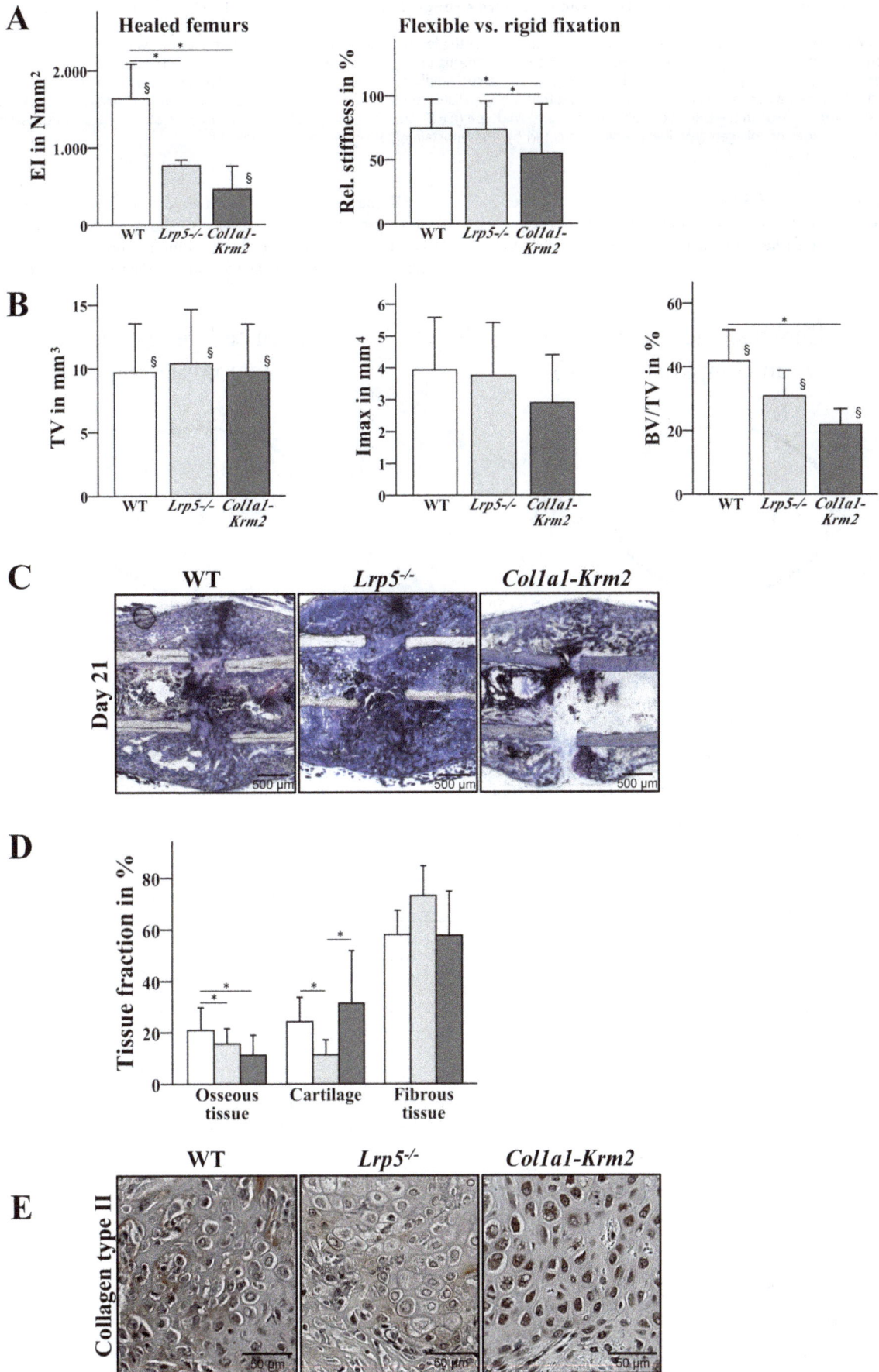

A

B

C

D

E

Figure 3. _Krm2_ overexpression in osteoblasts lead to a more strongly impaired healing than Lrp5 deficiency. The fractured femurs of wildtype, _Col1a1-Krm2_ and _Lrp5_$^{-/-}$ mice were stabilized using a flexible fixator in order to induce delayed healing as described in the Material and Methods section. (A) In order determine the mechanical competence of the femurs the stiffness of the fractured femurs was measured. (B) μCT analysis was performed to measure callus volume (TV), maximum moment of inertia (Imax) and bone volume fraction (BV/TV). Wildtype (n = 5), _Lrp5_$^{-/-}$ (n = 4), _Col1a1-Krm2_ (n = 7) ± SD. * p<0.05 versus wildtype. § p<0.05 versus rigidly fixated group. (C) For histological analysis, sections of methacrylate embedded calli were stained with Paragon at day 21 post fracture. (D) Histomorphometric evaluation was performed to quantify total osseous tissue, cartilage, and fibrous tissue in the calli at day 21 post fracture. Wildtype (n = 5), _Lrp5_$^{-/-}$ (n = 4), _Col1a1-Krm2_ (n = 5) ± SD. * p<0.05 versus wildtype. (E) Representative images of collagen type II expression detected by immunostaining at day 10 post fracture.

regeneration in _Col1a1-Krm2_ transgenic mice, as the bone trabeculae appeared crude and less branched and the osteoblasts covering the bone surfaces displayed an irregular morphology.

We have previously shown that both external fixators, which were used in the present study, allowed fracture healing under controlled rigid and flexible conditions, and that the more flexible fixation resulted in delayed bone healing compared to the more

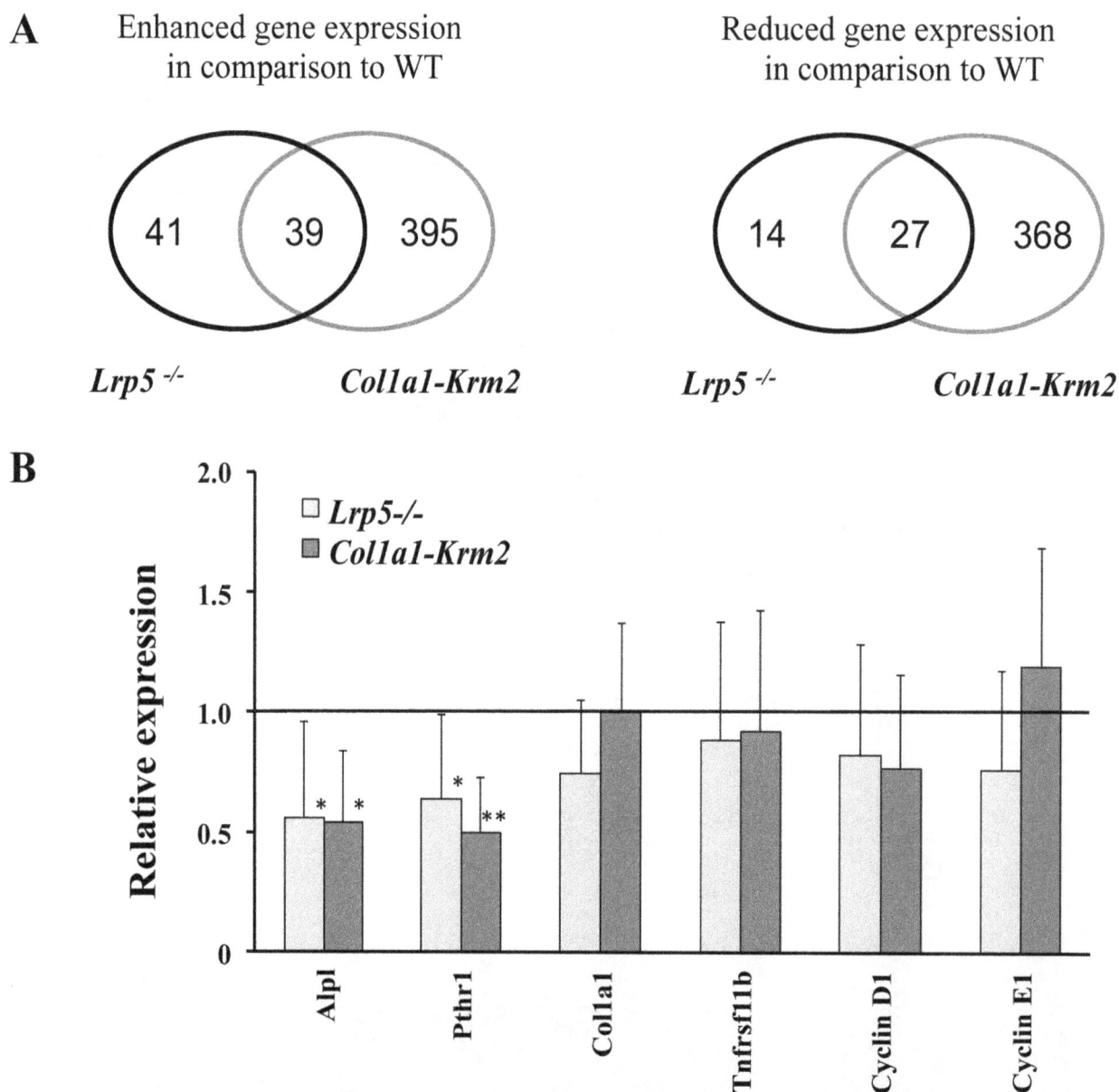

A Enhanced gene expression in comparison to WT

Reduced gene expression in comparison to WT

B

Figure 4. _Krm2_ overexpression in osteoblasts has a stronger effect on gene expression than _Lrp5_ deficiency. (A) The numbers indicate the number of gene products with significantly differential expression in calli of _Col1a1-Krm2_ and _Lrp5-/-_ mice in comparison to WT mice (for gene names see Table S1). (B) Relative changes in gene expression of osteoblast associated genes and Wnt target genes. QPCR was performed with samples prepared from callus tissue under semi-rigid fixation 10 days post-fracture. Gene expression in _Col1a1-Krm2_ mice and _Lrp5_$^{-/-}$ mice are expressed as fold change relative to wildtype mice. Wildtype (n = 6), _Lrp5_$^{-/-}$ (n = 6), _Col1a1-Krm2_ (n = 5) ± SD. * p<0.05, ** p<0.01.

Table 3. Candidate genes for impaired fracture healing in *Col1a1-Krm2* and *Lrp5*$^{-/-}$ mice.

| | | Microarray | | | | |
| | | | Col1a1-Krm2 (n = 3) | | Lrp5$^{-/-}$ (n = 3) | |
Gene	Gene Title	Probe set ID	FC	SD	FC	SD
Bone/Ossification						
Alpl	alkaline phosphatase, liver/bone/kidney	1423611_at	0.57	0.24	0.66	0.23
Cd276	CD276 antigen	1417599_at	0.58	0.19	_	_
Col13a1	collagen, type XIII, alpha 1	1422866_at	0.61	0.28	_	_
Col1a2	collagen, type I, alpha 2	1446326_at	0.66	0.27	_	_
Ctse	cathepsin E	1418989_at	4.22	2.38	_	_
Egfr	epidermal growth factor receptor	1435888_at	0.62	0.17	_	_
Fgfr2	fibroblast growth factor receptor 2	1433489_s_at	0.61	0.26	_	_
Lrrc17	leucine rich repeat containing 17	1429679_at	0.62	0.15	_	_
Mmp14	matrix metallopeptidase 14	1416572_at	0.54	0.21	_	_
Mmp2	matrix metallopeptidase 2	1439364_a_at	0.63	0.25	_	_
Pbx1	pre B-cell leukemia transcription factor 1	1440037_at	1.91	0.59	_	_
Phex	phosphate regulating gene with homologies to endopeptidases on the X chromosome	1421979_at	0.71	0.24	_	_
Pth1r	parathyroid hormone 1 receptor	1417092_at	0.60	0.39	0.66	0.33
Smpd3	sphingomyelin phosphodiesterase 3, neutral	1422779_at	0.52	0.18	_	_
Tgfb2	transforming growth factor, beta 2	1450923_at	0.56	0.26	_	_
Cartilage						
Aspn	asporin	1416652_at	0.55	0.16	_	_
Col11a1	collagen, type XI, alpha 1	1449154_at	_	_	0.77	0.23

Differential gene expression in callus tissue was analyzed 10 days post-fracture by microarray analysis (n = 3). Only gene products that fulfilled criteria for significant gene expression changes (see methods) are listed.
FC: mean value of fold changes of the cross-wise comparisons with wildtype callus (n = 3) as determined by microarray analysis.
SD: standard deviation.
_ no significantly differential expression when compared to wildtype callus (n = 3) as determined by microarray analysis.

rigid fixation [21]. In the present study the differences in healing between the two genotypes became particularly evident in mice in which the more flexible fixation was used. The more flexible fixation revealed a significantly reduced bone tissue fraction in *Col1a1-Krm2* mice compared to wild-type mice. These results are consistent with our histological findings regarding the amount of bone that was significantly more reduced in *Col1a1-Krm2* mice than in *Lrp5*$^{-/-}$ mice compared to wild-type mice, when using the more flexible fixation and consistent with the observation that *Col1a1-Krm2* mice exhibited a significantly more severe osteoporotic phenotype than *Lrp5*$^{-/-}$ mice that has been shown to be due to increased bone resorption as well as disturbed osteoblast maturation and bone formation [6,7]. Our data from the flexible group at day 21 indicated that cartilage tissue was significantly more increased in *Col1a1-Krm2* than in *Lrp5*$^{-/-}$ mice. We assume that in *Col1a1-Krm2* mice less bone tissue might result, at least in part, from increased cartilage production and mainly from reduced intramembranous bone formation. The differentiation of osteoblast precursor cells into the osteogenic lineage should be impaired by osteoblast-specific *Krm2* overexpression and instead these cells could convert into chondrogenic cells. These assumptions are in line with previous studies demonstrating that in osteoblast precursors lacking β-catenin osteogenic differentiation is inhibited and these cells develop into chondrocytes [17].

Ex vivo studies on *Col1a1-Krm2* osteoblasts suggested a cell-autonomous differentiation defect underlying the osteoporotic phenotype of *Col1a1-Krm2* mice and indicated a reduced Wnt3a-dependent activation of canonical Wnt signaling among other by decreased total β-catenin levels in *Col1a1-Krm2* osteoblasts compared to wild-type osteoblasts.

The latter finding is in line with the results of the present study because immunohistological validation of active β-catenin levels in the callus tissue revealed less active β-catenin in the calli of *Col1a1-Krm2* mice than in calli of wild-type mice. Active β-catenin was predominantly detected in cells surrounding the cartilage, in prehypertrophic chondrocytes as well as in osteoblasts lining the periosteum and the woven bone. Hypertrophic chondrocytes and osteoblasts, more deeply embedded in the bone matrix did not reveal significantly active β-catenin staining. The callus tissue of *Lrp5*$^{-/-}$ mice revealed a similar staining distribution to that in wild-type mice. However, in *Lrp5*$^{-/-}$ mice, overall active β-catenin staining was lower than in wild-type mice.

These findings are consistent with the results from a former study on bone regeneration in mice which provided evidence of active canonical Wnt signaling in intramembranous and endochondral ossification [37] and possibly account for the decreased intramembranous bone formation in *Col1a1-Krm2* and *Lrp5*$^{-/-}$ mice as well as the significantly diminished endochondral bone formation that was seen especially in *Lrp5*$^{-/-}$ mice with the more flexible fixation in the present study. Cartilage tissue was not significantly altered in *Lrp5*$^{-/-}$ mice treated with the more rigid fixation at day 10 of healing compared to *Col1a1-Krm2* and

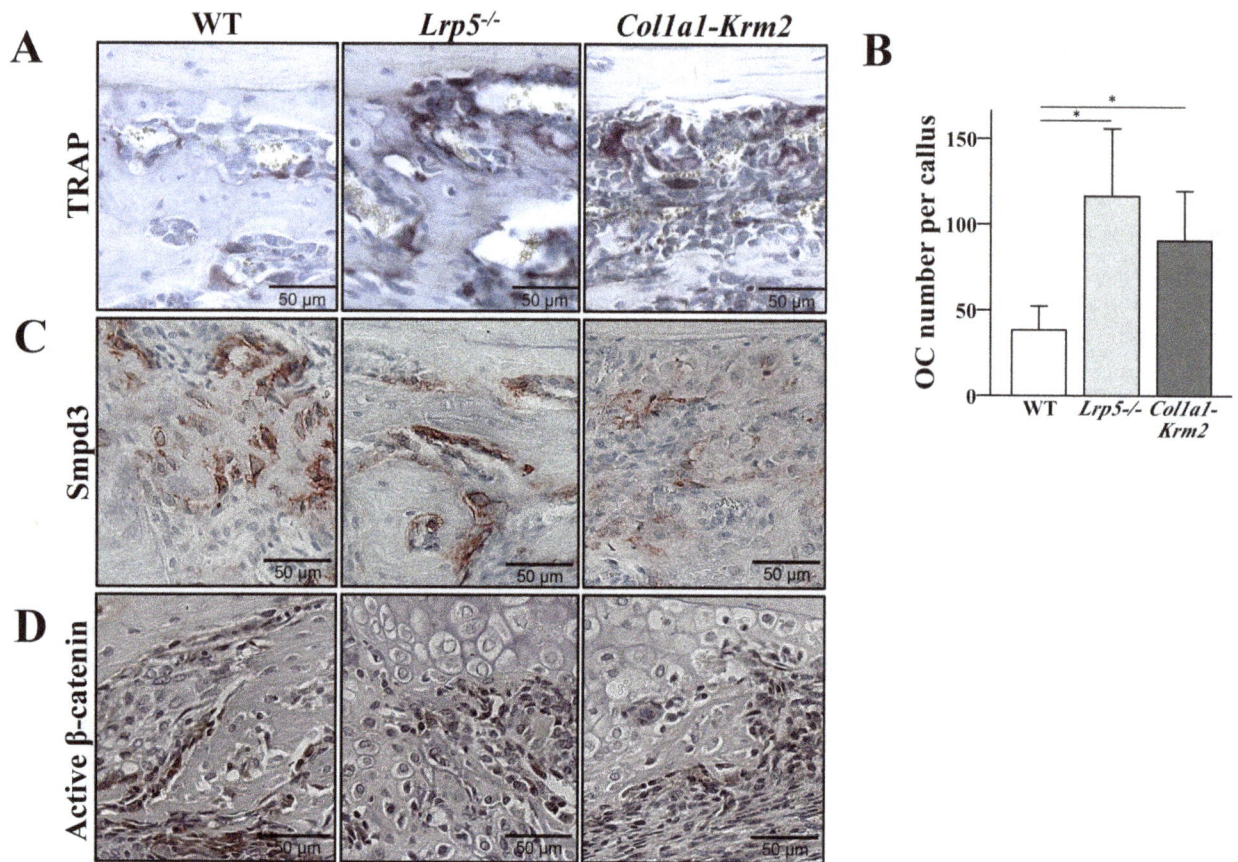

Figure 5. *Krm2* overexpression and *Lrp5* deficiency result in increased osteoclast number. (A) Osteoclasts were identified by histochemical staining of tartrat-resistant acid phosphatase (TRAP) at day 10 post fracture. (B) Osteoclast number was determined in the peripheral callus at day 10 post fracture. Wildtype (n = 6), *Lrp5*$^{-/-}$ (n = 4), *Col1a1-Krm2* (n = 5) ± SD. * p<0.05 versus wildtype. Representative images of (C) Smpd3 expression and (D) active β-catenin levels detected by immunostaining at day 10 post fracture.

wildtype mice. However, in *Lrp5*$^{-/-}$ mice with the flexible fixation cartilage tissue at day 21 was signficantly decreased compared to *Col1a1-Krm2* as well as to wildtype mice. This result suggests that *Lrp5* deficiency did not result in increased or prolonged cartilage production compared to *Col1a1-Krm2* and wildtype mice. Reduced bone tissue in these mice seemed to be due to decreased endochondral as well as intramembranous bone formation. This is in line with previous studies demonstrating that mice conditionally expressing β-catenin null alleles had a lack of bone as well as cartilage and showed immature mesenchymal cells persisting at the fracture sites [13]. Mesenchymal cells that begin to show phenotypic features of either chondrocyte or osteoblast precursors exhibit β-catenin mediated transcription [13]. Thus, *Lrp5*$^{-/-}$ mice that are characterized by mesenchymal stem cells with less β-catenin signaling due to Lrp5 deficiency showed less chondogenic as well as osteogenic tissue with the flexible fixation in the present study. We detected less staining of collagen type II in prechondrogenic mesenchymal stem cells and chondogenic cells in the calli of *Lrp5*$^{-/-}$ mice compared to *Col1a1-Krm2* and wildtype mice. The latter finding together with the altered staining for active β-catenin detected in the calli of *Lrp5*$^{-/-}$ mice suggests an important role for *Lrp5* as Wnt-coreceptor in endochondral bone formation.

It has been shown that Kremen proteins decrease Wnt/β-catenin signaling by binding to Dkk1 [9] and that Tnfrsf11b, the gene encoding the osteoclast-inhibitory factor Opg, being known

to be induced by canonical Wnt signaling in osteoblasts [28], is downregulated in *Col1a1-Krm2* mice [6], explaining the increased bone resorption and osteolytic lesions in the lower extremities in these mice. In contrast, bone resorption seemed to be unaffected in *Lrp5*$^{-/-}$ mice [7] and studies on mice expressing a mutant Lrp5 gene associated with high bone mass (HBM) demonstrated no significant changes in osteoclast number and function [4], suggesting that Lrp5 is not directly involved in regulating osteoclastogenesis and osteoclast activity. However, a more recent study showed an increase of the osteoclast surface in mice with a lack in Lrp5, implying that bone resorption might be affected by Lrp5 deficiency [38]. This would be consistent with our findings, which did not only reveal the expected significantly increased osteoclast number in the calli of *Col1a1-Krm2* mice, but also in the calli of *Lrp5*$^{-/-}$ mice, as assessed by histochemical staining of TRAP positive cells. In line with the results of Schulze et al. [6] regarding the expression of the sphingomyelinase *Smpd3*, that has been identified as an inhibitory factor of bone resorption [31] and has been shown to be downregulated in *Col1a1-Krm2* osteoblasts [6], we detected less expression of *Smpd3* in the calli of *Col1a1-Krm2* mice as verified by immunohistochemistry and microarray expression analysis. However, *Smpd3* expression did not seem to be decreased in the calli of *Lrp5*$^{-/-}$ mice. Nevertheless, the altered staining for active β-catenin in the fracture calli of *Lrp5*$^{-/-}$ mice suggests that *Lrp5* acts on canonical Wnt signaling in osteoblasts, which is compatible with the finding of a systemic influence of

Lrp5 on bone formation. Interestingly, patients suffering from a non-classical form of osteopetrosis, the autosomal dominant osteopetrosis type I (ADOI), which is caused by a specific gain-of-function mutation in the LRP5 gene and is associated with a high bone mass phenotype, have abnormally low number of osteoclasts *in vivo* [39]. Results from later studies on osteoclasts from theses patients strongly suggested that the specific ADOI phenotype is caused by the reduced ability of osteoblasts to support osteoclast development due to increased β-catenin-dependent *Opg* expression [40], implying that *Lrp5* might regulate canonical Wnt signaling and indirectly osteoclast differentiation by modulation *Opg* expression.

Skeletal defects in mice caused by *Lrp5* loss-of-function mutations manifest primarily during the postnatal period [7], whereas *Lrp6*-deficient mice are not viable, underlining the particular role of *Lrp6* in embryogenesis [41]. However, it has already been shown that *Lrp5* and *Lrp6* exert overlapping functions in the control of postnatal bone mass accrual [42–44], and since *Lrp5* and *Lrp6* are highly homologous and are coexpressed in primary osteoblasts it can be assumed that *Lrp6* is able to compensate for *Lrp5* function during some stages of osteoblast differentiation [35]. This compensation might be the reason for the less impaired healing that was observed in *Lrp5⁻/⁻* mice compared to *Col1a1-Krm2* mice in our study. Since *Krm2* is acting by binding to *Dkk1* that can inhibit Wnt signaling through a direct interaction with both, *Lrp5* and *Lrp6*, a poorer healing in *Col1a1-Krm2* mice might be expected due to a more pronounced decrease of bone formation and increased bone resorption in these mice. To address this hypothesis we performed microarray analysis, using RNA from calli of each mouse genotype to identify genes that might be responsible for the observed differences in healing in the two genotypes. In the calli of both mouse genotypes we observed a significantly decreased expression of genes associated with osteogenesis, including *Alpl* and *Col1α2*, however, more ossification-related genes showed decreased expression in the calli of *Col1a1-Krm2* mice. Moreover, expression of the gene, encoding the gastric aspartyl protease cathepsin E (*Ctse*) that has also been found to be expressed in active osteoclasts [32], was significantly upregulated only in the calli of *Col1a1-Krm2* mice, an observation that is in line with our finding of enhanced osteoclast

number in *Col1a1-Krm2* mice. The latter finding and the reduced expression of more osteogenesis-associated genes might at least be in part responsible for the more impaired bone healing observed in *Col1a1-Krm2* mice compared to *Lrp5⁻/⁻* mice.

In conclusion, our data underscore the important role of canonical Wnt signaling in bone formation as well as in drug targeting approaches, both in low bone mass diseases and in impaired fracture healing. Moreover, our data confirmed that activation of canonical β-catenin signaling as a therapy for fracture healing improvement should be restricted to mesenchymal precursor cells already committed to the osteogenic lineage. Since *Krm2* plays a crucial role in regulating bone formation, antagonizing KRM2 during a defined time of fracture healing might be an interesting option to improve fracture healing under compromised conditions, such as osteoporosis.

Supporting Information

Table S1 Differentially expressed gene products in fracture calli of *Col1a1-Krm2* and *Lrp5⁻/⁻* mice. Differential gene expression in callus tissue under semi-rigid fixation was analyzed 10 days post-fracture by microarray analysis (n = 3 each). Only gene products that fulfilled criteria for significant gene expression changes (see methods) are listed. FC: mean value of fold changes of the cross-wise comparisons with wildtype callus. SD: standard deviation. _ no significantly differential expression when compared to wildtype callus.

Acknowledgments

The authors thank Marion Tomo, Helga Bach, Jutta Meißner-Weigl and Melanie Krug for their skillful technical assistance.

Author Contributions

Conceived and designed the experiments: AI VR AL TS FJ. Performed the experiments: VR AL PB LKH. Analyzed the data: AL VR TS PB LKH JKL FJ AI. Contributed reagents/materials/analysis tools: AL VR TS PB RE LKH FJ JKL MA AI. Wrote the paper: AL AI.

References

1. Baron R, Kneissel M (2013) WNT signaling in bone homeostasis and disease: from human mutations to treatments. Nat Med 19: 179–192.
2. Gong Y, Slee RB, Fukai N, Rawadi G, Roman-Roman S, et al. (2001) LDL receptor-related protein 5 (LRP5) affects bone accrual and eye development. Cell 107: 513–523.
3. Zhang Y, Wang Y, Li X, Zhang J, Mao J, et al. (2004) The LRP5 high-bone-mass G171V mutation disrupts LRP5 interaction with Mesd. Mol Cell Biol 24: 4677–4684.
4. Babij P, Zhao W, Small C, Kharode Y, Yaworsky PJ, et al. (2003) High bone mass in mice expressing a mutant LRP5 gene. J Bone Miner Res 18: 960–974.
5. Hoeppner LH, Secreto FJ, Westendorf JJ (2009) Wnt signaling as a therapeutic target for bone diseases. Expert Opin Ther Targets 13: 485–496.
6. Schulze J, Seitz S, Saito H, Schneebauer M, Marshall RP, et al. (2010) Negative regulation of bone formation by the transmembrane Wnt antagonist Kremen-2. PLoS One 5: e10309.
7. Kato M, Patel MS, Levasseur R, Lobov I, Chang BH, et al. (2002) Cbfa1-independent decrease in osteoblast proliferation, osteopenia, and persistent embryonic eye vascularization in mice deficient in Lrp5, a Wnt coreceptor. J Cell Biol 157: 303–314.
8. van der Horst G, van der Werf SM, Farih-Sips H, van Bezooijen RL, Lowik CW, et al. (2005) Downregulation of Wnt signaling by increased expression of Dickkopf-1 and -2 is a prerequisite for late-stage osteoblast differentiation of KS483 cells. J Bone Miner Res 20: 1867–1877.
9. Mao B, Wu W, Davidson G, Marhold J, Li M, et al. (2002) Kremen proteins are Dickkopf receptors that regulate Wnt/beta-catenin signalling. Nature 417: 664–667.
10. Ellwanger K, Saito H, Clement-Lacroix P, Maltry N, Niedermeyer J, et al. (2008) Targeted disruption of the Wnt regulator Kremen induces limb defects and high bone density. Mol Cell Biol 28: 4875–4882.
11. Whyte JL, Smith AA, Helms JA (2012) Wnt signaling and injury repair. Cold Spring Harb Perspect Biol 4: a008078.
12. Chen Y, Alman BA (2009) Wnt pathway, an essential role in bone regeneration. J Cell Biochem 106: 353–362.
13. Chen Y, Whetstone HC, Lin AC, Nadesan P, Wei Q, et al. (2007) Beta-catenin signaling plays a disparate role in different phases of fracture repair: implications for therapy to improve bone healing. PLoS Med 4: e249.
14. Boland GM, Perkins G, Hall DJ, Tuan RS (2004) Wnt 3a promotes proliferation and suppresses osteogenic differentiation of adult human mesenchymal stem cells. J Cell Biochem 93: 1210–1230.
15. Ling L, Nurcombe V, Cool SM (2009) Wnt signaling controls the fate of mesenchymal stem cells. Gene 433: 1–7.
16. Hill TP, Spater D, Taketo MM, Birchmeier W, Hartmann C (2005) Canonical Wnt/beta-catenin signaling prevents osteoblasts from differentiating into chondrocytes. Dev Cell 8: 727–738.
17. Rodda SJ, McMahon AP (2006) Distinct roles for Hedgehog and canonical Wnt signaling in specification, differentiation and maintenance of osteoblast progenitors. Development 133: 3231–3244.
18. Li X, Grisanti M, Fan W, Asuncion FJ, Tan HL, et al. (2011) Dickkopf-1 regulates bone formation in young growing rodents and upon traumatic injury. J Bone Miner Res 26: 2610–2621.
19. Secreto FJ, Hoeppner LH, Westendorf JJ (2009) Wnt signaling during fracture repair. Curr Osteoporos Rep 7: 64–69.

20. Claes L, Augat P, Schorlemmer S, Konrads C, Ignatius A, et al. (2008) Temporary distraction and compression of a diaphyseal osteotomy accelerates bone healing. J Orthop Res 26: 772–777.

21. Rontgen V, Blakytny R, Matthys R, Landauer M, Wehner T, et al. (2010) Fracture healing in mice under controlled rigid and flexible conditions using an adjustable external fixator. J Orthop Res 28: 1456–1462.

22. Pfaffl MW (2001) A new mathematical model for relative quantification in real-time RT-PCR. Nucleic Acids Res 29: e45.

23. Zhang X, Siclari VA, Lan S, Zhu J, Koyama E, et al. (2011) The critical role of the epidermal growth factor receptor in endochondral ossification. J Bone Miner Res 26: 2622–2633.

24. Mansukhani A, Ambrosetti D, Holmes G, Cornivelli L, Basilico C (2005) Sox2 induction by FGF and FGFR2 activating mutations inhibits Wnt signaling and osteoblast differentiation. J Cell Biol 168: 1065–1076.

25. Mosig RA, Martignetti JA (2012) Loss of MMP-2 in osteoblasts upregulates osteopontin and bone sialoprotein expression in a circuit regulating bone homeostasis. Dis Model Mech.

26. Filanti C, Dickson GR, Di Martino D, Ulivi V, Sanguineti C, et al. (2000) The expression of metalloproteinase-2, -9, and -14 and of tissue inhibitors-1 and -2 is developmentally modulated during osteogenesis in vitro, the mature osteoblastic phenotype expressing metalloproteinase-14. J Bone Miner Res 15: 2154–2168.

27. Xu L, Zhang G, Zhou Y, Chen Y, Xu W, et al. (2011) Stimulation of B7-H3 (CD276) directs the differentiation of human marrow stromal cells to osteoblasts. Immunobiology 216: 1311–1317.

28. Glass DA, 2nd, Bialek P, Ahn JD, Starbuck M, Patel MS, et al. (2005) Canonical Wnt signaling in differentiated osteoblasts controls osteoclast differentiation. Dev Cell 8: 751–764.

29. The HYP Consortium (1995) A gene (PEX) with homologies to endopeptidases is mutated in patients with X-linked hypophosphatemic rickets. Nat Genet 11: 130–136.

30. Aubin I, Adams CP, Opsahl S, Septier D, Bishop CE, et al. (2005) A deletion in the gene encoding sphingomyelin phosphodiesterase 3 (Smpd3) results in osteogenesis and dentinogenesis imperfecta in the mouse. Nat Genet 37: 803–805.

31. Takeda H, Ozaki K, Yasuda H, Ishida M, Kitano S, et al. (1998) Sphingomyelinase and ceramide inhibit formation of F-actin ring in and bone resorption by rabbit mature osteoclasts. FEBS Lett 422: 255–258.

32. Yoshimine Y, Tsukuba T, Isobe R, Sumi M, Akamine A, et al. (1995) Specific immunocytochemical localization of cathepsin E at the ruffled border membrane of active osteoclasts. Cell Tissue Res 281: 85–91.

33. Li Y, Lacerda DA, Warman ML, Beier DR, Yoshioka H, et al. (1995) A fibrillar collagen gene, Col11a1, is essential for skeletal morphogenesis. Cell 80: 423–430.

34. Yadav VK, Ryu JH, Suda N, Tanaka KF, Gingrich JA, et al. (2008) Lrp5 controls bone formation by inhibiting serotonin synthesis in the duodenum. Cell 135: 825–837.

35. Cui Y, Niziolek PJ, MacDonald BT, Zylstra CR, Alenina N, et al. (2011) Lrp5 functions in bone to regulate bone mass. Nat Med 17: 684–691.

36. Kim KA, Wagle M, Tran K, Zhan X, Dixon MA, et al. (2008) R-Spondin family members regulate the Wnt pathway by a common mechanism. Mol Biol Cell 19: 2588–2596.

37. Zhong N, Gersch RP, Hadjiargyrou M (2006) Wnt signaling activation during bone regeneration and the role of Dishevelled in chondrocyte proliferation and differentiation. Bone 39: 5–16.

38. Iwaniec UT, Wronski TJ, Liu J, Rivera MF, Arzaga RR, et al. (2007) PTH stimulates bone formation in mice deficient in Lrp5. J Bone Miner Res 22: 394–402.

39. Bollerslev J, Marks SC, Jr., Pockwinse S, Kassem M, Brixen K, et al. (1993) Ultrastructural investigations of bone resorptive cells in two types of autosomal dominant osteopetrosis. Bone 14: 865–869.

40. Henriksen K, Gram J, Hoegh-Andersen P, Jemtland R, Ueland T, et al. (2005) Osteoclasts from patients with autosomal dominant osteopetrosis type I caused by a T253I mutation in low-density lipoprotein receptor-related protein 5 are normal in vitro, but have decreased resorption capacity in vivo. Am J Pathol 167: 1341–1348.

41. Pinson KI, Brennan J, Monkley S, Avery BJ, Skarnes WC (2000) An LDL-receptor-related protein mediates Wnt signalling in mice. Nature 407: 535–538.

42. Riddle RC, Diegel CR, Leslie JM, Van Koevering KK, Faugere MC, et al. (2013) Lrp5 and Lrp6 exert overlapping functions in osteoblasts during postnatal bone acquisition. PLoS One 8: e63323.

43. Holmen SL, Giambernardi TA, Zylstra CR, Buckner-Berghuis BD, Resau JH, et al. (2004) Decreased BMD and limb deformities in mice carrying mutations in both Lrp5 and Lrp6. J Bone Miner Res 19: 2033–2040.

44. Holmen SL, Zylstra CR, Mukherjee A, Sigler RE, Faugere MC, et al. (2005) Essential role of beta-catenin in postnatal bone acquisition. J Biol Chem 280: 21162–21168.

19

Raloxifene Prevents Skeletal Fragility in Adult Female Zucker Diabetic Sprague-Dawley Rats

Kathleen M. Hill Gallant[1,2]*, Maxime A. Gallant[1], Drew M. Brown[1], Amy Y. Sato[1], Justin N. Williams[1], David B. Burr[1]

1 Department of Anatomy and Cell Biology, Indiana University School of Medicine, Indianapolis, Indiana, United States of America, 2 Department of Nutrition Science, Purdue University, West Lafayette, Indiana, United States of America

Abstract

Fracture risk in type 2 diabetes is increased despite normal or high bone mineral density, implicating poor bone quality as a risk factor. Raloxifene improves bone material and mechanical properties independent of bone mineral density. This study aimed to determine if raloxifene prevents the negative effects of diabetes on skeletal fragility in diabetes-prone rats. Adult Zucker Diabetic Sprague-Dawley (ZDSD) female rats (20-week-old, n = 24) were fed a diabetogenic high-fat diet and were randomized to receive daily subcutaneous injections of raloxifene or vehicle for 12 weeks. Blood glucose was measured weekly and glycated hemoglobin was measured at baseline and 12 weeks. At sacrifice, femora and lumbar vertebrae were harvested for imaging and mechanical testing. Raloxifene-treated rats had a lower incidence of type 2 diabetes compared with vehicle-treated rats. In addition, raloxifene-treated rats had blood glucose levels significantly lower than both diabetic vehicle-treated rats as well as vehicle-treated rats that did not become diabetic. Femoral toughness was greater in raloxifene-treated rats compared with both diabetic and non-diabetic vehicle-treated ZDSD rats, due to greater energy absorption in the post-yield region of the stress-strain curve. Similar differences between groups were observed for the structural (extrinsic) mechanical properties of energy-to-failure, post-yield energy-to-failure, and post-yield displacement. These results show that raloxifene is beneficial in preventing the onset of diabetes and improving bone material properties in the diabetes-prone ZDSD rat. This presents unique therapeutic potential for raloxifene in preserving bone quality in diabetes as well as in diabetes prevention, if these results can be supported by future experimental and clinical studies.

Editor: Carlos M. Isales, Georgia Regents University, United States of America

Funding: This project was funded by a National Institutes of Health grant (AR047838) to DBB. The funders had no role in study design, data collection and analysis, decision to publish, or preparation of the manuscript.

Competing Interests: Raloxifene was provided by Eli Lilly and Co., Indianapolis, IN. DBB has received grants/research support from Eli Lilly and Co., and Amgen, served as a consultant/scientific advisor for PharmaLegacy, Wright Medical, Agnovos, and AbbieVie, and served as a speaker for the Japan Implant Practice Society. AYS has a family member who is a retired employee of Eli Lilly and Co. KMHG, MAG, DMB and JNW have no competing interests to declare. This does not alter the authors' adherence to PLOS ONE policies on sharing data and materials.

* Email: hillgallant@purdue.edu

Introduction

People with type 2 diabetes mellitus have a greater risk for bone fragility fractures compared with healthy adults, despite normal or higher bone mineral density [1–5]. This suggests that bone quality, not quantity, is responsible for the increase in fracture risk in diabetes. Raloxifene is a selective estrogen receptor modulator (SERM) used clinically in women to treat post-menopausal osteoporosis. Our group has previously shown that dogs treated with raloxifene have greater femoral and vertebral toughness, despite no significant effect on bone mineral density [6,7]. Similarly, in post-menopausal women, raloxifene decreases risk of fracture with little effect on bone mineral density [8–10]. This indicates that raloxifene improves bone resistance to fracture by affecting bone quality, and may therefore be an agent with potential to improve bone properties in diabetes where fracture risk is higher apparently due to reduced bone quality rather than reduced bone mass.

The Zucker Diabetic Sprague-Dawley (ZDSD) rat is a recently developed rodent model of type 2 diabetes crossbred from the diet-induced-obesity CD (Sprague-Dawley-derived) and lean Zucker Diabetic Fatty rats (ZDF$^{fa/+}$) [11]. Unlike the diabetic obese ZDF$^{fa/fa}$ rats, ZDSD rats do not have a leptin receptor mutation, and both sexes develop a type 2 diabetes phenotype of polygenic origin more gradually with age or by induction with a high-fat diet, thus reflecting more closely the pathogenesis of human type 2 diabetes [11,12]. This study aimed to test the effects of raloxifene on bone quality and strength in adult female ZDSD rats. Although we have shown positive effects of raloxifene on bone material properties in normoglycemic animals, no studies have been performed in a model subject to diabetes to determine whether raloxifene in a hyperglycemic environment will prevent increased skeletal fragility.

Materials and Methods

Animals and Experimental Design

Twenty-week-old female (n = 24) Zucker Diabetic Sprague Dawley (ZDSD) rats (PreClinOmics, Indianapolis, IN) were randomized (n = 12/group) to receive daily subcutaneous injections of raloxifene (0.5 mg/kg, Eli Lilly Co., Indianapolis, IN) or vehicle (10% cyclodextrin, Sigma-Aldrich) for 12 weeks, and all rats were fed a diabetogenic high-fat diet (48% fat; 5SCA, TestDiet, Richmond, IN) for the duration of the study. The high-fat diet is used to synchronize diabetes induction. Additionally, in contrast to male ZDSD rats that will develop diabetes with age even while on a normal rat diet[11], female ZDSD rats are more resistant to developing diabetes and require the high-fat diet for diabetes induction and to maintain the diabetic state. Blood glucose was measured weekly by glucometer (AlphaTRAK, Abbott Laboratories, Abbott Park, IL) and diabetes was defined as blood glucose $\geq$ 250 mg/dL for 2 consecutive weeks. Whole blood and serum samples were collected at baseline and sacrifice. Glycated hemoglobin (HbA1c,%) was measured in whole blood by immunological assay (Daytona Chemistry Anlayzer, Randox Laboratories, Kearneysville, WV). Serum insulin was measured by ELISA (Mercodia Inc., Winston Salem, NC) and serum triglycerides were measured by colorimetric assays (Daytona Chemistry Analyzer, Randox Laboratories, Kearneysville, WV). Serum c-telopeptide of type I collagen was measured by ELISA (Biotang Inc., Lexington, MA). Prior to sacrifice, rats were double-labeled by intraperitoneal injections of calcein (5 mg/kg; Sigma-Alrich, St. Louis, MO) with a 7-day interlabel period and a 3-day period for incorporation and washout (i.e. 1-7-1-3). Bones (femora, lumbar vertebrae) were collected at the time of sacrifice when rats were 32-weeks-old. Femora and L4 vertebrae were wrapped in saline-soaked gauze and frozen at −20°C for storage prior to bone imaging and mechanical testing; L5 vertebrae were cleaned of soft tissue and fixed in 10% phosphate-buffered formalin for 48 h, then transferred to 70% ethanol, dehydrated in a graded series of ethanol from 70–100%, then embedded (undecalcified and unstained) in methyl-methacrylate with 3% dibutyl phthalate (Sigma-Aldrich, St. Louis, MO) for dynamic histomorphometry. This protocol was approved by the Indiana University Animal Care and Use Committee, and all institutional and national guidelines for the care and use of laboratory animals were followed.

Bone Imaging

Dual-energy x-ray absorptiometry (DXA, GE Lunar PixiMus, Madison, WI) was performed on excised right femora and L4 vertebrae for measures of areal bone mineral density (aBMD g/cm^2), bone mineral content (BMC, g) and area (cm^2). Peripheral quantitative computed tomography (pQCT, XCT Research SA+, Stratec Medizintechnik GmbH, Pforzheim, Germany) was performed on the right femur midshaft for cortical bone morphometric properties (volumetric BMD (vBMD), BMC, cortical area and thickness, periostal and endosteal circumferences and x-axis cross-sectional moment of inertia). Micro-computed tomography (µCT, Brucker Skyscan 1172, Kontich, Belgium) was performed on L4 vertebral bodies and the right distal femur for cancellous bone morphometric properties. Scans were done at 8 µm resolution, 65 kV and 120 µA using a 0.7° rotation step. Reconstructed µCT images (NRecon software) were analyzed using CT Analyzer software (Skyscan, Kontich, Belgium). The same parameters/thresholds were used for each site for reconstruction and analysis. Outcome measurements included whole vertebral body bone volume (BV, mm^3), trabecular bone volume

fraction (BV/TV,% [where TV is tissue volume]), trabecular number (Tb.N, mm^{-1}), trabecular thickness (Tb.Th, mm), trabecular separation (Tb.Sp, mm), connectivity density (Conn.D, mm^{-3}), and structural model index (SMI).

Mechanical Testing

Mechanical properties of the femur mid-diaphysis were determined by three-point bending using standard methods [13]. Briefly, bones were thawed to room temperature, and placed posterior side down on the bottom support (18 mm wide) of a servohydraulic test system (100P225 Modular Test Machine, TestResources, Shakopee, MN), so that the descending probe contacted the central anterior surface. Bones were loaded to failure using a displacement rate of 2 mm/min. Force vs. displacement data was collected at 10 Hz. Material properties were calculated based on standard equations using structural mechanical properties and geometric measures from pQCT [13]. Reduced platen compression (RPC) was used to determine mechanical properties of cancellous bone on a 2 mm thick slab of distal femur (100P225 Modular Test Machine, TestResources, Shakopee, MN). For RPC, platen size was set at 70% of the maximum circle diameter to include only cancellous bone [6], which was determined by uCT scanning of the samples prior to mechanical testing. Tests were performed at 0.5 mm/min and data collected at 2 Hz until sample failure.

Mechanical properties of L4 vertebrae were determined by axial compression after removal of vertebral processes using a dremel tool with a minisaw attachment, and removal of the cranial and caudal endplates parallel to each other using a low-speed bone saw (Isomet, Buehler, Lake Bluff, IL). L4 vertebral bodies (+/- 3.5 mm height) were loaded at a rate of 0.5 mm/min until failure (100P225 Modular Test Machine) and data were collected at 10 Hz.

Structural mechanical properties of femoral cortical bone, L4 vertebrae and cancellous bone from the RPC testing were determined from the load-deformation curves using standard definitions. Material properties were calculated based on standard equations using structural mechanical properties and geometric measures from caliper measurements and pQCT (cortical bone) or µCT [13].

Bone Turnover

Bone turnover was measured by serum C-terminal telopeptides of type I collagen (Ctx) by EIA (RatLaps™, IDS, Inc.), and by dynamic histomorphometry of L5 vertebrae. Thin sections (approximately 6 µm) of the L5 vertebra were cut longitudinally with a microtome (Reichert-Jung SuperCut). Approximately 5 mm^2 of cancellous bone tissue 0.5 mm from the endocortical surface was analyzed from one section. Measurements were made at 200x magnification using a fluorescent microscope (Nikon Optiophot 2, Nikon, Inc., Garden City, NY) and images were analyzed using the Bioquant system (R&M Biometrics, Nashville, TN). All measurements and calculations were performed following the guidelines of the American Society for Bone and Mineral Research Histomorphometry Nomenclature Committee [14]. Parameters measured included single-label perimeter (sL.Pm), double-label perimeter (dL.Pm), and interlabel width (Ir.L.Wi). From these primary measurements, the following outcome parameters were calculated: mineral apposition rate (MAR = Ir.L.Wi/7 days [µm/day]); mineralizing surface (MS/BS = (0.5*sL.Pm + dl.Pm)/B.Pm*100 [%]); and bone formation rate (BFR/BS = MAR*MS/BS*365 [µm^3/µm^2/year]).

Statistical analyses

The planned two-way analysis of variance (diabetes and raloxifene as factors) was not possible because none of the raloxifene-treated rats became diabetic. Thus, one-way analysis of variance with Tukey's posthoc analysis was used to detect differences in means among the three groups: raloxifene-treated (RAL), vehicle-treated non-diabetic (VEH-ND), and vehicle-treated diabetic rats (VEH-D). Body weight was tested as a covariate for all measures and used for DXA variables and L4 BV/TV. Diabetes induction was analyzed by log-rank test of Kaplan-Meier survival curves and Fisher's exact tests. Statistical analyses were performed using SAS 9.2 software (Cary, NC) and significance was set at α 0.05. Values are presented as least squares means $\pm$ SEM unless otherwise noted.

Results

Rats randomized to receive raloxifene injections and vehicle injections had similar baseline body weight (mean $\pm$ SD: 342$\pm$14 and 348$\pm$23 g, respectively), blood glucose (mean $\pm$ SD: 114$\pm$7 and 112$\pm$12 mg/dL, respectively), HbA1c (mean $\pm$ SD: 4.5$\pm$0.3 [n = 11] and 4.5$\pm$0.1% [n = 9], respectively), serum insulin (mean $\pm$ SD: 0.50$\pm$0.26 [n = 6] and 0.47$\pm$0.36 [n = 10], respectively) and serum triglycerides (mean $\pm$ SD: 3.37$\pm$1.39 [n = 7] and 2.73$\pm$1.01 [n = 9]). After 12 weeks, none of the 12 rats treated with raloxifene became diabetic whereas 4 out of 12 rats that received vehicle injections became diabetic. By Fisher's exact test, the difference in diabetes frequency did not reach statistical significance (p = 0.09). However, by survival analysis of Kaplan-Meier curves, raloxifene significantly reduced diabetes induction (p = 0.03) (**Fig. 1a**).

At the time of sacrifice, vehicle-treated non-diabetic (VEH-ND) rats weighed more than both vehicle-treated diabetic (VEH-D) (p<0.0001) and raloxifene-treated (RAL) (p<0.0001) rats (**Table 1**).VEH-D rats had higher blood glucose over the course of the study, as determined by area-under-the-curve (AUC) compared with RAL or VEH-ND rats (p<0.0001) (**Fig. 1b,c**). Additionally, RAL-treated rats had lower cumulative blood glucose over the course of the study (AUC) than VEH-ND rats (p = 0.048) (**Fig. 1c**), but endpoint values were not significantly different between RAL-treated and VEH-ND rats (**Table 1**). At sacrifice, HbA1c was higher in VEH-D (p<0.0001) compared with RAL and VEH-ND rats. Serum insulin tended to be lower in the VEH-D rats compared with the VEH-ND and RAL-treated rats, but this was not significant. Serum triglycerides were higher in VEH-D rats compared with the RAL-treated rats (p = 0.02) (**Table 1**). Bone resorption measured by serum Ctx was similar among VEH-ND, VEH-D, and RAL-treated rats. However, dynamic histomorphometry showed non-significant trends for lower MS/BS (−28%) and BFR/BS (−26%) but higher MAR (+10%) in RAL-treated rats versus VEH-ND rats. Additionally, diabetic rats (VEH-D) had significantly lower MAR and non-significant trends for lower MS/BS and BFR/BS compared to the non-diabetic animals (VEH-ND or RAL-treated) (**Table 1**).

Areal bone mineral density and bone mineral content of the whole femur were lower in VEH-D compared with the other two groups (**Table 2**). There were no significant differences among groups for pQCT measures of the femoral midshaft. In the distal femur, bone volume normalized to tissue volume, trabecular thickness, and trabecular number were lower, and trabecular separation was higher in VEH-D rats compared with the other two groups, and structure model index was higher (more rod-like) in VEH-D compared with RAL rats (**Table 2**). There were no

significant differences among groups for DXA or μCT measures of L4 vertebrae (**Table 2**).

RAL-treated rats had greater energy to failure and post-yield energy to failure in femoral cortical bone compared with VEH-ND and VEH-D rats (**Table 3**). Correspondingly, the material-level properties of femoral toughness and post-yield toughness were also higher in RAL-treated rats (**Table 3**). There were no differences among groups in structure-level or material-level mechanical properties from vertebral axial compression (**Table 3**). RPC of the distal femur cancellous bone revealed greater energy to ultimate force in RAL versus VEH-D rats, and non-significant trends for greater toughness in RAL rats versus VEH-ND (p = 0.07) and VEH-D (p = 0.06) rats. Ultimate stress was significantly greater in RAL rats compared with VEH-D rats (**Table 3**). VEH-D rats had lower ultimate force and stiffness compared with RAL and VEH-ND, but the corresponding material property of modulus was not different among groups.

Discussion

This study showed that raloxifene treatment in female ZDSD rats improved blood glucose levels and showed a trend for prevention of type 2 diabetes while imparting a beneficial effect on bone material properties. While the frequency of diabetes between vehicle and raloxifene treated animals was not statistically different by Fisher's exact test, there was a significant difference by survival analysis using Kaplan-Meier curves. This is not conclusive but at least suggestive of a benefit of raloxifene for prevention of diabetes. The finding that raloxifene might prevent the onset of type 2 diabetes in ZDSD rats was an unexpected outcome of this study. A randomized controlled trial [15] found that raloxifene did not improve insulin sensitivity or glycemic control in postmenopausal women who had type 2 diabetes, and a post-hoc analysis [16] of the Multiple Outcomes of Raloxifene Evaluation (MORE) trial found no effect of raloxifene on glycemic control in postmenopausal women with or without diabetes, although a beneficial effect was found on serum lipids. However, these two studies did not evaluate the effect of raloxifene on diabetes onset. Conversely, our results are supported by experimental evidence on the effect of raloxifene on glucose homeostasis and diabetes: it has been shown that estradiol prevents pancreatic β-cell failure in diabetic rats fed a high-fat diet by suppressing fatty acid synthesis and accumulation within the β-cells through estrogen receptor signaling [17], and the same research group found similar results with raloxifene in an in vitro study [18]. Therefore, a potential mechanism by which raloxifene could prevent the onset or slow the progression of diabetes is by preventing pancreatic β-cell failure. Additionally, two recent clinical studies [19,20] found a beneficial effect of raloxifene on serum lipids in women with type 2 diabetes, further supporting a role beyond bone for raloxifene to improve health in people with diabetes.

The fact that none of the raloxifene treated animals became diabetic, while an interesting outcome in itself, was a limitation of this study as it precluded our ability to analyze the effects of raloxifene on bone in rats with established diabetes. However, we were able to show a benefit of raloxifene on bone toughness in a diabetes-prone rat model. While we have previously reported a positive effect of raloxifene on bone toughness in non-diabetic canines [6,7], this effect has not been previously shown in bones of normal rats [21,22]. It is possible the predisposition to diabetes in the ZDSD rats creates a therapeutic window for an effect of raloxifene on bone toughness that is not present in normal rats.

Another possible limitation of our study is that we did not include a ZDSD group on a normal diet. However, this would not

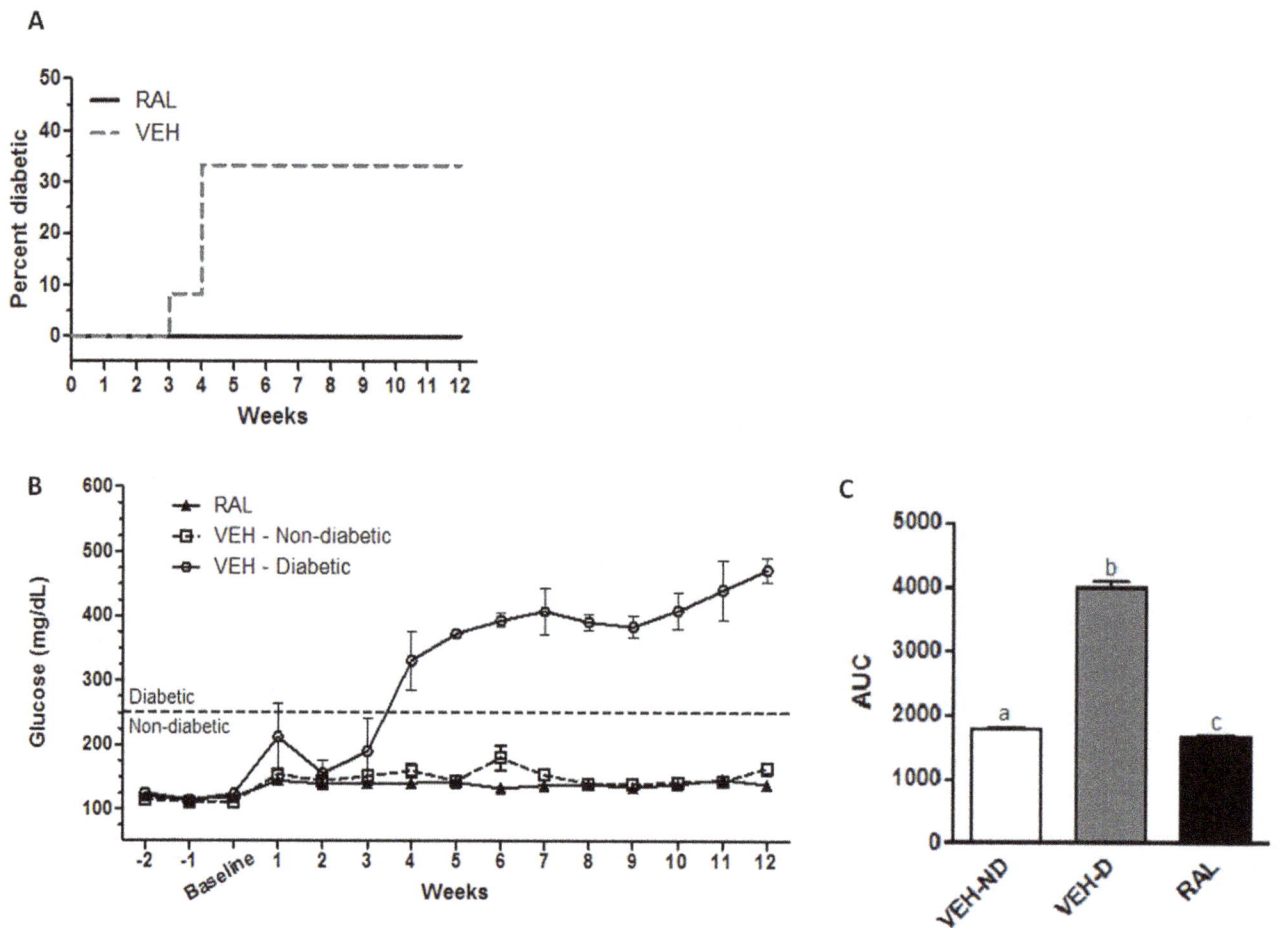

Figure 1. Diabetes Incidence and Glucose Levels in Raloxifene and Vehicle-Treated Rats. Panel A) Female ZDSD rats treated with raloxifene (RAL) had lower incidence of diabetes compared with vehicle treated rats (VEH) by survival analysis (p = 0.03) (shown), but by Fisher's exact test, the frequency of diabetes in VEH and RAL treated rats did not reach statistical significance (p = 0.09). Panels B,C) Over the course of the study, blood glucose was lowest in raloxifene treated rats (RAL), and highest in vehicle-injected rats that became diabetic (VEH-D), as assessed by area-under-the-curve (AUC). Different letters indicate differences in means with p<0.05.

Table 1. Body weight, metabolic parameters and bone turnover at end of study[a].

	VEH-ND (n = 8)		VEH-D (n = 4)[b]		RAL (n = 12)	
Body weight, g	532.5 (10.9)	a	411.0 (15.4)	b	417.8 (8.9)	b
Serum glucose, mg/dL	163.8 (8.0)	a	472.3 (11.3)	b	138.9 (6.5)	a
Blood HbA1c,%	4.8 (0.2)	a	10.3 (0.2)	b	4.7 (0.1)	a
Serum triglycerides, mg/dL	5.7 (0.7)	ab	7.7 (1.0)	a	4.4 (0.6)	b
Serum insulin, μg/L	3.6 (0.6)	a	1.8 (0.9)	a	3.2 (0.5)	a
Serum Ctx, ng/mL	19.6 (5.0)	a	34.9 (7.0)	a	23.9 (4.1)	a
L5 Histomorphometry						
MAR, μm/day	1.03 (0.11)	a	0.43 (0.18)	b	1.13 (0.10)	a
MS/BS,%	4.60 (0.85)	a	1.07 (1.39)	a	3.33 (0.76)	a
BFR/BS, μm³/μm²/year	18.27 (3.78)	a	2.13 (6.18)	a	13.52 (3.38)	a

[a]Different letters in each row indicate differences among groups by Tukey's post-hoc comparisons, p<0.05.
[b]n = 3 for VEH-D for the L5 histomophometry measures due to unavailable sample from 1 rat.

Table 2. Bone mass and microarcitecture of the femur and L4 vertebra from female ZDSD rats[a].

	VEH-ND (n = 8)		VEH-D (n = 4)		RAL (n = 12)	
Total Femur DXA						
aBMD, g/cm^2	0.249 (0.005)	a	0.224 (0.004)	b	0.246 (0.003)	a
BMC, g	0.626 (0.010)	a	0.574 (0.009)	b	0.619 (0.006)	a
Area, cm^2	2.51 (0.03)	a	2.56 (0.03)	a	2.51 (0.02)	a
Midshaft femur pQCT						
Ct. vBMD, mg/cm^3	1473 (2)	a	1467 (3)	a	1475 (2)	a
Ct. BMC, mg/mm	10.2 (0.1)	a	10.1 (0.1)	a	10.2 (0.1)	a
Ct.Ar, mm^3	6.90 (0.06)	a	6.89 (0.08)	a	6.90 (0.05)	a
Ct.Th, mm	0.86 (0.01)	a	0.85 (0.01)	a	0.85 (0.01)	a
Periosteal Circumference, mm	10.7 (0.08)	a	10.9 (0.11)	a	10.7 (0.07)	a
Endosteal Circumference, mm	6.02 (0.08)	a	5.99 (0.11)	a	6.01 (0.06)	a
Distal Femur μCT						
BV/TV,%	42.2 (2.2)	a	27.9 (3.2)	b	42.3 (1.8)	a
Tb.Th, mm	0.112 (0.003)	a	0.092 (0.005)	b	0.110 (0.003)	a
Tb.Sp, mm	0.170 (0.008)	a	0.206 (0.011)	b	0.171 (0.006)	a
Tb.N, #	3.75 (0.13)	a	3.02 (0.19)	b	3.83 (0.11)	a
Conn.Dn, #/mm^3	126.9 (6.4)	a	116.7 (9.1)	a	135.7 (5.3)	a
SMI, units	0.50 (0.20)	ab	1.32 (0.28)	b	0.39 (0.16)	a
L4 DXA						
aBMD, g/cm^2	0.127 (0.004)	a	0.125 (0.003)	a	0.129 (0.002)	a
BMC, g	0.025 (0.002)	a	0.024 (0.002)	a	0.025 (0.001)	a
L4 μCT						
BV/TV,%	38.6 (2.5)	a	40.7 (2.2)	a	42.6 (1.5)	a
Tb.Th, mm	0.102 (0.001)	a	0.097 (0.002)	a	0.102 (0.001)	a
Tb.Sp, mm	0.197 (0.008)	a	0.197 (0.011)	a	0.194 (0.006)	a
Tb.N, #	4.04 (0.14)	a	4.06 (0.19)	a	4.08 (0.11)	a
Conn.Dn, #/mm^3	97.2 (7.1)	a	96.8 (10.0)	a	100.4 (5.8)	a
SMI, units	0.22 (0.10)	a	0.22 (0.14)	a	0.18 (0.08)	a

[a]Different letters in each row indicate differences among groups by Tukey's post-hoc comparisons, $p < 0.05$.

have been a true control for the diabetes-prone rats because the effects of the different dietary composition on bone's material properties are not known. Moreover, we did not use CD rats which are sometimes used as non-diabetic controls. CD rats are not prone to diabetes even on a high fat diet, but are prone to obesity, and would introduce additional weight-related variables that could affect BMD or other mechanical properties of bone.

The effect of raloxifene on bone toughness was significant only for the femur, representing an effect on cortical bone, but a near-significant trend for greater toughness with raloxifene treatment was also observed for the distal femur by RPC, indicating a possible effect on cancellous bone as well. Our previous canine studies showed a beneficial effect of raloxifene on toughness in both cortical and cancellous bone [6,7]. Because cortical bone turnover is relatively slow [23], the effect of raloxifene on cortical bone toughness implies a direct effect of raloxifene on the existing bone material, rather than on newly formed bone. Furthermore, intracortical remodeling does not normally occur in rats and does not occur in the ZDSD rats. One mechanism by which raloxifene may improve toughness is by altering the hydration of the bone. We have shown that bone beams carved from human and dog cortical bone, when soaked in a raloxifene solution, have greater

toughness and that this is associated with higher water content of the bone [24]. Greater toughness and hydration were also observed in cortical bone beams from dogs treated *in vivo* with raloxifene for 1 year [24].

Additionally, our previous canine study showed no effect of raloxifene on BMD, which corresponds to clinical data from raloxifene trials in which fracture risk is reduced with little change in BMD [8–10]. Similarly, in the present study of diabetes-prone ZDSD rats, treatment with raloxifene resulted in greater femoral toughness without an effect on BMD, suggesting that raloxifene affects bone strength by improving bone quality rather than quantity. Because people with type 2 diabetes often have normal or high bone mineral density, the increased fracture risk observed in these patients appears to be due to impaired bone quality rather than reduced bone quantity. However, in this study, diabetic rats actually had lower bone density and mass compared with non-diabetic rats. This difference between human type 2 diabetes and the ZDSD rat model might be explained as follows: in humans with type 2 diabetes, overweight and obesity often persist after the onset of diabetes, and excess body weight may be protective of bone mass through mechanical loading or the positive effects of leptin and estrogen produced by adipose tissue. Conversely,

Table 3. Structure-level and material-level mechanical properties of femoral cortical and cancellous bone and L4 cancellous bone from female ZDSD rats[a].

	VEH-ND (n = 8)[b]		VEH-D (n = 4)		RAL (n = 12)[c]	
Femur 3-point bending (cortical bone)						
Structure-level						
Ultimate Force, N	135.1(2.7)	a	135.6 (3.6)	a	142.7 (2.1)	a
Stiffness, N/mm	342.4 (11.1)	a	346.8 (14.7)	a	342.4 (8.5)	a
Energy to Failure, mJ	46.0 (2.9)	a	43.7 (3.8)	a	57.4 (2.2)	b
Post-Yield Energy to Failure, mJ	26.5 (3.0)	a	23.5 (4.0)	a	36.6 (2.3)	b
Post-Yield Displacement, mm	0.210 (0.023)	a	0.187 (0.030)	a	0.275 (0.017)	a
Material-level						
Ultimate Stress, MPa	61.4 (1.6)	a	61.3 (2.1)	a	65.0 (1.2)	a
Elastic Modulus, MPa	2683 (92)	a	2724 (122)	a	2691 (70)	a
Toughness, mJ/m^3	1.21 (0.08)	a	1.13 (0.10)	a	1.51 (0.06)	b
Post-Yield Toughness, mJ/m^3	0.69 (0.07)	a	0.61 (0.10)	a	0.96 (0.06)	b
Distal femur RPC (cancellous bone)[b]						
Structure-level						
Ultimate Force, N	21.5 (2.3)	a	7.3 (3.1)	b	23.7 (1.9)	a
Stiffness, N/mm	239.4 (16.8)	a	142.6 (22.3)	b	249.1 (14.1)	a
Energy to Ultimate Force, mJ	1.41 (0.89)	ab	0.26 (1.18)	a	4.16 (0.75)	b
Material-level						
Ultimate Stress, MPa	20.6 (2.5)	ab	13.6 (3.4)	a	27.6 (2.1)	b
Modulus, MPa	400.7 (51.6)	a	474.5 (68.3)	a	534.8 (43.2)	a
Toughness, mJ/m^3	0.68 (0.55)	a	0.25 (0.73)	a	2.40 (0.46)	a
L4 axial compression (cancellous bone)						
Structure-level						
Ultimate Force, N	369.9 (18.9)	a	317.3 (25.0)	a	350.4 (15.1)	a
Stiffness, N/mm	1739 (117)	a	1476 (155)	a	1793 (93)	a
Energy to Ultimate Force, mJ	46.6 (3.2)	a	40.9 (4.2)	a	41.1 (2.5)	a
Material-level						
Ultimate Stress, MPa	2.27 (0.12)	a	2.11 (0.16)	a	2.22 (0.10)	a
Modulus, MPa	1175 (93)	a	1060 (123)	a	1269 (74)	a
Toughness, mJ/mm^3	2.51 (0.13)	a	2.28 (0.17)	a	2.31 (0.10)	a

[a]Different letters in each row indicate differences among groups by Tukey's post-hoc comparisons, $p < 0.05$.
[b]n = 7 for VEH-ND for distal femur RPC, L4 axial compression, and femur 3-point bending measures, due to specimens breaking during preparation or unavailable sample.
[c]n = 10 for RAL for the distal femur RPC measures and n = 11 for RAL for L4 axial compression measures, due to specimens breaking during preparation.

ZDSD rats gain weight with the high fat diet until the onset of diabetes, after which they begin to lose body weight due to the catabolic state produced by the diabetes. Indeed, diabetic rats in the present study had significantly lower body weight at the time of sacrifice compared with non-diabetic animals, and this may be associated with their lower BMD.

The results did not show lower bone resorption as measured by serum CTX in the raloxifene treated rats. However, the numerically lower BFR/BS and MS/BS with raloxifene treatment (−26% and −27% respectively in RAL versus VEH-ND rats) supports that the raloxifene treatment had an effect on reducing bone turnover. The non-significant differences are not surprising given this study was not powered to detect differences in these outcomes, and that raloxifene is a relatively weak antiresorptive agent [25]. However, the magnitude of the difference in BFR/BS with raloxifene treatment is similar to what we previously observed in dogs [7]. Additionally, the rats in this study were not ovariectomized, which also may have reduced our ability to detect a significant antiresorptive effect of raloxifene. The rats that became diabetic (VEH-D) had a lower bone formation rate, which is consistent with reduced bone observed in humans and animals with diabetes [26]. Despite the lack of significant differences in bone turnover measures with raloxifene treatment, our results show that raloxifene improves bone material properties, potentially through direct action of raloxifene on the bone matrix, and may prevent the induction of diabetes in female ZDSD rats. The risk of diabetes increases with age [27], as does the risk for bone fragility fractures [28]. If these results are supported by future experimental and clinical studies, they suggest that raloxifene could be a useful drug to prevent skeletal fragility in diabetes with an added benefit of ameliorating the diabetic condition.

Author Contributions

Conceived and designed the experiments: KMGH MAG DBB. Performed the experiments: KMHG MAG DBB AYS JNW. Analyzed the data: KMGH MAG DBB. Contributed reagents/materials/analysis tools: DBB. Wrote the paper: KMHG MAG DMB AYS JNW DBB.

References

1. Janghorbani M, Feskanich D, Willett WC, Hu F (2006) Prospective study of diabetes and risk of hip fracture: the Nurses' Health Study. Diabetes Care 29: 1573–1578.
2. Janghorbani M, Van Dam RM, Willett WC, Hu FB (2007) Systematic review of type 1 and type 2 diabetes mellitus and risk of fracture. Am J Epidemiol 166: 495–505.
3. Strotmeyer ES, Cauley JA, Schwartz AV, Nevitt MC, Resnick HE, et al. (2005) Nontraumatic fracture risk with diabetes mellitus and impaired fasting glucose in older white and black adults: the health, aging, and body composition study. Arch Intern Med 165: 1612–1617.
4. Yamamoto M, Yamaguchi T, Yamauchi M, Kaji H, Sugimoto T (2009) Diabetic patients have an increased risk of vertebral fractures independent of BMD or diabetic complications. J Bone Miner Res 24: 702–709.
5. Schwartz AV, Sellmeyer DE, Ensrud KE, Cauley JA, Tabor HK, et al. (2001) Older women with diabetes have an increased risk of fracture: a prospective study. J Clin Endocrinol Metab 86: 32–38.
6. Allen MR, Hogan HA, Hobbs WA, Koivuniemi AS, Koivuniemi MC, et al. (2007) Raloxifene enhances material-level mechanical properties of femoral cortical and trabecular bone. Endocrinology 148: 3908–3913.
7. Allen MR, Iwata K, Sato M, Burr DB (2006) Raloxifene enhances vertebral mechanical properties independent of bone density. Bone 39: 1130–1135.
8. Delmas PD, Ensrud KE, Adachi JD, Harper KD, Sarkar S, et al. (2002) Efficacy of raloxifene on vertebral fracture risk reduction in postmenopausal women with osteoporosis: four-year results from a randomized clinical trial. J Clin Endocrinol Metab 87: 3609–3617.
9. Ettinger B, Black DM, Mitlak BH, Knickerbocker RK, Nickelsen T, et al. (1999) Reduction of vertebral fracture risk in postmenopausal women with osteoporosis treated with raloxifene: results from a 3-year randomized clinical trial. Multiple Outcomes of Raloxifene Evaluation (MORE) Investigators. Jama 282: 637–645.
10. Siris ES, Harris ST, Eastell R, Zanchetta JR, Goemaere S, et al. (2005) Skeletal effects of raloxifene after 8 years: results from the continuing outcomes relevant to Evista (CORE) study. J Bone Miner Res 20: 1514–1524.
11. Reinwald S, Peterson RG, Allen MR, Burr DB (2009) Skeletal changes associated with the onset of type 2 diabetes in the ZDF and ZDSD rodent models. Am J Physiol Endocrinol Metab 296: E765–774.
12. Fajardo RJ, Karim L, Calley VI, Bouxsein ML (2014) A review of rodent models of type 2 diabetic skeletal fragility. J Bone Miner Res 29: 1025–1040.
13. Turner CH, Burr DB (1993) Basic biomechanical measurements of bone: a tutorial. Bone 14: 595–608.
14. Dempster DW, Compston JE, Drezner MK, Glorieux FH, Kanis JA, et al. (2013) Standardized nomenclature, symbols, and units for bone histomorphometry: a 2012 update of the report of the ASBMR Histomorphometry Nomenclature Committee. J Bone Miner Res 28: 2–17.
15. Andersson B, Johannsson G, Holm G, Bengtsson BA, Sashegyi A, et al. (2002) Raloxifene does not affect insulin sensitivity or glycemic control in postmeno-
pausal women with type 2 diabetes mellitus: a randomized clinical trial. J Clin Endocrinol Metab 87: 122–128.
16. Barrett-Connor E, Ensrud KE, Harper K, Mason TM, Sashegyi A, et al. (2003) Post hoc analysis of data from the Multiple Outcomes of Raloxifene Evaluation (MORE) trial on the effects of three years of raloxifene treatment on glycemic control and cardiovascular disease risk factors in women with and without type 2 diabetes. Clin Ther 25: 919–930.
17. Tiano JP, Delghingaro-Augusto V, Le May C, Liu S, Kaw MK, et al. (2011) Estrogen receptor activation reduces lipid synthesis in pancreatic islets and prevents beta cell failure in rodent models of type 2 diabetes. J Clin Invest 121: 3331–3342.
18. Tiano J, Mauvais-Jarvis F (2012) Selective estrogen receptor modulation in pancreatic beta-cells and the prevention of type 2 diabetes. Islets 4: 173–176.
19. Matsumura M, Monden T, Nakatani Y, Shimizu H, Domeki N, et al. (2010) Effect of raloxifene on serum lipids for type 2 diabetic menopausal women with or without statin treatment. Med Princ Pract 19: 68–72.
20. Mori H, Okada Y, Kishikawa H, Inokuchi N, Sugimoto H, et al. (2013) Effects of raloxifene on lipid and bone metabolism in postmenopausal women with type 2 diabetes. J Bone Miner Metab 31: 89–95.
21. Diab T, Wang J, Reinwald S, Guldberg RE, Burr DB (2011) Effects of the combination treatment of raloxifene and alendronate on the biomechanical properties of vertebral bone. J Bone Miner Res 26: 270–276.
22. Sato M, Bryant HU, Iversen P, Helterbrand J, Smietana F, et al. (1996) Advantages of raloxifene over alendronate or estrogen on nonreproductive and reproductive tissues in the long-term dosing of ovariectomized rats. J Pharmacol Exp Ther 279: 298–305.
23. Burr DB, Diab T, Koivunemi A, Koivunemi M, Allen MR (2009) Effects of 1 to 3 years' treatment with alendronate on mechanical properties of the femoral shaft in a canine model: implications for subtrochanteric femoral fracture risk. J Orthop Res 27: 1288–1292.
24. Gallant MA, Brown DM, Hammond M, Wallace J, Du J, et al. (2014) Bone cell-independent benefits of raloxifene on the skeleton: A novel mechanism for improving bone material properties. Bone 61: 191–200.
25. Sambrook PN, Geusens P, Ribot C, Solimano JA, Ferrer-Barriendos J, et al. (2004) Alendronate produces greater effects than raloxifene on bone density and bone turnover in postmenopausal women with low bone density: results of EFFECT (Efficacy of FOSAMAX versus EVISTA Comparison Trial) International. J Intern Med 255: 503–511.
26. Vestergaard P (2011) Risk of newly diagnosed type 2 diabetes is reduced in users of alendronate. Calcif Tissue Int 89: 265–270.
27. Narayan KM, Boyle JP, Thompson TJ, Sorensen SW, Williamson DF (2003) Lifetime risk for diabetes mellitus in the United States. Jama 290: 1884–1890.
28. Melton LJ, 3rd, Kan SH, Wahner HW, Riggs BL (1988) Lifetime fracture risk: an approach to hip fracture risk assessment based on bone mineral density and age. J Clin Epidemiol 41: 985–994.

20

Low Intensity Pulsed Ultrasound Enhanced Mesenchymal Stem Cell Recruitment through Stromal Derived Factor-1 Signaling in Fracture Healing

Fang-Yuan Wei[1], Kwok-Sui Leung[1,2], Gang Li[1], Jianghui Qin[1], Simon Kwoon-Ho Chow[1], Shuo Huang[1], Ming-Hui Sun[1], Ling Qin[1,2], Wing-Hoi Cheung[1,2]*

1 Department of Orthopaedics and Traumatology, Clinical Sciences Building, The Chinese University of Hong Kong, Shatin, New Territories, Hong Kong SAR, China, **2** Translational Medicine Research & Development Center, Institute of Biomedical and Health Engineering, Shenzhen Institutes of Advanced Technology, Chinese Academy of Sciences, Shenzhen, China

Abstract

Low intensity pulsed ultrasound (LIPUS) has been proven effective in promoting fracture healing but the underlying mechanisms are not fully depicted. We examined the effect of LIPUS on the recruitment of mesenchymal stem cells (MSCs) and the pivotal role of stromal cell-derived factor-1/C-X-C chemokine receptor type 4 (SDF-1/CXCR4) pathway in response to LIPUS stimulation, which are essential factors in bone fracture healing. For *in vitro* study, isolated rat MSCs were divided into control or LIPUS group. LIPUS treatment was given 20 minutes/day at 37°C for 3 days. Control group received sham LIPUS treatment. After treatment, intracellular CXCR4 mRNA, SDF-1 mRNA and secreted SDF-1 protein levels were quantified, and MSCs migration was evaluated with or without blocking SDF-1/CXCR4 pathway by AMD3100. For *in vivo* study, fractured 8-week-old young rats received intracardiac administration of MSCs were assigned to LIPUS treatment, LIPUS+AMD3100 treatment or vehicle control group. The migration of transplanted MSC to the fracture site was investigated by *ex vivo* fluorescent imaging. SDF-1 protein levels at fracture site and in serum were examined. Fracture healing parameters, including callus morphology, micro-architecture of the callus and biomechanical properties of the healing bone were investigated. The *in vitro* results showed that LIPUS upregulated SDF-1 and CXCR4 expressions in MSCs, and elevated SDF-1 protein level in the conditioned medium. MSCs migration was promoted by LIPUS and partially inhibited by AMD3100. *In vivo* study demonstrated that LIPUS promoted MSCs migration to the fracture site, which was associated with an increase of local and serum SDF-1 level, the changes in callus formation, and the improvement of callus microarchitecture and mechanical properties; whereas the blockade of SDF-1/CXCR4 signaling attenuated the LIPUS effects on the fractured bones. These results suggested SDF-1 mediated MSCs migration might be one of the crucial mechanisms through which LIPUS exerted influence on fracture healing.

Editor: Amarjit S. Virdi, Rush University Medical Center, United States of America

Funding: This research project was supported by an AO Grant (Ref: S-11-10C) and partially by OTC Foundation Research Fund (Ref: 2009-WHLG). The funders had no role in study design, data collection and analysis, decision to publish, or preparation of the manuscript.

Competing Interests: The authors have declared that no competing interests exist.

* Email: louis@ort.cuhk.edu.hk

Introduction

Millions of fractures occur annually as a result of traumatic injuries or pathological conditions. Although most fractures will successfully heal within a few months, a considerable proportion of fracture cases still result in delayed healing [1], which may prolong treatment period and increase morbidity of the patients.

Mesenchymal stem cells (MSCs) are multipotent stromal cells able to differentiate into many cell types and contribute to the regeneration of musculoskeletal tissues such as bone, cartilage, tendon, adipose, and muscle [2–4]. It is widely accepted that MSCs are normally retained in the special niches of different adult tissues. In stressful situations such as injury, when there is a need for tissue repair and to maintain tissue homeostasis, MSCs can be recruited to the site of injury and contribute to the repair process. When bone integrity is disrupted after fracture, the bone tissue

would enter a healing process that is generally divided into three overlapping phases including the inflammation, soft and hard callus formation, and the callus remodeling [5]. The damage of blood vessel and other tissues lead to local tissue bleeding and hypoxia. This process will trigger the inflammatory cascade [6]. In this early inflammatory phase of fracture healing, many types of cytokines, such as interleukin 6 (IL-6) and stromal cell-derived factor-1 (SDF-1), released from the damaged bone facilitate the egress of MSCs from the periosteum and bone marrow into the blood stream, which rapidly accumulate and engraft at fracture site, and initiate bone regeneration process [3,7,8]. Although the interactions between cytokines and MSCs in bone repair remain controversial, many studies found that MSCs expressed both SDF-1 and CXCR4 genes [9–11], and SDF-1/CXCR4 signaling is critical for the recruitment of MSCs to the fracture site during fracture healing. Granero-Molto *et al.* found that implanted MSCs were recruited to the fracture site in an exclusively CXCR4-dependent manner [12]. Kitaori *et al.* showed that SDF-1 level was elevated in the periosteum of injured bone, which recruited MSCs homing to the graft bone at the fracture site and promoted endochondral bone formation [8].

Low intensity pulsed ultrasound (LIPUS) has been reported to be effective in promoting fracture healing in both animal models and clinical trials [13–16]. In brief, the beneficial effects of LIPUS on fracture healing include the decrease in healing time at the tissue level, and the increase in the cellular responses including osteogensis-related gene expression [17], protein synthesis and cell proliferation [18]. The mechanical stimulation produced by the pressure waves of LIPUS on bone can result in series of biochemical events at cellular level [19,20]. However, the detailed mechanism through which LIPUS stimulates tissues remains unclear. Although osteocytes have been considered as the primary mechanosensors in bone, convincing data show that MSCs also have the ability to sense and respond to physical stimuli [21–23]. To date, very little is known about how physical stimuli affect MSCs mobilization. One possible mechanism through which LIPUS enhances fracture healing is through the enhancement in MSC recruitment. A recent report has demonstrated that LIPUS was able to enhance MSC recruitment from a parabiotic source at the fracture site in a surgically conjoined mice pair model. The report also suggested the involvement of SDF-1/CXCR4 signaling pathway by an apparent increase immuno-detection of the two proteins [24].

In this study, we attempted to investigate that under LIPUS treatment, (a) the migration of MSCs to the fracture site; (b) the role of SDF-1/CXCR4 in regulating the recruitment of MSCs; (c) the MSCs engraftment and fracture healing. The aim of the first part of this study was to evaluate the direct influence of LIPUS on MSCs migration and intracellular SDF-1/CXCR4 signaling *in vitro*. The second part was to investigate the effects of LIPUS on MSCs recruitment and femoral fracture repair in a rat model, with or without blocking SDF-1/CXCR4 pathway.

Materials and Methods

2.1. MSCs Isolation and Identification

2.1.1. MSCs Isolation. All experiments were approved by the Animal Experimentation Ethics Committee (AEEC) of the authors' institution (Ref: 10/007/GRF-5). MSCs were isolated from two 8-week female Sprague-Dawley (SD) rats, following protocol previously established in our laboratory [25]. Briefly, intact tibiae and femora were collected from euthanized healthy 8-week SD rats and carefully dissected free of muscles in the Petri dish containing sterile phosphate-buffered saline (PBS) and 1% penicillin-streptomycin (Invitrogen Corporation, Carlsbad, California, US). The bones were rinsed once in sterile $1 \times$ PBS before being transferred to the biosafety cabinet hood in the culture

room. After rinsed once with sterile $1 \times$ PBS, the bone ends were cut with bone clipper. With the cut surface facing the bottom of the centrifuge tube, the tube was spun at 2000 rpm for 1 minute (most of the bone marrow (BM) was collected at the bottom of the tube). Mononuclear cells were then isolated by density gradient centrifugation (850 g, 30 minutes) using Lymphoprep (1.077 g/ml; AXIS-SHIELD PoC AS, Oslo, Norway), and re-suspended in complete culture medium containing alpha minimum essential medium (α-MEM) (Gibco, Grand Island, NY, US), 10% fetal bovine serum (FBS) (Gibco, Grand Island, NY, US), 100 U/ml penicillin, 100 µg/ml streptomycin and 2 mM L-glutamine (Invitrogen, Carlsbad, California, US). These mononuclear cells were plated at an optimal low cell density (10^5 cells/cm^2) to isolate stem cells and cultured at 37°C, 5% CO_2/20% O_2 to form colonies. When colonies reached 80–90% confluence, the MSCs were sub-cultured and re-plated for further expansion. Medium was changed every three days. Cells at passage 3 were used for all the experiments. The surface marker expression and multi-lineage differentiation potential of MSCs were characterized before being used for the further experiments.

2.1.2. MSCs Characterization. The methods of the characterization of MSCs in this study were mainly based on the minimal criteria for human MSCs suggested by the Mesenchymal and Tissue Stem Cell Committee of the International Society for Cellular Therapy [26].

Flow Cytometry Assay. The surface marker expression of MSCs isolated from healthy rats, including CD90, CD44, CD45, CD31 and CD34, was analyzed by flow cytometry assay as described in the previous study [27]. Briefly, the MSCs at passage 3 were harvested by trypsinization, washed twice in PBS, then pelleted by centrifugation at 350 g for 5 minutes at room temperature and re-suspended in the staining buffer (Becton Dickson, Franklin Lakes, NJ, US) at 2×10^6/ml for 15 minutes at 4°C. One-hundred microliters cell suspension was incubated with primary antibodies against rat CD90 and CD44 (Abcam, Cambridge, UK) conjugated with phycoerythrin (PE), CD31 (Abcam, Cambridge, UK) and CD34 (Santa Cruz Biotechnology, Santa Cruz, CA, US) conjugated with fluorescein isothiocyanate (FITC), CD45 (Abcam, Cambridge, UK) without conjugation for 15 minutes at 4°C. Unbound antibodies were washed away by adding ice-cold staining buffer. The cell pellet was re-suspended in the staining buffer containing goat anti-rabbit immunoglobulin G (IgG) conjugated with FITC (Santa Cruz Biotechnology, Santa Cruz, CA, US) for CD45 detection for at least 15 minutes at 4°C. The cells were washed with ice-cold PBS containing 2% bovine serum albumin (BSA) before analysis using the LSRFortessa flow cytometer (Becton Dickinson, San Jose, CA, US). PE-conjugated isotype-matched mouse IgG1 (R&D systems Inc, Minneapolis, MN, US) was used as isotype control for both CD90 and CD44; FITC-conjugated isotype-matched mouse IgG1 (R&D systems, Inc, Minneapolis, MN, US) was used as isotype control for both

Table 1. Primer sequences of the target genes.

Gene	Primer nucleotide sequence	Product Size (bp)	Ta (°C)
SDF-1	Forward: 5'-TTGCCAGCACAAAGACACTCC-3' Reverse: 5'-CTCCAAAGCAAACCGAATACAG-3'	225	58
CXCR4	Forward: 5'-TCCGTGGCTGACCTCCTCTT-3' Reverse: 5'-CAGCTTCCTCGGCCTCTGGC-3'	210	56
GAPDH	Forward: 5'-AACTCCCATTCCTCCACCTT-3' Reverse: 5'-GAGGGCCTCTCTCTTGCTCT-3'	200	57

GAPDH = glyceraldehide-3-phosphate dehydrogenase.

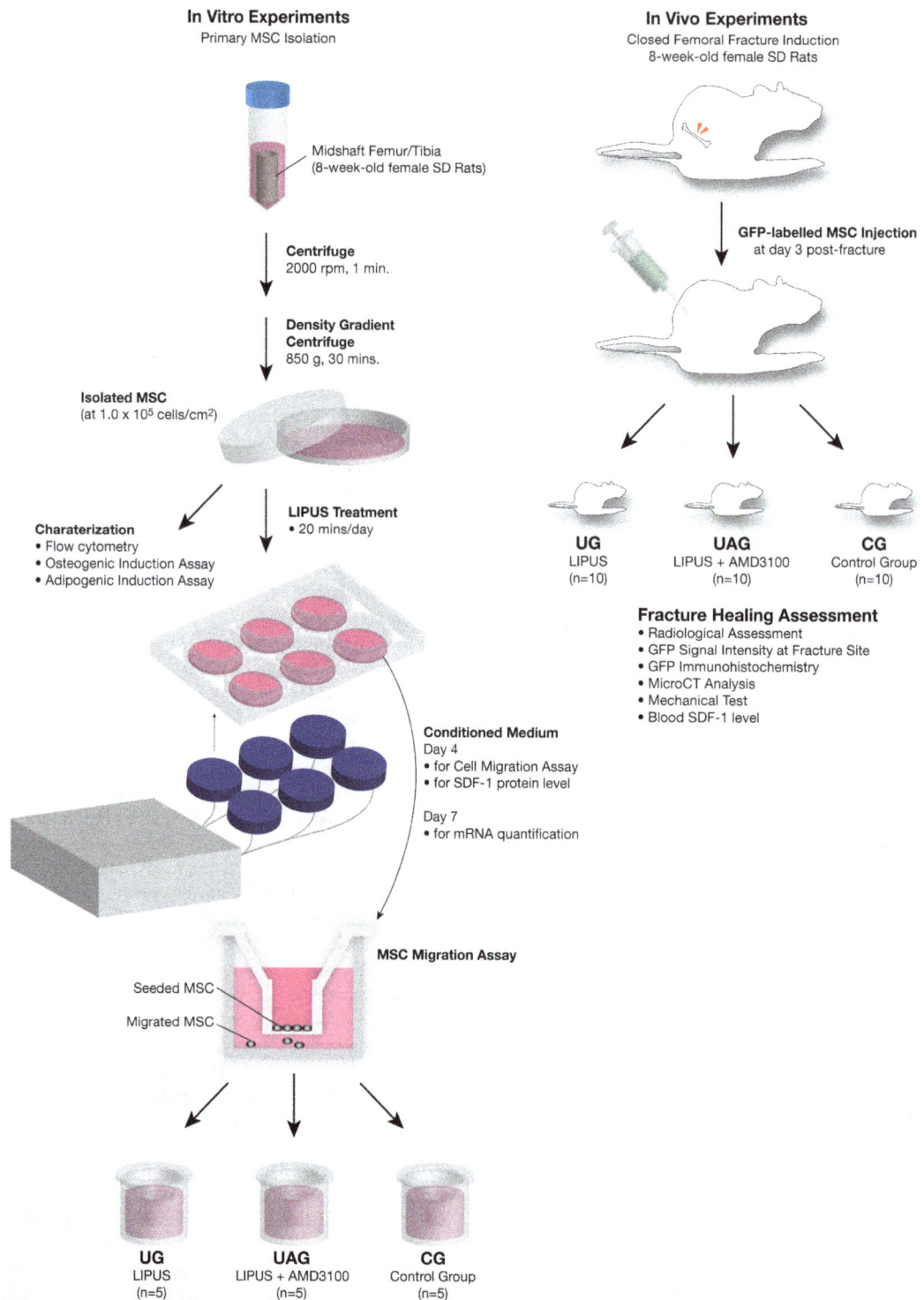

Figure 1. Flowchart of the study design. MSCs were isolated from two 8-week-old female SD rats and characterized by flow cytometry assay, osteogenic induction assay and adipogenic induction assay. In the in vitro experiments (n = 5), the SDF-1 protein and mRNA expression levels in condition medium were compared between control (CG) and LIPUS treatment (UG) groups, the MSCs migration ability was compared among CG, UG and LIPUS plus AMD3100 treatment (UAG) groups. In the in vivo experiments, closed femoral fractured rats were randomly divided into CG, UG and UAG groups (n = 10). GFP-labeled MSCs were intracardiac injected to all the rats on day 3 post-fracture and recruitment effects by LIPUS were compared among groups.

CD31 and CD34; and rabbit polyclonal IgG (Epitomics, Burlingame, CA, US) was used as isotype control for CD45.

Osteogenic Induction Assay and Alizarin Red S Staining. The methods have been described previously [25]. Briefly, MSCs at passage 3 were trypsinized and re-plated in a six-

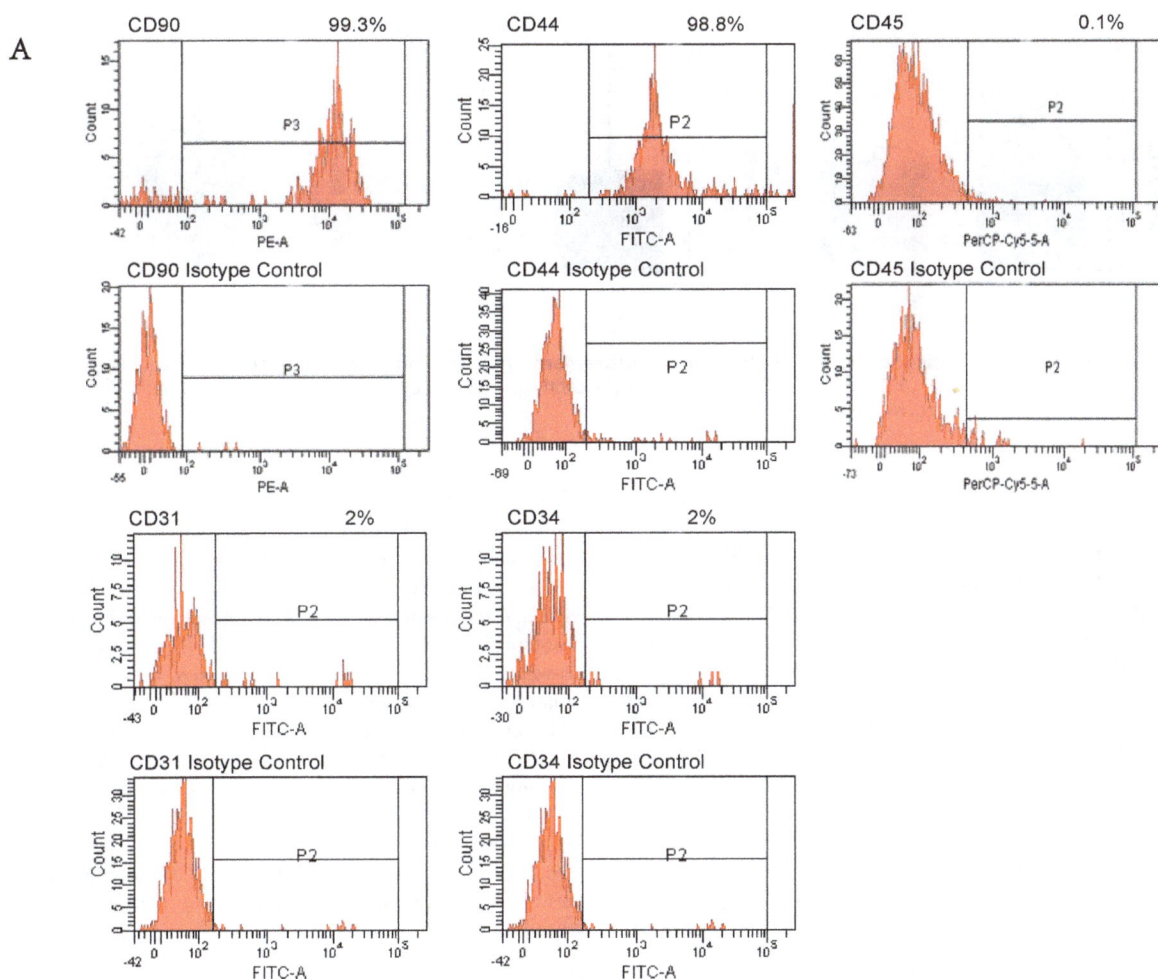

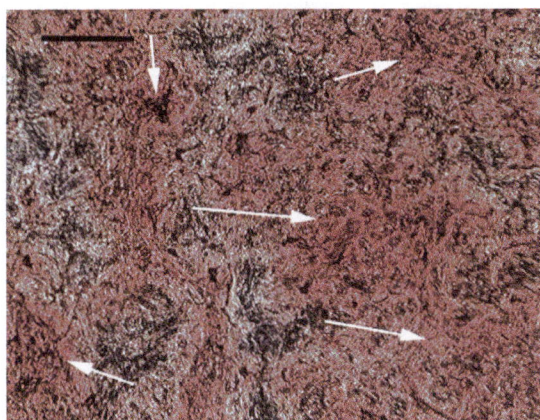

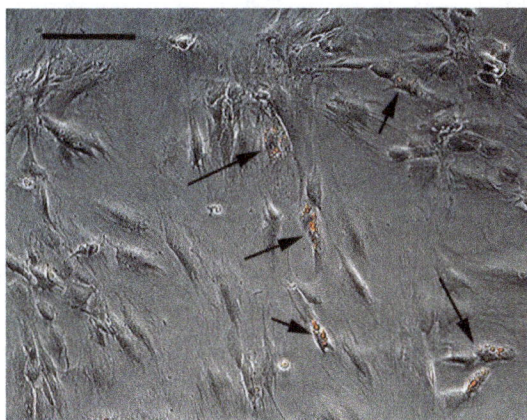

Figure 2. MSCs characterization. (A) The expressions of selected surface markers on the isolated cells from BM of SD rats. This figure shows the expressions of mesenchymal stem cell markers (CD90 and CD44), endothelial cell marker (CD31) and hematopoietic cell markers (CD34 and CD45) on the isolated cell colonies. **(B)** Representative microphotograph of Alizarin Red S-stained cells isolated from BM of SD rats. White arrows indicate the obvious calcium deposition areas in the matrix. Scale bar = 100 μm. **(C)** Representative microphotograph of Oil Red O-stained cells isolated from BM of SD rats. The black arrows indicate the adipose-differentiated cells. The small red bubbles in cells are lipids. Scale bar = 100 μm.

well plate at a concentration of 1×10^5 cells per well, and cultured in complete culture medium for three days. These cells were then incubated in osteogenic induction medium (OIM) containing 100 nmol/L dexamethasone, 10 mmol/L beta-glycerophosphate, and 0.05 mmol/L L-ascorbic acid-2-phosphate. The OIM was changed every three days for 21 days. Cell and matrix layer was washed with PBS, fixed with 70% ethanol for 10 minutes, and

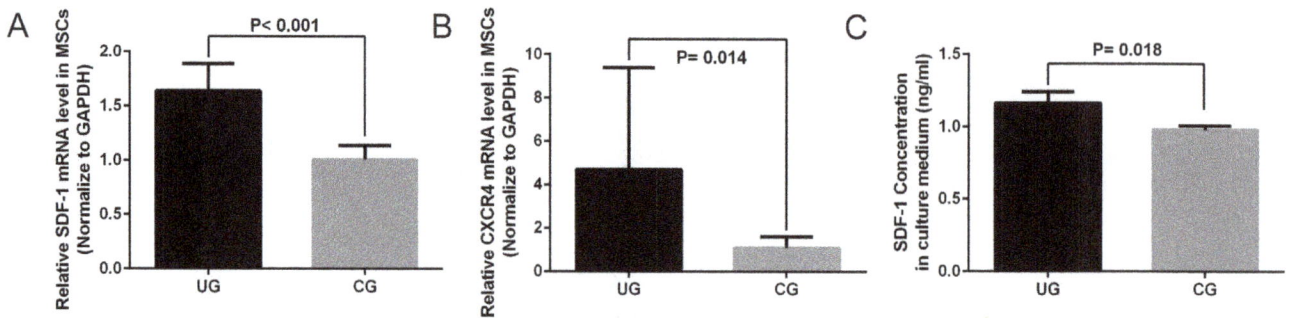

Figure 3. Target genes quantification and SDF-1 protein measurement. (**A**) LIPUS enhanced SDF-1 gene expression in MSCs significantly (p<0.0001), and (**B**) LIPUS enhanced CXCR4 gene expression in MSCs significantly (p = 0.014). (**C**) ELISA assay showed increased SDF-1 protein level in the culture medium of MSCs treated with LIPUS (p = 0.018).

stained with 0.5% Alizarin Red S (pH 4.1, Sigma, St. Louis, MO, US) for 30 minutes.

Adipogenic Induction Assay and Oil Red-O Staining. The method has been described previously [25]. MSCs were trypsinized and re-plated in a six-well plate at the same concentration as that for the osteogenic assay. The cells were cultured in the complete culture medium for three days, and were then incubated in adipogenic induction medium (AIM) containing 10% FBS, 1 μM dexamethasone, 10 μg/ml insulin, 50 μM indomethacin, and 0.5 mM isobuthyl-methylxanthine. The cells were cultured for an additional 21 days for assessment of the presence of oil droplets, which was confirmed by staining the cells with 0.3% fresh Oil Red-O solution (Sigma-Aldrich, St. Louis, MO, US) for 2 hours after fixation with 70% ethanol for 10 minutes.

2.2. LIPUS Treatment of MSCs

The isolated rat MSCs were divided into control (CG) or LIPUS treatment (UG) group (n = 5). The procedure of LIPUS treatment on cells was based on our previous protocol [19,28]. Briefly, LIPUS was provided by a Sonic Accelerated Fracture Healing System (Smith & Nephew, Memphis, TN, US) for cell culture. The 6-well culture plate (Corning, Lowell, MA, US) was placed on the matched ultrasound transducers with a thin layer of coupling gel. The ultrasound energy was calibrated by the manufacturer and tested with the output checker before use. For UG, LIPUS treatment (unfocused plane waves, frequency 1.5 MHz, duty cycle 1:4, spatial average-temporal average intensity 30 mW/cm^2, pulse repetition frequency 1 kHz for pulse duration of 200 μs) was given from the bottom of the culture plate for 20 minutes/day in open air at 37°C for 3 days. CG received sham LIPUS treatment, with

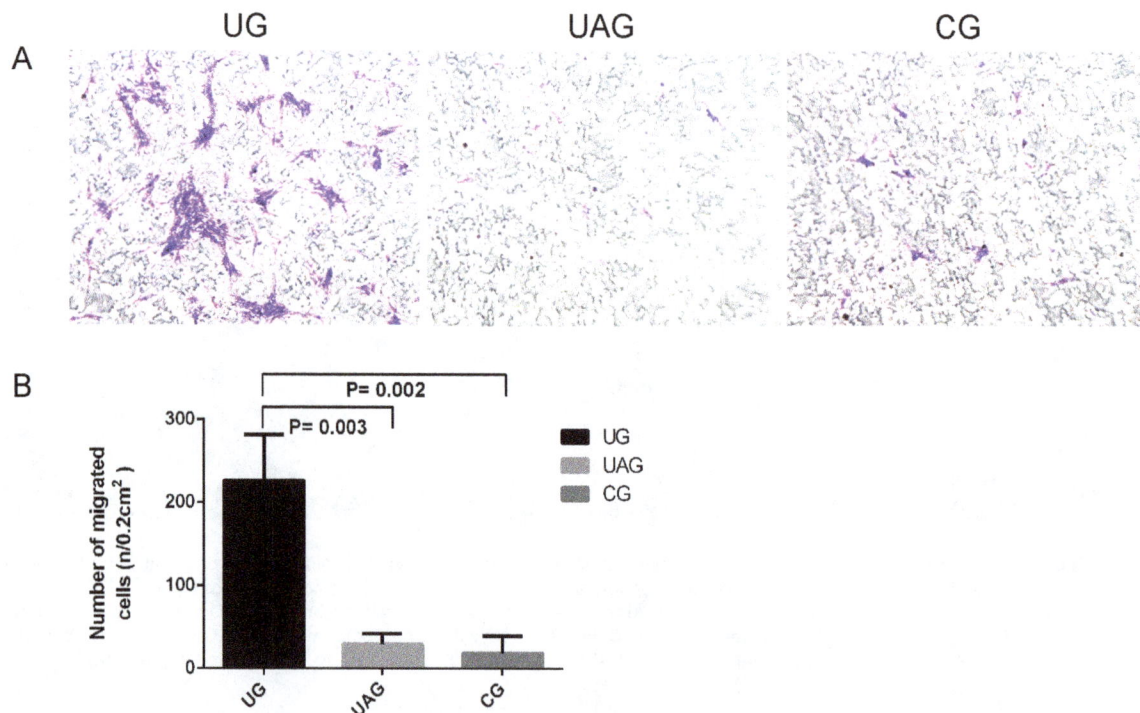

Figure 4. MSCs migration assay. (**A**) The migrated MSCs on the exterior of the insert in UG (left) were remarkably increased compared with UAG (middle) and CG (right) at ×100 magnification. (**B**) The number of migrated cells in UG was increased 12.1 times than in CG (p = 0.002); the number of migrated cells in UAG was decreased by 87.2% as compared to UG (p = 0.003).

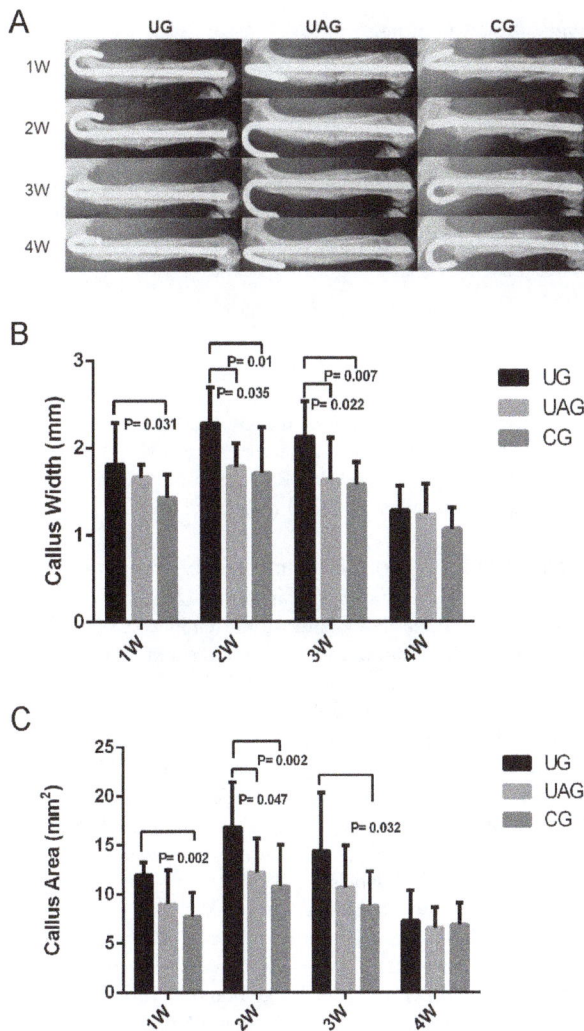

Figure 5. Radiographic analysis of fracture healing in young rats. (**A**) Series of representative radiographies showed better callus bridging in UG and UAG, compared with in CG at different time points. (**B**) The measurement of callus width (CW) showed: CW in UG was larger by 26.8% at week 1 (p = 0.031), by 33.6% at week 2 (p = 0.01) and by 35.0% at week 3 (p = 0.007) post-fracture than in CG, and by 27.8% at week 2 (p = 0.035) and by 30.0% at week 3 (p = 0.022) post-fracture than in UAG. (**C**) The quantitative measurement of callus area (CA) showed: CA was significantly larger in UG by 55.1% at week 1 (p = 0.002), by 55.5% at week 2 (p = 0.002), by 64.0% at week 3 (p = 0.032) than in CG, and was significantly larger by 37.7% at week 2 than in UAG (p = 0.047).

the culture plate placed on the transducers (with coupling gel) yet without ultrasound. On day 4, after changing the medium, the old conditioned medium from each group was collected for SDF-1 protein level analysis and cell migration assay; on day 7, the MSCs were harvested for real-time RT-PCR analysis.

2.3. Real-time RT-PCR Analysis

After 6 days of treatment, total RNA was isolated based on the established protocol [17]. The mRNA was then reverse-transcribed and amplified (Applied Biosystems, CA, USA). The synthesized cDNA was used as the template to quantify the relative content of mRNA by using LightCycler Real-Time PCR System (Roche Diagnostics, Penzberg, Germany). The glyceraldehyde 3-phosphate dehydrogenase (GAPDH) was used as the

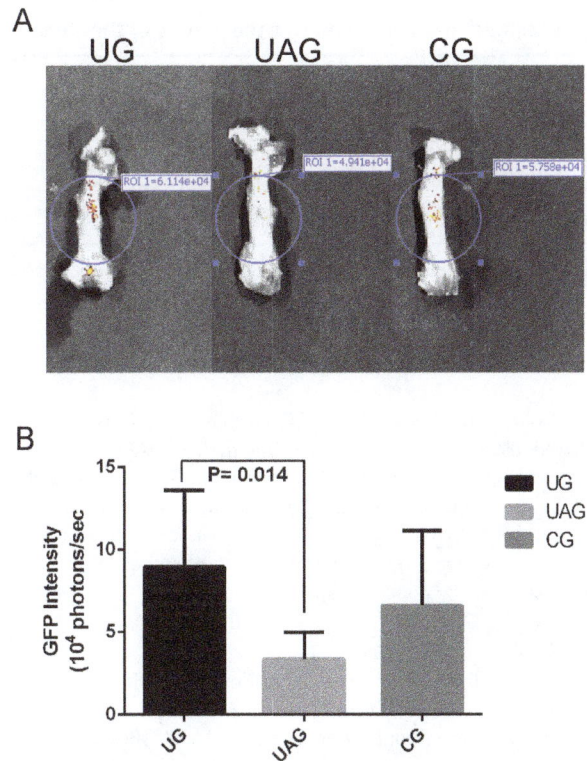

Figure 6. *Ex vivo* GFP intensity measurement. (**A**) On the representative image of each group, blue circles indicate the region of interest (ROI) for fluorescent imaging analysis. GFP signals in UG (left) was much higher than in UAG (middle) and CG (right). (**B**) Semi-quantitative GFP intensity of fracture callus in UG was increased 2.66 times than in UAG (p = 0.014), although no significant differences were found among other groups.

internal control. Primer sequences used in the experiments are summarized in Table 1 (all from Invitrogen, Carlsbad, CA, USA).

2.4. SDF-1 Protein Level Measurement

The culture medium was collected from UG and CG after 3 days of treatment. Protein level of SDF-1α was quantified using Quantikine SDF-1α enzyme immunoassay kit (R&D System,

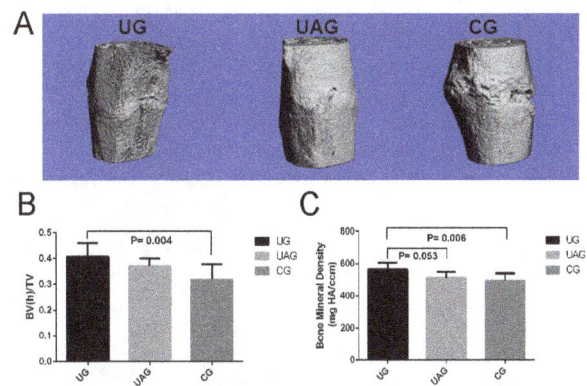

Figure 7. μCT measurement. (**A**) Representative 3D reconstructed micro-CT images of the three groups at week 4 post-fracture showed improved fracture healing in UG and UAG. (**B**) BVh/TV in UG was increased by 27.9% than in CG (p = 0.004). (**C**) BMD in UG was higher by 10% than in UAG (p = 0.053) and by 14.5% than in CG (p = 0.006).

Table 2. Mechanical properties of the femurs of the three groups at week 4 post-fracture.

Parameters	UG	UAG	CG
Ultimate Load (N)	126.2±7.0[a, b]	96.9±10.4[c]	62.9±26.9
Stiffness (N/mm)	53.5±7.2[b]	44.9±12.4	38.7±10.9
Energy to Failure (j)	0.05±0.02	0.03±0.01	0.03±0.02

UG, LIPUS treatment group; UAG, LIPUS+AMD3100 treatment group; CG, control group received sham treatment.
[a]$p < 0.05$ between UG and UAG;
[b]$p < 0.05$ between UG and CG;
[c]$p < 0.05$ between UAG and CG.

Minneapolis, Minnesota, USA). Colorimetric density of the developed plates was determined using BioTek μQuant Microplate Spectrophotometer (Bio-Tek Instruments Inc, Winooski, VT, US) at 450 nm wavelength. The enzyme-linked immunosorbent assay (ELISA) assay was performed in duplicate. A standard curve was constructed by plotting the mean absorbance for each standard against the concentration.

2.5. Cell Migration Assay

QCM 24-Well colorimetric cell migration assay (Millipore, MA, US) was used to study the migration of MSCs under LIPUS treatment, with or without the presence of AMD3100 (Sigma, St Louis, MO, US), in comparison with sham control [29]. AMD3100 is a specific antagonist of CXCR4 and not cross-reactive with other chemokine receptors [30]. MSCs at passage 3 were starved in serum-free medium for 1 day, washed twice with PBS and incubated in Harvesting Buffer at 37°C for 15 minutes. 20 ml Quenching Medium was added and cells were centrifuged at 1500 rpm for 5 minutes. The pellet was re-suspended in Quenching Medium, and brought to a final concentration at 5.0×10^5 cells/ml. 300 μl cell suspension were added to each insert (8 μm pore size). [31] These inserts then were randomly divided into 3 groups (n = 5), including LIPUS treatment group (UG), LIPUS plus AMD3100 treatment group (UAG) and sham control group (CG). For UAG, an additional 1 μM AMD3100 was added to the insert. LIPUS treatment was applied with the same custom-built platform designed for 6-well plated as described above, then 500 μl of old serum-free conditioned medium collected after 3 days of LIPUS treatment were added to the lower chambers in UG and UAG; 500 μl of old serum-free conditioned medium collected after 3 days of sham treatment was added to the lower chamber in CG. MSCs were incubated at 37°C in 5% CO_2/20% O_2 for 18 hours. The remaining cell suspension was removed; the migration insert was placed into a clean well containing 400 μl of Cell Stain and incubated for 20 minutes at room temperature. The insert was rinsed in water several times, and non-migratory cells were carefully removed from the interior of the insert. The migrated cells on the exterior of the insert were counted manually under the microscope (Leica DM IRB, Heerbrugg, Switzerland), and the images were taken at ×100 magnification.

2.6. Animal Model, Groupings and LIPUS Treatment

Thirty 8-week-old female SD rats were obtained from the Laboratory Animal Services Center of the Chinese University of Hong Kong. Closed femoral fractures were created at femur shaft based on our established protocol [32,33]. Postoperative radiographies were used to confirm the quality of fracture.

On day 3 post-fracture, the rats were anaesthetized by intraperitoneal injection of a mixture of ketamine (50 mg/kg) and xylazine (10 mg/kg). 1.0×10^6 GFP-labelled MSCs (RASMX-01101, Cyagen, Guangzhou, China) in 500 μl PBS were transplanted by intracardiac injection as previous described [34,35]. Briefly, the GFP-labeled MSCs were sub-cultured to the fifth passage, and then were trypsinized and diluted in 0.9% normal saline. Under anaesthesia, the rat was placed supine, kept firmly on the desk holding the chest between the thumb and forefinger. After removing the air in the liquid, a 23G needle was inserted through the thoracic wall at a point left to the sternum on a line connecting the left axillary pivot with the caudal tip of the sternum. In the meantime, the syringe containing MSCs suspension was aspirated; the injection of the MSCs suspension was performed by gently pressing the piston of the syringe. The position of needle was confirmed by an ultrasound system (Vevo 770, VisualSonics, ON, Canada) under B-mode (brightness mode).

After MSCs injection, the rats were randomly assigned to the following groups: 1) LIPUS group (UG, n = 10) in which LIPUS treatment (Exogen 3000+, Smith & Nephew Inc, Memphis, TN, USA) was applied 20 minutes/day, 5 days/week, after the cell injection. During treatment, the rats were laid on the ventral side under general anaesthesia and a 2.5 cm diameter ultrasound transducer was placed on the lateral side of the fracture site. The ultrasound signal consisting of a 200 μs burst of 1.5 MHz sine

Table 3. Histomorphometric analysis of femoral microarchitecture at week 4 post-fracture.

Parameters	UG	UAG	CG
Cl.Ar (mm²)	5.0±0.6	4.0±1.9	5.3±2.7
Cg.Ar (mm²)	0.0±0.0	0.1±0.0	0.9±0.9
Cg.Ar/Cl.Ar (%)	0.0±0.0[a]	0.0±0.0	0.1±0.1

UG, LIPUS treatment group; UAG, LIPUS treatment plus AMD3100 treatment group; CG, control group received sham treatment, Cl.Ar, total callus area; Cg.Ar, cartilage area; Cg.Ar/Cl.Ar, the percentage of cartilage area.
[a]$p = 0.038$ between UG and CG.

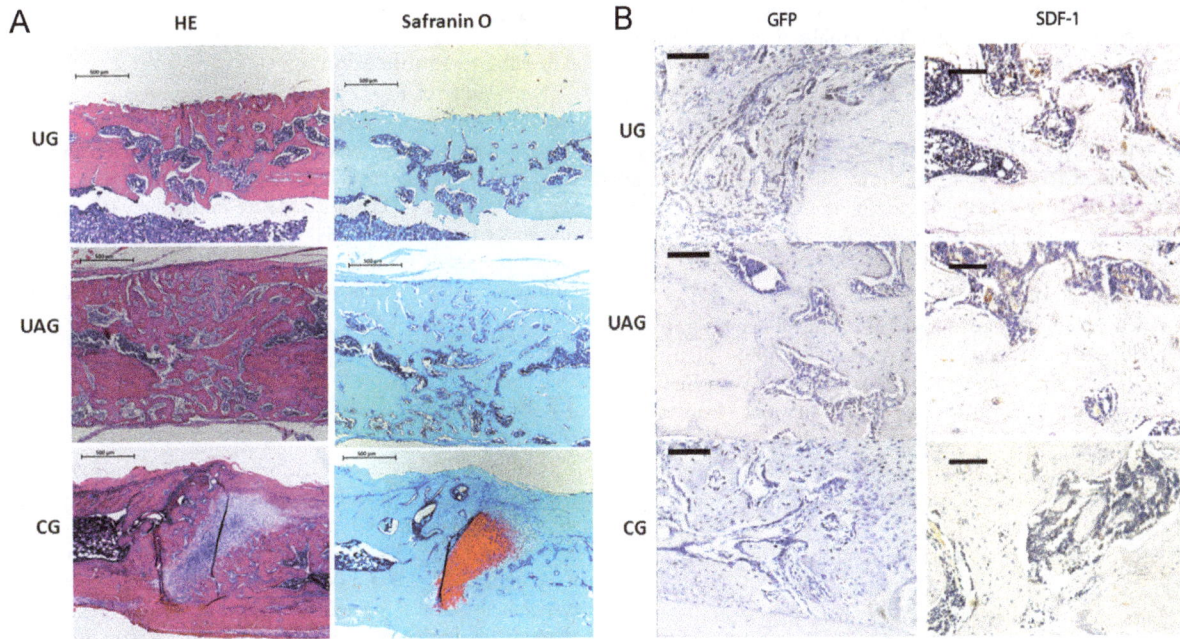

Figure 8. Histological and immunohistochemical results. (**A**) Representative H&E and safranin-O/fast green staining showed that in UG and UAG, there were large amounts of woven bone formation in the fracture areas, with almost no chondroid tissues (stained red by safranin-O), whereas lots of chondroid and fibrous tissues still existed at the fracture site in CG at week 4. Scale bars, 50 μm. (**B**, left) Representative immunohistochemistry for GFP showed that a large number of the GFP positive cells engrafted in the fracture area in UG, whereas fewer GFP positive cells were detected in CG, and even fewer GFP positive cells were found in UAG. Scale bars at ×100, 200 μm. (**B**, right) Representative images of SDF-1 staining of callus at week 4 post-fracture for young rats. Brown color indicates positive staining. SDF-1 was located mainly in the blood vessels or sinusoid-like regions. Scale bars at ×200, 100 μm.

wave repeating at 1.0 kHz with 30.0 ± 5.0 mW/cm^2 spatial average and temporal average incident intensity was given. 2) LIPUS+AMD3100 group (UAG, n = 10) in which daily LIPUS treatment was applied (same as UG), AMD3100 was resolved in saline to a final concentration of 1 mg/ml for injection and administered (1 mg/kg/day, intraperitoneal) [36] 30 minutes before LIPUS treatment. 3) Sham control group (CG, n = 10) in which the daily sham treatment (LIPUS machine turned off) was applied. Both UG and CG groups received vehicle injections of 0.9% normal saline (1 ml/kg/day, intraperitoneal). Animals were allowed full weight bearing, free cage activity, and food and water ad libitum. At week 4 post-fracture, animals were euthanized by overdosed sodium pentobarbital; the femora and blood were collected for the end-point assessments.

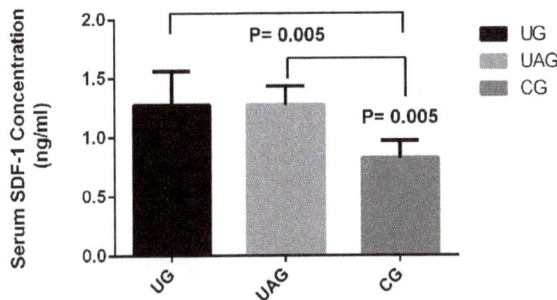

Figure 9. Serum SDF-1 protein concentration. The serum SDF-1 protein level measured by ELISA assay in UG was increased by 1.55 times than in CG (p = 0.005); the serum SDF-1 level in UAG was increased by 1.55 times than in CG (p = 0.005).

2.7. Radiological Assessment

Two-dimensional digital radiographs (MX-20, Faxitron, Lincolnshire, IL, USA) were taken weekly post-fracture to confirm the quality and degree of fracture healing. The quantified temporal changes of callus morphology were evaluated by using the Metamorph Image Analysis System (Universal Imaging Corporation, Downingtown, PA, USA) according to our previous established protocol [37], where callus width (CW) was defined as the maximal outer diameter of the mineralized callus (d2) minus the outer diameter of the femur (d1); and callus area (CA) was calculated as the sum of the areas of the external mineralized callus.

2.8. Ex Vivo GFP Signal Intensity Analysis

Animals were euthanized at week 4 post-fracture. The *ex vivo* fluorescent images were taken by the Xenogen Imaging System (IVIS 200; Caliper Life Sciences, Hopkinton, MA, USA), immediately after the femur was harvested with removal of soft tissues and K-wire. The GFP signals at callus area were acquired and measured by using the live image 2.5 software of Xenogen Imaging System with the settings of exposure time at 5 seconds, binning at 8 and f/stop at f/16 [12,35]. A standard circular region of interest (ROI) with a diameter of 1 cm at the callus area was selected for the measurements. The fluorescent image data was displayed in units of photons. The tissue autofluorescence was subtracted by using GFP background filter with the excitation passband at 440 nm, and emission passband at 550 nm.

2.9. μCT Analysis

Ex vivo micro-computed tomography scans (μCT40, Scanco Medical, Brüttisellen, Switzerland) were performed at 4 weeks post-fracture based on our established protocol [32,38]. The femora were positioned vertically with normal saline-soaked gauze in the sample holder during scanning. The newly formed bone (low-density bone, threshold = 165–350) and highly mineralized bone (high-density bone, threshold = 350–1000) were reconstructed separately [16,32]. The ratios of low-density bone volume over total tissue volume (BVl/TV), high-density bone volume over total tissue volume (BVh/TV), total bone volume fraction (BVt/TV) and bone mineral density (BMD) were calculated.

2.10. Mechanical Testing

A complete healing of closed femoral fracture in young rat was reported taking place around week 4 post-surgery [39]. After μCT scanning, the fractured femora were subjected to mechanical testing as previously described [32,37]. The ultimate load (UL), stiffness, and the energy to failure were calculated from load displacement curves using built-in software (QMAT Professional Material testing software).

2.11. Histomorphometric and Immunohistochemical Analysis

The harvested samples were performed hematoxylin–eosin (H&E) and safranin-O/fast green staining for histomorphometric analysis. The images were taken at ×50 magnification under microscope (Leica DMRB DAS; Leica, Heerbrugg, Switzerland). Quantitative assessment of the safranin-O-positive cartilage at the region of 1.5 mm proximal and distal to the fracture line was performed by using ImageJ (NIH, MD, USA). Cartilage area (Cg.Ar), callus area (Cl.Ar) and their ratio (Cg.Ar/Cl.Ar) were measured.

Immunohistochemical staining was carried out on deparaffinized sections using a rabbit ABC staining system (Santa Cruz Biotechnology, Santa Cruz, CA, USA). The sections were incubated overnight at 4°C in 1:500 rabbit anti-GFP polyclonal antibody (Abcam, Cambridge, MA, USA) or 1:200 rabbit anti-SDF-1 polyclonal antibody (Abcam, Cambridge, MA, USA), followed by incubation with biotinylated secondary antibody and color development according to the manufacturer's instructions. Images were captured using bright field microscopy at ×100 and ×200 magnification (Leica DMRB DAS; Leica, Heerbrugg, Switzerland).

2.12. Blood Collection and Serum SDF-1 Analysis

Five milliliter of blood was collected by cardiac puncture shortly before the animals were euthanized. The blood was centrifuged at 1,800 g for 10 minutes, and the separated serum samples were then stored at −80°C until analysis. The level of SDF-1 in the serum was measured by using the same SDF-1α ELISA kit and microplate reader settings used for culture medium testing as described above. All the serum samples were run in duplicate. A flowchart of the study design was shown in Fig. 1.

2.13. Statistical Analysis

All quantitative data were expressed as mean ± standard deviation and analyzed with SPSS version 20.0 software (IBM, NY, USA). Independent student's t test and one-way analysis of variance (ANOVA) with Tukey's post-hoc test were used for two-group or multiple-group comparisons respectively, as time since fracture induction was not considered as independent variable due to known temporal changes for our measured parameters. Statistical significance was set at $p < 0.05$.

Results

3.1. MSCs Identification

The results of flow cytometry demonstrated that over 99.3% and 98.8% of the mononucleated cell colonies isolated from BM of SD rats were positive for the fibroblastic marker CD90 and MSC marker CD44 respectively. They were negative for the endothelial stem cell marker CD31 and negative for the hematopoietic lineage markers, including CD34 and CD45 (Fig. 2A). Osteogenic induction assay showed abundant calcium deposits in the cell culture (Fig. 2B). Adipogenic induction assay indicated that a number of isolated cells were positively stained by Oil Red O (Fig. 2C).

3.2. Real-time RT-PCR and SDF-1 Protein Level Measurement

Real-time RT-PCR and ELISA results demonstrated that gene expression of SDF-1 and CXCR4 were significantly upregulated in UG, as compared with CG (p<0.0001 and p=0.014, respectively) (Fig. 3A, B). The SDF-1 and CXCR4 mRNA levels were increased 1.6 times and 4.3 times in UG than in CG respectively. SDF-1 protein level in the culture medium was also significantly increased in UG than CG (p = 0.018) (Fig. 3C).

3.3. Cell Migration Assay

Under light microscopy, abundant MSCs were found on the exterior of the inserts in UG (Fig. 4A, left); whereas only a small number of MSCs were observed on the exterior of the inserts in both UAG (Fig. 4A, middle) and CG (Fig. 4A, right).

Quantitatively, the number of migrated MSCs in UG was significantly increased than in UAG and CG (p = 0.003, p = 0.002, respectively) (Fig. 4B). No significant difference was observed in the number of migrated cells between UAG and CG.

3.4 Radiological Assessment

Radiographic analysis demonstrated that both UG and UAG showed earlier fracture healing than CG, as indicated by earlier callus bridging occurred at week 2, whereas callus bridging started from week 3 in CG (Fig. 5A). Quantitative measurement of callus morphometry showed that CW was significantly larger in UG than in CG at week 1, 2 and 3 (p = 0.031 for week 1, p = 0.01 for week 2, p = 0.007 for week 3, respectively); CW was significantly larger in UG than in UAG at week 2 (p = 0.035) and week 3 (p = 0.022) (Fig. 5B). CA was significantly larger in UG than in CG at week 1, 2 and 3 (p = 0.002 for week 1, 2; p = 0.032 for week 3); CA was significantly larger in UG than in UAG at week 2 (p = 0.047) (Fig. 5C).

3.5. Ex Vivo GFP Signal Intensity Analysis

GFP intensity in UG was significantly higher than in UAG (p = 0.014). Higher GFP intensity was found in UG as compared with CG, and in CG as compared with UAG, but no significance was found between these groups (Fig. 6).

3.6. μCT Analysis

3D reconstructed μCT images of the three groups at week 4 post-fracture showed that the fracture healing in UG and UAG were much faster than in CG, as indicated by early closure of fracture gap (Fig. 7A). The BVh/TV in UG was significantly higher than in CG (p = 0.004) (Fig. 7B); BMD in UG was higher than in UAG (p = 0.053) and CG (p = 0.006) (Fig. 7C). For BVl/TV and BVt/TV, no significant differences were found among groups.

3.7. Mechanical Testing

Femora in UG were significantly stronger than in other two groups (Table 2). The ultimate load of the fractured femur in UG was significantly greater than those in UAG and CG (p<0.05, p< 0.05 respectively). The stiffness of the fractured femur in UG was also marginally higher than that of CG (p = 0.065).

3.8. Histomorphometric and Immunohistochemical Analysis

Histological evaluation using hematoxylin–eosin (H&E) and safranin-O/fast green staining demonstrated enhanced fracture healing in UG and UAG at week 4, as reflected by newly formed woven bone with better bridging of fracture gap, whereas newly formed woven bone was observed to some extent in CG at week 4 but there were still many chondroid tissues in the fracture area (Fig. 8A). Quantitative analysis showed that Cg.Ar/Cl.Ar (%) in UG was significantly lower than in CG (Table 3).

Immunohistochemical analysis of GFP and SDF-1 demonstrated that at week 4 post-fracture, many GFP positive cells could be found in the callus area in all three groups, where the number of GFP positive cells in UG was remarkably increased than those in UAG and CG. In UAG, only a scarce number of GFP-positive cells could be found in the fracture area, as compared with UG and CG (Fig. 8B, left). SDF-1 protein in the callus area of UG and UAG was higher than in CG respectively (Fig. 8B, right).

3.9. Serum SDF-1 Protein Level Measurement

At week 4, the serum SDF-1 protein levels in UG and UAG were significantly increased, as compared with CG (p = 0.005 for both), while the level of SDF-1 in serum was comparable between UG and UAG (Fig. 9).

Discussion

Fracture healing is a complex and well-orchestrated biological process composed of three phases: inflammation, repair and remodeling. In the inflammation and repair phases, SDF-1/CXCR4 signaling participates in bone repair mainly by acting as a regulator of MSCs trafficking to fracture site [40]. In this study, we confirmed that LIPUS applied on the fractured bone promoted MSCs recruitment and that SDF-1/CXCR4 played a very important role in this process. Blocking of SDF-1 signaling with AMD3100 inhibited the migration of MSCs, and also reduced the promoting effect of LIPUS on fracture healing. The present study demonstrates that the enhanced MSCs migration mediated by SDF-1/CXCR4 pathway may be one of the crucial mechanisms through which LIPUS promotes fracture healing.

A major finding of the current study is that physical stimulation in form of LIPUS, can promote MSCs migration *in vitro* and during bone fracture healing *in vivo*. Mechanical stimuli are very important for the development and maintenance of bone [41]. Recently, increasing studies have shown that mechanical stimulation is crucial for regulating MSCs activities during bone repair. Luu *et al.* reported that low magnitude mechanical signals could significantly increase the proliferation and osteogenic differentiation of MSCs in the bone marrow of male C57BL/6J mice [42]; Lai *et al.* further demonstrated that LIPUS could increase osteogenic differentiation of human MSCs [43]. However, the role of mechanical signals in regulating MSCs migration is not reported. Our results revealed that mechanical signals might work in several ways to regulate MSCs behavior and functions. From *in vitro* study, the spontaneous migration capacity of the isolated rat MSCs in CG was observed. Similar phenomenon was observed by Adriana *et al.* in an *in vitro* migration study, which

demonstrated a low spontaneous migration capacity of BM-derived MSCs in the presence of medium alone (without growth factors or chemokines), after overnight incubation of the transwells at 37°C, 5%CO_2 [44]. It was most likely that the conditioned medium in the lower chamber of CG contained many bio-active factors that served as chemoattractant and induced the spontaneous migration of MSCs [45–48]. Our data found that LIPUS stimulation enhanced the migration of cultured MSCs, as indicated by the increased number of migrated cells at the exterior of inserts from UG, compared with those in CG. The effect of LIPUS on cell migration has been reported by several studies. Takao *et al.* studied the migration of osteoblast-like cell (MC3T3-E1 cells) under LIPUS treatment by using a wound healing assay. They found that after 20 minutes LIPUS treatment, the migration of MC3T3-E1 osteoblastic cells was significantly increased than the control group, as indicated by the distance between the wound line and the migration front at 6 h, 12 h and 20 h after wounding [49]. The upregulated SDF-1 and CXCR4 expression by LIPUS may be responsible for the enhanced motility of MSCs observed in cell migration assay in two possible ways. First, the enhanced CXCR4 expression of MSCs could lead to the increased MSCs migration. Shyam *et al.* isolated and cultured MSCs from healthy volunteers and transduced them with a retroviral vector containing either CXCR4 and GFP or GFP alone. They used a transwell migration system to study MSC migration to SDF-1, and found that MSCs transduced with CXCR4 showed significantly more migration toward SDF-1, with 3-fold greater at 3 h and more than 5-fold greater at 6 h [50]. Second, the upregulated SDF-1 expression, especially the increased SDF-1 protein level in the conditioned medium, promoted MSCs migration. Previously Son *et al.* used a chemoinvasion assay to evaluate the ability of MSCs to cross the reconstituted basement membrane Matrigel. After 24 hours of incubation at 37°C, 5% CO_2, the number of migrated MSCs toward the lower compartment containing SDF-1 was significantly higher than that in control [51]. Our results indicated that the enhanced cell migration may be due to the combined effects as described above. BM-derived MSCs are able to express CXCR4 and secrete SDF-1 simultaneously. The present study further demonstrated that after treating MSCs with AMD3100, the antagonist of SDF-1/CXCR4 pathway, the migration of MSCs under LIPUS treatment was strikingly reduced. This indicates the LIPUS-induced MSC migration is CXCR4-dependent. Although we still found a very small number of migrated cells in the combined treatment group (UAG), when compared with that in CG, there was no statistical significance. It suggested that AMD3100 might almost completely block the effect of LIPUS on MSC migration, since SDF-1 may not be the only chemokine in the conditioned medium of MSCs. Other bioactive factors secreted by MSCs may also influence MSC migration to some extent [45–48]. *In vivo*, the transplanted GFP-labeled MSCs were found to migrate to the callus, as indicated by the GFP intensity measured by fluorescent imaging and immunohistochemistry. Our findings confirmed that in young rat model, after 4 weeks of LIPUS treatment, both the serum and local SDF-1 protein levels in the callus of UG were increased than in CG, together with the higher GFP intensity from *ex vivo* fluorescent imaging, and increased GFP-positive cells in the callus of UG as detected by immunohistochemistry. Our findings were also substantiated by a similar report by Kumagai *et al.* demonstrating a positive effect in the recruitment of GFP-positive cells from a parabiotic mouse to the fracture site of another surgically conjoined mouse [24]. Therefore, there are sufficient evidence to conclude that there exist a strong relationship between LIPUS stimulation and MSCs migration.

This study demonstrated LIPUS treatment could activate SDF-1/CXCR4 pathway, which were substantiated by a few previous studies. Carlet *et al.* observed an intense expression of SDF-1 in the compression side of periodontal ligament during orthodontic tooth movement [52]; Li *et al.* also reported that cyclic stretch could upregulate SDF-1/CXCR4 axis in human saphenous vein smooth muscle cells [53]. Kumagai et al. also detected increased protein expression of both SDF-1 and CXC-R4 in the fracture site in the LIPUS treatment group as compared to the control group [24]. However, the mechanisms responsible for mechanical stimuli induced SDF-1/CXCR4 signaling in these cells are largely unknown. Integrins are the main receptors that connect the cytoskeleton to the extracellular matrix (ECM) [54]. They transmit mechanical stresses across the plasma membrane that enables the tractional forces developed in the cytoskeleton to be conveyed to the ECM [55]. Integrins also regulates signaling pathways [56,57]. Many recent studies have demonstrated the important interactions between SDF-1/CXCR4 pathway and integrins in regulating cellular activities in different cell types, including MSCs [58–61]. Thus, the effect we observed might be the downstream of LIPUS's interactions with the transmembrane integrins on the MSCs.

The direct regulatory effect of LIPUS on MSCs found *in vitro* may not fully reflect the complexity of the *in vivo* situation. During fracture repair, SDF-1 was found not only in MSCs, but also in other cell types, including endothelial cells [62,63], periosteal cells [28,64], chondrocytes [65], and osteoblasts [66,67] etc. Many previous studies have shown these cells might also secrete SDF-1 and contribute to the recruitment of MSCs. Given the fact that mechanical signals provided by LIPUS could be sensed and transduced by many cell types, which has been extensively studied in the past [68–73], it is most likely that LIPUS may act on these cells through different ways. LIPUS might promote SDF-1 secretion from different cells through physical interactions [74,75] and integrins signal transductions [76–79] in the site of injury; simultaneously, LIPUS enhances CXCR4 expression on the surface of MSCs from circulation or the adjacent BM, thus promoting these cells to migrate toward the SDF-1 gradient and engraft in the fracture site.

In the rat model, LIPUS promoted early callus formation, as indicated by weekly radiographic analysis. In all the groups, the temporal changes of CW and CA followed the similar pattern, i.e. from week 1 to week 2, both CW and CA increased gradually; from week 2 to week 4, both CW and CA decreased rapidly. The largest callus size was generally found at week 2, which indicated the most active callus formation; whereas the smallest callus size was found at week 4, which represented the callus remodeling. Significantly increased callus size in UG, in comparison with CG, was observed from week 1 to week 3 post-fracture, which reflected the promoting effect of LIPUS on callus formation in the early phase of fracture healing. Another finding of the radiographic analysis was that the callus bridging in UG was accelerated, which started at week 2, in contrast to CG at week 3. The present findings were consistent with many previous researches. In 1983, Dyson *et al.* applied therapeutic ultrasound on the complete bilateral transverse fibular fractures in adult female Wistar rats, and found that ultrasound therapy was most effective during the first two weeks after injury [80]. Later, by using bilateral closed femoral shaft fracture rat model, Wang *et al.* [81] and Yang *et al.* [82] demonstrated increased callus size after 7 daily 15-minute exposures to LIPUS treatment, compared with the contralateral controls. Our recent studies on LIPUS effects in rat closed fracture

healing substantiated these early works and demonstrated the promoted early callus formation [17,35,38,74].

LIPUS was also found to promote callus mineralization and remodeling in rats. As described earlier, from the radiographic analysis, the callus size of all the groups decreased rapidly, after reaching the peak value at week 2. It represented the start of the remodeling phase, overlapping significantly with the reparative phase, characterized by the slow modeling and remodeling of the fracture callus from woven to mature lamellar bone, and ultimately, the restoration of the bone to normal or near normal morphology and mechanical strength [83]. Among all the groups, the callus size in UG reduced more rapidly from week 2 to week 4 post-fracture, which suggested an accelerated remodeling process. The radiographic findings were supported by the results from μCT, which reflected the microstructure and mineralization of the callus. At week 4 post-fracture, we found BVh/TV and BMD in UG was significantly increased than in CG. Both BVh/TV and BMD are important tools for reflecting the degree of mineralization in callus. BMD of the callus has been used for the quantitative evaluation of the mechanical properties of healing bone [84–86]. The present results suggested LIPUS might accelerate the maturation process of callus. We also observed the apparent trend in the reduction of TV, BVl and BVl/TV in the callus of UG at week 4, as compared to in CG, although the differences were not statistically significant. These parameters reflected the reduced callus size and unmineralized tissue in the callus of UG, which was consistent with the radiographic analysis. The mechanical testing results further demonstrated the improved mechanical properties of callus under LIPUS treatment, as indicated by the higher UL and increased stiffness in UG at week 4. These findings were substantiated by the histological analysis, which showed the enhanced endochondral ossification in UG, in which fracture gap was better bridged at week 4 and filled with woven bone, whereas chondroid tissues were still present in the fracture area in CG.

Disrupting SDF1/CXCR4 signaling pathway by daily administration of AMD3100 on the rats receiving LIPUS treatment resulted in the significantly reduced GFP-positive cells in the fracture area, reduced callus size and less cartilage volume during fracture healing. These findings were supported by several previous studies. Toupadakis *et al.* examined the effect of AMD3100 on bone repair by using a murine fracture model. They found that the administration of AMD3100 led to a significantly reduced hyaline cartilage volume, callus volume and mineralized bone volume, associated with reduction of genes expression related to endochondral ossification [40]. Recently, Zhou found that in a traumatic brain injury/closed femoral fracture mice model, following AMD3100 treatment, the MSC migration was inhibited, and new bone formation was significantly reduced by 47% at the fracture sites in comparison with the controls treated with PBS [87]. However, when comparing to CG, UAG showed slightly better fracture healing, as shown by the early callus bridging (started from week 2), less chondroid tissues at fracture site and higher ultimate load. Taken together, these data suggest that SDF-1/CXCR4 signaling plays a very important role in fracture healing. Disrupting the SDF/CXCR4 pathway during LIPUS treatment could partially reduce, but not fully abolish LIPUS-induced fracture healing, indicating that other factors or signaling pathways might also be involved in this accelerated fracture repair process, such as increased blood circulation [88], upregulated osteogenic genes [89], and gap junctional cell-to-cell intercellular communication in rat MSCs [69].

The limitation of our study is that we used transplanted GFP-labeled allogenic MSCs to explore the migration activities of endogenous MSCs *in vivo*, which might not fully reflect the exact pattern of MSCs recruitment during facture healing. Further research may be necessary to understand the possible roles of endogenous MSCs in participating in tissue repair process.

Conclusion

In conclusion, our study demonstrated that the application of LIPUS treatment could enhance SDF-1 signaling pathway, promote MSCs migration towards the fracture site, and accelerate fracture healing. This is the first evidence showing the micro-mechanical stimulation produced by LIPUS's pressure waves can regulate MSCs migration through SDF-1/CXCR4 pathway in fracture healing. It provides novel insights into comprehensive mechanisms, through which LIPUS promotes fracture healing, and will potentially lead to the development of LIPUS enhanced MSC therapies for improving bone regeneration in a wide range of orthopaedic conditions.

Author Contributions

Conceived and designed the experiments: FYW KSL GL LQ WHC. Performed the experiments: FYW SH JHQ SKHC MHS. Analyzed the data: FYW WHC. Wrote the paper: FYW WHC.

References

1. Claes L, Recknagel S, Ignatius A (2012) Fracture healing under healthy and inflammatory conditions. Nat Rev Rheumatol 8: 133–143.
2. Caplan AI (1991) Mesenchymal stem cells. Journal of orthopaedic research : official publication of the Orthopaedic Research Society 9: 641–650.
3. Minguell JJ, Erices A, Conget P (2001) Mesenchymal stem cells. Exp Biol Med (Maywood) 226: 507–520.
4. Short B, Brouard N, Occhiodoro-Scott T, Ramakrishnan A, Simmons PJ (2003) Mesenchymal stem cells. Arch Med Res 34: 565–571.
5. Schindeler A, McDonald MM, Bokko P, Little DG (2008) Bone remodeling during fracture repair: The cellular picture. Semin Cell Dev Biol 19: 459–466.
6. Kolar P, Gaber T, Perka C, Duda GN, Buttgereit F (2011) Human early fracture hematoma is characterized by inflammation and hypoxia. Clin Orthop Relat Res 469: 3118–3126.
7. Bastian O, Pillay J, Alblas J, Leenen L, Koenderman L, et al. (2011) Systemic inflammation and fracture healing. J Leukoc Biol 89: 669–673.
8. Kitaori T, Ito H, Schwarz EM, Tsutsumi R, Yoshitomi H, et al. (2009) Stromal cell-derived factor 1/CXCR4 signaling is critical for the recruitment of mesenchymal stem cells to the fracture site during skeletal repair in a mouse model. Arthritis Rheum 60: 813–823.
9. Ponomaryov T, Peled A, Petit I, Taichman RS, Habler L, et al. (2000) Induction of the chemokine stromal-derived factor-1 following DNA damage improves human stem cell function. J Clin Invest 106: 1331–1339.
10. Ma M, Ye JY, Deng R, Dee CM, Chan GC (2011) Mesenchymal stromal cells may enhance metastasis of neuroblastoma via SDF-1/CXCR4 and SDF-1/CXCR7 signaling. Cancer Lett 312: 1–10.
11. Houthuijzen JM, Daenen LG, Roodhart JM, Voest EE (2012) The role of mesenchymal stem cells in anti-cancer drug resistance and tumour progression. Br J Cancer 106: 1901–1906.
12. Granero-Molto F, Weis JA, Miga MI, Landis B, Myers TJ, et al. (2009) Regenerative effects of transplanted mesenchymal stem cells in fracture healing. Stem Cells 27: 1887–1898.
13. Duarte LR (1983) The stimulation of bone growth by ultrasound. Arch Orthop Trauma Surg 101: 153–159.
14. Kristiansen TK, Ryaby JP, McCabe J, Frey JJ, Roe LR (1997) Accelerated healing of distal radial fractures with the use of specific, low-intensity ultrasound. A multicenter, prospective, randomized, double-blind, placebo-controlled study. The Journal of bone and joint surgery American volume 79: 961–973.
15. Leung KS, Lee WS, Tsui HF, Liu PP, Cheung WH (2004) Complex tibial fracture outcomes following treatment with low-intensity pulsed ultrasound. Ultrasound Med Biol 30: 389–395.
16. Fung CH, Cheung WH, Pounder NM, de Ana FJ, Harrison A, et al. (2012) Effects of different therapeutic ultrasound intensities on fracture healing in rats. Ultrasound in medicine & biology 38: 745–752.
17. Cheung WH, Chow SK, Sun MH, Qin L, Leung KS (2011) Low-intensity pulsed ultrasound accelerated callus formation, angiogenesis and callus remodeling in osteoporotic fracture healing. Ultrasound Med Biol 37: 231–238.
18. Khan Y, Laurencin CT (2008) Fracture repair with ultrasound: clinical and cell-based evaluation. J Bone Joint Surg Am 90 Suppl 1: 138–144.
19. Tam KF, Cheung WH, Lee KM, Qin L, Leung KS (2008) Osteogenic effects of low-intensity pulsed ultrasound, extracorporeal shockwaves and their combination - an in vitro comparative study on human periosteal cells. Ultrasound Med Biol 34: 1957–1965.
20. Wang YX, Leung KC, Cheung WH, Wang HH, Shi L, et al. (2010) Low-intensity pulsed ultrasound increases cellular uptake of superparamagnetic iron oxide nanomaterial: results from human osteosarcoma cell line U2OS. J Magn Reson Imaging 31: 1508–1513.
21. Arnsdorf EJ, Tummala P, Kwon RY, Jacobs CR (2009) Mechanically induced osteogenic differentiation-the role of RhoA, ROCKII and cytoskeletal dynamics. J Cell Sci 122: 546–553.
22. Li YJ, Batra NN, You L, Meier SC, Coe IA, et al. (2004) Oscillatory fluid flow affects human marrow stromal cell proliferation and differentiation. J Orthop Res 22: 1283–1289.
23. Kasper G, Glaeser JD, Geissler S, Ode A, Tuischer J, et al. (2007) Matrix metalloprotease activity is an essential link between mechanical stimulus and mesenchymal stem cell behavior. Stem Cells 25: 1985–1994.
24. Kumagai K, Takeuchi R, Ishikawa H, Yamaguchi Y, Fujisawa T, et al. (2012) Low-intensity pulsed ultrasound accelerates fracture healing by stimulation of recruitment of both local and circulating osteogenic progenitors. J Orthop Res 30: 1516–1521.
25. Xu L, Song C, Ni M, Meng F, Xie H, et al. (2012) Cellular retinol-binding protein 1 (CRBP-1) regulates osteogenenesis and adipogenesis of mesenchymal stem cells through inhibiting RXRalpha-induced beta-catenin degradation. Int J Biochem Cell Biol 44: 612–619.
26. Dominici M, Le Blanc K, Mueller I, Slaper-Cortenbach I, Marini F, et al. (2006) Minimal criteria for defining multipotent mesenchymal stromal cells. The International Society for Cellular Therapy position statement. Cytotherapy 8: 315–317.
27. Rui YF, Lui PP, Li G, Fu SC, Lee YW, et al. (2010) Isolation and characterization of multipotent rat tendon-derived stem cells. Tissue Eng Part A 16: 1549–1558.
28. Leung KS, Cheung WH, Zhang C, Lee KM, Lo HK (2004) Low intensity pulsed ultrasound stimulates osteogenic activity of human periosteal cells. Clin Orthop Relat Res: 253–259.
29. Wynn RF, Hart CA, Corradi-Perini C, O'Neill L, Evans CA, et al. (2004) A small proportion of mesenchymal stem cells strongly expresses functionally active CXCR4 receptor capable of promoting migration to bone marrow. Blood 104: 2643–2645.
30. Fricker SP, Anastassov V, Cox J, Darkes MC, Grujic O, et al. (2006) Characterization of the molecular pharmacology of AMD3100: a specific antagonist of the G-protein coupled chemokine receptor, CXCR4. Biochem Pharmacol 72: 588–596.
31. Guo Y, Hangoc G, Bian H, Pelus LM, Broxmeyer HE (2005) SDF-1/CXCL12 enhances survival and chemotaxis of murine embryonic stem cells and production of primitive and definitive hematopoietic progenitor cells. Stem Cells 23: 1324–1332.
32. Leung KS, Shi HF, Cheung WH, Qin L, Ng WK, et al. (2009) Low-magnitude high-frequency vibration accelerates callus formation, mineralization, and fracture healing in rats. J Orthop Res 27: 458–465.
33. Sun MH, Leung KS, Zheng YP, Huang YP, Wang LK, et al. (2012) Three-dimensional high frequency power Doppler ultrasonography for the assessment of microvasculature during fracture healing in a rat model. J Orthop Res 30: 137–143.
34. Furlani D, Li W, Pittermann E, Klopsch C, Wang L, et al. (2009) A transformed cell population derived from cultured mesenchymal stem cells has no functional effect after transplantation into the injured heart. Cell Transplant 18: 319–331.
35. Cheung WH, Chin WC, Wei FY, Li G, Leung KS (2013) Applications of exogenous mesenchymal stem cells and low intensity pulsed ultrasound enhance fracture healing in rat model. Ultrasound Med Biol 39: 117–125.
36. De Clercq E (2003) The bicyclam AMD3100 story. Nat Rev Drug Discov 2: 581–587.
37. Shi HF, Cheung WH, Qin L, Leung AH, Leung KS (2010) Low-magnitude high-frequency vibration treatment augments fracture healing in ovariectomy-induced osteoporotic bone. Bone 46: 1299–1305.
38. Cheung WH, Chin WC, Qin L, Leung KS (2012) Low intensity pulsed ultrasound enhances fracture healing in both ovariectomy-induced osteoporotic and age-matched normal bones. J Orthop Res 30: 129–136.
39. Ekeland A, Engesoeter LB, Langeland N (1982) Influence of age on mechanical properties of healing fractures and intact bones in rats. Acta Orthop Scand 53: 527–534.
40. Toupadakis CA, Wong A, Genetos DC, Chung DJ, Murugesh D, et al. (2012) Long-term administration of AMD3100, an antagonist of SDF-1/CXCR4 signaling, alters fracture repair. J Orthop Res 30: 1853–1859.
41. Carter DR, Van Der Meulen MC, Beaupre GS (1996) Mechanical factors in bone growth and development. Bone 18: 5S–10S.
42. Luu YK, Capilla E, Rosen CJ, Gilsanz V, Pessin JE, et al. (2009) Mechanical stimulation of mesenchymal stem cell proliferation and differentiation promotes osteogenesis while preventing dietary-induced obesity. J Bone Miner Res 24: 50–61.
43. Lai CH, Chen SC, Chiu LH, Yang CB, Tsai YH, et al. (2010) Effects of low-intensity pulsed ultrasound, dexamethasone/TGF-beta1 and/or BMP-2 on the

transcriptional expression of genes in human mesenchymal stem cells: chondrogenic vs. osteogenic differentiation. Ultrasound Med Biol 36: 1022–1033.

44. Ponte AL, Marais E, Gallay N, Langonne A, Delorme B, et al. (2007) The in vitro migration capacity of human bone marrow mesenchymal stem cells: comparison of chemokine and growth factor chemotactic activities. Stem Cells 25: 1737–1745.

45. Nagaya N, Kangawa K, Itoh T, Iwase T, Murakami S, et al. (2005) Transplantation of mesenchymal stem cells improves cardiac function in a rat model of dilated cardiomyopathy. Circulation 112: 1128–1135.

46. Caplan AI, Dennis JE (2006) Mesenchymal stem cells as trophic mediators. J Cell Biochem 98: 1076–1084.

47. Walter MN, Wright KT, Fuller HR, MacNeil S, Johnson WE (2010) Mesenchymal stem cell-conditioned medium accelerates skin wound healing: an in vitro study of fibroblast and keratinocyte scratch assays. Exp Cell Res 316: 1271–1281.

48. Meirelles Lda S, Fontes AM, Covas DT, Caplan AI (2009) Mechanisms involved in the therapeutic properties of mesenchymal stem cells. Cytokine Growth Factor Rev 20: 419–427.

49. Iwai T, Harada Y, Imura K, Iwabuchi S, Murai J, et al. (2007) Low-intensity pulsed ultrasound increases bone ingrowth into porous hydroxyapatite ceramic. J Bone Miner Metab 25: 392–399.

50. Bhakta S, Hong P, Koc O (2006) The surface adhesion molecule CXCR4 stimulates mesenchymal stem cell migration to stromal cell-derived factor-1 in vitro but does not decrease apoptosis under serum deprivation. Cardiovasc Revasc Med 7: 19–24.

51. Son BR, Marquez-Curtis LA, Kucia M, Wysoczynski M, Turner AR, et al. (2006) Migration of bone marrow and cord blood mesenchymal stem cells in vitro is regulated by stromal-derived factor-1-CXCR4 and hepatocyte growth factor-c-met axes and involves matrix metalloproteinases. Stem Cells 24: 1254–1264.

52. Garlet TP, Coelho U, Repeke CE, Silva JS, Cunha Fde Q, et al. (2008) Differential expression of osteoblast and osteoclast chemmoatractants in compression and tension sides during orthodontic movement. Cytokine 42: 330–335.

53. Li F, Guo WY, Li WJ, Zhang DX, Lv AL, et al. (2009) Cyclic stretch upregulates SDF-1alpha/CXCR4 axis in human saphenous vein smooth muscle cells. Biochem Biophys Res Commun 386: 247–251.

54. Ernstrom GG, Chalfie M (2002) Genetics of sensory mechanotransduction. Annu Rev Genet 36: 411–453.

55. Huang S, Ingber DE (1999) The structural and mechanical complexity of cell-growth control. Nat Cell Biol 1: E131–138.

56. Schwartz MA, Assoian RK (2001) Integrins and cell proliferation: regulation of cyclin-dependent kinases via cytoplasmic signaling pathways. J Cell Sci 114: 2553–2560.

57. Katsumi A, Orr AW, Tzima E, Schwartz MA (2004) Integrins in mechanotransduction. J Biol Chem 279: 12001–12004.

58. Peled A, Kollet O, Ponomaryov T, Petit I, Franitza S, et al. (2000) The chemokine SDF-1 activates the integrins LFA-1, VLA-4, and VLA-5 on immature human CD34(+) cells: role in transendothelial/stromal migration and engraftment of NOD/SCID mice. Blood 95: 3289–3296.

59. Jing D, Fonseca AV, Alakel N, Fierro FA, Muller K, et al. (2010) Hematopoietic stem cells in co-culture with mesenchymal stromal cells–modeling the niche compartments in vitro. Haematologica 95: 542–550.

60. Cencioni C, Capogrossi MC, Napolitano M (2012) The SDF-1/CXCR4 axis in stem cell preconditioning. Cardiovasc Res 94: 400–407.

61. Cheng M, Qin G (2012) Progenitor cell mobilization and recruitment: SDF-1, CXCR4, alpha4-integrin, and c-kit. Prog Mol Biol Transl Sci 111: 243–264.

62. Yamaguchi J, Kusano KF, Masuo O, Kawamoto A, Silver M, et al. (2003) Stromal cell-derived factor-1 effects on ex vivo expanded endothelial progenitor cell recruitment for ischemic neovascularization. Circulation 107: 1322–1328.

63. Dar A, Goichberg P, Shinder V, Kalinkovich A, Kollet O, et al. (2005) Chemokine receptor CXCR4-dependent internalization and resecretion of functional chemokine CXCL-1 by bone marrow endothelial and stromal cells. Nat Immunol 6: 1038–1046.

64. Kitaori T, Ito H, Schwarz EM, Tsutsumi R, Yoshitomi H, et al. (2009) Stromal cell-derived factor 1/CXCR4 signaling is critical for the recruitment of mesenchymal stem cells to the fracture site during skeletal repair in a mouse model. Arthritis and rheumatism 60: 813–823.

65. Murata K, Kitaori T, Oishi S, Watanabe N, Yoshitomi H, et al. (2012) Stromal cell-derived factor 1 regulates the actin organization of chondrocytes and chondrocyte hypertrophy. PLoS One 7: e37163.

66. Jung Y, Wang J, Schneider A, Sun YX, Koh-Paige AJ, et al. (2006) Regulation of SDF-1 (CXCL12) production by osteoblasts; a possible mechanism for stem cell homing. Bone 38: 497–508.

67. Katayama Y, Battista M, Kao WM, Hidalgo A, Peired AJ, et al. (2006) Signals from the sympathetic nervous system regulate hematopoietic stem cell egress from bone marrow. Cell 124: 407–421.

68. Azuma Y, Ito M, Harada Y, Takagi H, Ohta T, et al. (2001) Low-intensity pulsed ultrasound accelerates rat femoral fracture healing by acting on the various cellular reactions in the fracture callus. J Bone Miner Res 16: 671–680.

69. Sena K, Angle SR, Kanaji A, Aher C, Karwo DG, et al. (2011) Low-intensity pulsed ultrasound (LIPUS) and cell-to-cell communication in bone marrow stromal cells. Ultrasonics 51: 639–644.

70. Sun JS, Hong RC, Chang WH, Chen LT, Lin FH, et al. (2001) In vitro effects of low-intensity ultrasound stimulation on the bone cells. J Biomed Mater Res 57: 449–456.

71. Li JK, Chang WH, Lin JC, Ruaan RC, Liu HC, et al. (2003) Cytokine release from osteoblasts in response to ultrasound stimulation. Biomaterials 24: 2379–2385.

72. Naruse K, Miyauchi A, Itoman M, Mikuni-Takagaki Y (2003) Distinct anabolic response of osteoblast to low-intensity pulsed ultrasound. J Bone Miner Res 18: 360–369.

73. Sant'Anna EF, Leven RM, Virdi AS, Sumner DR (2005) Effect of low intensity pulsed ultrasound and BMP-2 on rat bone marrow stromal cell gene expression. J Orthop Res 23: 646–652.

74. Fung CH, Cheung WH, Pounder NM, de Ana FJ, Harrison A, et al. (2012) Effects of different therapeutic ultrasound intensities on fracture healing in rats. Ultrasound Med Biol 38: 745–752.

75. Mehta S, Antich P (1997) Measurement of shear-wave velocity by ultrasound critical-angle reflectometry (UCR). Ultrasound Med Biol 23: 1123–1126.

76. Hsu HC, Fong YC, Chang CS, Hsu CJ, Hsu SF, et al. (2007) Ultrasound induces cyclooxygenase-2 expression through integrin, integrin-linked kinase, Akt, NF-kappaB and p300 pathway in human chondrocytes. Cell Signal 19: 2317–2328.

77. Pounder NM, Harrison AJ (2008) Low intensity pulsed ultrasound for fracture healing: a review of the clinical evidence and the associated biological mechanism of action. Ultrasonics 48: 330–338.

78. Yang R-S, Lin W-L, Chen Y-Z, Tang C-H, Huang T-H, et al. (2005) Regulation by ultrasound treatment on the integrin expression and differentiation of osteoblasts. Bone 36: 276–283.

79. Whitney NP, Lamb AC, Louw TM, Subramanian A (2012) Integrin-mediated mechanotransduction pathway of low-intensity continuous ultrasound in human chondrocytes. Ultrasound in medicine & biology.

80. Dyson M, Brookes M (1983) Stimulation of bone repair by ultrasound. Ultrasound Med Biol Suppl 2: 61–66.

81. Wang SJ, Lewallen DG, Bolander ME, Chao EY, Ilstrup DM, et al. (1994) Low intensity ultrasound treatment increases strength in a rat femoral fracture model. J Orthop Res 12: 40–47.

82. Yang KH, Parvizi J, Wang SJ, Lewallen DG, Kinnick RR, et al. (1996) Exposure to low-intensity ultrasound increases aggrecan gene expression in a rat femur fracture model. J Orthop Res 14: 802–809.

83. Hadjiargyrou M, McLeod K, Ryaby JP, Rubin C (1998) Enhancement of fracture healing by low intensity ultrasound. Clinical orthopaedics and related research 355: S216–S229.

84. Augat P, Merk J, Genant HK, Claes L (1997) Quantitative assessment of experimental fracture repair by peripheral computed tomography. Calcif Tissue Int 60: 194–199.

85. Dai K-R, Hao Y-Q (2007) Quality of healing compared between osteoporotic fracture and normal traumatic fracture. Advanced Bioimaging Technologies in Assessment of the Quality of Bone and Scaffold Materials: Springer. 531–541.

86. Nyman JS, Munoz S, Jadhav S, Mansour A, Yoshii T, et al. (2009) Quantitative measures of femoral fracture repair in rats derived by micro-computed tomography. Journal of biomechanics 42: 891–897.

87. Liu X, Zhou C, Li Y, Ji Y, Xu G, et al. (2013) SDF-1 promotes endochondral bone repair during fracture healing at the traumatic brain injury condition. PLoS One 8: e54077.

88. Rawool NM, Goldberg BB, Forsberg F, Winder AA, Hume E (2003) Power Doppler assessment of vascular changes during fracture treatment with low-intensity ultrasound. J Ultrasound Med 22: 145–153.

89. Favaro-Pipi E, Bossini P, de Oliveira P, Ribeiro JU, Tim C, et al. (2010) Low-intensity pulsed ultrasound produced an increase of osteogenic genes expression during the process of bone healing in rats. Ultrasound Med Biol 36: 2057–2064.

21

Trunk Muscle Activity Is Modified in Osteoporotic Vertebral Fracture and Thoracic Kyphosis with Potential Consequences for Vertebral Health

Alison M. Greig[1], Andrew M. Briggs[2,3], Kim L. Bennell[4], Paul W. Hodges[5]*

1 Department of Physical Therapy, University of British Columbia, Vancouver, Canada, **2** School of Physiotherapy and Exercise Science, Curtin University, Perth, Australia, **3** Arthritis and Osteoporosis Victoria, Melbourne, Australia, **4** Centre for Health, Exercise and Sports Medicine, The University of Melbourne, Melbourne, Australia, **5** The University of Queensland, Centre for Clinical Research Excellence in Spinal Pain, Injury and Health, School of Health and Rehabilitation Sciences, Brisbane, Australia

Abstract

This study explored inter-relationships between vertebral fracture, thoracic kyphosis and trunk muscle control in elderly people with osteoporosis. Osteoporotic vertebral fractures are associated with increased risk of further vertebral fractures; but underlying mechanisms remain unclear. Several factors may explain this association, including changes in postural alignment (thoracic kyphosis) and altered trunk muscle contraction patterns. Both factors may increase risk of further fracture because of increased vertebral loading and impaired balance, which may increase falls risk. This study compared postural adjustments in 24 individuals with osteoporosis with and without vertebral fracture and with varying degrees of thoracic kyphosis. Trunk muscle electromyographic activity (EMG) associated with voluntary arm movements was recorded and compared between individuals with and without vertebral fracture, and between those with low and high thoracic kyphosis. Overall, elderly participants in the study demonstrated co-contraction of the trunk flexor and extensor muscles during forwards arm movements, but those with vertebral fractures demonstrated a more pronounced co-contraction than those without fracture. Individuals with high thoracic kyphosis demonstrated more pronounced alternating flexor and extensor EMG bursts than those with less kyphosis. Co-contraction of trunk flexor and extensor muscles in older individuals contrasts the alternating bursts of antagonist muscle activity in previous studies of young individuals. This may have several consequences, including altered balance efficacy and the potential for increased compressive loads through the spine. Both of these outcomes may have consequences in a population with fragile vertebrae who are susceptible to fracture.

Editor: Dominique Heymann, Faculté de médecine de Nantes, France

Funding: This study was supported by a Program Grant from the National Health and Medical Research Council (NHMRC) of Australia. PH was supported by a Senior Principal Research Fellowship (APP1002190) from the NHMRC. KB was supported by a Future Fellowship from the Australian Research Council (ARC). The funders had no role in study design, data collection and analysis, decision to publish, or preparation of the manuscript.

Competing Interests: The authors have declared that no competing interests exist.

* Email: p.hodges@uq.edu.au

Introduction

Osteoporosis is a significant public health problem particularly in women, with vertebral fractures recognised as one of the hallmarks of the condition. The "vertebral fracture cascade" refers to the 4–7 fold increased risk of subsequent vertebral fractures and increased risk of fracture in the appendicular skeleton (e.g. odds ratio of 2.8 for developing a fracture at the femoral neck [1]), after an incident fracture is sustained [2]. Physical impairments, psychosocial morbidity and health care costs increase similarly as the frequency of fractures increase [3,4]. Identification of individuals at risk of sustaining an incident vertebral fracture, or recurrent fractures, is a priority.

Low bone mineral density alone is an unreliable predictor of vertebral fracture at the individual patient level [5]. This suggests other factors moderate fracture risk. A comprehensive review identified several non-osseous factors as potential contributors to the fracture cascade. These include neurophysiologic properties such as trunk muscle activation (which may increase spinal load) and compromised balance (which may increase falls risk) [2]. Despite limited research, some data suggest balance impairments

in populations with osteoporosis, particularly those with greater thoracic kyphosis [6,7]. However, as the presence of existing vertebral fractures was not investigated in the osteoporotic populations in these studies, it is not possible to determine whether balance deficits were mediated by postural change or the presence of fractures. Our recent study showed that balance impairment is related to vertebral fracture rather than thoracic kyphosis among women with osteoporosis [8]. A further complication for investigation of factors that contribute to fracture risk is the differentiation between the presence of a vertebral fracture and normal age-related changes in vertebral morphology. It is necessary to disentangle the relative contribution of thoracic kyphosis and fracture to functional changes associated with osteoporosis to guide appropriate selection of interventions.

Changes in trunk muscle activation could underlie both the increased fracture risk and balance deficits. Preliminary evidence shows greater activation of paraspinal (extensor) muscles, which increase spinal load, in individuals with vertebral fractures than those without [9]. From other populations, decreased spinal mobility related to increased back muscle activation has been linked to compromised balance [10,11]. However, several

Table 1. Descriptive statistics for fracture groups expressed as mean (SD).

	Fracture (n = 10)	No Fracture (n = 14)	
Height (cm)	158.9 (5.4)	157.5 (4.1)	p = 0.486
Mass (kg)	67.0 (10.8)	59.8 (9.2)	p = 0.092
Age (years)	68.1 (7.1)	64.0 (8.9)	p = 0.239
BMI (kg/m²)	26.6 (4.5)	24.5 (3.8)	p = 0.235
Kyphosis - Cent 4–9 (deg)	34.1 (9.4)	32.5 (7.6)	p = 0.660
Kyphosis - Cobb 4–9 (deg)	44.5 (9.8)	38.5 (8.4)	p = 0.125
PASE[†]	164.4 (50.6)	156.7 (54.5)	p = 0.738

[†]Physical Activity Scale for the Elderly.

questions remain unanswered. First, activity of other trunk muscles remains unexplored in people with osteoporosis, and if co-activation of trunk flexor and extensor muscles is increased this substantially increases spinal load, as is common in back pain [12]. Second, changes in trunk muscle activity could be related to the degree of thoracic kyphosis or the presence of vertebral fracture [8], and these have not been differentiated.

Investigation of postural adjustments is an ideal model to investigate changes in trunk muscle activation in osteoporosis. Analysis of anticipatory postural adjustments in association with arm movements [13–15] provides an opportunity to investigate the pre-programmed strategy initiated by the nervous system to counteract predictable challenges to balance. Anticipatory postural adjustments are affected by a number of factors that are associated with osteoporosis and fracture, including posture [16], pain [17–19], and fear of falling [20]; these latter two effects are known to be mediated by increased co-contraction of antagonist flexor and extensor trunk muscles during the postural adjustments [20,21].

This study aimed to investigate differences in activity of the trunk muscles using electromyography (EMG) during postural adjustments in older individuals with primary osteoporosis. Participants were divided into groups based on; (i) the presence or absence of osteoporotic vertebral fractures, and (ii) the magnitude of thoracic kyphosis (high vs. low).

Materials and Methods

Participants

Twenty-four community-dwelling women with primary osteoporosis and more than five years post menopause were recruited for this study. Women were recruited from the community via local advertising (newspapers, posters) and by approaching osteoporosis peer support groups in metropolitan Melbourne. Participants were also recruited from local private medical specialist clinics and public outpatient clinics and bone densitometry units at the Royal Melbourne Hospital and Broadmeadows Hospital.

Subject to meeting the inclusion criteria (diagnosis of primary osteoporosis, pain <4/10, age ≥55 years and more than 5 years post menopause), participants were divided into fracture (n = 10), and no-fracture (n = 14) groups. Participants were also independently grouped based on low (n = 12) and high (n = 12) thoracic kyphosis. Exclusion criteria included any other medical conditions that affect bone metabolism or balance, or participation in any high intensity exercise that could affect trunk control. Physical activity was assessed using the Physical Activity Scale for the Elderly (PASE) [22]. Pain immediately prior to and during testing, was assessed using an 11-point numerical rating scale (NRS)

anchored with "no pain" and "worst pain imaginable". Pain of less than 4/10 was required for participation in this study in order to ensure comfort and safety of participants and overcome the potentially moderating influence of pain on EMG responses.

Osteoporosis was diagnosed from bone densitometry results using World Health Organization criteria [23], and vertebral fractures were diagnosed from standardised lateral radiographs (lumbar and thoracic spine) using conservative classification criteria [24] as reduction in anterior vertebral height of ≥30% compared to posterior height and the posterior height of the adjacent superior or inferior vertebral body. Compression fractures were identified from qualitative reviews of spinal radiographs, consistent with an accepted semi-quantitative method [25]. Lateral spine radiographs were used to measure thoracic kyphosis using the vertebral centroid angle (T4 to T9). Reliability and validity for the centroid measure have been established, and this measure is considered superior to traditional methods such as the Cobb angle [26,27]. Nonetheless, traditional Cobb angles (T 4–9) were also measured according to Goh and colleagues [28], for comparison to previous literature.

Participants were grouped into two categories based on the: i) presence of vertebral fracture; and ii) degree of thoracic kyphosis. For the first analysis, based on fracture, there were no differences in demographic characteristics between groups categorised in this manner (all p>0.092) (Table 1). Seventeen anterior wedge fractures were identified in the fracture group at vertebral levels T4 (17.6%), T5 (11.8%), T6 (23.5%), T7 (11.8%), T8 (23.5%), T9 (5.9%) and T12 (5.9%). Thoracic kyphosis was not different

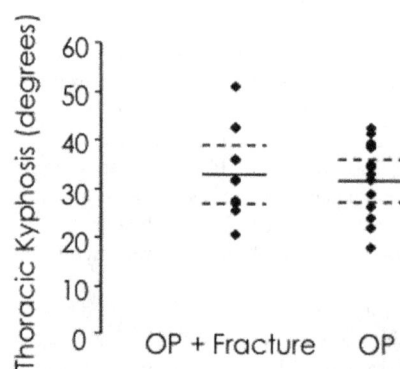

Figure 1. Magnitude of thoracic kyphosis based on fracture group. Mean and 95% confidence interval for each group (fracture and no-fracture) is shown. Thoracic kyphosis was not significantly different between groups (p = 0.660).

between fracture groups based on either the centroid ($p = 0.660$) or Cobb ($p = 0.125$) measurements (Fig. 1). For the second analysis participants were divided by the median centroid angle of $35°$ in to low and high thoracic kyphosis groups. We elected to divide the group into these high and low categories using a median split in the data rather than using clinical thresholds for thoracic hyperkyphosis (determined by traditional Cobb-based measurement approaches), as the Cobb method is particularly prone to measurement error in populations with osteoporosis. For example, the Cobb angle predominantly reflects endplate tilt of vertebrae between selected limits of the curve, and may not reveal changes regionally within the curve, nor true intervertebral curvature relative to vertical [26,27]. Although the vertebral centroid method has been used previously in a population with osteoporosis and measurement properties established [26], there is currently no agreement regarding a threshold for classification of hyperkyphosis. Although the median-split approach arbitrarily categorized participants into "high" and "low" groups, it enabled valid statistical comparison between equal-sized groups and comparable variance based on visual inspection of the spread of the data. When considering the traditional Cobb angle method for measuring thoracic kyphosis, we observed a Cobb angle between T4-9 of greater than $40°$ (hyper-kyphosis) in 12 (50%) participants. There were no differences in demographic parameters between kyphosis groups (all $p > 0.103$) (Table 2). Pain was $< 2/10$ for all participants during testing and was not different between groups ($p > 0.05$). Ethical approval was granted by the Institutional Human Research Ethics Committee and all participants provided written, informed consent.

Electromyography

Electromyographic activity (EMG) was recorded using pairs of Ag/AgCl adhesive electrodes (1 cm discs, Meditrace, Kendall LTP, MA, USA), placed along the muscle (inter-electrode distance - 2 cm). Recordings were made of obliquus internus (OI), and externus abdominis (OE), rectus abdominis (RA), and erector spinae (ES) at L3 and T7 EMG [29,30]. EMG electrodes were placed over the anterior and posterior deltoid, and a ground electrode was placed over the right iliac crest. EMG data were amplified 1000x, band pass filtered between 20–1000 Hz (2nd order Butterworth 12dB/octave filter) and sampled at 2000 Hz. A notch filter was used at 50 Hz. Data were recorded and stored using a Power1401 data acquisition system and Spike 2 (v 4.10) software (Cambridge Electronic Design Limited, Cambridge, England), and exported for analysis with Matlab 6.5.0 (The Mathworks, Natick, MA, USA).

Task Protocol – Anticipatory Postural Adjustments

Participants rapidly moved their right arm to disturb balance while standing with feet shoulder-width apart, toes aligned forward, and equal weight through both feet. Participants move their arm forward (shoulder flexion to $\sim 60°$) or backwards (shoulder extension to $\sim 40°$) as rapidly as they could in response to a light that indicated the direction of movement. Participants were instructed to relax between arm movements. The light was triggered manually and recorded with EMG data. Direction of arm movements was randomized for 10 trials in each direction (forward or backward), resulting in a total of 20 unique arm movements performed in a random sequence. An accelerometer (Crossbow Technology Inc, San Jose, CA, USA) was fixed to the dorsum of the right hand to provide information regarding movement onset and arm displacement. Five practice trials were undertaken with each participant to ensure they understood the protocol.

Data Analysis

Deltoid EMG provided information about the direction and timing of arm movements to which trunk EMG could be related. The time of onset of deltoid EMG was identified visually as this method has been shown to be reliable and less affected by background EMG than many statistical based methods [31]. We elected to characterise the pattern of the EMG activity of the trunk muscles based on analysis the activity of each muscle, averaged over participants, within epochs/time intervals either side of the onset of deltoid EMG rather than analysis of the onsets of EMG of each of the trunk muscles. The main reason underpinning this decision was the difficulty in to identify the onset of EMG, particularly of the thoracic extensor muscles, when there is ongoing tonic activity. This approach has been successfully used to characterise postural patterns of muscle activation in earlier studies [32]. Root mean square (RMS) EMG amplitude was calculated for each trunk muscle in ten 50-ms epochs (from 250 ms before to 250 ms after deltoid EMG onset). Maximum voluntary contractions were not performed in this study for EMG normalisation due to risks associated with vertebral fragility. Normalisation to a submaximal task is also not appropriate as this would lead to inaccurate conclusions if the different groups perform the submaximal task differently. Due to these limitations, EMG data were analysed in two alternate ways. First, EMG data were normalised to the peak activity recorded for each muscle, across all epochs and trials. This approach to normalisation enables a valid comparison in EMG amplitude between epochs and between arm movement directions for a given muscle. Given this approach does

Table 2. Descriptive statistics for thoracic kyphosis groups expressed as mean (SD).

	Low Kyphosis (n = 12)	High Kyphosis (n = 12)	
Height (cm)	157.9 (5.3)	158.2 (4.0)	$p = 0.905$
Mass (kg)	59.3 (10.3)	66.2 (9.6)	$p = 0.103$
Age (years)	64.8 (6.9)	66.6 (9.7)	$p = 0.615$
BMI (kg/m^2)	24.3 (4.4)	26.5 (3.8)	$p = 0.203$
Kyphosis - Cent 4–9 (deg)	26.4 (4.7)	39.9 (4.6)	$p < 0.001^a$
Kyphosis - Cobb 4–9 (deg)	35.1 (6.5)	46.8 (8.0)	$p < 0.001^a$
PASE†	154.0 (47.1)	166.0 (58.5)	$p = 0.591$

^{a}significant difference.
†Physical Activity Scale for the Elderly.

not use a between-muscle normalisation, such as maximum voluntary contraction across muscles, the method precludes valid comparison of EMG amplitude between muscles and between participant groups. This approach to normalisation has been used previously [9]. Second, non-normalised EMG amplitude was used for comparison of each muscle between groups. This analysis is affected by differences in electrode placement and filtering by subcutaneous tissue. However, as there was no difference in BMI between fracture groups ($p = 0.232$) or groups based on thoracic kyphosis ($p = 0.203$) we had no reason to suspect any systematic difference in subcutaneous tissue between groups. We argue that, with some caution, interpretation using the non-normalised EMG data could be made for an exploratory analysis in conjunction with the analysis of EMG pattern from data normalised to peak EMG.

Statistical Analysis

Repeated measures analysis of variance (ANOVA) was used to compare normalised EMG amplitude between Epochs and arm movement Directions for each muscle. This analysis provided detailed information about the *pattern* of muscle activation and enabled identification of the epochs during which EMG activity increased above baseline (*epoch 0*). The pattern of trunk muscle activation was qualitatively compared between groups. In addition we undertook an exploratory analysis on non-normalised EMG data to compared EMG amplitude between groups for each muscle and each arm movement using independent t-tests. As this study was exploratory in nature, it was not considered appropriate to apply adjustments for multiple comparisons as this has been argued to mask potentially important differences [33]. Statistical analyses were conducted using SPSS for windows (v 11.0.1; SPSS Inc, Chicago, Illinois, USA) and significance was set at $p < 0.05$.

Results

Electromyography during arm movement

When participants moved their arm forwards, bursts of EMG activity of the trunk flexor and extensor muscles were initiated almost simultaneously. Such overlapping activity of antagonist muscles (up-going panels in Fig. 2) is consistent with a trunk co-contraction pattern. In general, during arm flexion, EMG amplitude increased above baseline ($p < 0.05$, filled shapes in Fig. 2) during *epochs 3 to 5* (150-0 ms prior to deltoid) for both trunk flexor and extensor muscles.

Backwards movement of the arm was not accompanied by co-contraction of the trunk muscles. Instead, there was a burst of trunk flexor muscle EMG and either no change or decreased activity of the extensor muscles (down-going panels in Fig. 2). Activity of OE and RA increased above baseline (filled shapes in Fig. 2) during *epochs 6 to 7* (from deltoid onset, to 100 ms after).

Association with fracture

Some differences in muscle activation were evident between fracture and no-fracture groups (Fig. 2). Irrespective of fracture status, EMG of OI and OE increased above baseline in epoch 4 (100–50 ms prior to deltoid onset). RA EMG only increased above baseline in the no-fracture group and this also occurred in epoch 4 (100–50 ms prior to deltoid onset). During forward arm movements ES EMG at L3 and T7 increased during a later epoch in the fracture group compared with no-fracture group (*epoch 4* vs. *3*).

During backwards arm movements, OI EMG did not change from baseline in the fracture group, but reduced from baseline during *epochs 5 to 7* (50 ms prior to and 100 after deltoid onset) in the no-fracture group. RA EMG increased from baseline during *epochs 7 to 10* (100 to 250 ms after deltoid) in the fracture group,

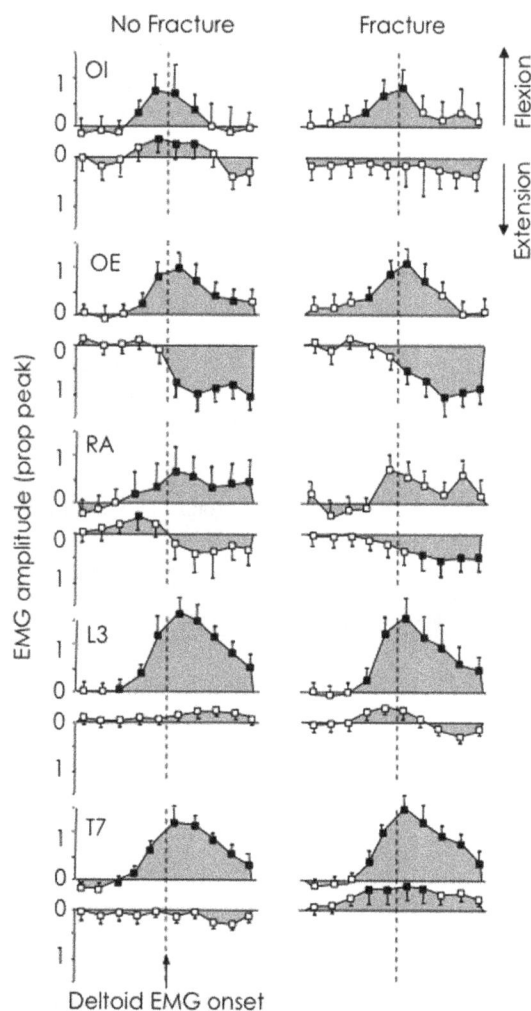

Figure 2. Average normalised EMG amplitude of trunk muscles for 10 epochs (250 ms before and after onset of deltoid EMG). Up-going panels and down-going panels demonstrate forwards and backwards arm movements, respectively. Filled shapes denote values that differ significantly ($p < 0.05$) in amplitude from the baseline, and unfilled shapes denote values that are not different from baseline. Abdominal (OI, OE and RA) and back (Erector spinae at L3 and T7) increased during the same epoch during arm flexion rather than the predicted earlier onset of back muscle activity.

but there was a decrease in RA EMG in *epoch 4* in the no-fracture group. Activity of ES T7 decreased below baseline during *epochs 3 to 6* (150 ms prior to and 50 ms after deltoid onset) in the fracture group, while there was no change in ES T7 activity from baseline in the no-fracture group. Non-normalised EMG amplitudes was not different between fracture groups (Fig. 3; all $p > 0.116$).

Association with thoracic kyphosis

When participants were grouped based on the magnitude of thoracic kyphosis, activity of trunk flexor muscles (up-going panels, Fig. 4) and extensor muscles (down-going panels, Fig. 4) showed a similar overlapping pattern, consistent with co-contraction. When participants in both groups moved their arm forwards, OI and OE EMG increased above baseline in *epochs 4* and *5*, respectively. ES L3 and T7 EMG increased during an earlier epoch in the high

Trunk Muscle Activity Is Modified in Osteoporotic Vertebral Fracture and Thoracic Kyphosis...

201

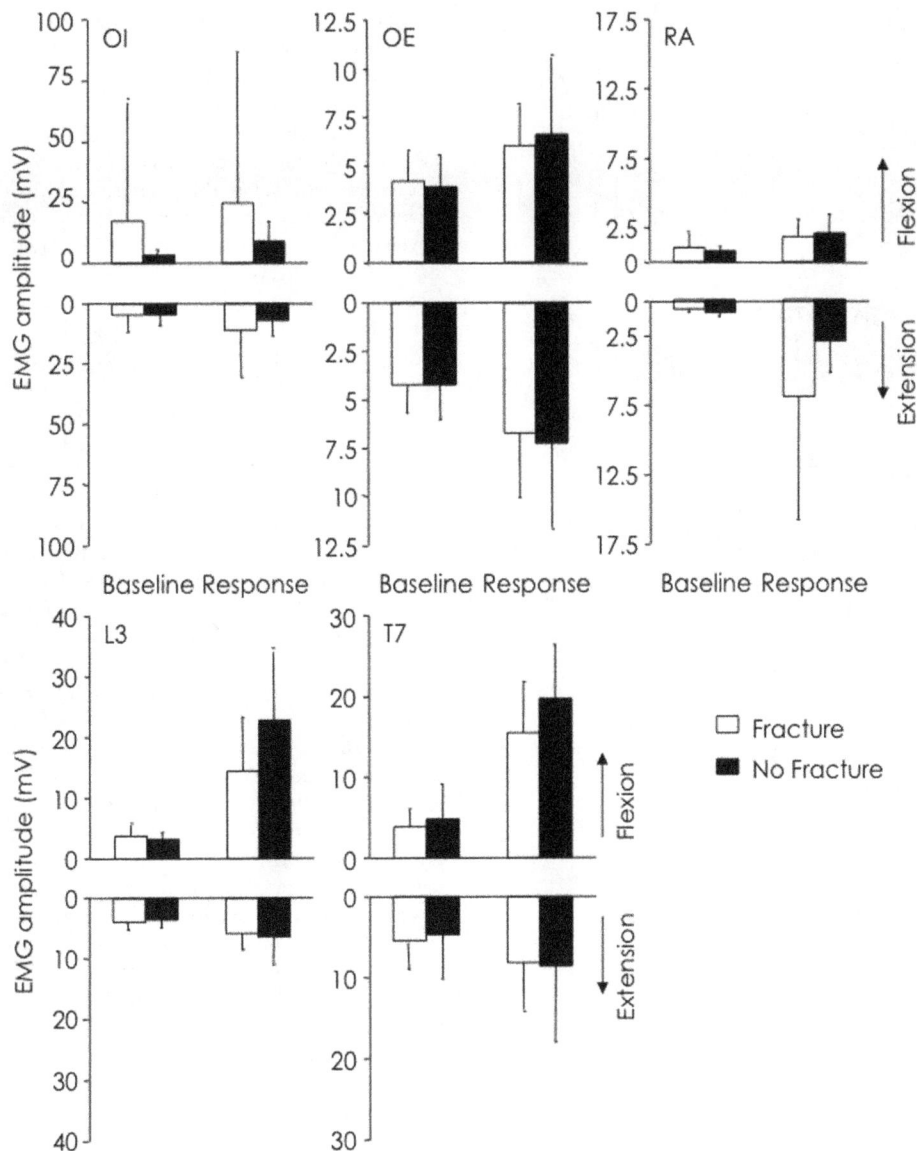

Figure 3. EMG amplitude based on fracture grouping. EMG amplitude at baseline (*epoch* 0) and during response (*epochs* 6–10) for fracture and no-fracture groups during forwards (up-going) and backwards (down-going) arm movements. There was no difference between groups for any muscle.

kyphosis group compared with low kyphosis group (*epoch 3* vs. *4*, respectively).

Backwards arm movements were associated with bursts of trunk flexor EMG activity. In the high kyphosis group OE and RA EMG increased above baseline in *epochs 6* and *7*, respectively, but there was no change in trunk extensor muscle EMG. In the group with low kyphosis, OE EMG activity also increased above baseline in *epoch 6*, but there were no other changes in EMG activity in either trunk flexor or extensor muscles.

Analysis of non-normalised EMG amplitude revealed less OE EMG in the group with high kyphosis, compared to low kyphosis ($p = 0.029$; Fig. 5). There were no other differences between groups for any muscle, but there was a non-significant trend toward lower RA EMG in the group with high kyphosis ($p = 0.067$).

Discussion

The results of this study demonstrate that in this elderly population with established primary osteoporosis, unlike younger individuals reported previously [13,34], arm flexion is associated with co-contraction of trunk flexor and extensor muscles. Here, we refer to our cohort as "elderly" as the majority of studies with comparable methods have sampled younger adults, and thus we refer to elderly in relative terms. Trunk co-contraction may have several consequences, including increased spinal compression and compromised postural recovery with implications for balance and falls risk. Both of these consequences may have negative implications in a population with increased vertebral fragility. Differences in trunk muscle activity were identified based on grouping by the presence of vertebral fracture or thoracic kyphosis. As there was no difference in thoracic kyphosis between

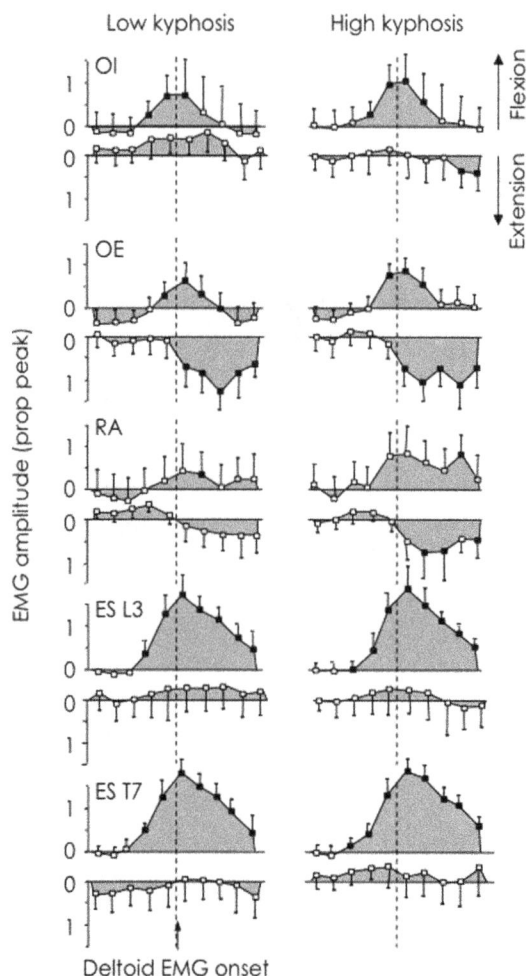

Figure 4. Average normalised EMG amplitude of trunk muscles for 10 epochs (250 ms before and after onset of deltoid EMG). Up-going panels and down-going panels demonstrate forwards and backwards arm movements, respectively. Filled shapes denote values that differ significantly ($p<0.05$) in amplitude from the baseline, and unfilled shapes denote values that are not different from baseline. Activity of back muscles (erector spinae at L3 and T7 increased earlier than flexors (OE and RA) during the forward arm movement.

the fracture groups in this cohort, influences of fracture and thoracic kyphosis appear to be independent.

Co-contraction of the trunk antagonist muscles is increased in older individuals

A new observation in this elderly population was that antagonist trunk muscles co-contracted in association with voluntary forwards arm movements. This contrasts data from younger individuals that indicate a triphasic response of alternating antagonist trunk muscle activity to counteract the perturbation from arm movement [13,32].

Alternating bursts of trunk muscle activity induces spine movement in advance of the arm movement [34]. Recent work in people with low back pain indicates reduced spine movement (which would be expected to accompany co-contraction) is associated with compromised quality of postural control [35]. Increased co-contraction of antagonist muscles (stiffening) in other body regions has also been reported in elderly populations. For example, ankle stiffness in standing is increased in the elderly

population [36], and older individuals demonstrate longer durations of lower leg and trunk muscle co-contraction during external perturbations [37].

Stiffening strategies may be employed to maintain a tighter control of the body's centre of mass (COM) within the base of support [20], and to compensate for narrowed limits of stability associated with aging [38]. Thus, trunk stiffening may be an adaptive strategy of the neuromuscular system in the elderly. Given this study is cross-sectional in nature; we are unable to speculate conclusively on the drivers underpinning this trunk stiffening response. Although self-report physical activity data for our cohort suggest moderate to high levels of current physical activity as measured with the PASE instrument [22], we did not collect historic physical activity data to make inferences about how activity history and agility may influence the trunk motor control strategies. Nonetheless, the moderate to high levels of current physical activity point to our sample as active and imply that the trunk stiffening response is not secondary to inactivity and disuse which could impact the neuromotor system's strategies to maintain balance and control the trunk. Data from several studies suggest stiffening may be associated with fear of falling. Elderly individuals, who are less stable, demonstrate an increased tendency to stiffen their trunk in response to a tilting support surface [21], and lower leg stiffness is increased when moving to higher-threat conditions [20]. Although increased trunk stiffening may be an adaptation to improve postural control in static conditions, it may not be an optimal strategy when responding to perturbations of greater magnitude that require coordinated movement of the trunk to restore balance [15,34]. Furthermore, increased loading from trunk muscle co-contraction [12,39] may have negative consequences in individuals with spinal osteoporosis who have increased vertebral fragility. To our knowledge no physiologically-representative data are available which unequivocally identify the minimum forces required from trunk muscle co-activation to cause vertebral fracture, hence this suggestion remains speculative. Indeed, this may be an important area for future research.

Although co-contraction was increased in forwards arm movements across groups, this overlapping pattern of flexor and extensor muscle activity was not evident during backwards arm movements. This finding may be related to the argument that a forwards arm movements induces a riskier perturbation, as it creates a posterior displacement of the COM. Several authors argue posterior COM displacement induces greater falls risk because of compromised ability to generate ankle torque to counteract the COM displacement in that direction [40]. Taken together, co-contraction with forwards arm movements and evidence of increased stiffness in situations of high threat, suggest perturbation in this direction is more risky for the elderly individuals.

Trunk muscle activity is altered in individuals with vertebral fracture

In the present study, the participants with vertebral fracture demonstrated differences in trunk muscle activation compared with those without fracture (Fig. 6A). This finding agrees with a previous study of paraspinal muscle control in this population [9]. During forwards arm movements, individuals with fracture concurrently increased activity of both flexor and extensor muscles, whereas the no-fracture group activated trunk extensor muscles prior to trunk flexor muscles. The latter pattern is more representative of the triphasic response observed in young individuals [13,34]. This finding highlights a more pronounced co-contraction strategy in individuals with fracture. The co-

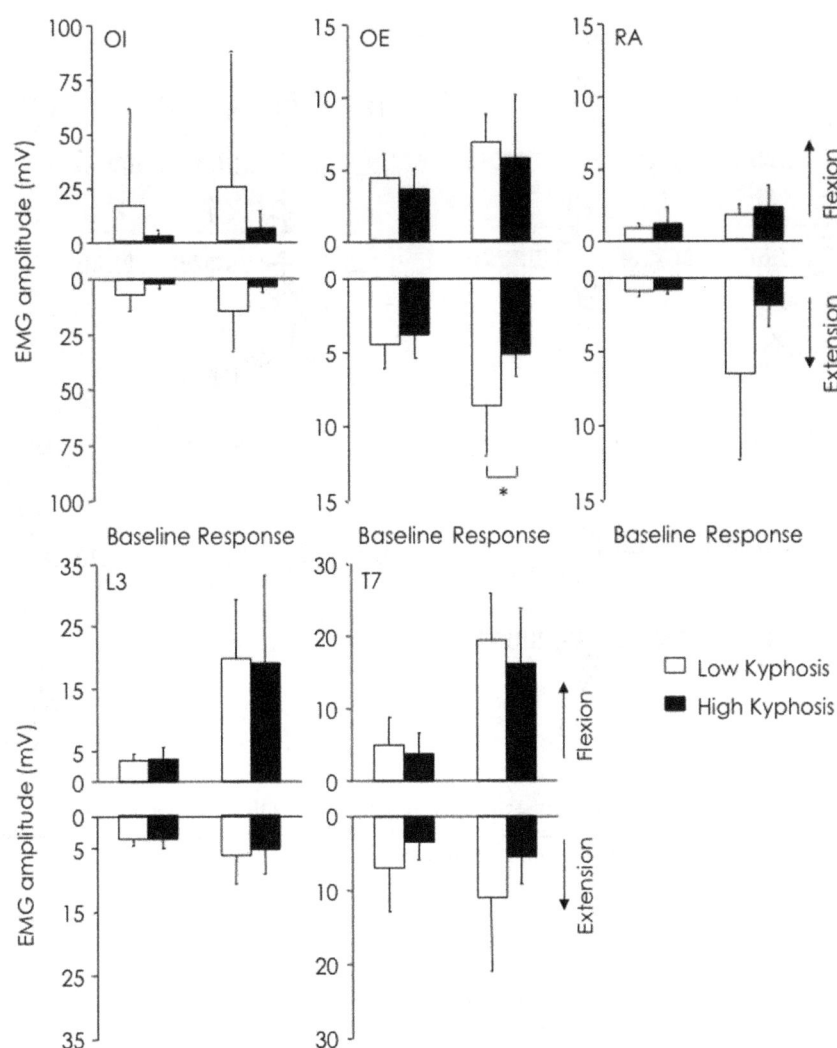

Figure 5. EMG amplitude based on kyphosis grouping. EMG amplitude at baseline (*epoch* 0) and during response (*epochs* 6–10) for thoracic kyphosis groups during forwards (up-going) and backwards (down-going) arm movements. Note significantly lower (*-P<0.05) OE EMG and a trend toward lower RA EMG in the group with least kyphosis.

contraction response may indicate greater vertebral loading [12] during dynamic tasks. Taken together with increased vertebral loading observed in this population in a static situation [41], this may help explain, in part, the vertebral fracture cascade. The combination of increased static postural loading and the potential for further increases in loading during dynamic tasks may substantially increase vertebral fracture risk. Studies using EMG-driven biomechanical models would be required to clarify this issue.

During backwards arm movements the fracture group reduced paraspinal muscle activity at T7 to below the baseline amplitude (Fig. 6B). This reduction in back extensor muscle activity during a less risky perturbation direction may be an adaptation to reduce spinal compressive loads through fragile vertebral bodies, or reduce muscle activation around a previously painful fracture site. It is also possible that back extensor weakness, which is associated with fracture [42], may have forced individuals to use different trunk control strategies compared to the individuals without fracture.

Trunk muscle activity is altered in individuals with greater thoracic kyphosis

When participants were grouped according to kyphosis angle the co-contraction strategy during forwards arm movements was evident in both low and high kyphosis groups (Fig. 6A). However, unlike the grouping based on fracture, the onsets of activity of the antagonist muscle groups were not simultaneous: trunk extensor EMG increased above baseline prior to arm movement, followed by trunk flexor muscles after arm movement onset. The most obvious differences between kyphosis groups was earlier onset of ES L3 and T7 in the group with high thoracic kyphosis and lower non-normalised OE EMG amplitude. These changes in the high kyphosis group may be explained by changes in mechanical demand for thorax control because of differences in posture. Increased forward spinal curvature and more anteriorly displaced COM from increased thoracic kyphosis places greater demand on the extensor muscles and reduced demand on flexors [7,43]. The more anterior COM position also provides the main contribution to increased compression and shear at the spine in osteoporosis [41]. Prior to a forwards arm movement, the trunk extensor

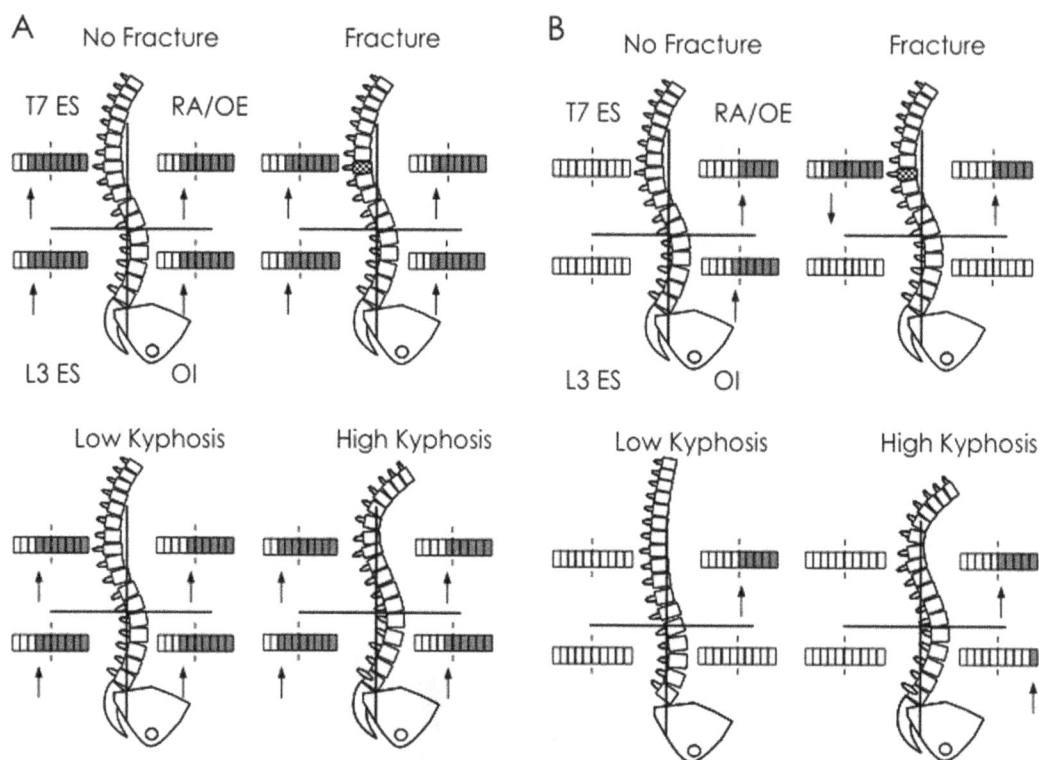

Figure 6. Summary of temporal differences in muscle activity in participants with osteoporosis grouped by presence or not of fracture and low and high kyphosis in (A) forwards and (B) backwards arm movements. Filled boxes indicate epoch in which muscle activity changes (" ↑ " increase and " ↓ " decrease). Boxes without fill indicate no change in activity from baseline.

muscles create an extension moment and the COM moves posteriorly [44,45]. In individuals with an already anteriorly displaced COM, the demand for extensor activity would be increased, and that of OE reduced. There were no marked differences in muscle activity recruitment patterns during backwards arm movements (Fig. 6B), but, variability in muscle activity within the groups may have obscured small differences.

Methodological issues

Thoracic spine curvature did not differ between those with and without fracture using two radiographic measures of kyphosis (e.g. Cobb, centroid). This was surprising as thoracic curvature is expected to increase with fracture. One interpretation is that existing methods lack sensitivity to detect small differences in curvature, and thus alternative measurement approaches have been proposed [26].

The main EMG analysis involved normalisation to the peak EMG among trials. This provides a sensitive measure of pattern of activity and formed the primary analysis. In addition, we compared the non-normalised EMG amplitude. Although this has the potential for error due to differences in electrode placement and properties of subcutaneous tissues [46] between individuals, we argue the alternative methods of normalisation to maximal or submaximal efforts are either not possible in this group or introduce errors due to potential differences in strategy to perform submaximal tasks in a system with a complex array of muscles available to generate torque. The main risk from analysis of non-normalised data is lack of sensitivity to detect differences between individuals due to inherent variability. We believe the analysis of non-normalised data is justified and the identification of

differences in amplitude between groups provides further context to interpret the changes in neuromuscular strategy as a secondary analysis.

Conclusion

The results of this study demonstrate postural adjustments of trunk muscles activity with arm movements differ in elderly participants with osteoporosis and patterns of trunk muscle responses varied according to the presence of vertebral fracture and degree of thoracic kyphosis. The tendency to increase trunk muscle co-contraction in this elderly cohort may be detrimental for vertebral loading, especially in individuals with compromised bone strength. Further research is required to establish a temporal relationship between vertebral fracture and differences in trunk control strategies to determine cause and effect. In addition, future research is needed to evaluate whether rehabilitation of trunk control strategies to reduce reliance on trunk stiffening is clinically effective in prevention of subsequent vertebral fractures and falls.

Acknowledgments

The authors gratefully acknowledge the in kind support provided by the Densitometry Unit at the University of Melbourne Department of Medicine, Royal Melbourne Hospital, Victoria.

Author Contributions

Conceived and designed the experiments: AG AB KB PH. Performed the experiments: AG AB PH. Analyzed the data: AG AB KB PH. Wrote the paper: AG AB KB PH.

References

1. Black DM, Arden NK, Palermo L, Pearson J, Cummings SR (1999) Prevalent vertebral deformities predict hip fractures and new vertebral deformities but not wrist fractures. Study of Osteoporotic Fractures Research Group. J Bone Miner Res 14: 821–828.

2. Briggs AM, Greig AM, Wark JD (2007) The vertebral fracture cascade in osteoporosis: a review of aetiopathogenesis. Osteoporos Int 18: 575–584.

3. Ensrud KE, Black DM, Harris F, Ettinger B, Cummings SR (1997) Correlates of kyphosis in older women. The Fracture Intervention Trial Research Group. J Am Ger Soc 45: 682–687.

4. Gabriel SE, Tosteson AN, Leibson CL, Crowson CS, Pond GR, et al. (2002) Direct medical costs attributable to osteoporotic fractures. Osteoporos Int 13: 323–330.

5. Marshall D, Johnell O, Wedel H (1996) Meta-analysis of how well measures of bone mineral density predict occurrence of osteoporotic fractures. Brit Med J 312: 1254–1259.

6. Cook C (2002) The relationship between posture and balance disturbances in women with osteoporosis. Phys Occ Ther Ger 20: 37–49.

7. Lynn SG, Sinaki M, Westerlind KC (1997) Balance characteristics of persons with osteoporosis. Arch Phys Med Rehabil 78: 273–277.

8. Greig AM, Bennell KL, Briggs AM, Wark JD, Hodges PW (2007) Balance impairment is related to vertebral fracture rather than thoracic kyphosis in individuals with osteoporosis. Osteoporos Int 18: 543–551.

9. Briggs AM, Greig AM, Bennell KL, Hodges PW (2007) Paraspinal muscle control in people with osteoporotic vertebral fracture. Eur Spine J 16: 1137–1144.

10. Mok NW, Brauer SG, Hodges PW (2007) Failure to use movement in postural strategies leads to increased spinal displacement in low back pain. Spine 32: E537–543.

11. Gruneberg C, Bloem BR, Honegger F, Allum JH (2004) The influence of artificially increased hip and trunk stiffness on balance control in man. Exp Brain Res 157: 472–485.

12. Marras WS, Davis KG, Ferguson SA, Lucas BR, Gupta P (2001) Spine loading characteristics of patients with low back pain compared with asymptomatic individuals. Spine 26: 2566–2574.

13. Aruin AS, Latash ML (1995) Directional specificity of postural muscles in feed-forward postural reactions during fast voluntary arm movements. Exp Brain Res 103: 323–332.

14. Hodges PW, Richardson CA (1999) Transversus abdominis and the superficial abdominal muscles are controlled independently in a postural task. Neurosci Lett 265: 91–94.

15. Horak F, Nashner LM (1986) Central programming of postural movements: Adaptation to altered support-surface configurations. J Neurophysiol 55: 1369–1381.

16. van der Fits IB, Klip AW, van Eykern LA, Hadders-Algra M (1998) Postural adjustments accompanying fast pointing movements in standing, sitting and lying adults. Exp Brain Res 120: 202–216.

17. Hodges PW, Moseley GL, Gabrielsson A, Gandevia SC (2003) Experimental muscle pain changes feedforward postural responses of the trunk muscles. Exp Brain Res 151: 262–271.

18. Hodges PW, Richardson CA (1996) Inefficient muscular stabilisation of the lumbar spine associated with low back pain: A motor control evaluation of transversus abdominis. Spine 21: 2640–2650.

19. Moseley GL, Nicholas MK, Hodges PW (2003) Pain differs from non-painful attention-demanding or stressful tasks in its effect on postural control patterns of trunk muscles. Exp Brain Res 156: 64–71.

20. Carpenter MG, Frank JS, Silcher CP, Peysar GW (2001) The influence of postural threat on the control of upright stance. Exp Brain Res 138: 210–218.

21. Maki BE, Holliday PJ, Fernie GR (1990) Aging and postural control. A comparison of spontaneous- and induced-sway balance tests. J Am Ger Soc 38: 1–9.

22. Washburn RA, Smith KW, Jette AM, Janney CA (1993) The Physical Activity Scale for the Elderly (PASE): development and evaluation. J Clin Epidemiol 46: 153–162.

23. NIH Consensus Development Panel on Osteoporosis Prevention, Diagnosis, and Therapy (2001) Osteoporosis prevention, diagnosis, and therapy. JAMA 285: 785–795.

24. McCloskey EV, Spector TD, Eyres KS, Fern ED, O'Rourke N, et al. (1993) The assessment of vertebral deformity: a method for use in population studies and clinical trials. Osteoporos Int 3: 138–147.

25. Genant HK, Jergas M, Palermo L, Nevitt M, Valentin RS, et al. (1996) Comparison of semiquantitative visual and quantitative morphometric assessment of prevalent and incident vertebral fractures in osteoporosis The Study of Osteoporotic Fractures Research Group. J Bone Miner Res 11: 984–996.

26. Briggs AM, Wrigley TV, Tully EA, Adams PE, Greig AM, et al. (2007) Radiographic measures of thoracic kyphosis in osteoporosis: Cobb and vertebral centroid angles. Skeletal Radiol 36: 761–767.

27. Harrison DE, Harrison DD, Cailliet R, Troyanovich SJ, Janik TJ, et al. (2000) Cobb method or Harrison posterior tangent method: which to choose for lateral cervical radiographic analysis. Spine 25: 2072–2078.

28. Goh S, Price RI, Leedman PJ, Singer KP (2000) A comparison of three methods for measuring thoracic kyphosis: implications for clinical studies. Rheumatol 39: 310–315.

29. Ng JK, Kippers V, Richardson CA (1998) Muscle fibre orientation of abdominal muscles and suggested surface EMG electrode positions. Electromyogr Clin Neurophysiol 38: 51–58.

30. Schultz A, Andersson GBJ, Örtengren R, Bjork R, Nordin M (1982) Analysis and quantitative myoelectric measurements of loads on the lumbar spine when holding weights in standing postures. Spine 7: 390–397.

31. Hodges PW, Bui B (1996) A comparison of computer based methods for the determination of onset of muscle contraction using electromyography. Electroencephalogr Clin Neurophysiol 101: 511–519.

32. Lee LJ, Coppieters MW, Hodges PW (2009) Anticipatory postural adjustments to arm movement reveal complex control of paraspinal muscles in the thorax. J Electromyogr Kinesiol 19: 46–54.

33. Perneger TV (1998) What's wrong with Bonferroni adjustments. Bmj 316: 1236–1238.

34. Hodges PW, Cresswell AG, Thorstensson A (1999) Preparatory trunk motion accompanies rapid upper limb movement. Exp Brain Res 124: 69–79.

35. Mok N, Brauer S, Hodges P (2011) Changes in lumbar movement in people with low back pain are related to compromised balance. Spine 36: E45–52.

36. Laughton CA, Slavin M, Katdare K, Nolan L, Bean JF, et al. (2003) Aging, muscle activity, and balance control: physiologic changes associated with balance impairment. Gait Posture 18: 101–108.

37. Tang PF, Woollacott MH (1998) Inefficient postural responses to unexpected slips during walking in older adults. J Gerontol A Biol Sci Med Sci 53: M471–480.

38. Robinovitch SN, Cronin T (1999) Perception of postural limits in elderly nursing home and day care participants. J Gerontol A Biol Sci Med Sci 54: B124–130.

39. Van Dieen JH, Cholewicki J, Radebold A (2003) Trunk muscle recruitment patterns in patients with low back pain enhance the stability of the lumbar spine. Spine 28: 834–841.

40. Carpenter MG, Allum JH, Honegger F, Adkin AL, Bloem BR (2004) Postural abnormalities to multidirectional stance perturbations in Parkinson's disease. J Neurol Neurosurg Psychiatry 75: 1245–1254.

41. Briggs AM, Wrigley TV, van Dieen JH, Phillips B, Lo SK, et al. (2006) The effect of osteoporotic vertebral fracture on predicted spinal loads in vivo. Eur Spine J 15: 1785–1795.

42. Sinaki M, Khosla S, Limburg PJ, Rogers JW, Murtaugh PA (1993) Muscle strength in osteoporotic versus normal women. Osteoporos Int 3: 8–12.

43. Horak FB, Diener HC, Nashner LM (1989) Influence of central set on human postural responses. J Neurophysiol 62: 841–853.

44. Bouisset S, Zattara M (1981) A sequence of postural adjustments precedes voluntary movement. Neurosci Lett 22: 263–270.

45. Hodges PW, Cresswell AG, Daggfeldt K, Thorstensson A (2000) Three dimensional preparatory trunk motion precedes asymmetrical upper limb movement. Gait Posture 11: 92–101.

46. Smith MD, Coppieters MW, Hodges PW (2007) Postural activity of the pelvic floor muscles is delayed during rapid arm movements in women with stress urinary incontinence. Int Urogynecol J Pelvic Floor Dysfunct 18: 901–911.

22

MCP/CCR2 Signaling Is Essential for Recruitment of Mesenchymal Progenitor Cells during the Early Phase of Fracture Healing

Masahiro Ishikawa[1,2], Hiromu Ito[1]*, Toshiyuki Kitaori[1], Koichi Murata[1], Hideyuki Shibuya[1], Moritoshi Furu[1,2], Hiroyuki Yoshitomi[3], Takayuki Fujii[1], Koji Yamamoto[4], Shuichi Matsuda[1]

1 Department of Orthopaedic Surgery, Kyoto University Graduate School of Medicine, Kyoto, Japan, 2 Department of the Control for Rheumatic Disease, Kyoto University Graduate School of Medicine, Kyoto, Japan, 3 The Center for Innovation in Immunoregulative Technology and Therapeutics, Kyoto University Graduate School of Medicine, Kyoto, Japan, 4 Center for the Promotion of Interdisciplinary Education and Research, Kyoto University, Kyoto, Japan

Abstract

Objective: The purpose of this study was to investigate chemokine profiles and their functional roles in the early phase of fracture healing in mouse models.

Methods: The expression profiles of chemokines were examined during fracture healing in wild-type (WT) mice using a polymerase chain reaction array and histological staining. The functional effect of monocyte chemotactic protein-1 (MCP-1) on primary mouse bone marrow stromal cells (mBMSCs) was evaluated using an *in vitro* migration assay. MCP-1$^{-/-}$ and C-C chemokine receptor 2 (CCR2)$^{-/-}$ mice were fractured and evaluated by histological staining and micro-computed tomography (micro-CT). RS102895, an antagonist of CCR2, was continuously administered in WT mice before or after rib fracture and evaluated by histological staining and micro-CT. Bone graft exchange models were created in WT and MCP-1$^{-/-}$ mice and were evaluated by histological staining and micro-CT.

Results: *MCP-1* and *MCP-3* expression in the early phase of fracture healing were up-regulated, and high levels of MCP-1 and MCP-3 protein expression observed in the periosteum and endosteum in the same period. MCP-1, but not MCP-3, increased migration of mBMSCs in a dose-dependent manner. Fracture healing in MCP-1$^{-/-}$ and CCR2$^{-/-}$ mice was delayed compared with WT mice on day 21. Administration of RS102895 in the early, but not in the late phase, caused delayed fracture healing. Transplantation of WT-derived graft into host MCP-1$^{-/-}$ mice significantly increased new bone formation in the bone graft exchange models. Furthermore, marked induction of MCP-1 expression in the periosteum and endosteum was observed around the WT-derived graft in the host MCP-1$^{-/-}$ mouse. Conversely, transplantation of MCP-1$^{-/-}$ mouse-derived grafts into host WT mice markedly decreased new bone formation.

Conclusions: MCP-1/CCR2 signaling in the periosteum and endosteum is essential for the recruitment of mesenchymal progenitor cells in the early phase of fracture healing.

Editor: Federico Quaini, University-Hospital of Parma, Italy

Funding: This work was supported by Grant-in-Aids from the Ministry of Education of Japan (No. 19591756, 21591942). The funders had no role in study design, data collection and analysis, decision to publish, or preparation of the manuscript.

Competing Interests: The authors have declared that no competing interests exist.

* Email: hiromu@kuhp.kyoto-u.ac.jp

Introduction

The prevalence of osteoporosis is increasing with the aging of society. In particular, osteoporotic fractures are a major public health problem with a low one-year patient's survival rate [1,2]. Management of the fracture is difficult because of poor bone quality, and there is a high risk of fixation failure and nonunion. To avoid these difficulties, numerous attempts have been made to develop techniques to improve fracture healing, including addition or injection of bone-forming factors or cells such as mesenchymal stem/progenitor cells [3,4]. However, treatment options remain below expectations despite vigorous attempts to find new useful therapies. One major reason is that the mechanisms responsible for fracture healing are complex and not fully understood. Hence, elucidating the mechanisms involved in fracture healing is fundamental to developing novel therapeutic strategies to improve fracture healing.

Normal fracture healing follows a unique, distinct healing process, which can be divided into three overlapping phases: inflammation, repair and remodeling [5]. Among these three phases, the repair and remodeling phases largely recapitulate the process of normal bone development [6]. In contrast, the inflammation phase is a unique process that is not observed in the organogenesis of bone and develops after birth to induce bone repair. Previous studies have shown that inflammation plays a pivotal role in fracture healing [7,8] and that mesenchymal stem/progenitor cells are systemically or locally recruited to the fracture site in the early inflammatory phase [5,9]. Many proinflammatory cytokines and chemokines are released from the fracture site in the early inflammatory phase [9,10]. Chemokines are small, chemoattractant cytokines that play key roles in the recruitment of leukocytes to sites of inflammation and injury. Studies have shown that stem/progenitor cell migration and organ-specific recruitment are regulated by chemokines and their receptors [11–13]. In addition, mesenchymal stem/progenitor cells express a variety of chemokine receptors [14], and chemokine-mediated mesenchymal stem/progenitor cell migration has been shown *in vitro* and *in vivo* [15,16].

Over the past decade, attention has focused on stem/progenitor cells because of their pivotal role in tissue regeneration. Mesenchymal stem/progenitor cells exhibit extensive tropism for tissue injury sites [17]. These cells differentiate into mesenchymal lineage cells when exposed to appropriate environmental cues and can promote tissue repair of many organs, including bone. In addition, mesenchymal stem/progenitor cells appear to exist in almost all tissues, including bone marrow, muscle and the periosteum, and if not present, can reach tissues via the blood circulation [18]. Therefore, mesenchymal stem/progenitor cells can be recruited from the circulation or surrounding tissues and participate in the repair of the injured organs [12,19].

Several studies have shown that systemically infused mesenchymal stem/progenitor cells can migrate to, and participate in, the repair of injured tissue [20–22]. We have previously demonstrated in a bone graft model that stromal cell-derived factor-1 (SDF-1) is induced in the periosteum of fracture sites and promotes endochondral bone repair by recruiting C-X-C chemokine receptor 4 (CXCR4)-expressing mesenchymal stem/progenitor cells [23]. Thus, mesenchymal stem/progenitor cell therapy may be a novel therapeutic strategy to improve fracture healing. To develop an efficient therapy, it is crucial to elucidate the precise mechanisms for recruitment of mesenchymal stem/progenitor cells to the fracture site. However, these mechanisms, especially during the early inflammatory phase, are largely unknown.

To identify the factor(s) essential for normal fracture healing, we used a polymerase chain reaction (PCR) array and mouse rib fracture model in which cell potential is non-impaired by surgical intramedullary fixation. We also used an exchange-graft model to show gain- or loss-of-function. We demonstrate herein that the expression level of monocyte chemotactic protein-1 (MCP-1) is up-regulated exclusively in the early fracture phase and that MCP-1 is expressed at the periosteum and endosteum of the fractured bones. Gain- and loss-of-function studies showed that the MCP-1/C-C chemokine receptor 2 (CCR2) axis is crucial in the early phase of fracture healing. In summary, these results indicate that the MCP-1/CCR2 axis provides essential signaling for normal bone healing and may be a novel, potent therapeutic target for fracture healing.

Materials and Methods

Reagents

Recombinant mouse MCP-1 and MCP-3 were purchased from Abcam (Cambridge, MA, USA). CCR2 antagonist (RS102895) was purchased from Sigma (St. Luis, MO, USA).

Mouse rib fracture model

All animal studies were conducted in accordance with principles and procedures approved by the Kyoto University Committee of Animal Resources. Surgeries were undergone under anesthesia with diethylether, and mice were euthanatized with cervical dislocation upon sacrifice. Mouse rib fracture models were created using 6-week-old C57BL/6 wild-type (WT), MCP-1$^{-/-}$ and CCR2$^{-/-}$ mice, as described previously [24]. Five mice from each fracture group were sacrificed 0, 1, 2, 3, 5, 7, 10, 14, 21, and 25 days after fracture. To evaluate the inhibitory effect of the receptor antagonist, the mice received continuous administration of the selective CCR2 antagonist, RS102895. RS102895 was dissolved in dimethyl sulfoxide (DMSO) and via an osmotic pump (model 1002; Durect, Cupertino, CA, USA), was delivered to a total of 10 mg/kg/day, beginning 2 days before or 4 days after rib fracture, and until day 12. In the control group, DMSO alone was administered for 14 days.

Femoral segmental bone graft transplantation model

A mouse segmental bone graft model was created using 6-week-old C57BL/6 WT and MCP-1$^{-/-}$ mice as described previously [25]. Briefly, 4-mm of mid-diaphyseal segmental bone was removed from the femur of the donor mouse. The graft was dissected carefully to remove the muscle and bone marrow without compromising the periosteum, and segmental bone derived from a WT or MCP-1$^{-/-}$ mouse was transplanted immediately into a 4-mm segmental defect in a host WT or MCP-1$^{-/-}$ mouse. Four groups of segmental bone graft models were used: MCP-1$^{-/-}$ donor to MCP-1$^{-/-}$ host [knockout (KO)-to-KO], WT donor to MCP-1$^{-/-}$ host (WT-to-KO), WT donor to WT host (WT-to-WT), and MCP-1$^{-/-}$ donor to WT host (KO-to-WT). The bone graft was stabilized using a 25 G stainless pin placed through the intramedullary marrow cavity, and the mice were sacrificed on day 21 after the surgery for RNA extraction and histological analysis.

Micro-CT analysis

Mice were sacrificed postoperatively for micro-computed tomography (micro-CT) imaging on days 7 (femoral bone graft model) and 21 (rib fracture model). The rib and femur were scanned using a micro-CT system (SMX-100CT-SV3; Shimadzu, Tokyo, Japan) at 2400 views, five frames per view, 40 kV, and 40 μA. Three-dimensional (3D) images were rendered and evaluated using VG Studio MAX (Nihon Visual Science Software, Tokyo, Japan). The newly formed callus was spatially segmented from the native cortical bone in the two-dimensional (2D) tomograms, the 3D images of the callus were rendered, and the total volume was measured on the digitally extracted callus tissue. The newly formed calluses in a region of interest covering the entire length of the bone graft, including 1 mm of the host bone at both proximal and distal bone graft junctions, were analyzed to determine bone graft healing.

RNA extraction, quantitative real-time PCR and PCR array

Total RNA was extracted from mouse rib and femoral bone graft specimens as described previously [26]. A PCR array was performed to measure mRNA levels for chemokines during the fracture healing process. Two micrograms of RNA was processed using an RT2 First Strand Kit (SA Biosciences, Frederick, MD, USA) according to the manufacturer's specifications. Quantitative PCR analysis for chemokines and receptors was assessed using a chemokine array (Chemokines & Receptors PCR Array, Mouse, PAMM-022, SA Biosciences). We analyzed the data using the RT2 profiler PCR Array Data Analysis software (SA Biosciences). The change in gene expression level determined by PCR array analysis was confirmed by quantitative real-time PCR. All gene

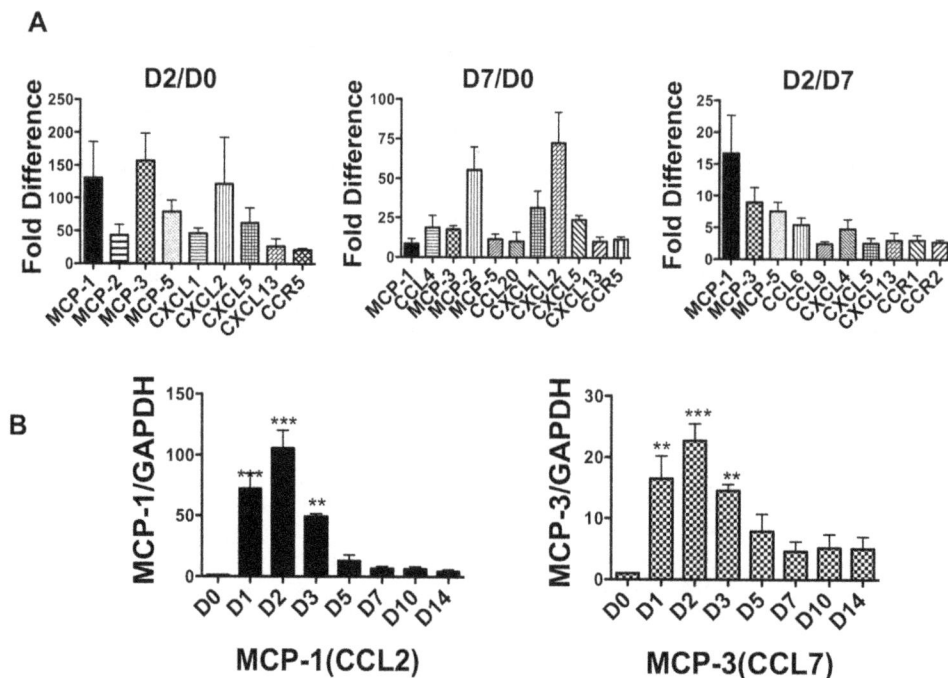

Figure 1. The expression profiles of chemokines and their receptors during fracture healing. Expression levels during fracture healing were examined using a rib fracture model. **A**: PCR array data for up-regulated chemokines and their receptors during fracture healing are shown. Expression levels were compared between days 0 and 2, days 0 and 7, and days 2 and 7. **B**: Time course of *MCP-1* and *MCP-3* mRNA expression in a rib fracture model, as analyzed by real-time PCR. Expression levels are the fold change from day 0 levels. Values are means ± SEM of more than four separate experiments. **P<0.01 ***P<0.001 compared with the day 0 group.

expression data were normalized against glyceraldehyde phosphate dehydrogenase (GAPDH).

Histological analysis

Rib and femur specimens were processed as paraffin-embedded sections and stained with hematoxylin and eosin and were subjected to immunohistochemical analyses as described previously [23,24].

In vitro chemotaxis assay

In vitro cell migration of primary mouse bone marrow stromal cells (mBMSCs) (1.0×10^5 cells/100 μl) was assessed using Transwell inserts with an 8-μm pore membrane, as described previously [23]. For the chemotaxis assay, different concentrations of MCP-1 or MCP-3 (0, 10, or 100 ng/ml) in 500 μl of medium were applied to the lower chambers. For the inhibition assay, RS102895 (400 nM) was also applied to the lower chambers. After 24 h of incubation, the migrated cells were counted under light microscopy.

Primary cell culture, cell line, osteogenesis and chondrogenesis assay

For the osteogenesis assay, mBMSCs were harvested and cultured as described previously [23]. mBMSCs were cultured with osteogenic base media (R&D Systems, Minneapolis, MN, USA) for 2 days. On reaching 70% confluence, the medium was replaced with osteogenic differentiation medium and was changed every 3 days thereafter. In some experiments, recombinant mouse MCP-1 (200 ng/ml) was added every 3 days with each medium change. On day 14 after plating, cells were harvested for alizarin red staining and gene expression analysis. For the chondrogenesis

assay, ATDC5 cells were cultured and maintained in Dulbecco's Modified Eagles Medium (DMEM) and Ham's F-12 at a 1:1 ratio with 5% fetal bovine serum (FBS) supplemented with insulin (10 mg/mL, Sigma), transferrin (5.5 mg/mL, Sigma), and sodium selenite (5 ng/mL, Sigma) to induce chondrocyte differentiation as described previously [27]. The medium was changed every 2 days thereafter. In some experiments, MCP-1 (0, 20, 100 or 200 ng/ml) was simultaneously added every 2 days with the medium change. On day 28 after plating, cells were harvested for gene expression analysis.

Statistical analysis

Data are presented as means ± standard error of the mean (SEM). We analyzed the data using GraphPad Prism Version 5.00 (GraphPad software). Statistical comparisons between two groups were performed using a Student's two-tailed *t* test. Differences between three groups were analyzed using the Bonferroni method. *P* values <0.05 were considered significant.

Results

Chemokine expression profile in the early phase of fracture healing

We first used PCR array to investigate the expression profile of chemokines during fracture healing in the WT mouse rib fracture model. The PCR array analysis showed that the expression levels of *MCP-1* and *MCP-3* were significantly higher on day 2 compared with days 0 and 7 (Figure 1A). *MCP-1* and *MCP-3* expression levels were more than 100 times higher on day 2 than on day 0. *MCP-1* and *MCP-3* expression levels on day 2 were five times higher than those on day 7. To confirm the PCR array data, we next examined the gene expression levels for *MCP-1* and

MCP-3 during the fracture healing process. Consistent with the PCR array analysis, the expression of *MCP-1* and *MCP-3* increased during the early phase of fracture healing (Figure 1B). *MCP-1* and *MCP-3* were expressed on day 1 and their expression peaked on day 2. By day 7, expression of both genes had declined markedly.

In vivo expression of MCP-1 during the early inflammatory phase of fracture healing

Because CCR2 is the major and common receptor for MCP-1 and MCP-3, we focused on the expression of MCP-1, MCP-3 and CCR2 in fracture healing, especially during the early inflammatory phase. To confirm the localization of MCP-1, MCP-3 and CCR2 expression during the early inflammatory phase of fracture healing, we used immunohistochemistry to examine rib fracture healing in WT mice. Low expression levels of MCP-1 and MCP-3 were observed at the periosteum in the unfractured rib, (Figures S1A, B) and high levels of MCP-1 and MCP-3 protein were observed at the periosteum and endosteum on day 3 in the fractured rib (Figure 2A, B). Conversely, little or no CCR2 staining was detected in the unfractured rib (Figure S1C), and on day 3, CCR2-positive cells were found predominantly within the bone marrow and surrounding tissues (Figure 2C).

MCP-1 induces mBMSCs migration *in vitro*

To examine the functional roles of MCP-1 and MCP-3 signaling in fracture healing, we first examined whether MCP-1 and MCP-3 could induce the migration of mBMSCs. MCP-1 significantly increased mBMSC migration in a dose-dependent manner, whereas MCP-3 did not (Figure 3A). Because MCP-1 and MCP-3 act through their receptor CCR2, we examined the expression of CCR2 in these cells. Consistent with a previous report [30], RT-PCR analysis showed that CCR2 was expressed in mBMSCs (Figure 3B). We also examined whether CCR2 mediates MCP-1-induced migration of mBMSCs. RS102895 (400 nM) effectively inhibited the MCP-1-induced migration of mBMSCs (Figure 3A). Because MCP-3 did not affect migration of the cells, we therefore focused on MCP-1. To further investigate possible roles of MCP-1, we next examined osteogenic differentiation of mBMSCs in response to MCP-1. Isolated mBMSCs were capable of spontaneously differentiating into alizarin red-positive cells and showed increased levels of *Runx2, osterix* and *alkaline phosphatase (ALP)* in the osteoinduction media on day 14. However, alizarin red staining revealed no difference between osteoinduced mBMSCs with or without MCP-1 (Figure S2A). Similarly, no difference in the gene expression of *Runx2, osterix, or ALP* was observed in cells treated with or without MCP-1 (Figure S2A). Because MCP-1 did not affect the osteogenic differentiation of mBMSCs, we also examined whether MCP-1 affects chondrogenic differentiation using ATDC5 cells *in vitro*. Alcian blue staining showed that the presence of MCP-1 was not associated with any obvious differences in cells treated with or without MCP-1 on day 28. Moreover, *SOX9, Col-2* and *Col-10* showed similar expression patterns in cells treated with or without MCP-1 (Figure S2B).

In vivo roles of MCP-1 and CCR2 during the early inflammatory phase of fracture healing

To investigate the functional roles of MCP-1 and CCR2 in fracture healing, rib fracture healing was assessed in WT and KO mice. Fracture calluses were examined by micro-CT and histological analysis. Histological analyses showed a smaller proportion of cartilage in the callus in MCP-1$^{-/-}$ mice compared

with WT mice on day 7 (Figure S3A). By day 21, fractures had healed in the WT mice and cartilage was almost completely replaced by bone in the callus (Figure 4A). Conversely, the healing processes progressed incompletely in MCP-1$^{-/-}$ and CCR2$^{-/-}$ mice by day 21, and the central area of the cartilaginous callus remained (Figure 4A). By day 25, a bridging callus was apparent in MCP-1$^{-/-}$ and CCR2$^{-/-}$ mice, and was similar in appearance to that observed in WT mice on 21 day (Figure S3B). The callus volume was significantly smaller in both MCP-1$^{-/-}$ and CCR2$^{-/-}$ mice than in WT mice on day 21 (Figure 4B, C).

Next, to elucidate whether the MCP-1/CCR2 axis is involved during the early phase of fracture healing, we continuously administered RS102895 before (pre-treatment) or after (post-treatment) rib fracture. Micro-CT analysis showed delayed fracture healing in the pre-treatment group compared with both the control and post-treatment groups. On day 21, the callus volume was significantly smaller in the pre-treatment group than in the control and post-treatment groups (Figures 5A, B). Histological analysis showed that fractures in both the control and post-treatment groups had healed by day 21 and that cartilaginous tissue was absent in the callus. Conversely, less cartilaginous tissue was observed in the callus in the pre-treatment group on day 7 (Figure 5C), and cartilaginous tissue in a central area of the callus was observed on day 21 (Figure S3C). These results indicate that the MCP-1/CCR2 axis is an essential component during the early phase of fracture healing.

Periosteal bone formation in grafts from WT mice implanted into MCP-1-deficient mice: gain-of-function

To examine the roles of MCP-1 at the periosteum and endosteum during fracture healing, we performed gain-of-function studies using a segmental bone graft transplantation model. A segmental bone graft was transplanted from an MCP-1$^{-/-}$ mouse to another MCP-1$^{-/-}$ mouse (KO-to-KO). Micro-CT and histological analysis were used to quantify new bone formation on day 21. Radiologic and micro-CT analyses showed that KO-to-KO transplantation caused a delay in fracture healing on day 21 (Figure 6A). Minimal periosteal bone formation was observed along the surface of the bone graft because of the lack of periosteal bone formation. We next created bone graft exchanging models between MCP-1$^{-/-}$ and WT mice, in which a segmental bone derived from a WT mouse was transplanted into a host MCP-1$^{-/-}$ mouse (WT-to-KO). In contrast to KO-to-KO bone graft transplantation, transplantation of the WT-derived graft into the host KO mouse significantly increased new bone formation and led to marked recovery of periosteal bone formation on day 21 (Figures 6A, B). Histological analysis further revealed marked and localized induction of MCP-1 expression in the callus and endosteum around the WT-derived graft in the host MCP-1$^{-/-}$ mouse (Figure 6C). By contrast, no MCP-1 expression was observed in the callus and endosteum of the host bone in the same section.

Reduction in periosteal bone formation in grafts from MCP-1-deficient mice implanted into WT mice: loss-of-function

To confirm whether MCP-1 is a crucial chemokine in the fracture healing process, we performed loss-of-function studies using WT-to-WT and KO-to-WT bone graft models. Transplantation of a WT donor graft into a WT host mouse led to abundant new bone formation and a bridging callus around the WT-derived graft on day 21 (Figures 6D, E). By contrast, transplantation of a KO-derived graft into a WT host markedly reduced the amount of periosteal bone formation in the donor graft.

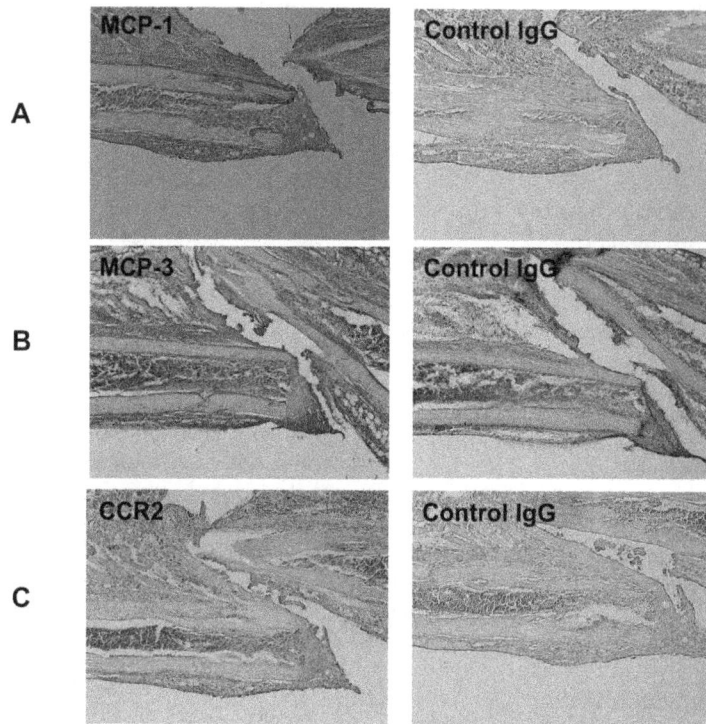

Figure 2. Immunohistochemical analysis of WT rib fracture on day 3. A, B, Protein expression levels of MCP-1 (**A**) and MCP-3 (**B**) were identified at the periosteum and endosteum on day 3. **C**, CCR2-positive cells were predominantly found within the bone marrow and surrounding tissues on day 3. Original magnification, 40×. Middle panel, high-magnification views (original magnification, 200×). The result is representative of three separate experiments.

Discussion

Our data highlight crucial roles of the MCP-1/CCR2 axis in the early phase of fracture healing. Compared with no fracture, the expression levels of many inflammatory chemokines increased on day 3 after fracture. In particular, *MCP-1* and *MCP-3*

expression were temporarily up-regulated in the early phase of fracture healing (Figure 1). Then, we found that deletion of either MCP-1 or CCR2 caused delayed fracture healing (Figure 4), and that, blockade of CCR2 only in the early phase of healing caused delayed fracture healing (Figure 5). Taken together, these results

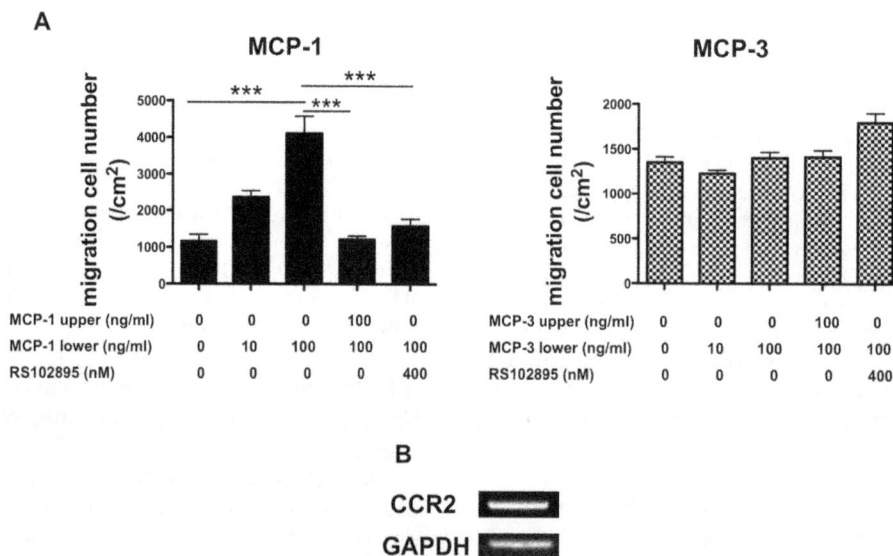

Figure 3. Effect of MCP-1 on cell migration. A: *In vitro* migration assay. mBMSCs were stimulated by MCP-1 or MCP-3 at indicated doses and RS102895 at 400 nM. Cells that migrated to the undersurface of the membrane were counted. Numbers of cells are represented as cell number per cm². Values are means ± SEM ($n = 5$, respectively). **B**: Expression of *CCR2* mRNA in mBMSCs. Data are shown as means ± SEM. *$P < 0.05$.

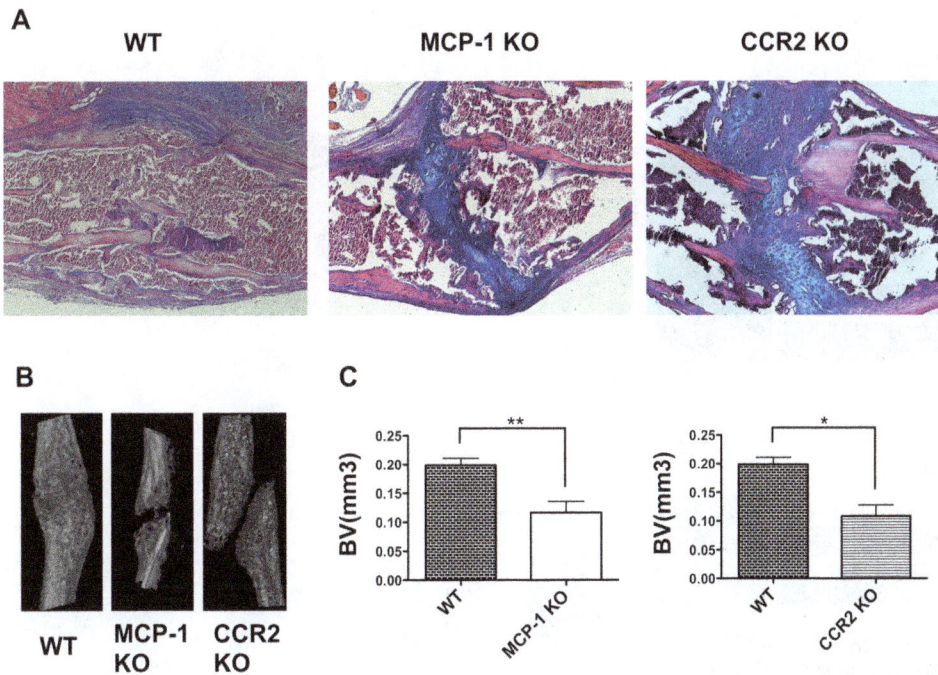

Figure 4. MCP-1$^{-/-}$ and CCR2$^{-/-}$ mice displayed delayed fracture healing *in vivo*. A: Histology of the fracture callus stained by hematoxylin-eosin/alcian-blue staining on day 21. **B**: Representative 3D micro-CT image of a fractured rib on day 21. **C**: Newly formed callus volume in the MCP-1$^{-/-}$ and CCR2$^{-/-}$ mice on day 21 was quantified using micro-CT.

suggest that the temporary increase of MCP-1, MCP-3 and CCR2 expression in the early inflammatory phase may play a pivotal role for successful fracture healing. A recent study reported that

deletion of CCR2 induces delayed fracture healing because of a decreased ability to resorb bone by osteoclasts in the remodeling phase [28]. The persistent cartilage fracture healing phenotype

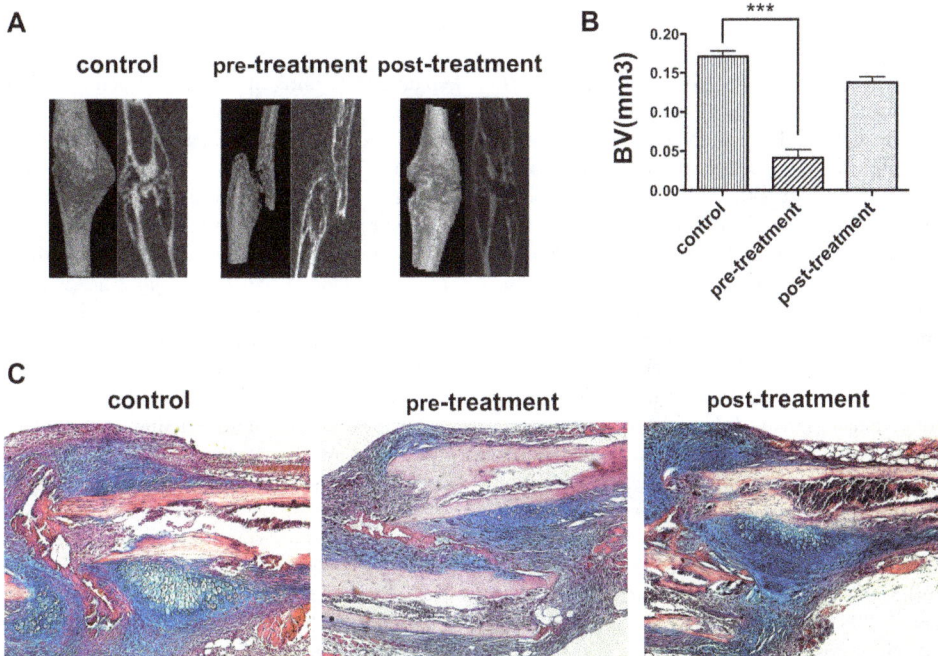

Figure 5. Blockade of CCR2 in the early phase displayed delayed fracture healing *in vivo*. A: WT mice received continuous administration of CCR2 antagonist, RS102895, or DMSO (controls) until day 12, beginning 2 days before or 4 days after rib fracture. In the control group, DMSO was administered as a control for 14 days. Representative micro-CT image of a fractured rib on day 21. **B**: Newly formed callus volume on day 21 in the pre-treatment or post-treatment group was quantified using micro-CT. **C**: Histology of the fracture callus stained by hematoxylin-eosin/alcian-blue staining on day 7.

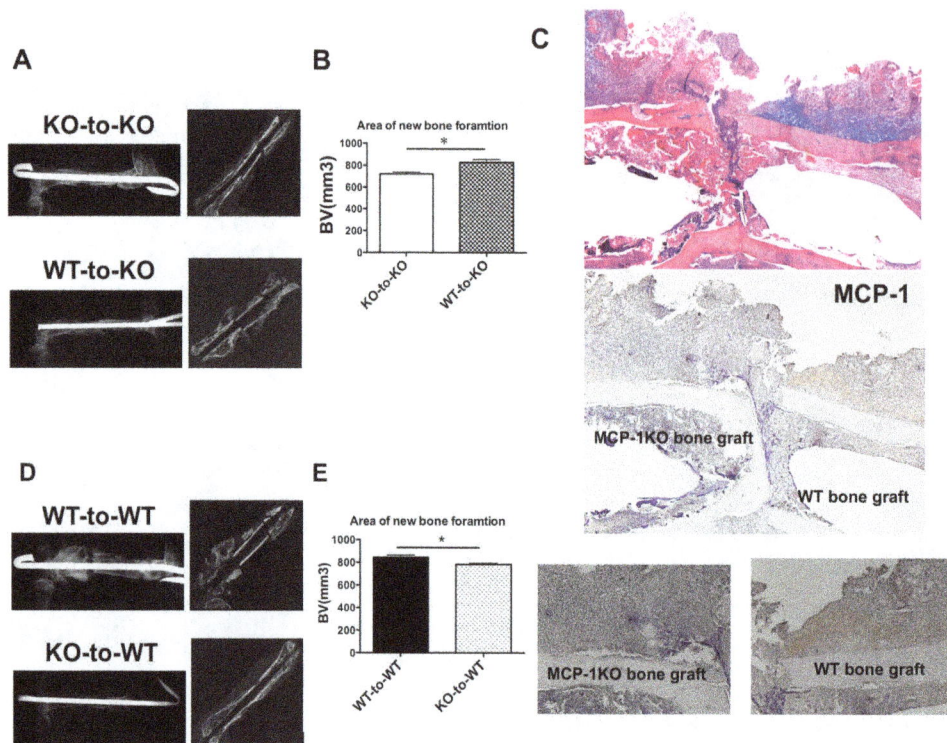

Figure 6. Femoral segmental bone graft exchanging model. Bone exchange surgeries were performed between WT and MCP-1$^{-/-}$ mice as described in the Methods section. Samples were harvested on day 21 for micro-CT and histological analyses. **A and B**, Representative micro-CT images and quantitative analyses demonstrate that WT mouse-derived bone graft caused a significant increase of new bone formation compared with KO mouse-derived bone graft. **C**, Immunohistochemical staining for MCP-1 in MCP-1$^{-/-}$ mice is shown. Pronounced MCP-1 expression at the periosteum and endosteum in the WT graft was observed in the host MCP-1$^{-/-}$ mouse. **D**, Representative micro-CT images and quantitative analyses demonstrate that MCP-1$^{-/-}$ mouse-derived bone graft caused a significant decrease of new bone formation compared with WT mouse-derived bone graft. Values are means $\pm$ SEM of more than three separate experiments. *$P<0.05$.

could be caused by defects in chondroclast/osteoclast chemotaxis that delays vascular invasion, calcification and/or remodeling. However, MCP-1 expression is known to induce the early inflammatory phase [29], when osteoclasts do not play major roles in fracture healing. Consistent with the findings of previous studies, our data show that *MCP-1* and *MCP-3* mRNA were up-regulated on day 3 (Figure 1) and that localized MCP-1 and MCP-3 expression were increased in the periosteum and endosteum in the early phase of fracture healing (Figure 2A). This suggests that increased MCP-1 and MCP-3 expression in the early inflammatory phase may be essential for normal fracture healing.

MCP-1 and its receptor CCR2 are involved in recruitment of various cells, including leukocytes, BMSCs and hematopoietic stem cells [30–33], and in the regeneration of damaged tissues [34,35]. As established in earlier developmental studies, CCR2 is necessary for organ-specific homing of bone marrow-derived pluripotent mesenchymal stem cells into damaged tissues [36,37]. Consistent with this finding, our data showed that *CCR2* mRNA was induced in the mBMSCs derived from WT mice (Figure 3B). We also found that MCP-1, but not MCP-3, induced the migration of mBMSCs in a dose-dependent manner and that *in vitro* migration was markedly inhibited by a CCR2 antagonist (Figure 3A). Therefore, this axis may be a potent candidate in the development of stem/progenitor cell-based therapy for improving fracture healing.

We have previously demonstrated that SDF-1 is induced in the periosteum during bone injury and promotes endochondral bone repair by recruiting mesenchymal stem/progenitor cells to the site of injury. In the PCR array, an increased level of SDF-1 was not observed during fracture healing in this current study, especially in the early inflammatory phase. This inconsistency may be explained partly by the differences between the presence of the unimpaired bone marrow in simple fracture healing and bone graft healing with an intramedullary nail. Moreover, the previous study investigated allograft healing, in which the surgical site is greatly avascular, and under hypoxia this induces hypoxia-inducible factor-1 activation and subsequent SDF-1 up-regulation. Hence, we consider that the MCP-1/CCR2 axis is a crucial signaling pathway during the normal fracture healing process.

Previous studies have demonstrated that damage to the periosteum and bone marrow leads to impaired osteogenesis and chondrogenesis, and delays bone healing [38,39]. Thus, the periosteum and bone marrow seem to be important sources for recruiting mesenchymal stem/progenitor cells or osteogenic progenitor cells for promoting osteogenesis and chondrogenesis. In this study, we found that the expression of CCR2 increased transiently in the bone marrow in the early inflammatory phase and that the expression of MCP-1 also increased transiently in the periosteum and endosteum during the same period (Figure 2). We also found that WT mouse-derived bone graft markedly increased new bone formation and promoted successful fracture healing, whereas the MCP-1$^{-/-}$ mouse-derived bone graft caused less new bone formation and delayed fracture healing (Figure 6). Importantly, although other osteogenic factors were present at the fracture site, they could not compensate for the lack of MCP-1. Collectively, these findings indicate clearly that increased MCP-1 expression in the periosteum and endosteum recruits CCR2-expressing cells and is essential for successful fracture healing.

This study has several limitations. First, we did not fully analyze the functions of other ligands for CCR2, such as MCP-3 and MCP-5, which may have roles different from those of MCP-1 in fracture healing. However, CCR2 KO mice showed similar impairment of bone healing compared with MCP-1$^{-/-}$ mice. Therefore, it is reasonable to consider that other ligands may also have similar functions. Second, the MCP-1/CCR2 axis may have a function other than the recruitment of progenitor cells in the early phase of fracture healing, such as promoting angiogenesis. Several studies report the role of the MCP-1/CCR2 axis in angiogenesis, but not in fracture healing. This point should be clarified in the future. Lastly, we did not elucidate the cell source(s) of mesenchymal stem/progenitor cells for fracture healing in this study. Recent reports, including ours, indicate the periosteum is the key source of potent cells [19,40], but this requires further investigation.

In conclusion, we have shown that increased expression of MCP-1 in the early phase plays a pivotal role in fracture healing by recruiting CCR2-expressing cells derived from surrounding tissues. The MCP-1/CCR2 axis is a potential target for achieving successful fracture healing. Further studies are needed to understand the functional relevance of the MCP-1/CCR2 axis in fracture healing.

Supporting Information

Figure S1 Immunohistochemical analysis of WT un-fractured rib. A, B, C, Low expression levels of MCP-1, MCP-

3 and CCR2 were observed at the periosteum in the unfractured rib.

Figure S2 Effects of MCP-1 on osteogenesis, and chondrogenesis. A: mBMSCs were cultured in osteoinduction media with or without MCP-1 for 14 days and stained with alizarin red S. The expression of each gene was analyzed by quantitative RT-PCR. ($n = 5$, respectively). **B**: ATDC5 cells were induced chondrocyte differentiation. MCP-1 (0, 20, 100 or 200 ng/ml) was simultaneously added every 2 days with the medium change. On days 28 after plating, cells were harvested, and the expression of each gene was analyzed by quantitative RT-PCR. ($n = 6$, respectively).

Figure S3 A, C: Histology of the fracture callus stained by hematoxylin-eosin/alcian-blue staining on day 7 (A) or day 21(C). B: Histology of the fracture in MCP-1 or CCR2 KO stained by hematoxylin-eosin on day 25 (left panel) or 23 (right panel).

Acknowledgments

We are grateful to Drs. R. Tsutsumi, S. Tanida and K. Nishitani (Kyoto University Graduate School of Medicine) for their valuable technical assistance.

Author Contributions

Conceived and designed the experiments: MI HI SM. Performed the experiments: MI TK KM HS KY TF. Analyzed the data: MI HI HY MF. Contributed reagents/materials/analysis tools: MI TK. Contributed to the writing of the manuscript: MI HI TK.

References

1. Tsuboi M, Hasegawa Y, Suzuki S, Wingstrand H, Thorngren KG (2007) Mortality and mobility after hip fracture in Japan: a ten-year follow-up. J Bone Joint Surg Br 89: 461–466.
2. Bliuc D, Nguyen ND, Milch VE, Nguyen TV, Eisman JA, et al. (2009) Mortality risk associated with low-trauma osteoporotic fracture and subsequent fracture in men and women. JAMA 301: 513–521.
3. Griffin M, Iqbal SA, Bayat A (2011) Exploring the application of mesenchymal stem cells in bone repair and regeneration. J Bone Joint Surg Br 93: 427–434.
4. Hernigou P, Poignard A, Manicom O, Mathieu G, Rouard H (2005) The use of percutaneous autologous bone marrow transplantation in nonunion and avascular necrosis of bone. J Bone Joint Surg Br 87: 896–902.
5. Claes L, Recknagel S, Ignatius A (2012) Fracture healing under healthy and inflammatory conditions. Nat Rev Rheumatol 8: 133–143.
6. Vortkamp A, Pathi S, Peretti GM, Caruso EM, Zaleske DJ, et al. (1998) Recapitulation of signals regulating embryonic bone formation during postnatal growth and in fracture repair. Mech Dev 71: 65–76.
7. Glass GE, Chan JK, Freidin A, Feldmann M, Horwood NJ, et al. (2011) TNF-alpha promotes fracture repair by augmenting the recruitment and differentiation of muscle-derived stromal cells. Proc Natl Acad Sci U S A 108: 1585–1590.
8. Lange J, Sapozhnikova A, Lu C, Hu D, Li X, et al. (2010) Action of IL-1 beta during fracture healing. J Orthop Res 28: 778–784.
9. Dimitriou R, Tsiridis E, Giannoudis PV (2005) Current concepts of molecular aspects of bone healing. Injury 36: 1392–1404.
10. Mountziaris PM, Mikos AG (2008) Modulation of the inflammatory response for enhanced bone tissue regeneration. Tissue Eng Part B Rev 14: 179–186.
11. Sasaki M, Abe R, Fujita Y (2008) Mesenchymal stem cells are recruited into wounded skin and contribute to wound repair by transdifferentiation into multiple skin cell type. J Immunol 180: 2581–2587.
12. Schenk S, Mal N, Finan A, Zhang M, Kiedrowski M, et al. (2007) Monocyte chemotactic protein-3 is a myocardial mesenchymal stem cell homing factor. Stem Cells 25: 245–251.
13. Si Y, Tsou C, Croft K, Charo I (2010) CCR2 mediates hematopoietic stem and progenitor cell trafficking to sites of inflammation in mice. J Clin Invest 120: 1192–1203.
14. Docheva D, Haasters F, Schieker M (2008) Mesenchymal stem cells and their cell surface receptors. Curr Rheumatol Rev 4: 155–160.
15. Bielby R, Jones E, McGonagle D (2007) The role of mesenchymal stem cells in maintenance and repair of bone. Injury 38 Suppl 1: S26–32.
16. Augello A, Kurth TB, De Bari C (2010) Mesenchymal stem cells: a perspective from in vitro cultures to in vivo migration and niches. Eur Cell Mater 20: 121–133.
17. Caplan A (2009) Why are MSCs therapeutic? New data: new insight. J Pathol 217(2): 318–324.
18. Jones E, Yang X (2011) Mesenchymal stem cells and bone regeneration: current status. Injury 42: 562–568.
19. Ito H (2011) Chemokines in mesenchymal stem cell therapy for bone repair: a novel concept of recruiting mesenchymal stem cells and the possible cell sources. Mod Rheumatol 21: 113–121.
20. Granero-Moltó F, Weis JA, Miga MI, Landis B, Myers TJ, et al. (2009) Regenerative effects of transplanted mesenchymal stem cells in fracture healing. Stem Cells 27: 1887–1898.
21. Khosla S, Westendorf JJ, Mödder UI (2010) Concise review: Insights from normal bone remodeling and stem cell-based therapies for bone repair. Stem Cells 28: 2124–2128.
22. Kumar S, Wan C, Ramaswamy G, Clemens TL, Ponnazhagan S (2010) Mesenchymal stem cells expressing osteogenic and angiogenic factors synergistically enhance bone formation in a mouse model of segmental bone defect. Mol Ther 18: 1026–1034.
23. Kitaori T, Ito H, Schwarz EM, Tsutsumi R, Yoshitomi H, et al. (2009) Stromal cell-derived factor 1/CXCR4 signaling is critical for the recruitment of mesenchymal stem cells to the fracture site during skeletal repair in a mouse model. Arthritis Rheum 60: 813–823.
24. Ito H, Akiyama H, Shigeno C, Iyama K, Matsuoka H, et al. (1999) Hedgehog signaling molecules in bone marrow cells at the initial stage of fracture repair. Biochem Biophys Res Commun 262: 443–451.
25. Ito H, Koefoed M, Tiyapatanaputi P, Gromov K, Goater JJ, et al. (2005) Remodeling of cortical bone allografts mediated by adherent rAAV-RANKL and VEGF gene therapy. Nat Med 11: 291–297.
26. Murata K, Kitaori T, Oishi S, Watanabe N, Yoshitomi H, et al. (2012) Stromal cell-derived factor 1 regulates the actin organization of chondrocytes and chondrocyte hypertrophy. PLoS One 7: e37163.
27. Murata K, Ito H, Yoshitomi H, Yamamoto K, Fukuda A, et al. (2014) Inhibition of miR-92a enhances fracture healing via promoting angiogenesis in a model of stabilized fracture in young mice. J Bone Miner Res 29: 316–326.

28. Xing Z, Lu C, Hu D, Yu Y, Wang X, et al. (2010) Multiple roles for CCR2 during fracture healing. Dis Model Mech 3: 451–458.

29. Shireman PK, Contreras-Shannon V, Reyes-Reyna SM, Robinson SC, McManus LM (2006) MCP-1 parallels inflammatory and regenerative responses in ischemic muscle. J Surg Res 134: 145–157.

30. Qian BZ, Li J, Zhang H, Kitamura T, Zhang J, et al. (2011) CCL2 recruits inflammatory monocytes to facilitate breast-tumour metastasis. Nature 475: 222–225.

31. Zhang F, Tsai S, Kato K, Yamanouchi D, Wang C, et al. (2009) Transforming growth factor-beta promotes recruitment of bone marrow cells and bone marrow-derived mesenchymal stem cells through stimulation of MCP-1 production in vascular smooth muscle cells. J Biol Chem 284: 17564–17574.

32. Tsou C, Peters W, Si Y (2007) Critical roles for CCR2 and MCP-3 in monocyte mobilization from bone marrow and recruitment to inflammatory sites. J Clin Inv 117: 2–9.

33. Serbina NV, Pamer EG (2006) Monocyte emigration from bone marrow during bacterial infection requires signals mediated by chemokine receptor CCR2. Nat Immunol 7: 311–317.

34. Lu H, Huang D, Saederup N, Charo IF, Ransohoff RM, et al. (2011) Macrophages recruited via CCR2 produce insulin-like growth factor-1 to repair acute skeletal muscle injury. FASEB J 25: 358–369.

35. Shireman PK, Contreras-Shannon V, Ochoa O, Karia BP, Michalek JE, et al. (2007) MCP-1 deficiency causes altered inflammation with impaired skeletal muscle regeneration. J Leukoc Biol 81: 775–785.

36. Belema-Bedada F, Uchida S, Martire A, Kostin S, Braun T (2008) Efficient homing of multipotent adult mesenchymal stem cells depends on FROUNT-mediated clustering of CCR2. Cell Stem Cell 2: 566–575.

37. Van Linthout S, Stamm C, Schultheiss H-P, Tschöpe C (2011) Mesenchymal stem cells and inflammatory cardiomyopathy: cardiac homing and beyond. Cardiol Res Pract: ID 757154. DOI:10.4061/2011/757154

38. Colnot C (2009) Skeletal cell fate decisions within periosteum and bone marrow during bone regeneration. J Bone Miner Res 24: 274–282.

39. Utvåg SE, Grundnes O, Reikeraos O (1996) Effects of periosteal stripping on healing of segmental fractures in rats. J Orthop Trauma 10: 279–284.

40. Murao H, Yamamoto K, Matsuda S, Akiyama H (2013) Periosteal cells are a major source of soft callus in bone fracture. J Bone Miner Metab 31: 390–398.

23

N-Phenacylthiazolium Bromide Reduces Bone Fragility Induced by Nonenzymatic Glycation

Brian S. Bradke, Deepak Vashishth*

Department of Biomedical Engineering, Rensselaer Polytechnic Institute, Troy, New York, United States of America

Abstract

Nonenzymatic glycation (NEG) describes a series of post-translational modifications in the collagenous matrices of human tissues. These modifications, known as advanced glycation end-products (AGEs), result in an altered collagen crosslink profile which impacts the mechanical behavior of their constituent tissues. Bone, which has an organic phase consisting primarily of type I collagen, is significantly affected by NEG. Through constant remodeling by chemical resorption, deposition and mineralization, healthy bone naturally eliminates these impurities. Because bone remodeling slows with age, AGEs accumulate at a greater rate. An inverse correlation between AGE content and material-level properties, particularly in the post-yield region of deformation, has been observed and verified. Interested in reversing the negative effects of NEG, here we evaluate the ability of n-phenacylthiazolium bromide (PTB) to cleave AGE crosslinks in human cancellous bone. Cancellous bone cylinders were obtained from nine male donors, ages nineteen to eighty, and subjected to one of six PTB treatments. Following treatment, each specimen was mechanically tested under physiological conditions to failure and AGEs were quantified by fluorescence. Treatment with PTB showed a significant decrease in AGE content versus control NEG groups as well as a significant rebound in the post-yield material level properties ($p < 0.05$). The data suggest that treatment with PTB could be an effective means to reduce AGE content and decrease bone fragility caused by NEG in human bone.

Editor: Ryan K. Roeder, University of Notre Dame, United States of America

Funding: This work was supported by The Whitaker Foundation, NIH/NIA AG 20618, and NIH Training Grant T32GM067545. The funders had no role in study design, data collection and analysis, decision to publish, or preparation of the manuscript.

Competing Interests: The authors have declared that no competing interests exist.

* Email: vashid@rpi.edu

Introduction

Non-traumatic skeletal fractures are directly related to increased incapacitation, morbidity, and mortality and pose a serious health problem to an aging population [1–3]. Several age-related changes in bone morphology and composition have been identified and were subsequently linked to an increased risk of non-traumatic fracture [4–7]. One such change is the accumulation of advanced glycation end-products (AGEs) within the collagen network of cortical and cancellous bone [8–10].

AGEs are a series of post-translational modifications in the cross-link profile of long-lived proteins throughout the body [11]. These modifications are caused by the reaction of reducing sugars found in the extracellular space with amino groups of collagen through a process called non-enzymatic glycation (NEG). The resulting covalent, glucose-derived protein crosslinks are naturally occurring and can be replicated in-vitro by subjecting collagen to reducing sugars in solution [12].

Because collagen is a structural protein, altering its crosslink profile impacts the form and function of the constituent tissue. Bank et al. demonstrated that in-vivo NEG produces a stiffer organic matrix in normal human cartilage [12]. The biomechanical properties of human bone, which has an organic phase consisting primarily of type I collagen, are similarly affected by NEG [13,14].

The organic phase of bone is predominately responsible for the tissue's ductility and overall ability to absorb impact loading as it allows bone to deform and release energy before failure. Stiffening of the collagenous matrix due to NEG reduces the total strain the tissue is able to resist before ultimate failure. This reduction is measured as a decrease in post-yield and ultimate strain values via mechanical testing. Vashishth et al. [14] demonstrated that changes in bone quality resulting from NEG had a significant effect on post-yield properties and the tissue's overall ability to resist fracture. We have also demonstrated that AGEs in bone accumulate at an increased rate during bisphosphonate therapy for post-menopausal osteoporosis and this accumulation of AGEs is associated with changes in post-yield fracture properties [15].

Knowing that NEG contributes to increased bone fragility and increased fracture risk, we set out to identify a compound that cleaved the established AGE crosslinks in bone. In a 1996 publication, Vasan et al. reported that a novel, thiazolium-based nucleophile called "N-Phenacylthiazolium Bromide" (PTB) selectively cleaves AGE crosslinks in rat-tail tendon both in-vitro and in-vivo [16].

In particular, they administered PTB to Lewis rats with above-average AGE content due to laboratory-induced diabetes. Dissection and collagen extraction from the tail-tendon revealed a decrease in AGE crosslinks after 32 weeks of treatment, proving the feasibility of in-vivo treatment [16]. Our study expands upon their groundbreaking work in rat models, by treating human skeletal tissue with PTB in vitro and collecting mechanical data in addition to biochemical analysis. Bolstered by this previous research here we evaluated the effectiveness of PTB in reversing the effects of NEG on human cancellous bone in vitro.

Table 1. Outline of Control and Treatment Groups.

Group:	Control Group (C)	Ribosylated Group (R)	Experimental Group 1 (X1)	Experimental Group 2 (X2)	Experimental Group 3 (X3)	Experimental Group 4 (X4)
1st Treatment:	Buffered Saline Solution at 37°C for 7 days.	Buffered solution with 0.6 M Ribose at 37°C for 7 days.	Buffered solution with 0.6 M Ribose at 37°C for 7 days.	Buffered solution with 0.6 M Ribose at 37°C for 7 days.	Buffered solution with 0.6 M Ribose at 37°C for 7 days.	Buffered solution with 0.6 M Ribose at 37°C for 7 days.
2nd Treatment:	Buffered PBS solution at 37°C for 7 days	Buffered PBS solution at 37°C for 7 days	PBS solution with 0.015 M PTB at 37°C for 3 days	PBS solution with 0.015 M PTB at 37°C for 7 days	PBS solution with 0.15 M PTB at 37°C for 3 days	PBS solution with 0.15 M PTB at 37°C for 7 days

Materials and Methods

Cancellous bone cylinders were taken from the tibial plateaus of 9 male cadavers aged 19, 29, 39, 45, 48, 49, 50, 64 and 80. None of the donors were diagnosed with osteoarthritis, and they were also certified to be free of metabolic bone diseases, HIV, and hepatitis B (National Disease Research Interchange and International Institute for the Advancement of Medicine). No live human subjects were involved in this research study (IRB Waiver, Albany Medical College Hospital/Rensselaer Polytechnic Institute). Cadaveric human specimens used in the study were obtained the anatomical gift registry (National Diseases Research Interchange, Philadelphia PA).

The cylinders were obtained under wet-conditions using a three-eighths inch diameter, diamond-tipped, core drilling bit (Starlite Industries, Inc., www.starliteindustires.com) that was mounted in a standard bench-top drill press. The cylinders were then wet-machined to a specific length of ten millimeters using a variable speed diamond saw from Buehler Inc. (www.buehler. com). Specimens were excised from the donor's centralized tibial plateau, parallel to the longitudinal axis of the diaphysis, and were randomly assigned to the treatment groups described below.

A total of eighteen cylindrical specimens were obtained from each of the nine donors. Each specimen was thoroughly rinsed with and stored in normal calcium-buffered saline at −20°C until testing. Previous studies done in our laboratory have demonstrated

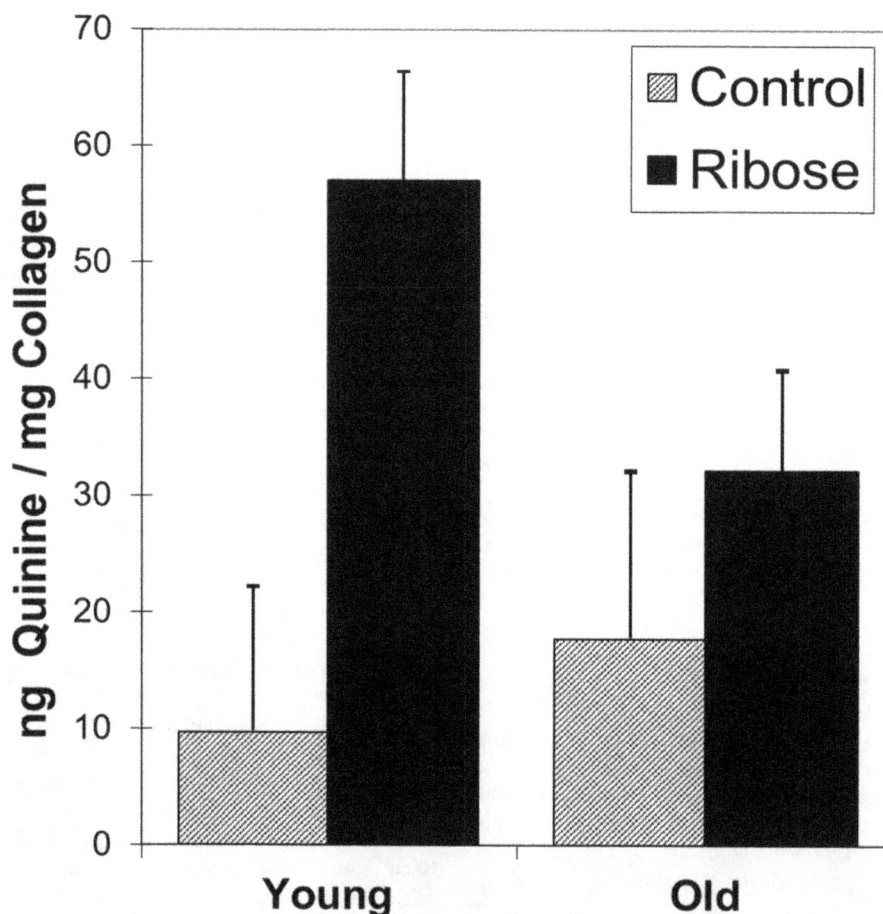

Figure 1. NEG Content for Control (shaded) and Ribosylated (solid black) specimens in Young and Old groups (p<0.05).

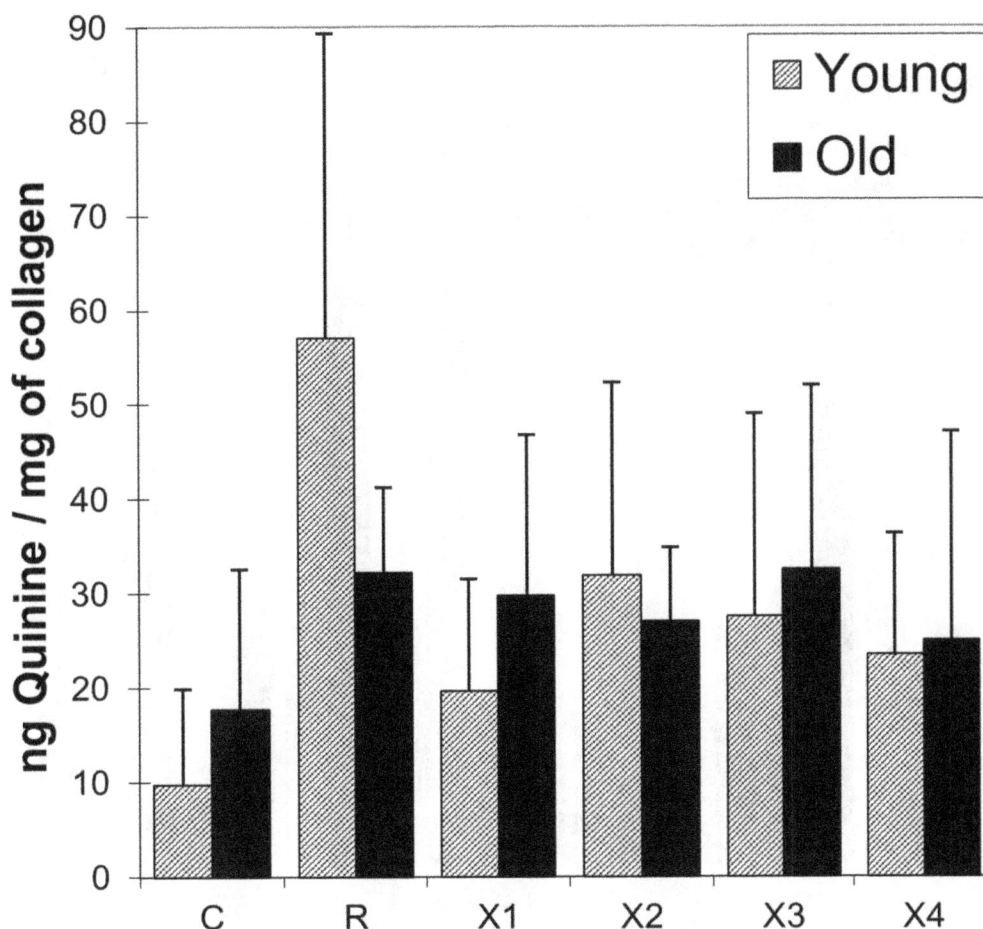

Figure 2. NEG content for Young (shaded) vs. Old (solid black) for all treatment groups C-control, R-ribosylated, X1 & X2 0.015 M PTB for 3 & 7 days, respectively and X3 & X4 0.15 M PTB for 3 & 7 days, respectively.

that this procedure preserves the mineral and organic matrix within the bone [14,17].

The bone specimens of each donor were randomly assigned to one of six treatment groups. The treatment groups consisted of a control (C), a glycated (ribosylated) control (R), and four treatment groups (X1-X4), each with a different concentration of PTB in a phosphate buffered saline solution. The specific treatment of each group is summarized in Table 1.

A base solution for glycation was prepared in Hanks buffer (Sigma Inc. Ref# H9269) with a final concentration of 25 mM E-amino-n-caproic acid (Sigma Inc. Ref# A2504), 5 mM Benzamidine (Fluka Chemika Ref#12072), 10 mM N-ethylmaleimide (Sigma Inc. Ref# E3876-5G), and 30 mM of Hepes buffer (Sigma Inc. Ref# H3375). One-sixth of this solution was set aside for the control group. D-ribose (Sigma Inc. Ref# R 7500) was added to the remainder of the base solution to create a 0.6 M ribose solution.

The control specimens (C) were submersed in the control (non-ribose) solution while the remaining specimens (R, X1, X2, X3 and X4) were submersed in the ribose solution at 37°C. The temperature was maintained at 37°C and, if necessary, the pH of the solution was adjusted and maintained between 7.2 and 7.6 using 0.5N NaOH or 0.5N HCl. We have previously demonstrated that this incubation protocol does not cause loss of mineral content from bone [14,17].

Two solutions of PTB [0.15 M and 0.015 M] were prepared in stock phosphate buffered saline (PBS). Experimental groups X1 and X2 were submersed in identical aliquots of 0.15 M PTB; the X1 for 3 days and the X2 for 7 days at 37°C. Experimental groups X3 and X4 were submersed in identical aliquots of 0.015 M PTB; the X3 for 3 days and the X4 for 7 days. The control and ribosylated groups were each submersed in a solution of PBS at 37°C. Since PTB has a short half-life in PBS [18], the PTB solution was replaced daily. The PBS solution was changed in the control and ribosylated groups every day as well. On the fourth day, experimental groups X1 and X3 were rinsed with PBS and were submersed in PBS in the same fashion as the control and ribosylated groups for the remainder of the seven days. At completion of the second treatment, all specimens were thoroughly rinsed with saline and subjected to mechanical testing.

Mechanical Testing

Cancellous bone cylinders, subjected to chemical treatments described above, were glued to a pair of precision-machined brass end-caps and tested using a Mini-Bionix Servo-Hydraulic tensile testing machine (Model 858; MTS Systems). For testing, the machine's actuator was brought into contact with the specimen and the specimen was allowed to rest for 2 minutes while being irrigated with normal saline. The specimen was then compressed to failure at a constant strain rate of 0.02 mm/sec while measuring force and displacement at a rate of 100 Hz.

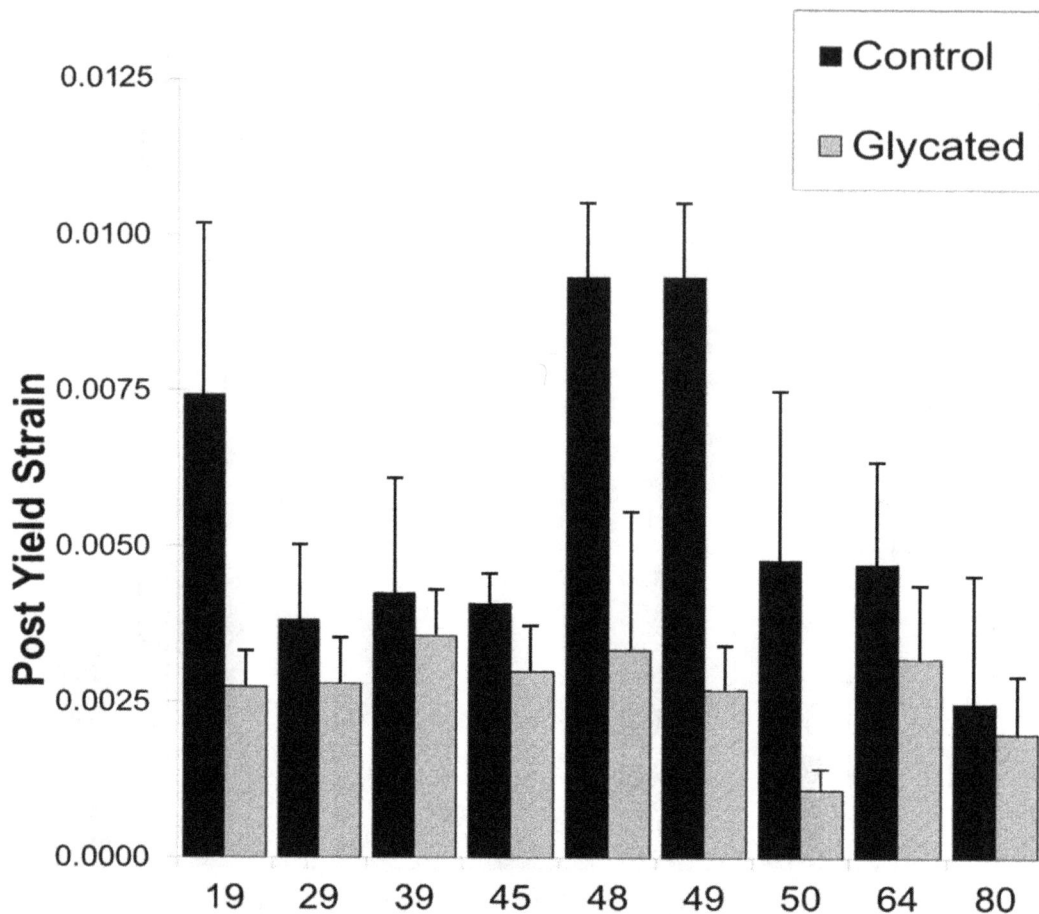

Figure 3. Post Yield Strain values of all donors are shown for Control specimens (solid black) against Ribosylated (grey) specimens. For all donors, post yield strain was significantly reduced (P<0.01).

The test data were converted to stress and strain and used for obtaining the following variables. Young's modulus was determined using the eleven-point regression method from the linear portion of the curve [19]. Yield stress and yield strain were determined from the point where the stress-strain curve deviated outside of the 95% confidence interval of the linear portion of the curve. Ultimate stress and ultimate strain were defined by the maximum stress observed during the compression test. The secant modulus was calculated by dividing the ultimate stress by the ultimate strain. The strain ratio (Ultimate Strain/Yield Strain), and post yield strain (Ultimate Strain – Yield Strain) were also calculated for each specimen.

AGE Analysis

After mechanical testing, each specimen was demineralized in 70% formic acid and complete demineralization was ensured by using a Poly No-Cal Endpoint Determination Kit (www. polysciences.com). One half of each demineralized bone specimen was papain digested in 0.4 mg/mL papain collagenase in 0.1 mM sodium acetate buffered to a pH of 6.0 for 16 hours at 65°C. AGE content was determined by fluorescence in an MR600 micro-plate reader using 370-nm excitation and 440-nm emission wavelength standardized against a serially-diluted quinine sulphate solution. The remaining halves of demineralized bone were dried. Collagen

content was determined by hydroxyproline assay using hydrolysates of the papain digested specimens [14,20].

Statistics

Because AGE content data exhibited large variability across age groups, the data was parsed in two groups- young (19–49) and old (>50) to reduce the variance of the means. The young versus old cutoff age was set at 50 years old based on previous laboratory observations showing that younger bone contains lower levels of in vivo AGEs and is therefore more susceptible to in-vitro NEG than old bone [21]. As such, the "Old" specimens exhibited a smaller percentage increase in NEG from control to ribosylated groups.

A univariate analysis of variance (1-way ANOVA) was performed on the response variables (yield strain, ultimate strain, and post-yield strain) for each control and experimental group for every donor. Post-yield strain and strain ratio were normalized within each group and averaged and displayed with standard deviations. Significance for the null hypothesis as shown was determined by 1-way ANOVA at $\alpha = 0.05$.

One-way ANOVA was selected over two-way because age was not considered a treatment variable. A student's t-test was only used when data was parsed into two paired groups of normalized data with equal variance. In that case, a two-tailed, paired, student's t-test was used.

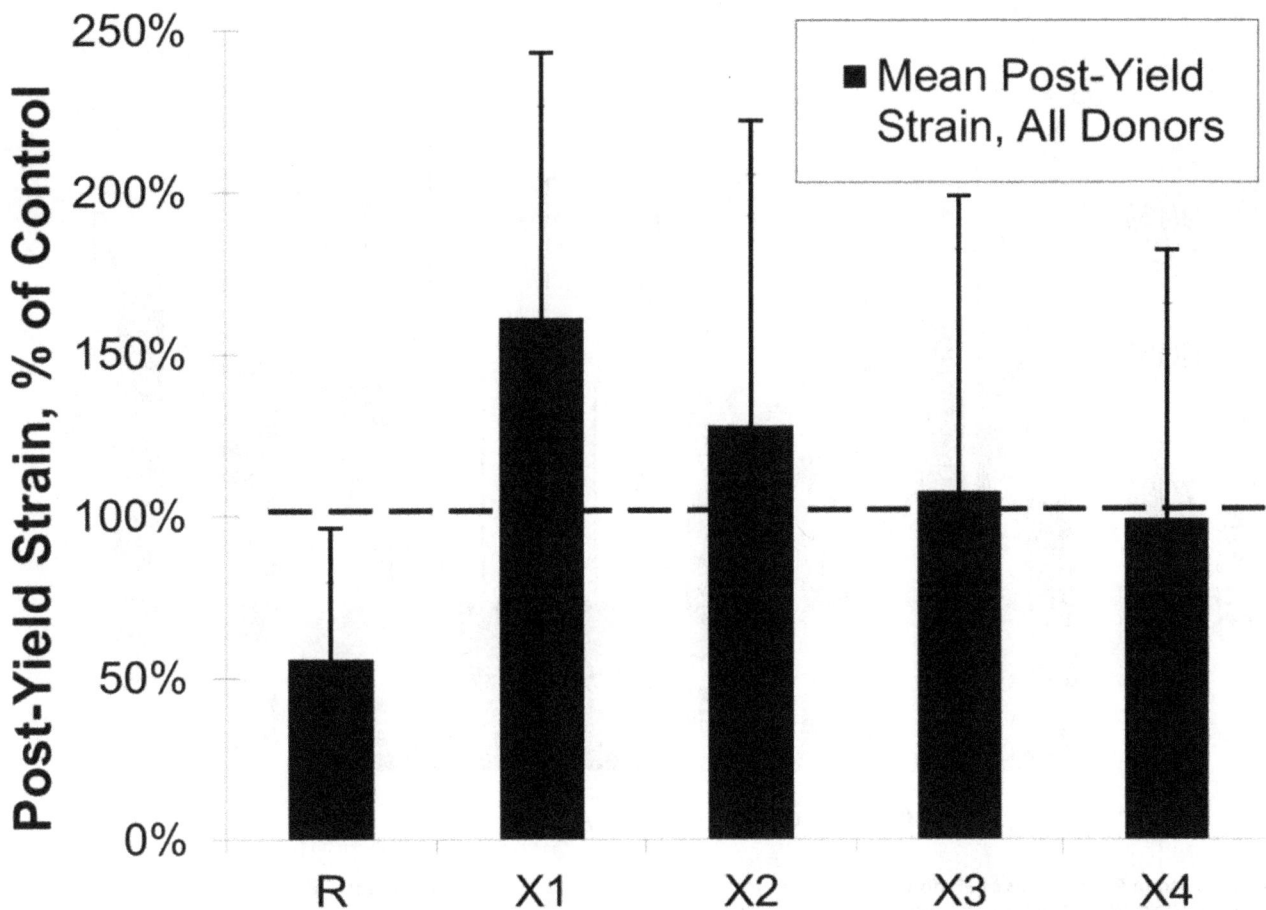

Figure 4. Effects of PTB on the Post-Yield Strain for all age groups is shown in black. R-ribosylated, X1 & X2 0.015 M PTB for 3 & 7 days, respectively and X3 & X4 0.15 M PTB for 3 & 7 days, respectively. Mean values of Post-Yield Strain were calculated and then normalized as a percentage of Control value. The dashed line represents control level. For all PTB treatments post-yield strain increased from the ribosylated value, (P<0.01).

Results

AGEs

Presence of AGEs was observed as a uniform color change of the bone specimen from white to brownish-yellow (Figure 1). For both Old and Young groups, AGE content, defined as nanograms of quinine-sulphate fluorescence per milligram of collagen, increased markedly (p<0.05) from control to ribosylated groups. The Old Control group had more AGEs than the Young Control group (p<0.01) which verifies the presence and increase of in-vivo AGEs with age.

As shown in Figure 2, the AGEs for all treatment groups were decreased after PTB treatment. PTB treatment was more effective for specimens taken from younger donors, but it also significantly decreased AGEs in the Old group (p<0.05). There was no clear correlation between the amount of AGE reduction and PTB treatment concentration, but the seven day treatment resulted in a greater reduction of AGEs than the three day treatment.

Mechanical Properties

Post-yield strain, an indicator of bone ductility, of Control and Ribosylated groups for all donors is shown in Figure 3. Ribosylated "R" groups exhibited a significant decrease in post-yield strain (p<0.01), which is consistent with brittle material behavior. The means for the normalized data from all donors are

shown in Figure 4 as a percentage of control value. The PTB treatment groups X1-X4 show a significant increase of post-yield strain versus the ribosylated group back to control levels (p<0.01).

The strain ratio for each specimen, calculated by dividing ultimate strain by yield strain, represents the amount of energy dissipated pre- and post-yield and amplifies any significant changes in post-yield behavior. As shown in Figure 5, strain ratio was increased by glycation for all donors (p<0.05). Values for strain ratio were normalized against controls and the mean for each treatment group was calculated. Figure 6 shows the means for the PTB experimental groups (X1-X4) against the ribosylated group (R). For all treatment groups, strain ratio decreased toward control levels as represented by the dashed line. All treatment groups had a significant reduction in the strain ratio as compared to the ribosylated group (X1&X2 p<0.001, X3&X4 p<0.05).

Discussion

One of the relevant age-related changes in bone quality is the accumulation of AGEs in bone's organic matrix [14,17,21–23]. At the macro-level, AGEs directly affect bone by reducing its post-yield material properties [17,21]. On a micro-level, AGEs indirectly affect bone by slowing the remodeling process, allowing micro-damage and AGEs to accumulate at a greater rate [21,24–26]. Here for the first time, we show the ability of n-

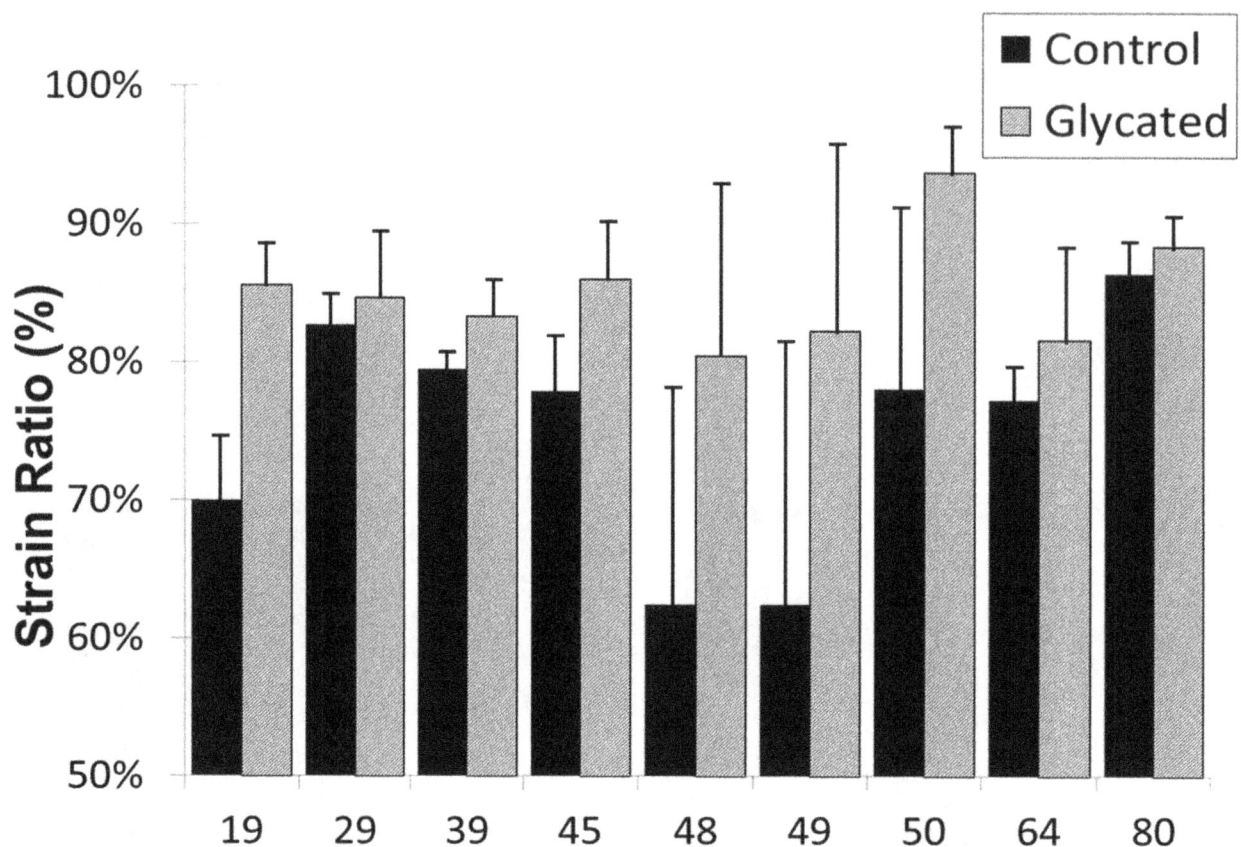

Figure 5. Strain Ratio values of all donors are shown for Control specimens (solid black) against Ribosylated (grey) specimens. For all donors, strain ratio was significantly increased (P<0.05) after glycation.

Phenacylthiazolium Bromide to improve the quality of existing bone matrix by cleaving established AGE crosslinks known to accumulate with aging, disease, and the anti-resorptive treatment of osteoporosis.

PTB was originally identified as a potential crosslink breaker because of the susceptibility of AP-ene-dione-derived protein crosslinks to cleavage by certain thiazolium salts [16,27]. PTB consists of nucleophilic centres at the thiazolium-2 position and the α-position of the N-substituent. These nucleophilic centres react with the carbonyl groups of an AGE crosslink to form a five-membered ring and thereby convert the carbonyl-group carbons to a tetrahedral geometry which facilitates spontaneous cleavage at physiological pH. When applied in practice, PTB was shown to selectively cleave established AGE crosslinks in vitro and in vivo by Vasan et al. [16]. Using their work as a baseline, we applied PTB to human bone previously subjected to non-enzymatic glycation. This resulted in a decrease in total AGE content, demonstrating the viability of PTB treatment for both old and young bone (Figure 2).

Post yield deformation is an important aspect of bone fracture specific to energy dissipation before failure. The amount of energy a bone can absorb before it breaks is dependent on its ability to first elastically deform (pre-yield), then to plastically deform in an effort to dissipate energy (post-yield) before ultimate failure. Glycation, both in vivo and in vitro, does not significantly alter pre-yield mechanics. However, it reduces the amount of energy the bone can dissipate post-yield and thereby increases fracture risk for otherwise benign traumas [14,17,21]. When alterations in post-yield material properties are combined with decreased bone

mass (osteoporosis), the risk of fracture is further amplified. Results of this study show that the removal of AGE crosslinks using PTB restores bone's post-yield properties and reduces fragility. Furthermore, we found that PTB treatment is effective across age groups which suggests that PTB is able to cleave AGE crosslinks in older and more mature bone tissue.

The ability of PTB to reverse AGE accumulation in bone is also important because of the interaction between AGEs and the natural remodeling process. Recent research has shown that glycated bone is less susceptible to osteoclastic digestion and consequently has a slower resorption rate than normal bone [23]. Thus, decreasing the AGE content of mature bone may initiate bone turnover and promote new bone formation. This finding is especially relevant for patients undergoing anti-resorptive therapies including bisphosphonate (BP) therapy. Since bone resorption is reduced, AGEs will accumulate at a faster rate with BP therapy [15,24]. If BP treatment is halted, or if an anabolic treatment like PTH is administered, the response of bone to the remodeling stimulus may still be reduced due to the increased AGE content and the inhibition of osteoclastic activity. PTB treatment during drug holidays, which are recommended throughout BP therapy, may improve bone quality in patients undergoing long term BP therapy or patients transitioning to PTH from BP [28,29].

The major limitation of the work presented is that it was conducted in vitro. In order to prove feasibility for human use, in-vivo animal and human studies need to be performed. It is noteworthy that PTB has previously been tested in an in vivo animal model and successfully cleaved AGE crosslinks in soft-tissue [16,27]. In light of these previous studies and the in-vitro

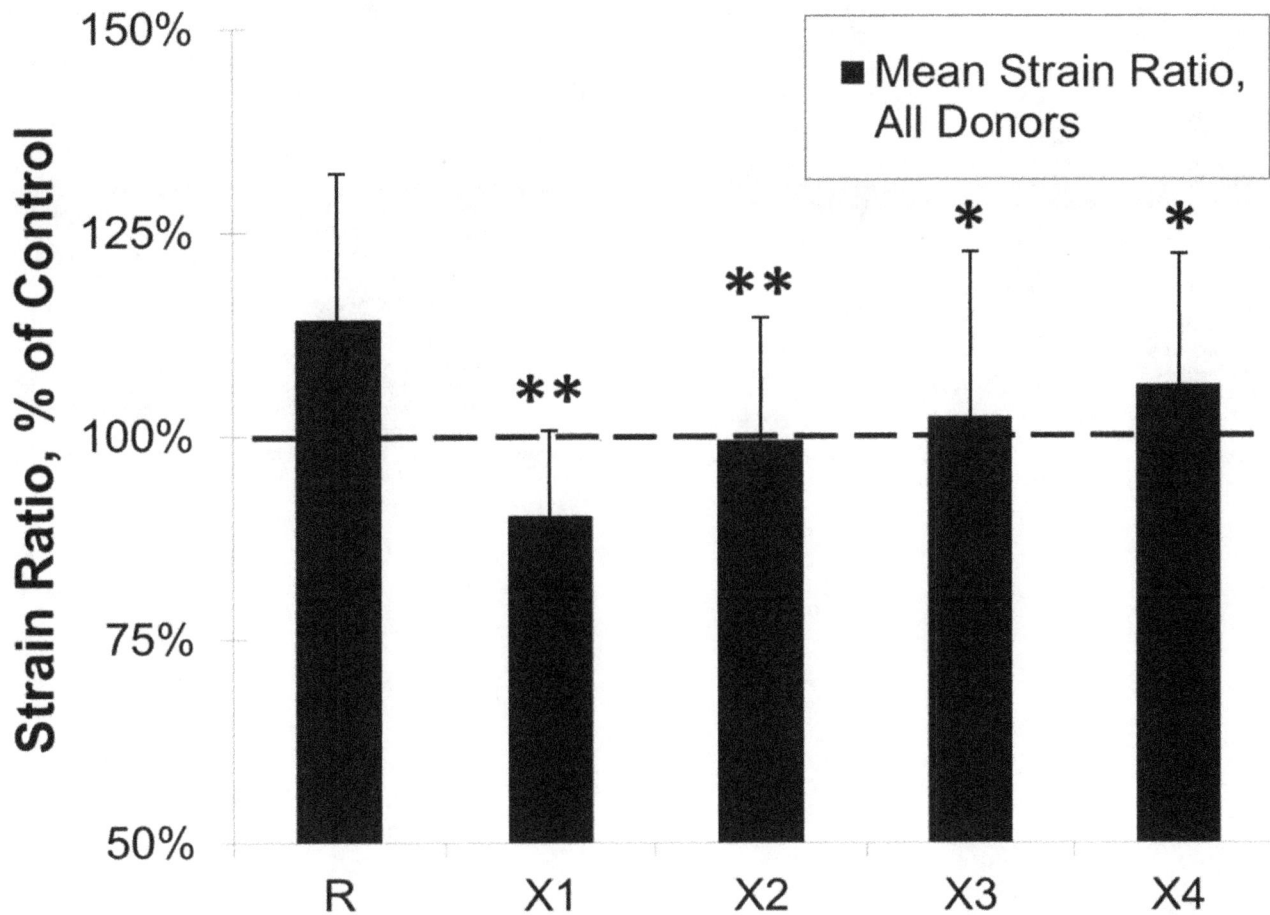

Figure 6. Effects of PTB on Strain Ratio for all age groups is shown in black. R-ribosylated, X1 & X2 0.015 M PTB for 3 & 7 days, respectively and X3 & X4 0.15 M PTB for 3 & 7 days, respectively. Mean values of Strain Ratio were calculated and then normalized as a percentage of Control value. The dashed line represents control level. For all PTB treatments strain ratio decreased from the ribosylated value, (*P<0.001, **P<0.05).

results presented in this study, we suggest that PTB or its derivatives may be suitable treatments for improving bone quality and warrants further investigation.

In summary, this study demonstrates that AGEs crosslinks in human bone are susceptible to cleavage by a thiazolium-based nucleophile and that reducing the AGE content in bone restores the material-level post-yield properties of the trabecular architecture. With this discovery, a pharmacological intervention for age-related changes in bone's organic structure may be possible.

Acknowledgments

We are grateful to Dr. Simon Tang for his assistance with laboratory procedures and to Mrs. Terry Peters for statistical analysis of the NEG results.

Author Contributions

Conceived and designed the experiments: BSB DV. Performed the experiments: BSB. Analyzed the data: BSB. Contributed reagents/materials/analysis tools: BSB DV. Wrote the paper: BSB DV.

References

1. Melton LJ 3rd, Kan SH, Wahner HW, Riggs BL (1988) Lifetime fracture risk: an approach to hip fracture risk assessment based on bone mineral density and age. J Clin Epidemiol 41: 985–994.
2. Ray NF, Chan JK, Thamer M, Melton LJ 3rd (1997) Medical expenditures for the treatment of osteoporotic fractures in the United States in 1995: report from the National Osteoporosis Foundation. J Bone Miner Res 12: 24–35.
3. Singer BR, McLauchlan GJ, Robinson CM, Christie J (1998) Epidemiology of fractures in 15,000 adults: the influence of age and gender. J Bone Joint Surg Br 80: 243–248.
4. Hui SL, Slemenda CW, Johnston CC Jr. (1988) Age and bone mass as predictors of fracture in a prospective study. J Clin Invest 81: 1804–1809.
5. Parfitt AM (1987) Trabecular bone architecture in the pathogenesis and prevention of fracture. Am J Med 82: 68–72.
6. Marcus R (1996) Clinical review 76: The nature of osteoporosis. J Clin Endocrinol Metab 81: 1–5.
7. Tanizawa T, Itoh A, Uchiyama T, Zhang L, Yamamoto N (1999) Changes in cortical width with bone turnover in the three different endosteal envelopes of the ilium in postmenopausal osteoporosis. Bone 25: 493–499.
8. Hedlund LJ, Maki DD, Griffiths HJ (1998) Calcaneal fractures in diabetic patients. J Diabetes Complications 12: 81–87.
9. Meyer HE, Tverdal A, Falch JA (1993) Risk factors for hip fracture in middle-aged Norwegian women and men. Am J Epidemiol 137: 1203–1211.
10. Seeley DG, Kelsey J, Jergas M, Nevitt MC (1996) Predictors of ankle and foot fractures in older women. The Study of Osteoporotic Fractures Research Group. J Bone Miner Res 11: 1347–1355.
11. Monnier VM, Sell DR, Abdul-Karim FW, Emancipator SN (1988) Collagen browning and cross-linking are increased in chronic experimental hyperglycemia. Relevance to diabetes and aging. Diabetes 37: 867–872.
12. Bank RA, Bayliss MT, Lafeber FP, Maroudas A, Tekoppele JM (1998) Ageing and zonal variation in post-translational modification of collagen in normal human articular cartilage. The age-related increase in non-enzymatic glycation affects biomechanical properties of cartilage. Biochem J 330 (Pt 1): 345–351.

13. Gundberg CM, Anderson M, Dickson I, Gallop PM (1986) "Glycated" osteocalcin in human and bovine bone. The effect of age. J Biol Chem 261: 14557–14561.

14. Vashishth D, Gibson GJ, Khoury JI, Schaffler MB, Kimura J, et al. (2001) Influence of nonenzymatic glycation on biomechanical properties of cortical bone. Bone 28: 195–201.

15. Tang SY, Sharan AD, Vashishth D (2008) Effects of collagen crosslinking on tissue fragility. Clin Biomech (Bristol, Avon) 23: 122–123; author reply 124–126.

16. Vasan S, Zhang X, Zhang X, Kapurniotu A, Bernhagen J, et al. (1996) An agent cleaving glucose-derived protein crosslinks in vitro and in vivo. Nature 382: 275–278.

17. Vashishth D (2005) Collagen glycation and its role in fracture properties of bone. J Musculoskelet Neuronal Interact 5: 316.

18. Price DL, Rhett PM, Thorpe SR, Baynes JW (2001) Chelating activity of advanced glycation end-product inhibitors. J Biol Chem 276: 48967–48972.

19. Fyhrie DP, Vashishth D (2000) Bone stiffness predicts strength similarly for human vertebral cancellous bone in compression and for cortical bone in tension. Bone 26: 169–173.

20. Chandrakasan G, Torchia DA, Piez KA (1976) Preparation of intact monomeric collagen from rat tail tendon and skin and the structure of the nonhelical ends in solution. J Biol Chem 251: 6062–6067.

21. Tang SY, Zeenath U, Vashishth D (2007) Effects of non-enzymatic glycation on cancellous bone fragility. Bone 40: 1144–1151.

22. Tang SY, Vashishth D (2010) Non-enzymatic glycation alters microdamage formation in human cancellous bone. Bone 46: 148–154.

23. Valcourt U, Merle B, Gineyts E, Viguet-Carrin S, Delmas PD, et al. (2007) Non-enzymatic glycation of bone collagen modifies osteoclastic activity and differentiation. J Biol Chem 282: 5691–5703.

24. Allen MR, Burr DB (2008) Changes in vertebral strength-density and energy absorption-density relationships following bisphosphonate treatment in beagle dogs. Osteoporos Int 19: 95–99.

25. Chesnut IC, Skag A, Christiansen C, Recker R, Stakkestad JA, et al. (2004) Effects of oral ibandronate administered daily or intermittently on fracture risk in postmenopausal osteoporosis. J Bone Miner Res 19: 1241–1249.

26. Giusti A, Hamdy NA, Dekkers OM, Ramautar SR, Dijkstra S, et al. (2011) Atypical fractures and bisphosphonate therapy: a cohort study of patients with femoral fracture with radiographic adjudication of fracture site and features. Bone 48: 966–971.

27. Rahbar S, Figarola JL (2002) Inhibitors and Breakers of Advanced Glycation Endproducts (AGEs): A Review. Current Medicinal Chemistry - Immunology, Endocrine & Metabolic Agents 2: 135–161.

28. Licata AA (2005) Discovery, clinical development, and therapeutic uses of bisphosphonates. Ann Pharmacother 39: 668–677.

29. Russell RG, Croucher PI, Rogers MJ (1999) Bisphosphonates: pharmacology, mechanisms of action and clinical uses. Osteoporos Int 9 Suppl 2: S66–80.

24

Gli1 Haploinsufficiency Leads to Decreased Bone Mass with an Uncoupling of Bone Metabolism in Adult Mice

Yoshiaki Kitaura[1,2], Hironori Hojo[1,2], Yuske Komiyama[1,2], Tsuyoshi Takato[1], Ung-il Chung[2,3], Shinsuke Ohba[2,3]*

1 Department of Sensory and Motor System Medicine, The University of Tokyo Graduate School of Medicine, Bunkyo-ku, Tokyo, Japan, **2** Division of Clinical Biotechnology, The University of Tokyo Graduate School of Medicine, Bunkyo-ku, Tokyo, Japan, **3** Department of Bioengineering, The University of Tokyo Graduate School of Engineering, Bunkyo-ku, Tokyo, Japan

Abstract

Hedgehog (Hh) signaling plays important roles in various development processes. This signaling is necessary for osteoblast formation during endochondral ossification. In contrast to the established roles of Hh signaling in embryonic bone formation, evidence of its roles in adult bone homeostasis is not complete. Here we report the involvement of *Gli1*, a transcriptional activator induced by Hh signaling activation, in postnatal bone homeostasis under physiological and pathological conditions. Skeletal analyses of *Gli1*$^{+/-}$ adult mice revealed that *Gli1* haploinsufficiency caused decreased bone mass with reduced bone formation and accelerated bone resorption, suggesting an uncoupling of bone metabolism. Hh-mediated osteoblast differentiation was largely impaired in cultures of *Gli1*$^{+/-}$ precursors, and the impairment was rescued by *Gli1* expression via adenoviral transduction. In addition, *Gli1*$^{+/-}$ precursors showed premature differentiation into osteocytes and increased ability to support osteoclastogenesis. When we compared fracture healing between wild-type and *Gli1*$^{+/-}$ adult mice, we found that the *Gli1*$^{+/-}$ mice exhibited impaired fracture healing with insufficient soft callus formation. These data suggest that *Gli1*, acting downstream of Hh signaling, contributes to adult bone metabolism, in which this molecule not only promotes osteoblast differentiation but also represses osteoblast maturation toward osteocytes to maintain normal bone homeostasis.

Editor: Pierre J. Marie, Inserm U606 and University Paris Diderot, France

Funding: This work was supported by a Grant-in-Aid for Young Scientists (#23689079), the Center for Medical System Innovation, the Graduate Program for Leaders in Life Innovation, Core-to-Core Program A (Advanced Research Networks), the Funding Program for World-Leading Innovative R&D on Science and Technology, the Center for NanoBio Integration, and the S-innovation Program. The funders had no role in study design, data collection and analysis, decision to publish, or preparation of the manuscript.

Competing Interests: The authors have declared that no competing interests exist.

* Email: ohba@bioeng.t.u-tokyo.ac.jp

Introduction

Hedgehog (Hh) signaling is a highly conserved pathway that plays important roles in various development processes. Hh signaling is indispensable for osteoblast formation in endochondral ossification, one of the two ossification processes in mammals, which forms bones in limbs, the trunk, and some head structures [1]. In this context, Indian hedgehog (Ihh) expressed in prehypertrophic chondrocytes is thought to act directly on progenitors in the perichondrium and the bone marrow to induce their differentiation into bone-forming osteoblasts [2–4]. The deletion of Ihh or smoothened (Smo), a transmembrane signaling transducer for Hh, caused no bone collar or primary spongiosa in mice [2,4]. These mutant mice lacked the expression of runt-related transcription factor 2 (*Runx2*), a key determinant for osteoblasts [5,6] and bone gamma-carboxyglutamate (gra) protein (osteocalcin; official gene symbol, *Bglap*), a bona fide marker for osteoblasts [1], in the perichondrium.

Gli transcription factors mediate the transcription of target genes downstream of Hh signaling. Gli1, a target gene of Hh signaling, acts as a transcriptional activator, whereas Gli2 and Gli3 can act as both activators and repressors [7]. The activator function of Gli2 and the repressor function of Gli3 were reported to mediate substantial aspects of the action of Ihh on bone development [8,9]. In addition, we found that Gli1 participated in the Hh-mediated osteoblast formation collectively with Gli2 and Gli3 [10,11].

Regarding postnatal roles of Hh signaling in bone metabolism, we reported that the haploinsufficiency of patched 1 (*Ptch1*), a transmembrane Hh receptor that represses signaling activity without Hh input, led to high bone mass in adult mice and humans [12]. Mice in which *Ptch1* was deleted in *Bglap*-positive mature osteoblasts showed low bone mass [13]. Although both of the mutants mentioned above had high bone turnover, where both osteoblastogenesis and osteoclastogenesis were enhanced, the balance shifted toward the opposite phenotypes. When an activator form of *Gli2* was forcibly expressed in osteoblast precursors expressing *Sp7* (osterix-Osx), another key determinant of osteoblasts, the skeleton was not affected at the fetal stage in mice. However, the mutants postnatally showed severe osteopenia with a decrease in osteoblast number, although the number of osteoclasts was not changed [14]. Thus, in contrast to the established roles of Hh signaling in embryonic bone formation, the evidence of its roles in adult bone homeostasis is not adequate. In particular, little is known about the roles of Gli1, a potent transcriptional activator induced by Hh signaling, in postnatal bone metabolism.

In the present study, we attempted to examine Hh signaling in the postnatal skeletal system, focusing on the functions of Gli1 in the bone metabolism. We analyzed skeletal phenotypes of *Gli1* heterozygous knockout mice postnatally *in vivo* and *in vitro*. We also compared fracture healing between mutant and wild-type (WT) mice. We report that *Gli1* haploinsufficiency affects adult bone metabolism, at least partly through the uncoupling of bone formation and bone resorption, leading to a decrease in bone mass and a delay in fracture healing in postnatal skeletons.

Materials and Methods

Animal Experiments

Wild-type C57BL/6J mice were obtained from Charles River Japan, and $Gli1^{+/-}$ mice were generated as previously described [15]. All experiments were performed in accord with the protocol approved by the Animal Care and Use Committee of The University of Tokyo (#KA13-5). Mice were kept in individual cages under controlled temperature and humidity with a 12-hr circadian rhythm. They were given *ad libitum* access to food and water. All efforts were made to minimize the suffering of the mice. Euthanasia of mice was performed with an overdose of barbiturates.

Reagents and Vectors

Smoothened agonist (SAG) was purchased from Calbiochem (San Diego, CA; 566660). Receptor activator of NF-kappa-B ligand (RANKL) was purchased from Pepro Tech (Rocky Hill, NJ; 184-01791). Sonic hedgehog (Shh) was purchased from R&D Systems (Minneapolis, MN; 1845-SH). Cyclopamine was purchased from Enzo Life Sciences (Farmingdale, NY; BML-GR3334). Plasmids expressing human *GLI1* were constructed as previously described [12]. The adenoviral vector expressing human *GLI1-Biotin-3xFLAG-IRES-dsRed* was constructed using the pAd/PL-DEST vector and ViraPower Adnoviral Expression System (Life Technologies, Carlsbad, CA), according to the manufacturer's instructions. In brief, human *GLI1* cDNA carrying Biotin-3xFLAG tag [16] was initially cloned into pCID vectors [17]; *GLI1-Biotin-3xFLAG-IRES-dsRed* was then transferred into the pENTR1A vector in conjunction with the CAGGS promoter and subjected to adenoviral vector construction using the Gateway system. The pAd/PL-DEST expressing the CAGGS promoter-driven *GLI1-Biotin-3xFLAG-IRES-dsRed* was linearized with Pac I and transfected into 293A cells. After amplification, the virus was stored at −80°C. The viral titer was determined by an end-point titer assay using 293A cells.

Cell Culture

C3H10T1/2 cells were obtained from the RIKEN Cell Bank (Ibaraki, Japan). Mouse primary bone marrow stromal cells were isolated from the long bones of 8-week-old male mice. Mouse primary osteoblast precursors were isolated from calvarias of mouse neonates. Cells were cultured in high-glucose Dulbecco's modified Eagle Medium (DMEM; Sigma-Aldrich, St. Louis, MO) containing 10% fetal bovine serum (FBS) and 1% penicillin/streptomycin. For osteogenic cultures, the cells were cultured in osteogenic media [18,19] supplemented with Smoothened agonist (SAG). Co-culture experiments using mouse primary bone marrow stromal cells and bone marrow macrophages were performed as

previously described [18]. The *in vitro* osteoclast differentiation of RAW264.7 cells was performed as previously described [20]. Adenoviruses expressing *GLI1-Biotin-3xFLAG-IRES-dsRed* (Ax-Gli1) or GFP (Ax-GFP) were used to infect cells at MOI (multiplicity of infection) 10. Alkaline phosphatase (ALP), von Kossa, and tartrate-resistant acid phosphatase (TRAP) staining were performed as previously described [12,18].

Real-Time RT-PCR

Total RNA extraction and real-time reverse transcription-polymerase chain reaction (RT-PCR) were performed as previously described [21]. All reactions were run in triplicate. The primer sequences are as follows: *β-actin*, AGATGTGGATCAG-CAAGCAG (forward) and GCGCAAGTTAGGTTTTGTCA (reverse); *Alp*, GCTGATCATTCCCACGTTTT (forward) and CTGGGCCTGGTAGTTGTTGT (reverse); *Ibsp*, CAGAGGA-GGCAAGCGTCACT (forward) and CTGTCTGGGTGCCAA-CACTG (reverse); *Bglap*, AAGCAGGAGGGCAATAAGGT (forward) and TTTGTAGGCGGTCTTCAAGC (reverse); *Gli1*, GCACCACATCAACAGTGAGC (forward) and GCGTCTT-GAGGTTTTCAAGG (reverse); *Gli2*, CTGAAGGATTCCTG-CTCGTG (forward) and ACAGTGTAGGCCGAGCTCAT (reverse); *Runx2*, CCGCACGACAACCGCACCAT (forward) and CGCTCCGGCCCACAAATCTC (reverse); *Sp7*, ACTCATCC-CTATGGCTCGTG (forward) and GGTAGGGAGCTGGGT-TAAGG (reverse); *Tnfsf11*, AGCCATTTGCACACCTCAC (forward) and CGTGGTACCAAGAGGACAGAGT (reverse); *Tbfrsf11b*, GTTTCCCGAGGACCACAAT (forward) and CCA-TTCAATGATGTCCAGGAG (reverse); *Dmp1*, CAGTGAG-GATGAGGCAGACA (forward) and TCGATCGCTCCTGG-TACTCT (reverse); *Sost*, AAGCCGGTCACCGAGTTGGT (forward) and GTGAGGCGCTTGCACTTGCA (reverse); *Ptch1*, CTGGACTCTGGCTCCTTGTC (forward) and CAA-CAGTCACCGAAGCAGAA (reverse); *Ctsk*, ACGGAGGCATC-GACTCTGAA (forward) and GATGCCAAGCTTGCGTC-GAT (reverse); and *Nfatc1*, CCTTCGGAAGGGTGCCTTTT (forward) and AGGCGTGGGGCCTCAGCAGG (reverse).

Luciferase Assay

Cells were plated onto 24-well plates and transfected with 0.4 µg of DNA in a mixture containing the reporter plasmids (8×3′-Gli BS-luc) [22], the control reporter plasmids encoding Renilla luciferase, and effector plasmids (pCMV-*myc-GLI1*) or adenoviral vectors expressing *GLI1*. A dual-luciferase assay was performed as previously described [12].

Immunoblot

Whole-cell lysates were isolated using RIPA buffer as previously described [23]. Sodium dodecyl sulfate-polyacrylamide gel electrophoresis (SDS-PAGE) and immunoblotting were performed using anti-Gli1 (sc-20687, 1:1000, Santa Cruz Biotechnology, Santa Cruz, CA) and HRP-conjugated anti-FLAG M2 antibodies (A8592-2MG, 1:500, Sigma-Aldrich) as previously described [12].

Radiological analysis

X-ray photographs of the left tibiae of WT and $Gli1^{+/-}$ mice (n = 10 each) were taken using a soft x-ray system (M-60; Softex Co., Tokyo). Micro-computed tomography (CT) scanning of the harvested femurs was performed using a microfocus X-ray CT system SMX-90CT (Shimadzu, Kyoto, Japan) under the following conditions: tube voltage, 90 kV; tube current, 110 µA; layer thickness, 5.3 mm; and field of view (XY), 10.4 mm. The resolution of one CT slice was 512×512 pixels. The three-

Gli1 Haploinsufficiency Leads to Decreased Bone Mass with an Uncoupling of Bone Metabolism...

225

dimensional construction software package TRI/3D-BON (Ratoc System Engineering, Tokyo) was used for quantitative analysis.

Histological analysis

We intraperitoneally injected calcein (0.16 mg per 10 g of body weight; Sigma) into mice 4 days and 1 day before sacrifice. We stained the undecalcified sections of the femur with toluidine blue, von Kossa, and TRAP as previously described [12]. Images were taken using an Axio Imager A1 (Carl Zeiss, Jena, Germany) and processed using AxioVision (Carl Zeiss). Histomorphometric analyses were performed using the HistometryRT CAMERA system. We analyzed five mice for each group.

Fracture model

Ten 8-week-old male mice were used in each group. Under general anesthesia with isofluorane in O_2, the left hind limb was shaved and sterilized for surgery. A 15-mm incision was made longitudinally, and a blunt dissection of the muscle was made to expose the tibia. A transverse osteotomy was performed using disk-shaped dental steel bars at the mid point of the tibia. The fracture was repositioned, and then the full-length of the bone marrow cavity was internally stabilized as previously described [24]. After irrigation with saline, the skin was closed with 4-0 nylon sutures. Fourteen days after surgery, the tibias were harvested from the euthanized mice.

Statistical analysis

The means of groups were compared by an analysis of variance (ANOVA), and the significances of the differences were determined by Student's t-test. P-values <0.05 were considered significant.

Results

Gli1 haploinsufficiency causes decreased bone mass in adult mice

As reported, we found that $Gli1^{-/-}$ mice had no gross abnormalities at birth [11,15]. Although $Gli1^{-/-}$ pups were born in Mendelian ratios, the number of $Gli1^{-/-}$ adults turned out to be approximately 10% of the total pups obtained because of their reduced survival rates during the first 10 days after birth (Table 1). In addition, the growth rate of the surviving $Gli1^{-/-}$ mice was significantly lower than those of both the wild-type (WT) or $Gli1^{+/-}$ mice, and the body weights of the 8-week-old $Gli1^{-/-}$ mice were approximately 20% lower than those of the WT and $Gli1^{+/-}$ mice (Figure S1).

These findings suggest that the $Gli1^{-/-}$ mice were largely affected by systemic abnormalities due to complete loss of $Gli1$ gene. Therefore, to investigate the roles of Gli1 in adult bone

metabolism as directly as possible, we analyzed the skeletal system in $Gli1^{+/-}$ male mice, which had weights and gross appearance comparable to those of the WT male mice. Micro-computed tomography (μ-CT) analyses of distal femurs revealed that the trabecular density of the 8-week-old $Gli1^{+/-}$ mice was reduced compared to that of WT mice (Figure 1A). The bone morphometric analysis using the micro-CT data supported the finding, as the $Gli1^{+/-}$ mice showed less bone mineral density (BMD) along with decreased parameters for bone formation (Figure 1B). These skeletal phenotypes were also observed in the $Gli1^{+/-}$ female mice (Figure S2). In contrast, there was no significant difference in the cortical bone between WT and $Gli1^{+/-}$ mice (Figure S3), suggesting differences between trabecular and cortical bones with regard to the contribution of Gli1.

The histological analyses of the distal femurs of 8-week-old mice showed that $Gli1^{+/-}$ mice had reduced trabecular bones compared to the WT mice (Figure 2A, see von Kossa), whereas the growth plate appeared normal (Figure 2A, see toluidine blue). Indeed, the bone volume/tissue volume (BV/TV) and trabecular thickness (Tb.Th) values were significantly decreased in $Gli1^{+/-}$ mice compared to WT mice, as observed in micro-CT-based analyses (Figure 2B). $Gli1^{+/-}$ mice also had significantly lower values of osteoid surface/bone surface (OS/BS) and single-labeled surface/bone surface (sLS/BS), which are parameters of the osteogenic capacity (Figure 2B).

Regarding bone resorption, the numbers of TRAP-positive osteoclasts were significantly higher in the $Gli1^{+/-}$ mice compared to the WT mice (Figure 2C and D, see N.Oc/B.Pm). Consistent with this finding, the $Gli1^{+/-}$ mice showed a trend toward increased bone resorption capacity parameters, compared to WT mice (Figure 2D, see ES/BS and Oc.S/BS). These data suggest that $Gli1$ haploinsufficiency causes an uncoupling of bone turnover in adult mice, which leads to decreased bone mass.

Osteoblast differentiation is impaired by Gli1 haploinsufficiency

To investigate whether $Gli1$ haploinsufficiency caused decreased osteogenic capacity through the impairment of osteoblast differentiation from precursors, we examined osteoblast differentiation in ex vivo cultures of primary bone marrow stromal cells (BMSCs) harvested from 8-week-old WT and $Gli1^{+/-}$ mice (Figure 3A and B) and primary osteoblast precursors (OPs) from neonates of each genotype (Figure 3C and D). Given that $Gli1$ expression is induced upon Hh signaling, we suspected that any difference resulting from the loss of one allele of $Gli1$ would be observed under Hh signaling-activated conditions. We therefore performed the experiments in the presence of Smoothened agonist (SAG), a small molecule that activates Hh signaling. The mRNA expression levels of osteoblast-related genes were lower in $Gli1^{+/-}$

Table 1. Survival rate of Gli1 mutant mice during postnatal 10 days.

Genotype	Postnatal day	
	1	**10**
$Gli1^{+/+}$	11 (30.6)	37 (28.5)
$Gli1^{+/-}$	16 (44.4)	81 (62.3)
$Gli1^{-/-}$	9 (25.0)	12 (9.2)
Total	36	130

Percentages are in parentheses.

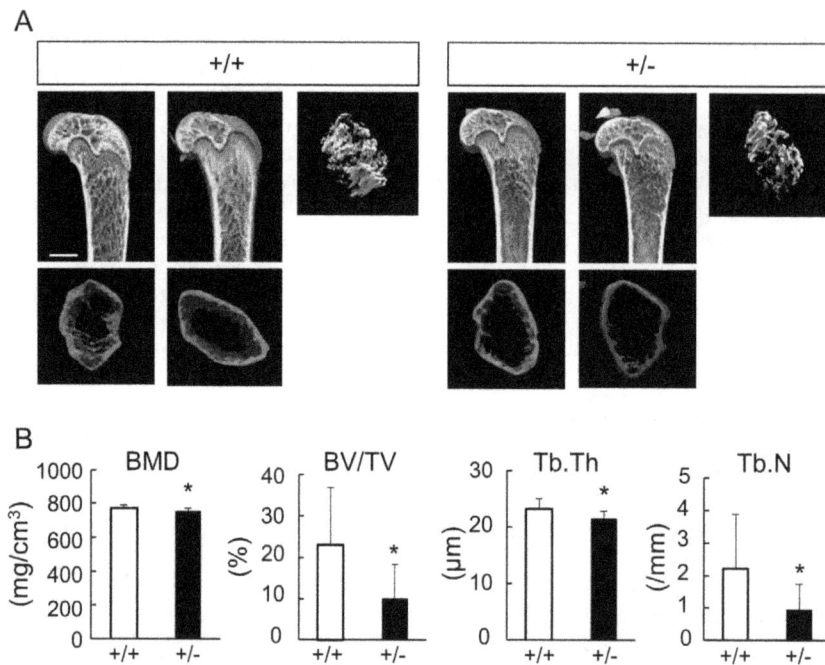

Figure 1. Radiological findings of long bones in wild-type (WT) and GliT$^{+/-}$ mice. (**A**) Three-dimensional micro-computed tomography (3D-micro-CT) images of the distal femurs of representative 8-week-old WT and Gli1$^{+/-}$ male mice. Sagittal sections, transverse sections, and 3D reconstruction images of the primary spongiosa are shown for each genotype. Bar, 1 mm. (**B**) Histomorphometric analyses of 3D-micro-CT data. BMD, bone mineral density; BV/TV, bone volume per tissue volume; Tb.Th, trabecular thickness; Tb.N trabecular number parameters. Data are means ± SDs of eight male mice per genotype. *p<0.05 vs. WT.

BMSCs than in WT BMSCs. In particular, alkaline phosphatase (*Alp*) and integrin-binding sialoprotein (*Ibsp*) expression levels were significantly reduced in the *Gli1*$^{+/-}$ BMSCs (Figure 3A), which was consistent with our previous finding that Gli1 directly induced the expression of these two genes [11]. ALP activity and matrix calcification, key features of osteoblasts, were also suppressed in the *Gli1*$^{+/-}$ BMSCs as evidenced by ALP and von Kossa staining (Figure 3B). The impaired osteoblast differentiation due to loss of one allele of *Gli1* was more prominent in the OPs. All of the genes tested here showed significantly lower expression levels in the *Gli1*$^{+/-}$ OPs compared to WT (Figure. 3C), and ALP activity and calcification were impaired in the *Gli1*$^{+/-}$ OPs (Figure 3D). Lastly, *Gli1* was reduced via the loss of one allele of *Gli1* in both cell types, although a significant reduction was observed only in the OPs (Figure 3A and C, see *Gli1*).

The data above suggest that *Gli1* haploinsufficiency affects osteoblast differentiation in a cell-autonomous manner. We then attempted to further verify the hypothesis by testing whether the recovery of *Gli1* expression would rescue the osteoblast phenotypes in *Gli1*$^{+/-}$ cells. We prepared an adenoviral vector expressing *Gli1* (Ax-*Gli1*) (Figure S4A). Gli1 protein expression induced by Ax-*Gli1* and its function were confirmed by western blotting using a specific antibody, luciferase reporter assays using the Gli-responsive element, and mRNA expression analyses of *Alp* and *Ibsp* in C3H10T1/2 cells (Figures S4B–D). As shown in Figure 3E, the introduction of *Gli1* into *Gli1*$^{+/-}$ OPs induced the expression of *Alp*, an early osteoblast marker, at a level comparable to that in WT OPs. The expression of *Bglap*, an osteoblast marker that is expressed at a later stage, was also upregulated but not fully recovered by *Gli1* introduction. Thus, *Gli1* haploinsufficiency in osteoblast precursors is likely to cause

impairment of their differentiation, which underlies reduced bone formation in *Gli1*$^{+/-}$ mice.

The Hh-Gli1 axis is involved in the capacity of osteoblasts/osteocytes to support osteoclastogenesis, but not in osteoclastogenesis itself

Bone homeostasis is achieved by the coupling of bone formation and bone resorption via cross-talk between osteoblasts/osteocytes and osteoclasts. Mature osteoblasts and osteocytes are known to support osteoclastogenesis by expressing the receptor activator of NF-kappa-B ligand (RANKL; official symbol, *Tnfsf11* - tumor necrosis factor (ligand) superfamily, member 11) and osteoprotegerin (OPG; official symbol, *Tnfrsf11b* - tumor necrosis factor receptor superfamily, member 11b), a stimulator and an inhibitor of osteoclastogenesis, respectively [25–28]. However, *Gli1*$^{+/-}$ mice exhibited impaired bone formation and accelerated bone resorption, suggesting an uncoupling state of bone metabolism.

To identify the cellular mechanism underlying the aberrant state in *Gli1*$^{+/-}$ bones, we conducted co-culture experiments using BMSC and bone marrow macrophages (BMMΦ) derived from either WT or *Gli1*$^{+/-}$ mice. The number of TRAP-positive multinucleated osteoclasts co-cultured with *Gli1*$^{+/-}$ BMMCs was significantly higher than those with WT BMMCs, regardless of the *Gli1* genotypes in the BMMΦ (Figure 4A and B). Thus, bone-forming cells and their progenitors, not osteoclastic cells, were likely to be responsible for the abnormalities in osteoclastogenesis of the *Gli1*$^{+/-}$ mice. This led us to analyze BMSCs in terms of their ability to support the osteoclastogenesis.

In BMSCs harvested from the femurs of 8-week-old *Gli1*$^{+/-}$ mice, the mRNA expression of RANKL (*Tnfsf11*) was significantly upregulated, whereas that of OPG (*Tnfrsf11b*) showed a trend toward downregulation compared to WT BMSCs (Fig-

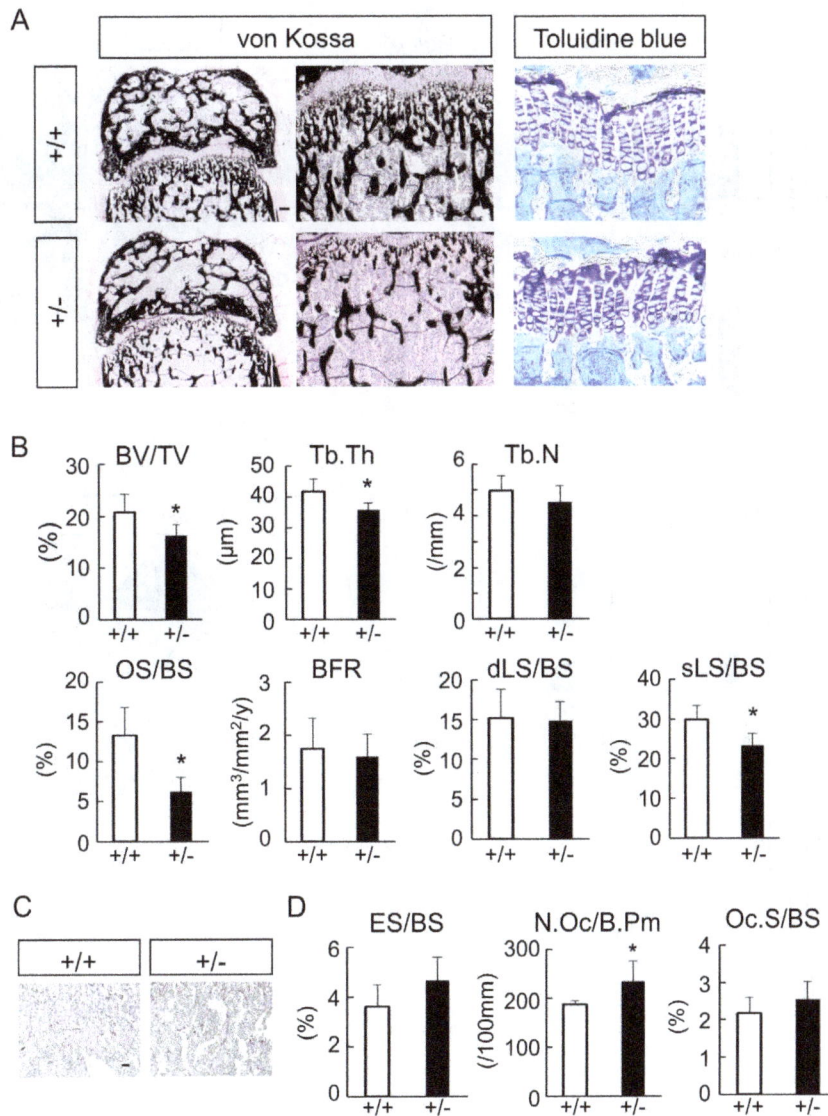

Figure 2. Histological findings of adult WT and *Gli1*$^{+/-}$ mice. (A) von Kossa staining and toluidine blue staining of the distal femur sections of representative 8-week-old WT and *Gli1*$^{+/-}$ male mice. Bar, 100 μm. **(B)** Histomorphometric analyses of bone volume and bone formation parameters in distal femurs from 8-week-old WT and *Gli1*$^{+/-}$ male mice. OS/BS, osteoid surface per bone surface; MAR, mineral apposition rate; BFR, bone formation rate per bone surface; dLS/BS, double-labeled surface per bone surface; sLS/BS, single-labeled surface per bone surface. Data are means ± SDs of five male mice per genotype. *p<0.05 vs. WT. **(C)** TRAP staining of the distal femur sections of representative 8-week-old WT and *Gli1*$^{+/-}$ male mice. Bar, 100 μm. **(D)** Histomorphometric analyses of bone resorption parameters in the distal femurs of 8-week-old WT and Gli1$^{+/-}$ male mice. ES/BS, eroded surface per bone surface; N. Oc/B. Pm, number of osteoclasts per 100 mm of bone perimeter; Oc. S/BS, osteoclast surface per bone surface. In **(B)** and **(D)**, data are means ± SDs of five mice per genotype. *p<0.05 vs. WT.

ure 4C). In addition, expression levels of dentin matrix acidic phosphoprotein 1 (*Dmp1*) and sclerostin (*Sost*), markers for osteocytes, were higher in the *Gli1*$^{+/-}$ BMSCs than in the WT (Figure 4C). This trend was also observed in OPs (Figure S5). Taken together with the downregulation of osteoblast marker genes in *Gli1*$^{+/-}$ BMSCs, these findings indicate that *Gli1* haploinsufficiency may promote a premature differentiation of osteoblast precursors into osteocytes, which have been reported as a major source of RANKL [25], and these results may indicate that the premature differentiation not only affects bone formation, but also stimulates bone resorption by inducing RANKL expression at a supraphysiological level. Given that the recovery of *Gli1* expression negated the upregulation of RANKL mRNA expression in *Gli1*$^{+/-}$ BMSCs (Figure S6), it is also possible that

Gli1 not only suppresses the differentiation of osteoblast precursors into osteocytes, but also negatively acts on the transcription of RANKL.

We next investigated the cell-autonomous effects of Hh signaling on osteoclastogenesis using RAW264.7 cells, which have been shown to differentiate into TRAP-positive osteoclasts in the presence of RANKL [20,29]. Treatment with neither Shh nor cyclopamine, an inhibitor of hedgehog signaling, affected the RANKL-induced osteoclast differentiation of RAW264.7 cells (Figures 4D and E) although the cells were responsive to Hh signaling, as indicated by the expression change of *Ptch1*, a readout of the Hh signaling, upon Shh and cyclopamine (Figure 4F). Finally, we analyzed osteoclastogenesis of primary BMMΦ harvested from 8-week-old WT or *Gli1*$^{+/-}$ mice.

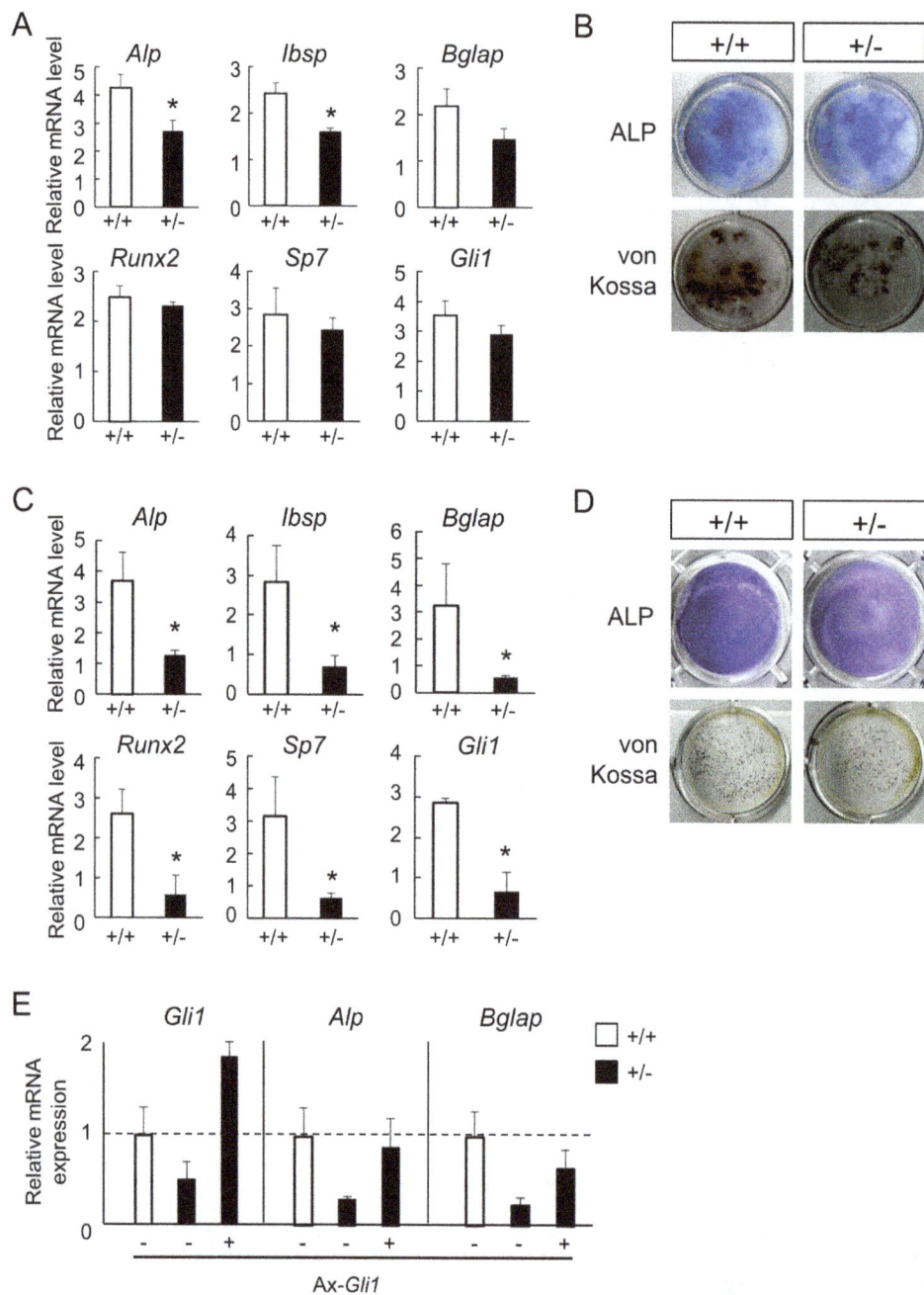

Figure 3. Osteoblast differentiation in cultures of precursor cells from WT and Gli1$^{+/-}$ mice. (**A**) mRNA expression of osteoblast marker genes in 14-day osteogenic cultures of BMSCs in the presence of the Smoothened agonist. mRNA expression was analyzed by real-time RT-PCR. (**B**) ALP and von Kossa stainings in 14-day osteogenic cultures of BMSCs in the presence of the Smoothened agonist. (**C**) mRNA expression of osteoblast marker genes in 7-day osteogenic cultures of osteoblast precursors (OPs) isolated from neonatal calvarias, in the presence of the Smoothened agonist. (**D**) ALP and von Kossa staining in 7-day osteogenic cultures of OPs in the presence of the Smoothened agonist. (**E**) Rescue of the expression levels of osteoblast marker genes in Gli1$^{+/-}$ OPs by the adenoviral overexpression of Gli1 in the presence of the Smoothened agonist. WT or Gli1$^{+/-}$ OPs were infected with Ax-GFP (−) or Ax-Gli1 (+) at MOI 10.

Expression levels of cathepsin K (*Ctsk*) and *Nfatc1*, markers for osteoclasts, were not affected by loss of *Gli1* in cultures of BMMΦ with M-CSF and RANKL (Figure 4G).

Thus, the Hh-Gli1 axis is unlikely to mediate osteoclastogenesis in a cell-autonomous manner, which further suggests that the accelerated bone resorption in *Gli1$^{+/-}$* mice is not caused by defects in osteoclastic cells. Abnormalities in osteoblast precursors due to *Gli1* haploinsufficiency may mediate all the aspects of the

disruption of bone homeostasis in *Gli1$^{+/-}$* bones, which explains why *Gli1$^{+/-}$* mice have a low bone mass phenotype.

Fracture healing was impaired by Gli1 haploinsufficiency

We next set out to examine the involvement of *Gli1* in postnatal bones under a pathological condition, comparing fracture healing between WT and *Gli1$^{+/-}$* mice in a model that was surgically created in the tibias of 8-week-old males. During the fracture

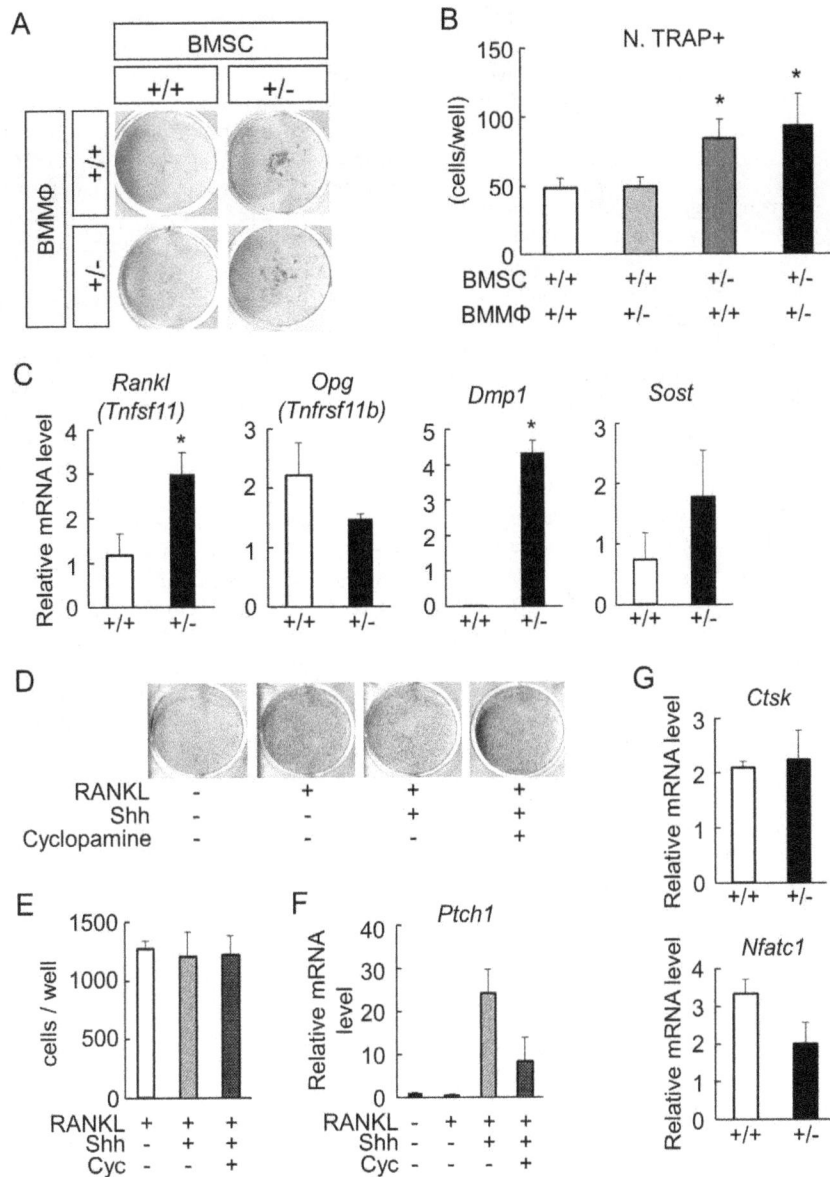

Figure 4. Osteoclast differentiation in cultures of bone marrow cells from WT and *Gli1⁺/⁻* mice. (**A**) Formation of TRAP-positive multinucleated osteoclasts by the co-culture of BMSCs and BMMΦ derived from WT or *Gli1⁺/⁻* mice. (**B**) The numbers of osteoclasts expressed as means ± SDs of 4 wells per group in (A). *p<0.05 vs. the control group (WT BMSC × WT BMMΦ). (**C**) mRNA expression of *Rankl*, *Opg*, *Dmp1*, and *Sost* in 14-day osteogenic cultures of BMSCs. The mRNA expression was analyzed by real-time RT-PCR. *Rankl*, receptor activator of nuclear factor-κB ligand; *Opg*, osteoprotegerin; *Dmp1*, dentin matrix acidic phosphoprotein 1; *Sost*, sclerostin. *p<0.05 vs. WT. (**D**) Formation of TRAP-positive multinucleated osteoclasts in 5-day cultures of RAW cells in the presence or absence of sonic hedgehog (Shh) and cyclopamine (Cyc). (**E**) The numbers of osteoclasts in (D) expressed as means ± SDs of 4 wells per group. (**F**) mRNA expression of *Ptch1* in cultured RAW cells in the presence or absence of Shh and cyclopamine (Cyc). Data are means ± SDs of 4 wells per group. (**G**) mRNA expression of cathepsin K (*Ctsk*) and *NFATc1* in osteoclasts derived from WT or *Gli1⁺/⁻* BMMΦ. Cells were cultured with recombinant M-CSF (10 ng/mL), RANKL (100 ng/mL), and Shh (25 nM). The mRNA expression was analyzed by real-time RT-PCR.

healing process, both intramembranous ossification and endochondral ossification are observed, and osteo-chondroprogenitor cells from the periosteum adjacent to fracture sites are major source of cells that contribute to the healing process [30,31]. Fracture healing was evaluated 2 weeks after the surgery, given that bony bridging at the fracture site was typically observed as early as the point [30,31]. In soft X-ray analyses, we observed impairment of callus formation and bone union in *Gli1⁺/⁻* mice compared to WT mice, as well as the variability and reproducibility of the fracture model itself (Figure 5A). Using 3D-micro-CT

analyses, we evaluated the areas of the calluses on horizontal cross-sections at the fracture lines and the volume of the callus. Both the areas and the volumes of the callus in the *Gli1⁺/⁻* mice were significantly lower than those in WT mice (Figures 5B and C).

We then performed histological analyses on sections stained with the hematoxylin-eosin (H–E) and alcian blue to identify differences in the healing process between WT and *Gli1⁺/⁻* mice (Figure 5D). In WT mice, large volumes of soft callus surrounded by hard calluses were observed around the fracture sites, as previously reported [32] (Figure 5D). However, in *Gli1⁺/⁻* mice, both the soft and hard calluses were reduced compared to those in the WT mice (Figure 5D), suggesting that both endochondral ossification and intramembranous ossification were affected by *Gli1* haploinsufficiency during the fracture healing process.

Discussion

The present study had six major findings. (1) Adult bone mass was affected by *Gli1* haploinsufficiency in mice, although body length and body weight were not. (2) The low bone mass phenotypes were accompanied by impaired bone formation and accelerated bone resorption, that is, an uncoupling of bone metabolism. (3) *Gli1* haploinsufficiency had a negative impact on Hh-mediated osteoblast differentiation in cultures of precursors. (4) Despite the impairment of osteoblast differentiation, the expression levels of *Dmp1* and *Rankl* were upregulated in cultures of *Gli1*$^{+/-}$ precursors, suggesting that *Gli1* haploinsufficiency induced the premature differentiation of osteoblasts into osteocytes, which have a greater ability to promote osteoclastogenesis than do osteoblasts. (5) Hh-Gli1 was not involved in osteoclastogenesis in a cell-autonomous manner in vitro. (6) *Gli1* haploinsufficiency affected fracture healing in adult mice. Based on these findings, we propose that Gli1, acting downstream of Hh signaling, not only promotes osteoblast differentiation but also acts as a repressor of osteoblast maturation toward osteocytes to maintain normal bone homeostasis in adult mice.

There are two possible mechanisms underlying the aberrant upregulation of osteocyte marker genes in *Gli1*$^{+/-}$ precursors. The first possibility is that the overall differentiation of osteoblast precursors is accelerated by *Gli1* haploinsufficiency, although the differentiation program is kept normal. The second possibility is that the program itself is disturbed by *Gli1* haploinsufficiency, and the disturbance may induce the premature differentiation of precursors into osteocytes by skipping proper phases of osteoblast differentiation. The second possibility is more likely, because osteocyte marker genes (*Dmp1* and *Sost*) were highly induced in *Gli1*$^{+/-}$ cells, despite downregulation of both early and late osteoblast marker genes (*Alp*, *Ibsp*, *Runx2*, *Sp7*, and *Bglap*). If the first possibility was the case, *Gli1*$^{+/-}$ precursors would show upregulation of both osteoblast and osteocyte marker genes.

It remains to be elucidated how *Gli1* haploinsufficiency disturbs the osteoblast differentiation program, which results in accelerated bone resorption as well as decreased bone formation, i.e., an uncoupling of bone metabolism in development. *Gli1*, collectively with *Gli2* and *Gli3*, is involved in the specification of osteochondroprogenitor cells in the perichondrium into an osteoblast lineage, and it promotes early osteoblast differentiation in a Runx2-independent manner [11]. The removal of *Smo* after the specification of *Sp7*-positive osteoblast precursors showed normal osteoblast development, suggesting that Hh signaling is not required for the differentiation of *Sp7*-positive osteoblast precursors into osteoblasts [33]. In contrast, the phenotypes of *Gli1*$^{+/-}$ mice suggest that Gli1 acts to repress the maturation of osteoblasts into osteocytes in postnatal bones directly or indirectly via a negative feedback loop-like mechanism, in addition to its specifier function. In addition to the repressive effects of Gli1 on the terminal differentiation of osteoblasts, Gli1-mediated negative regulation of *Rankl* transcription may also explain the enhanced osteoclastogenesis in *Gli1*$^{+/-}$ mice. An extensive search for Gli binding regions in the osteoblast genome will be useful for understanding the precise roles of Gli1 in bone metabolism.

Given that one copy of *Gli1* allele was removed in all the cells of the mice used in the present study, cells other than skeletal lineages may also be involved in the osteoblast phenotypes seen in the mutants via systemic factors or direct contact with osteoblastic cells. Indeed, the body weights of the 8-week-old *Gli1*$^{-/-}$ mice were about 20% less than those of the WT and *Gli1*$^{+/-}$ mice, suggesting systemic abnormalities upon complete loss of *Gli1*. Stage- and tissue-specific manipulation of *Gli1* using a floxed *Gli1* allele would clarify the distinct function of *Gli1* at different stages of osteoblast development, although such mutant mice are not yet available.

The involvement of Hh signaling in the regulation of bone metabolism has been debated. We previously found that *Ptch1*$^{+/-}$ mice and patients with nevoid basal cell carcinoma syndrome, in which Hh signaling was activated by the loss of one copy of the *Ptch1* allele, demonstrated high bone mass phenotypes [12], whereas Mak et al. reported that the disruption of the gene in *Bglap*-positive cells caused low bone mass [13]. At cellular levels, a common phenomenon underlies the contradictory phenotypes. Both osteoblastogenesis and osteoclastogenesis were enhanced in both mutants. Therefore, those different outcomes might be due to an alteration of the balance between enhanced bone formation and bone resorption. These studies and the present investigation have provided consistent evidence of the direct promotion of osteoblastogenesis by Hh signaling in adult mice.

In contrast, there are some arguments with respect to the involvement of Hh signaling in osteoclastogenesis. The studies mentioned above [12,13] and the present one support the concept that Hh signaling stimulates osteoclastogenesis indirectly via the augmentation of osteoblasts or osteocytes. Conversely, Heller et al. described that the inhibition of Smo suppressed osteoclastogenesis in a cell-autonomous manner [34]. The reasons for these conflicting findings should be elucidated with regard to cell type and culture conditions. Joeng et al. recently reported postnatal skeletal phenotypes in mice expressing a constitutively active form of *Gli2* in *Sp7*-positive cells. The mutants showed osteopenia with decreased bone formation and unaltered bone resorption, although osteoblast differentiation was enhanced in cultures of precursor cells isolated from the mutants [14]. Although *Gli1* is thought to be upregulated in the mutants as *Ptch1* upregulation was confirmed [14], their skeletal phenotypes are seemingly inconsistent with those in the *Gli1*$^{+/-}$ mice. The discrepancy may be caused by the difference in populations in which Hh signaling was manipulated or the difference in Gli factors that were manipulated between the studies. Overall, these results suggest that as Joeng et al. mentioned [14], the roles of Hh signaling in bone metabolism depend on its target population, the timing of its activation, and complex regulation by Gli factors downstream of the signaling; the roles are possibly modulated by non-skeletal cells or factors.

We demonstrated roles of Gli1 in the fracture healing process as well as in mouse adult bone homeostasis. A previous report on defects of bone healing in *Smo*-deleted mice [35] supports the impairment of callus formation in the *Gli1*$^{+/-}$ mice although the tested models are different between that study and our present investigation. Given that cartilage development was not largely affected by the complete loss of *Gli1* [11], the reduced size of soft calluses during fracture healing of the *Gli1*$^{+/-}$ mice was unexpected. In development, Gli3 repressor, rather than Gli activators, was shown to play a major role in the Hh-mediated control of cartilage formation [8]. Thus, it is possible that the involvement of *Gli1* in chondrogenesis and/or cartilage metabolism is different between embryos and adults or physiological conditions and pathological ones. Hh signaling may require a contribution from the Gli activators during fracture healing, where the rapid growth of cartilaginous tissues is likely to depend more on cellular proliferation than on increases in cellular volume or

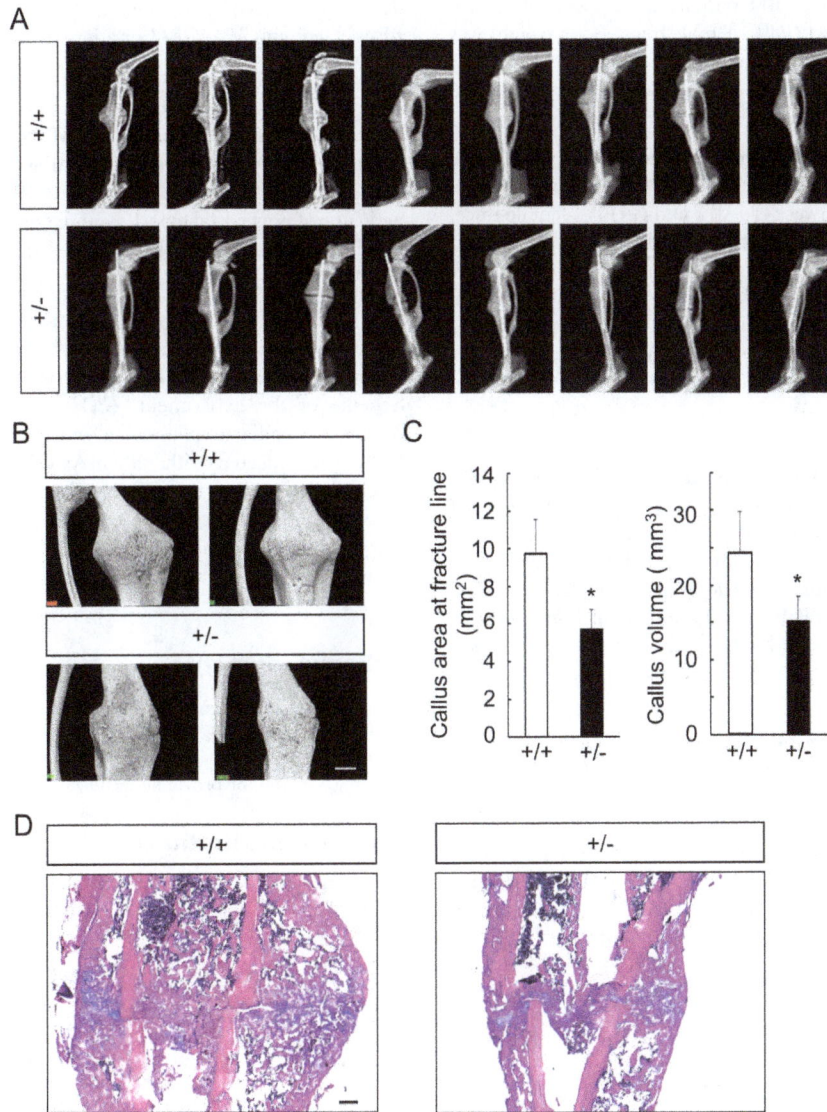

Figure 5. Comparison of bone fracture healing between 8-week-old WT and *Gli1*[+/−] mice. (**A**) Soft X-ray pictures of the fracture sites of all WT (n = 8) and *Gli1*[+/−] (n = 8) male mice tested at 2 weeks after the fracture. (**B**) Representative micro-CT images of the callus in WT and *Gli1*[+/−] male mice. Bar, 1 mm. (**C**) The areas of horizontal cross-sections at fracture lines (left) and the volume of the calluses (right) of WT and *Gli1*[+/−] mice, calculated using 3D-micro-CT data. Data are means ± SDs of eight mice per genotype. *p<0.05 vs. WT. (**D**) H&E and alcian blue double staining of the calluses 2 weeks after the fracture. Bar, 200 μm.

matrix deposition [32]. The promotion of proliferation is known to be a direct action of Hh signaling on chondrocytes [36].

When discussing the regulation of the adult skeleton by Hh-Gli signaling under physiological and pathological conditions, we should consider target cell types and sources of Hh ligands. Maeda et al. demonstrated that Ihh secreted from chondrocytes in the growth plate is required for the maintenance of trabecular bones in postnatal mice [37]. Type I collagen-positive cells in bone lining were shown to express Ihh in humans [38]. Both Ihh expressed in soft calluses [39] and sonic hedgehog (Shh) expressed in the periosteum [40] or osteoblasts/osteocytes [41] have been implicated in fracture healing. These findings imply that Gli1 is likely to contribute to adult bone metabolism upon the inputs of Ihh and Shh. In addition, given that Hh signaling acts to maintain the skeleton in adults, and some species close the growth plate after

puberty, skeletal components other than growth plate chondrocytes may produce Hh ligands in this context.

In conclusion, the results of the present study lead us to propose the involvement of *Gli1* in postnatal bone homeostasis under physiological and pathological conditions although further studies are necessary to obtain an integrative understanding of the roles of all Gli family members in this context. Collectively with previous studies, the present study also indicates the importance of tissue- and stage-specific manipulation of Hh signaling for the treatment of bone-related disease, as well as the need for a greater understanding of all the actions of Hh signaling on the skeletal tissue throughout life.

Supporting Information

Figure S1   Gross appearance of WT and *Gli1* mutant male mice. (**A**) Gross appearance of WT, *Gli1*[+/−], and *Gli1*[−/−]

male mice at 8 weeks of age. (**B**) Comparison of postnatal growth between WT, $Gli1^{+/-}$, and $Gli1^{-/-}$ male mice. Body weight was measured on the indicated dates after birth. *p<0.05 vs. WT or $Gli1^{+/-}$.

Figure S2 Radiological analyses of long bones in female WT and $Gli1^{+/-}$ mice. (**A**) 3D-micro-CT images of the distal femurs of representative 8-week-old WT and $Gli1^{+/-}$ female mice. Sagittal sections, transverse sections, and 3D reconstruction images of the primary spongiosa are shown for each genotype. Bar, 1 mm. (**B**) Histomorphometric analyses of the 3D-micro-CT data in (A). BMD, bone mineral density; BV/TV, bone volume per tissue volume; Tb.Th, trabecular thickness; Tb.N, trabecular number parameters. Data are means ± SDs of five female mice per genotype. *p<0.05 vs. WT.

Figure S3 Radiological analyses of cortical bones in WT and $Gli1^{+/-}$ mice. (**A**) 3D-micro-CT images of distal femurs of representative 8-week-old WT and $Gli1^{+/-}$ male mice. Transverse sections of the primary spongiosa are shown for each genotype. Bar, 500 μm. (**B**) Histomorphometric analyses of 3D-micro-CT data in (A). Cv/Av, cortical bone volume per all bone volume; Cvt, cortical bone thickness; BMD, bone mineral density. Data are means ± SDs of ten male mice per genotype.

Figure S4 Construction of adenoviral vector expressing $GLI1$. (**A**) Schematic representation of pAd/PL-DEST vectors expressing $GLI1$. (**B**) Luciferase reporter assay using the 8×3'-Gli BS-luc in combination with $dsRed$, Myc-$GLI1$, and the constructed adenoviral vector ($GLI1$-$IRES$-$deRed$). The luciferase assay was performed 48 hours after transfection in C3H10T1/2 cells. (**C**) Protein expression of GLI1 in C3H10T1/2 cells transfected with Myc-$GLI1$ or adenovirally transduced with $GLI1$-$IRES$-

$dsRed$. (**D**) mRNA expression of Alp and $Ibsp$ in C3H10T1/2 cells transfected with Myc-$GLI1$ or adenovirally transduced with $GLI1$-$IRES$-$dsRed$.

Figure S5 mRNA expression of $Rankl$, Opg, $Dmp1$, and $Sost$ in 7-day osteogenic cultures of OPs. The mRNA expression was analyzed by real-time RT-PCR. $Rankl$, receptor activator of nuclear factor-κB ligand; Opg, osteoprotegerin; $Dmp1$, dentin matrix acidic phosphoprotein 1; $Sost$, sclerostin. *p<0.05 vs. WT.

Figure S6 Suppression of $Rankl$ expression in response to the recovery of $Gli1$ expression in $Gli1^{+/-}$ BMSCs. (**A**) Scheme of the experiment. $Gli1^{+/-}$ BMSCs were cultured in osteogenic media supplemented with Smoothened agonist (SAG). Cells were infected with either Ax-GFP (control) or Ax-$GLI1$-$IRES$-$dsRed$ on Day 4 and cultured for another 7 days. (**B**) mRNA expression of $Rankl$ on days 0, 4, and 11. The mRNA expression was analyzed by real-time RT-PCR analyses. *p<0.05 vs. Ax-GFP.

Acknowledgments

We thank Drs. Alexandra L. Joyner, Chi-chung Hui, Gen Yamada, Andrew P. McMahon, and Hiroshi Sasaki for providing experimental materials. We are also grateful to Katsue Morii, Harumi Kobayashi, and Nozomi Nagumo for providing technical assistance.

Author Contributions

Conceived and designed the experiments: SO UI. Performed the experiments: Y. Kitaura HH SO. Analyzed the data: Y. Kitaura HH Y. Komiyama TT UI SO. Wrote the paper: Y. Kitaura SO.

References

1. Kronenberg HM (2003) Developmental regulation of the growth plate. Nature 423: 332–336.
2. St-Jacques B, Hammerschmidt M, McMahon AP (1999) Indian hedgehog signaling regulates proliferation and differentiation of chondrocytes and is essential for bone formation. Genes Dev 13: 2072–2086.
3. Chung UI, Schipani E, McMahon AP, Kronenberg HM (2001) Indian hedgehog couples chondrogenesis to osteogenesis in endochondral bone development. J Clin Invest 107: 295–304.
4. Long F, Chung UI, Ohba S, McMahon J, Kronenberg HM, et al. (2004) Ihh signaling is directly required for the osteoblast lineage in the endochondral skeleton. Development 131: 1309–1318.
5. Komori T, Yagi H, Nomura S, Yamaguchi A, Sasaki K, et al. (1997) Targeted disruption of Cbfa1 results in a complete lack of bone formation owing to maturational arrest of osteoblasts. Cell 89: 755–764.
6. Otto F, Thornell AP, Crompton T, Denzel A, Gilmour KC, et al. (1997) Cbfa1, a candidate gene for cleidocranial dysplasia syndrome, is essential for osteoblast differentiation and bone development. Cell 89: 765–771.
7. Ingham PW, McMahon AP (2001) Hedgehog signaling in animal development: paradigms and principles. Genes Dev 15: 3059–3087.
8. Hilton MJ, Tu X, Cook J, Hu H, Long F (2005) Ihh controls cartilage development by antagonizing Gli3, but requires additional effectors to regulate osteoblast and vascular development. Development 132: 4339–4351.
9. Joeng KS, Long FX (2009) The Gli2 transcriptional activator is a crucial effector for Ihh signaling in osteoblast development and cartilage vascularization. Development 136: 4177–4185.
10. Hojo H, Ohba S, Taniguchi K, Shirai M, Yano F, et al. (2013) Hedgehog-Gli Activators Direct Osteo-chondrogenic Function of Bone Morphogenetic Protein toward Osteogenesis in the Perichondrium. J Biol Chem 288: 9924–9932.
11. Hojo H, Ohba S, Yano F, Saito T, Ikeda T, et al. (2012) Gli1 Protein Participates in Hedgehog-mediated Specification of Osteoblast Lineage during Endochondral Ossification. Journal of Biological Chemistry 287: 17860–17869.
12. Ohba S, Kawaguchi H, Kugimiya F, Ogasawara T, Kawamura N, et al. (2008) Patched1 haploinsufficiency increases adult bone mass and modulates Gli3 repressor activity. Dev Cell 14: 689–699.
13. Mak KK, Bi Y, Wan C, Chuang PT, Clemens T, et al. (2008) Hedgehog signaling in mature osteoblasts regulates bone formation and resorption by controlling PTHrP and RANKL expression. Dev Cell 14: 674–688.
14. Joeng KS, Long F (2013) Constitutive activation of Gli2 impairs bone formation in postnatal growing mice. PLoS ONE 8: e55134.
15. Park HL, Bai C, Platt KA, Matise MP, Beeghly A, et al. (2000) Mouse Gli1 mutants are viable but have defects in SHH signaling in combination with a Gli2 mutation. Development 127: 1593–1605.
16. Zhang X, Peterson KA, Liu XS, McMahon AP, Ohba S (2013) Gene regulatory networks mediating canonical Wnt signal-directed control of pluripotency and differentiation in embryo stem cells. Stem Cells 31: 2667–2679.
17. Tenzen T, Allen BL, Cole F, Kang JS, Krauss RS, et al. (2006) The cell surface membrane proteins Cdo and Boc are components and targets of the Hedgehog signaling pathway and feedback network in mice. Dev Cell 10: 647–656.
18. Ogata N, Chikazu D, Kubota N, Terauchi Y, Tobe K, et al. (2000) Insulin receptor substrate-1 in osteoblast is indispensable for maintaining bone turnover. J Clin Invest 105: 935–943.
19. Akune T, Ogata N, Hoshi K, Kubota N, Terauchi Y, et al. (2002) Insulin receptor substrate-2 maintains predominance of anabolic function over catabolic function of osteoblasts. J Cell Biol 159: 147–156.
20. Ogasawara T, Katagiri M, Yamamoto A, Hoshi K, Takato T, et al. (2004) Osteoclast differentiation by RANKL requires NF-kappaB-mediated downregulation of cyclin-dependent kinase 6 (Cdk6). J Bone Miner Res 19: 1128–1136.
21. Ohba S, Ikeda T, Kugimiya F, Yano F, Lichtler AC, et al. (2007) Identification of a potent combination of osteogenic genes for bone regeneration using embryonic stem (ES) cell-based sensor. Faseb J 21: 1777–1787.
22. Sasaki H, Hui C, Nakafuku M, Kondoh H (1997) A binding site for Gli proteins is essential for HNF-3beta floor plate enhancer activity in transgenics and can respond to Shh in vitro. Development 124: 1313–1322.
23. Ogasawara T, Kawaguchi H, Jinno S, Hoshi K, Itaka K, et al. (2004) Bone morphogenetic protein 2-induced osteoblast differentiation requires Smad-mediated down-regulation of Cdk6. Mol Cell Biol 24: 6560–6568.
24. Kugimiya F, Kawaguchi H, Kamekura S, Chikuda H, Ohba S, et al. (2005) Involvement of endogenous bone morphogenetic protein (BMP) 2 and BMP6 in bone formation. J Biol Chem 280: 35704–35712.

25. Nakashima T, Hayashi M, Fukunaga T, Kurata K, Oh-Hora M, et al. (2011) Evidence for osteocyte regulation of bone homeostasis through RANKL expression. Nat Med 17: 1231–1234.

26. Takahashi N, Akatsu T, Udagawa N, Sasaki T, Yamaguchi A, et al. (1988) Osteoblastic cells are involved in osteoclast formation. Endocrinology 123: 2600–2602.

27. Suda T, Takahashi N, Udagawa N, Jimi E, Gillespie MT, et al. (1999) Modulation of osteoclast differentiation and function by the new members of the tumor necrosis factor receptor and ligand families. Endocr Rev 20: 345–357.

28. Udagawa N, Takahashi N, Yasuda H, Mizuno A, Itoh K, et al. (2000) Osteoprotegerin produced by osteoblasts is an important regulator in osteoclast development and function. Endocrinology 141: 3478–3484.

29. Yamamoto A, Miyazaki T, Kadono Y, Takayanagi H, Miura T, et al. (2002) Possible involvement of IkappaB kinase 2 and MKK7 in osteoclastogenesis induced by receptor activator of nuclear factor kappaB ligand. J Bone Miner Res 17: 612–621.

30. Shimoaka T, Kamekura S, Chikuda H, Hoshi K, Chung UI, et al. (2004) Impairment of bone healing by insulin receptor substrate-1 deficiency. J Biol Chem 279: 15314–15322.

31. Murao H, Yamamoto K, Matsuda S, Akiyama H (2013) Periosteal cells are a major source of soft callus in bone fracture. J Bone Miner Metab 31: 390–398.

32. Gerstenfeld LC, Cullinane DM, Barnes GL, Graves DT, Einhorn TA (2003) Fracture healing as a post-natal developmental process: molecular, spatial, and temporal aspects of its regulation. J Cell Biochem 88: 873–884.

33. Rodda SJ, McMahon AP (2006) Distinct roles for Hedgehog and canonical Wnt signaling in specification, differentiation and maintenance of osteoblast progenitors. Development 133: 3231–3244.

34. Heller E, Hurchla MA, Xiang J, Su X, Chen S, et al. (2012) Hedgehog signaling inhibition blocks growth of resistant tumors through effects on tumor microenvironment. Cancer Res 72: 897–907.

35. Wang Q, Huang C, Zeng F, Xue M, Zhang X (2010) Activation of the Hh pathway in periosteum-derived mesenchymal stem cells induces bone formation in vivo: implication for postnatal bone repair. Am J Pathol 177: 3100–3111.

36. Long F, Zhang XM, Karp S, Yang Y, McMahon AP (2001) Genetic manipulation of hedgehog signaling in the endochondral skeleton reveals a direct role in the regulation of chondrocyte proliferation. Development 128: 5099–5108.

37. Maeda Y, Nakamura E, Nguyen MT, Suva LJ, Swain FL, et al. (2007) Indian Hedgehog produced by postnatal chondrocytes is essential for maintaining a growth plate and trabecular bone. Proc Natl Acad Sci U S A.

38. Nakase T, Miyaji T, Kuriyama K, Tamai N, Horiki M, et al. (2001) Immunohistochemical detection of parathyroid hormone-related peptide, Indian hedgehog, and patched in the process of endochondral ossification in the human. Histochem Cell Biol 116: 277–284.

39. Vortkamp A, Pathi S, Peretti GM, Caruso EM, Zaleske DJ, et al. (1998) Recapitulation of signals regulating embryonic bone formation during postnatal growth and in fracture repair. Mech Dev 71: 65–76.

40. Miyaji T, Nakase T, Iwasaki M, Kuriyama K, Tamai N, et al. (2003) Expression and distribution of transcripts for sonic hedgehog in the early phase of fracture repair. Histochem Cell Biol 119: 233–237.

41. Horikiri Y, Shimo T, Kurio N, Okui T, Matsumoto K, et al. (2013) Sonic hedgehog regulates osteoblast function by focal adhesion kinase signaling in the process of fracture healing. PLoS One 8: e76785.

25

Long Bone Structure and Strength Depend on BMP2 from Osteoblasts and Osteocytes, but Not Vascular Endothelial Cells

Sarah H. McBride[1,2]*, Jennifer A. McKenzie[1], Bronwyn S. Bedrick[3], Paige Kuhlmann[1], Jill D. Pasteris[3], Vicki Rosen[4], Matthew J. Silva[1]

1 Department of Orthopaedic Surgery, Musculoskeletal Research Center, Washington University in St. Louis, St. Louis, Missouri, United States of America, 2 Department of Orthopaedic Surgery, Saint Louis University, St. Louis, Missouri, United States of America, 3 Department of Earth and Planetary Sciences, Washington University in St. Louis, St. Louis, Missouri, United States of America, 4 Department of Developmental Biology, Harvard School of Dental Medicine, Boston, Massachusetts, United States of America

Abstract

The importance of bone morphogenetic protein 2 (BMP2) in the skeleton is well known. BMP2 is expressed in a variety of tissues during development, growth and healing. In this study we sought to better identify the role of tissue-specific BMP2 during post-natal growth and to determine if BMP2 knockout affects the ability of terminally differentiated cells to create high quality bone material. We targeted BMP2 knockout to two differentiated cell types known to express BMP2 during growth and healing, early-stage osteoblasts and their progeny (osterix promoted Cre) and vascular endothelial cells (vascular-endothelial-cadherin promoted Cre). Our objectives were to assess post-natal bone growth, structure and strength. We hypothesized that removal of BMP2 from osteogenic and vascular cells (separately) would result in smaller skeletons with inferior bone material properties. At 12 and 24 weeks of age the osteoblast knockout of BMP2 reduced body weight by 20%, but the vascular knockout had no effect. Analysis of bone in the tibia revealed reductions in cortical and cancellous bone size and volume in the osteoblast knockout, but not in the vascular endothelial knockout. Furthermore, forelimb strength testing revealed a 30% reduction in ultimate force at both 12 and 24 weeks in the osteoblast knockout of BMP2, but no change in the vascular endothelial knockout. Moreover, mechanical strength testing of femurs from osteoblast knockout mice demonstrated an increased Young's modulus (greater than 35%) but decreased post-yield displacement (greater than 50%) at both 12 and 24 weeks of age. In summary, the osteoblast knockout of BMP2 reduced bone size and altered mechanical properties at the whole-bone and material levels. Osteoblast-derived BMP2 has an important role in post-natal skeletal growth, structure and strength, while vascular endothelial-derived BMP2 does not.

Editor: Gwendolen Reilly, University of Sheffield, United Kingdom

Funding: This work was funded by the following sources: Washington University T32 Metabolic Skeletal Disorders Training Program (NIH 1T32AR060719-01) (SM), National Institutes of Health/National Institute of Arthritis and Musculoskeletal and Skin Diseases (NIH/NIAMS) AR050211 (SM, JM, MJS), Washington University Musculoskeletal Research Center (NIH P30 AR057235), and Amgen Scholars Program (PK). The funders had no role in study design, data collection and analysis, decision to publish, or preparation of the manuscript.

Competing Interests: The authors have declared that no competing interests exist.

* E-mail: SMcBrid9@SLU.edu

Introduction

Bone morphogenetic protein 2 (BMP2) plays critical roles in the skeleton. Extensive research has focused on BMP2's ability to enable differentiation of precursor cells into osteoblasts and enhance osteoblast function[1–5]. BMP2 is highly expressed in osteoblasts[6–8], but little is known about how a deficiency of BMP2 affects differentiated osteogenic cells[9–11]. Furthermore, research has indicated that BMP2 is expressed in a variety of non-osseous tissues during development, growth, and healing [3,6,12,13]. It is unknown if a lack of BMP2 in these other tissue types affects post-natal bone growth.

BMP2 null mice are embryonic lethal due to defects in heart development and mesoderm [14]. Thus, conditional knockout mice must be used to study the effect of BMP2 deficiency on bone development and growth [9,10]. Tsuji and colleagues knocked out BMP2 in all osteo- and chondro-progenitor cells and their lineages

(e.g. chondrocytes, osteoblasts and osteocytes) using the limb specific promoter Prx1-Cre [10]. Surprisingly, these knockout mice were similar to wildtype mice at birth. However, as early as one week postnatally they began to exhibit defects in both cartilage and bone formation, and as they matured the phenotype worsened. Knockout mice had thinner, less dense bones that spontaneously fractured. However, it is unclear if one cell type (progenitor, chondrocyte, osteoblast, osteocyte) is the major contributor of BMP2 causing the phenotype or if the phenotype is a result of knockout from all chondro- and osteo- cells. Also, it is unknown if the spontaneous fractures were due solely to the smaller size of the knockout bones or if there was a defect in the bone material of knockout mice [9,10]. In support of the latter, a recent report indicates that BMP2 deletion in cells of the osteoblast lineage results in a brittle bone phenotype [15].

Bone development, growth, remodeling, and healing are dependent on vascular cells and angiogenesis. For example, mineralization of the cartilaginous template follows vascular invasion [16]. Also, the periosteum, the bilayer membrane surrounding bones that is responsible for circumferential growth through life, is well vascularized [17]. Inhibition of angiogenesis or vasodilation during bone healing decreases the generation of new bone [18–21]. Interestingly, there is also a strong connection between BMP2 and vascular cells. As previously mentioned, global loss of BMP2 results in severe heart development defects [14]. Mice lacking BMP2 expression in osteoblasts and osteocytes have a reduced vascular network [15]; and recent work from our lab and others have indicated that BMP2 is expressed in vascular cells during intramembranous bone healing (stress fracture healing and distraction osteogenesis) [12,13]. Moreover, there is a wealth of research linking arterial calcification with increased local BMP2 expression [22,23]. To our knowledge there are no studies that have investigated the role of vascular-derived BMP2 on the skeleton.

In this study we sought to better identify the role of tissue-specific BMP2 during post-natal skeletal growth and to determine if BMP2 knockout affects the ability of terminally differentiated cells to create normal quality bone material. We targeted BMP2 knockout to two differentiated cell types known to express BMP2 during growth and healing, early-stage osteoblasts (and their progeny) and vascular endothelial cells. We then assessed bone growth, structure and strength. We hypothesized that removal of BMP2 from osteogenic and vascular cells (separately) results in smaller skeletons with inferior bone material properties.

Methods

Ethics Statement

This study was carried out in strict accordance with the recommendations in the Guide for the Care and Use of Laboratory Animals of the National Institutes of Health. The protocol was approved by the IACUC of Washington University of St. Louis (Protocol Number: 20110209). All efforts were made to minimize suffering. Mice were maintained in standard housing with 12 hr light/dark cycles and food and water *ad libitum*. All dual energy X-ray absorptiometry, microCT, and forelimb loading experiments were performed on live animals under anesthesia (Ketamine & Xylazine – dual energy X-ray absorptiometry or 1–3% isofluorane – microCT and forelimb loading). Euthanasia was carried out by CO_2 asphyxiation. Three-point bending and Raman spectroscopy were performed post mortem on harvested bones.

Transgenic mice with the *Bmp2* gene floxed (obtained through materials transfer agreement with Harvard University) were crossed with either osterix-promoted Cre (Osx-Cre, B6.Cg-Tg(Sp7-tTA,tetO-EGFP/Cre)1Amc/J) [24] or vascular-endothelial-cadherin-promoted Cre (VEC-Cre, B6.Cg-Tg(Cdh5-Cre)7Mlia/J) [25]. Osx-Cre mice had a targeted deletion of BMP2 in early-stage osteoblasts, which continues as the cells develop into mature osteoblasts and osteocytes. VEC-Cre mice had a targeted deletion of BMP2 in vascular endothelial cells.

Male and female mice with the *Bmp2* floxed on one (fl/+, heterozygous) or two (fl/fl, homozygous) alleles were investigated. Throughout the paper mice with the genotype $Bmp2^{fl/fl}$; *Osx*-Cre+ are referred to as Osx-Cre cKO, while littermate mice with the genotype $Bmp2^{fl/fl}$ without Cre are referred to as Osx-Cre wildtype (WT). In addition, mice with the genotype $Bmp2^{fl/fl}$; *VEC*-Cre+ are referred to as VEC-Cre cKO, while littermate mice with the genotype $Bmp2^{fl/fl}$ without Cre are referred to as VEC-Cre WT.

Verification of Knockout

Tissue specific knockout of BMP2 was confirmed in two ways. First, the intended cell-specific Cre expression was verified. For the Osx-Cre a green fluorescent protein (GFP) tag was already attached to the Cre protein; cells currently producing Cre appear green. The VEC-Cre was crossed into an mTmG transgenic mouse $(Gt(ROSA)26Sor^{tm4(ACTB-tdTomato,-EGFP)Luo}/J)$ [26]. In an mTmG mouse all normal, non-Cre expressing cells produce a red fluorescent protein (RFP) in the cell membrane, whereas cells that have expressed Cre switch to produce a GFP instead of the RFP. For both mouse lines, forelimbs (ulna and radius with surrounding muscle) were harvested (n = 3–6/genotype), fixed in 10% neutral buffered formalin overnight, decalcified in 14% EDTA, and embedded in OCT media for cryosectioning. Transverse sections were examined near the ulnar midpoint. Before imaging, the slides were rinsed in water to remove the OCT media and coverslipped. They were then imaged with 10x, 20x and 40× objective magnification (IX51, Olympus, Center Valley, PA) using TRITC and FITC filters.

Second, diminished BMP2 protein expression in the target cells was verified. For both lines, forelimbs were harvested, fixed in 10% formalin overnight, decalcified in 14% EDTA and embedded in paraffin. Transverse sections were examined near the middle of the ulna (n = 3/genotype). Immunostaining was performed using goat ABC staining system (Santa Cruz, sc-2023, Santa Cruz, CA) with BMP2 antibody (Santa Cruz, sc-6895, 1:100 dilution overnight at 4°C) following manufacturers' instructions. After hydrating, antigen retrieval was performed using a decloaking chamber (Biocare Medical, 95°C, 10 min, Concord, CA) containing sodium citrate buffer (pH 6.0). To visualize protein DAB was applied for 5 min. Sections were not counterstained. Imaging was performed at 40× (BX51, Olympus).

Whole Body Measures

To measure growth body weight was recorded. *In vivo* dual energy X-ray absorptiometry (DXA, Lunar PIXImus GE) was used to measure percent fat, bone mineral content (BMC) and areal bone mineral density (aBMD) for the whole body of the mouse (excluding the head). Two separate cohorts of Osx-Cre mice were measured at 12 and 24 weeks of age (n = 4–10/group). A cohort of VEC-Cre mice were measured at 4, 8, 12, 16, 20, and 24 weeks of age (n = 4–5/group).

MicroCT

In vivo microCT was performed on the left tibia of mice to determine tibia length, cortical and cancellous bone measures (VivaCT 40, Scanco Medical, Wayne, PA; X-ray tube potential 70 kV, integration time 100 ms, X-ray intensity 114 µA, isotropic voxel size 21 um, frame averaging 1, projections 500, medium resolution scan) in accordance with published guidelines [27]. The following cortical bone measures were determined for 200 µm at the tibial midpoint: total volume (TV), bone volume (BV), bone volume to total volume (BV/TV), and tissue mineral density (TMD). The following cancellous bone measures were determined for 600 µm distal to the proximal growth plate: total volume (TV), bone volume (BV), bone volume to total volume (BV/TV), volumetric bone mineral density (vBMD), trabecular number (Tb.N), trabecular connectivity density (Conn.D), structure model index (SMI), trabecular thickness (Tb.Th), and trabecular separation (Tb.Sp). Two separate cohorts of Osx-Cre mice were measured at 12 and 24 weeks of age (n = 6–9/group). A cohort of VEC-Cre mice was measured at 8, 16, and 24 weeks of age (n = 4–5/group).

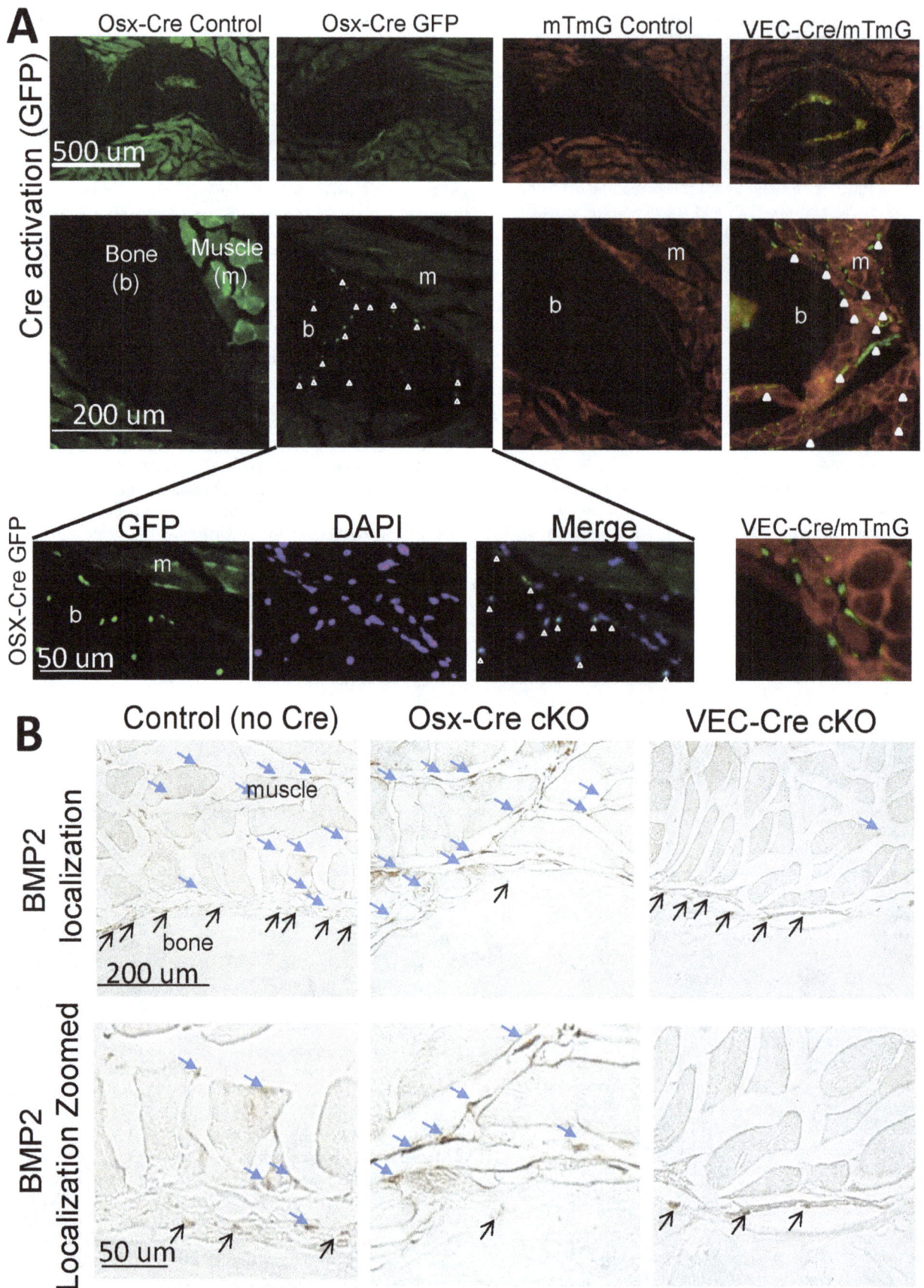

Figure 1. Deletion of BMP2 was evaluated in osteogenic cells (Osx-Cre) and vascular cells (VEC-Cre). (A) First, Cre activation was verified by examination of cortical bone (ulna) and muscle from transverse cross-sections through the mid-forelimb. In control samples the bone is

completely black. The Osx-Cre mouse has a GFP::Cre fusion protein which demonstrated the current expression of Cre in some osteocytes within the bone and osteoblasts lining the bone surface (open white arrowheads). The VEC-Cre mouse was crossed with mTmG reporter mouse and demonstrated Cre activation within muscle and periosteum compartments surrounding the bone (filled white arrowheads). (B) Confirmation of the BMP2 protein deletion was done using immunohistochemistry. In the control sample BMP2 expression was seen in the muscle (blue filled arrows) and bone-lining cells (thin black arrows). Using the Osx-Cre BMP2 expression was absent in the bone lining cells, but abundantly expressed throughout the muscle compartment (blue filled arrows). In contrast, using the VEC-Cre expression of BMP2 was limited to osteoblasts lining the bone surface (thin black arrows). Images are representative of 3–5 sections from 3–6 animals/group.

Mechanical Testing

To assess whole bone strength, mice forelimbs were loaded to failure using an established technique [28]. Briefly, mice were anesthetized and the elbow and wrist were held between two loading cups such that axial compressive loads create bending of the curved forelimb bones. The upper cup was displaced at a rate of 0.5 mm/s to compress the whole limb until complete fracture (DynaMight 8841, Instron, Norwood, MA). During displacement loading the force was recorded (LabVIEW, National Instruments, Austin, TX). Subsequent analysis identified the maximal force sustained by the whole forelimb. Two separate cohorts of Osx-Cre mice were loaded to fracture at 12 and 24 weeks old (n = 3–4/group). A cohort of VEC-Cre mice were loaded to fracture at 24 weeks old (n = 3–4/group). Mice were euthanized immediately following loading.

To assess both whole-bone strength and estimated material properties, the right and left femora of Osx-Cre mice were harvested post mortem and loaded in three-point bending (span length = 7 mm). Prior to testing, the midshaft of the femur (35 slices, 0.56 mm) was scanned using microCT (µCT40, Scanco Medical; X-ray tube potential 55 kVp, integration time 200 ms, X-ray intensity 145 µA, isotropic voxel size 16 um, frame averaging 1, projections 500, medium resolution scan). Femurs were loaded to failure at a rate of 0.1 mm/s (DynaMight 8841, Instron) while force and displacement data were collected (LabVIEW). Non-normalized properties were gathered from the force-displacement curve including stiffness, ultimate force, post-yield displacement, energy at ultimate force, and energy to fracture. Morphological parameters area and cortical thickness were calculated directly using the cross sectional microCT images. In addition, the area moment of inertia about the bending axis and the distance (c) to the farthest point of the cross section from the neutral axis were determined and used to calculate material properties of ultimate stress and Young's modulus. Two separate

cohorts of Osx-Cre mice were loaded at 12 and 24 weeks (n = 3–8/group).

Raman Spectroscopy

Eleven bilateral humeri from six 24-week-old mice and 11 unilateral femora from eleven 12-week-old mice were used for Raman spectroscopic analysis. The 24-week-old humeri were from a mixed group of male and female mice and intended as a pilot study (see supplemental data in Tables S1). The 12-week-old femora were the same bones used for three-point bending tests so that direct correlations between strength and composition could be made. The articulating ends of the humeri were removed and the samples were centrifuged to remove marrow. After three-point-bending, the uneven fracture surface of the femora specimens were removed using an Isomet saw (Buehler, Lake Bluff, IL) and then centrifuged at 12,000 rpm to remove marrow. If organic material such as blood or bone marrow still was visible, the specimen was rinsed with PBS. If a specimen was highly fluorescent under the laser, the specimen was soaked in PBS, dried, and re-analyzed. Therefore, the Raman spectra obtained and interpreted in this study showed relatively low fluorescence. Six spectra were collected for each humerus specimen: two near the inner edge of the cortex, two in the middle of the cortex, and two near the outer edge of the cortex. Examination of the spectra from the humeri indicated that the inner edge of the cortex had higher fluorescence than the other regions, probably due to the proximity of this region to the marrow cavity, and there were no substantial differences between the right and left humeri. Thus, for each femur specimen only four spectra were collected: two in the middle of the cortex and two near the outer edge. For each parameter, medians over all spectra taken on an individual specimen were obtained and used for the statistical analysis. Four femora spectra and six humeri spectra were determined to be abnormal and were not included in the statistical analysis.

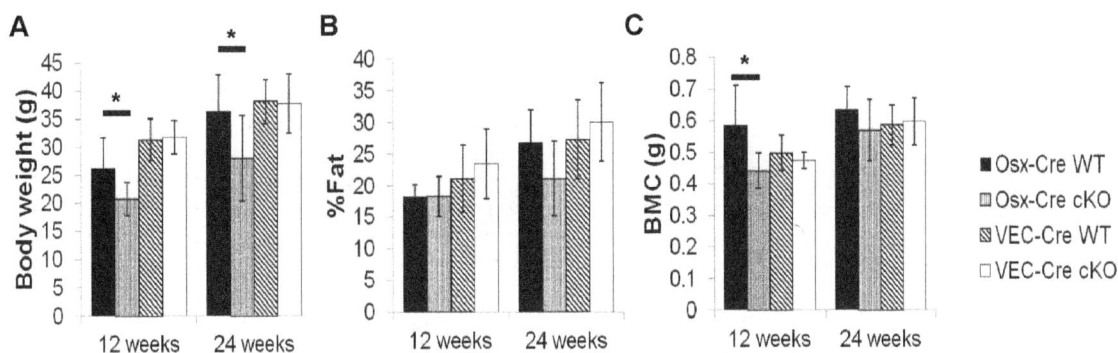

Figure 2. Whole body DXA results at 12 and 24 weeks for WT and cKO male mice. (A) Body weight was significantly reduced in the Osx-Cre cKO and unchanged for VEC-Cre mice. (B) Percent fat was not significantly reduced in the 12- and 24week old Osx-Cre cKO male mice (although it did reach significance at 24 weeks when male and female data were pooled (ANOVA)). (C) Osx-Cre cKO male mice showed a significant reduction in BMC at the 12-week time point, with a non-significant trend at 24 weeks (which was significant when male and female data were pooled (ANOVA)). BMC was unchanged for VEC-Cre mice at either time point.

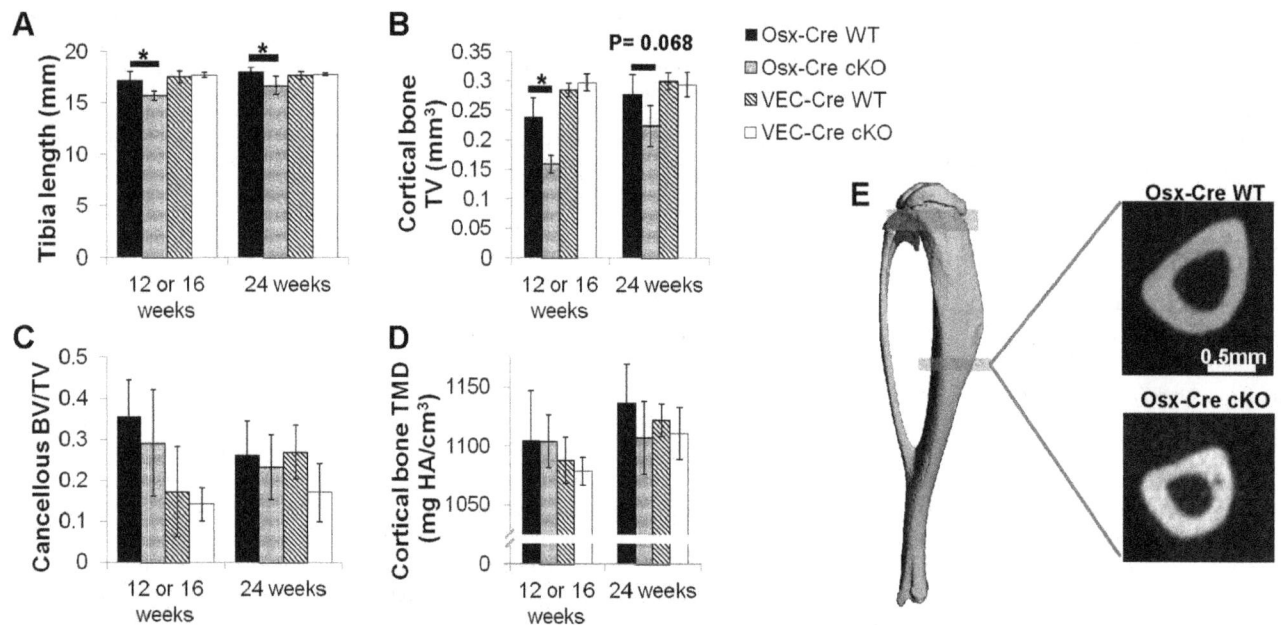

Figure 3. MicroCT was used to assess structural properties of the tibia at 12/16 and 24 weeks. (Osx-Cre data shown at 12 weeks, VEC-Cre data shown at 16 weeks.) Osx-Cre cKO mice had (A) shorter tibia and (B) reduced cortical bone volume with no change in (C) cancellous BV/TV or (D) cortical TMD. VEC-Cre mice showed no differences in any parameter. (E) Illustrations of cortical bone geometry show a smaller marrow cavity in the Osx-Cre cKO mice.

Spectra were collected using a HoloLab Series 5000 Raman microprobe (Kaiser Optical Systems Inc., Ann Arbor, MI). A laser of 532 nm excitation operated at 10 mW power (delivered to the sample surface) was focused by an $80\times$ objective lens (N.A. = 0.75) to a beam spot of approximately 1 μm diameter. A 2048-channel CCD detector monitored signal in the spectral range 100–4000 Δcm^{-1}. Each spectrum analyzed represents the average of 32 acquisitions of 4-seconds each.

Grams32^R (Galactic Software, Inc., Salem, NH) was used for all spectral processing. Baseline correction was performed on each spectrum. Spectral peaks were deconvolved into bands of best fit using a mixed Gaussian-Lorentzian algorithm. To assess the relative proportions of collagen and mineral, the 1003 Δcm^{-1} band was used to represent collagen and the 960 Δcm^{-1} band was used to represent mineral [29] The width of the 960 Δcm^{-1} band indicated the degree of crystalline organization of the mineral. To assess the degree of carbonate substitution in the mineral, the area of the 1070 Δcm^{-1} band (for Type-B carbonate substitution) was used to represent the proportion of carbonate and the area of the 960 Δcm^{-1} band to represent the apatite mineral [30].

Statistics

Data are presented as a mean ± standard deviation. DXA and microCT outcomes were analyzed using two-way ANOVA (factors: genotype and sex) (StatView v. 5.0, SAS Institute, Cary, NC). Individual ANOVAs were done for Osx-Cre and VEC-Cre strains, and for each timepoint. The p-values reported in the body of the text are based on these ANOVAs. If the main genotype effect was significant ($p<0.05$) post-hoc test Fischer's PLSD testing was performed. In general, males had larger bones than females, and the genotype effects were similar between sexes. Furthermore, heterozygous control mice (fl/+, Cre negative) were similar to homozygous controls (fl/fl, Cre negative) in both Cre strains. Outcomes for heterozygous Cre positive mice were either similar

to controls or were intermediate between the homozygous controls and homozygous knockouts. For conciseness, only data for homozygous male mice are presented in the main Tables and Figures for two timepoints (12 and 24 weeks for Osx-Cre; 16 and 24 weeks for VEC-Cre). (See the supplementary data in Tables S1 for all additional groups.) In the case of 3-point bending the right and left femur data were averaged and unpaired t-tests were performed on the pooled sets. For Raman spectroscopy differences between the two genotypes were assessed by two-sample t-tests of the spectral parameter means using Statistical Analysis System (SAS, Version 9.3 for Windows; SAS Institute, Cary, NC).

Results

BMP2 Deletion in Osteoblasts and Vascular Cells

BMP2 was successfully knocked down in our cells of interest, early stage osteoblasts and their progeny (including osteocytes), and vascular endothelial cells. The Osx- and VEC-Cres were expressed in the expected target tissues (Figure 1A, GFP signal). As seen in Figure 1A, the GFP signal of the OSX-Cre does not appear in all bone lining cells or osteocytes at any one time. This is because the GFP::Cre fusion protein is under that control of the Osterix promoter which is transiently expressed. Once the GFP::Cre protein is no longer created (i.e., Osterix is no longer being expressed) and all the GFP::Cre protein has been degraded, a cell will not fluoresce even though the knockout has occurred and the cell can no longer produce a functional BMP2 protein. The successful targeting of osteoblasts and osteocytes in post natal mice by this Osx-Cre has recently been reported [24,31] On the other hand, in the mTmG;VEC-Cre samples, GFP highlights any cell that has ever expressed Cre (under control of the VECAD promoter). The Cre recombination causes a switch in the production of a membrane protein from RFP to GFP. The GFP expression is maintained by the constitutive activity of the Rosa locus and thus is "on" for the remainder of the cell's life and that

Table 1. In vivo microCT results from tibia midshaft and metaphyseal regions.

Group	Genotype	Gender	Age (wk)	Number of mice	Cortical TV (mm³)	Cortical Bone BV/TV	Cortical Bone TMD (mg HA/cm³)	Trabecular TV (mm³)	Trabecular BV (mm³)	Trabecular vBMD (mg HA/cm³)	Trabecular Thickness (mm)	Trabecular Separation (mm)
Osx-Cre WT	BMP2 fl/fl; Osx-Cre−	Males	24	9	0.277±0.046	0.633±0.041	1140±32.4	1.43±0.145	0.377±0.149	235.9±57.7	0.071±0.008	0.189±0.040
Osx-Cre cKO	BMP2 fl/fl; Osx-Cre+	Males	24	6	0.224±0.057	0.679±0.046	1110±30.5	1.28±0.316	0.305±0.151	214.2±47.2	0.061[a] ±0.009	0.175±0.040
Osx-Cre WT	BMP2 fl/fl; Osx-Cre−	Males	12	11	0.245±0.044	0.665±0.052	1110±37.3	1.31±0.220	0.474±0.155	305.6±76.8	0.076±0.010	0.139±0.020
Osx-Cre cKO	BMP2 fl/fl; Osx-Cre+	Males	12	6	0.159[a] ±0.020	0.758[a] ±0.030	1100±22.5	0.970[a] ±0.240	0.279[a] ±0.078	256.7±46.8	0.061[a] ±0.006	0.138±0.030
Vec-Cre WT	BMP2 fl/fl; VEC-Cre−	Males	24	5	0.300±0.026	0.624±0.025	1120±13.8	1.47±0.163	0.388±0.075	257.7±41.3	0.071±0.006	0.187±0.030
Vec-Cre cKO	BMP2 fl/fl; VEC-Cre+	Males	24	4	0.294±0.032	0.582[z] ±0.017	1110±21.9	1.6±0.085	0.272±0.116	191.7±53.3	0.064±0.008	0.230±0.030

[z]$p<0.05$ BMP2 fl/fl; VEC-Cre+ vs. BMP2 fl/fl; VEC-Cre−.
[a]$p<0.05$ BMP2 fl/fl; Osx-Cre+ vs. BMP2 fl/fl; Osx-Cre−.

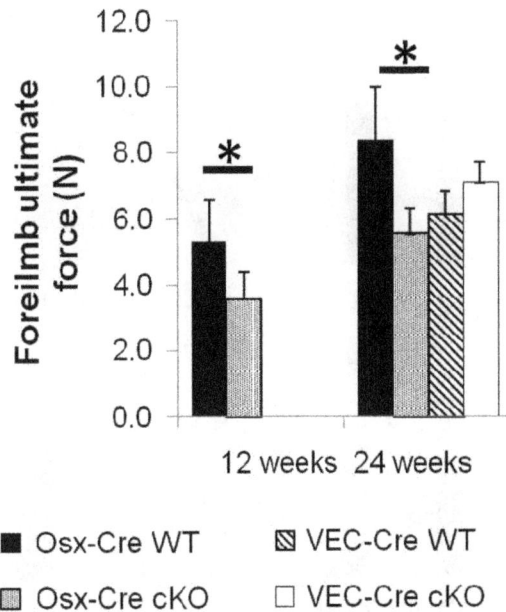

Figure 4. The forelimbs of mice were tested in axial compression. The ultimate force of the forelimb was significantly reduced in the Osx-Cre cKO mice at 12 and 24 weeks.

of any daughter cells. Immunohistochemistry showed BMP2 protein in both the muscle capillaries and bone lining cells of $Bmp2^{fl/fl}$ control mice (Figure 1B, control). BMP2 was absent in the bone lining cells of the Osx-Cre cKO mice but, as expected, remained in the muscle capillaries (Figure 1B). In contrast, BMP2 was absent in the muscle capillaries of VEC-Cre cKO mice but, as expected, remained in bone lining cells. While osteocyte expression of BMP2 was absent in all IHC samples, it is assumed that if successful BMP2 knockout in osteoblasts of the OSX-Cre line has occurred then it is also knocked out of osteocytes.

Osteoblast Knockout of BMP2 Reduces Bone Size, but Vascular Knockout does not

Osx-Cre cKO mice had 20% lower body weights at both 12 and 24 weeks age ($p = 0.04$ and 0.004, respectively) compared to littermate ($Bmp2^{fl/fl}$) controls. In contrast, VEC-Cre cKO and littermate control mice had similar weights at each timepoint (Figure 2A–12 & 24 week males, Table SA in Tables S1– All groups). At 12 weeks of age the OSX-Cre cKO mice had similar percent fat as controls, but by 24 weeks old the knockouts had 6% lower percent fat ($p = 0.03$). VEC-Cre mice had similar percent fat as controls at each time point (Figure 2B–12 & 24 week old males, Table SA in Tables S1– All groups). DXA measurements of aBMD and BMC were lower in 12 and 24 week old Osx-Cre cKO mice versus control ($p = 0.020$ and 0.005, respectively, at 12 weeks; $p = 0.009$ and 0.015, respectively, at 24 weeks). VEC-Cre cKO had no effect on aBMD or BMC at any time point (Figure 2C–12 & 24 week males, Table SA in Tables S1– All Groups).

Tibias of Osx-Cre cKO mice were shorter at both 12 and 24 weeks than controls ($p = 0.01$ and $p<0.0001$, respectively, Figure 3A–12 & 24 week males, Table SB in Tables S1– All groups). Osx-Cre cKO mice at 12 weeks had smaller bones as indicated by reduced cortical TV, cortical BV, cancellous TV, and cancellous BV versus control ($p = 0.006$, 0.02, 0.02, 0.06, respectively; Figure 3B, 3C and Table 1 – –12 & 24 week males, Tables SB & SC in Tables S1– All groups). Interestingly, cortical BV/TV was higher indicating a relatively smaller marrow cavity

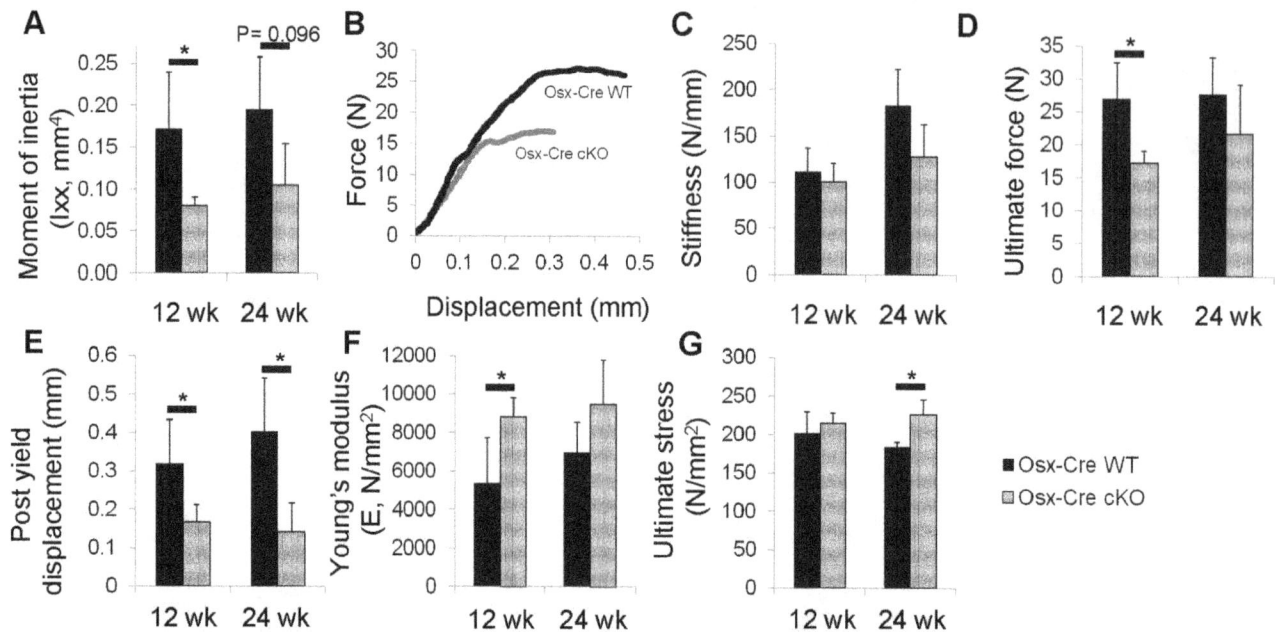

Figure 5. The femora of 12 and 24 week old Osx-Cre mice were tested in three-point bending. cKO mice had significantly reduced (A) moment of inertia compared to WT controls. (B) Example force-displacement curves for WT and cKO mice demonstrate the differences in structural properties (C) Stiffness was unchanged at either time point. However, (D) ultimate force and (E) post-yield displacement was decreased. (F) Young's modulus for cKO mice appears to be stiffer at both time points, but is only significant at 12 wks. Conversely, (G) ultimate stress is higher in cKO but only significant at 24 weeks.

(p = 0.005). Cancellous BV/TV was not affected, indicating normal spatial density of trabeculae. By 24 weeks similar differences for reduced cortical size remained in Osx-Cre cKO mice versus controls (p = 0.0005 for TV, and p = 0.017 for BV). However, cancellous BV and TV were now similar to controls. Cortical TMD of Osx-Cre cKO cortical bone was the same as littermate $Bmp2^{fl/fl}$ controls at both ages (Figure 3D). In the VEC-Cre mouse line the cKO mice had lower cortical bone BV/TV at 24 weeks (p = 0.016) and lower cancellous vBMD (p = 0.042), but in contrast to the Osx-Cre cKO, all other outcomes including those related to bone size were similar between VEC-Cre and control groups (Tables SB & SC in Tables S1– All groups).

Osx-Cre cKO Bones have Altered Mechanical Properties at Whole-bone and Material Levels

Whole forelimb strength was assessed by axial compression to failure. The ultimate force (a measure of strength of the entire structure) was significantly reduced in 12 and 24 week old Osx-Cre cKO mice (40% and 34%, p = 0.013 and 0.050 respectively) compared to littermate controls (Figure 4). There were no differences in ultimate force for the VEC-Cre cKO mice compared to WT.

Reduced strength of Osx-Cre forelimbs may be due to reduced bone size or reduced bone material properties. To assess these two factors, microCT and three-point bending were performed on femora of Osx-Cre mice. Given that the tibial structure and forelimb strength of VEC-Cre mice were not affected by BMP2 cKO, it was assumed unlikely there were any differences in the material properties and no further tests on VEC-Cre mice were performed.

MicroCT measurements of the femur midshaft corroborated findings from the tibia, confirming a smaller bone in Osx-Cre cKO versus WT (Figure 5, Table 2). In particular, Osx-Cre cKO femora had a lower bone area, and moment of inertia (p = 0.004

and 0.006, respectively; Figure 5A). Force-displacement data from three-point bending (Figure 5B) revealed that Osx-Cre cKO femora had normal whole-bone stiffness (Figure 5C), but reduced ultimate force (p = 0.004; Figure 5D) and dramatically decreased post-yield displacement (p = 0.002; Figure 5E). In combination these properties resulted in a significantly lower energy at ultimate force and energy to fracture (p = 0.004 and 0.002, respectively, Table 2), properties that reflect overall resistance to failure. Despite the inferior whole-bone mechanical properties, femora from Osx-Cre cKO mice actually had superior stiffness and strength at the material level (i.e., after accounting for size differences), as evidenced by the increased Young's modulus (p = 0.008; Figure 5F), and ultimate stress (p = 0.017 Figure 5G). Thus, at the material level Osx-Cre cKO bones are stiff and strong, but their reduced post-yield displacement indicates they are brittle. These material properties, when combined with their smaller size, result in a whole-bone that has normal stiffness but inferior strength and reduced energy to failure.

Raman Spectroscopy

To determine if the differences in material properties of Osx-Cre bones could be due to defects in the mineral or collagen aspect of bone, we performed Raman Spectroscopy. First, a set of humeri from 24-week old mice were analyzed as a pilot study. We then analyzed the same 12-week old femora that had been used for three-point bending (Table SD in Tables S1). Carbonated hydroxylapatite was the only mineral present in both the WT and the cKO specimens. The position of the deconvolved 960 Δcm^{-1} band ranged from 960.5 to 961.3 wavenumbers for the 12-week-old femora, which is normal for bone. This range indicate some variability in the chemical components of the bone, for instance by sodium incorporation as a result of carbonate substitution [32,33] However, the mean band positions were not statistically different between genotypes (p = 0. 92). Similarly, the

Table 2. Mechanical 3-point bending tests of mouse femora demonstrated reduced ductility in Osx-Cre cKO mice.

Group	Genotype	Gender	Age (wk)	Number mice	Average cortical thickness (mm)	Bone Area (mm2)	Distance from center of mass (c) (mm)	Energy at ultimate force (N*mm)	Energy at fracture force (N*mm)
Osx-Cre WT	BMP2 fl/fl; Osx-Cre−	Males	24	4 pairs	0.254±0.02	1.02±0.12	0.73±0.11	6.971±1.0	10.39±2.70
Osx-Cre cKO	BMP2 fl/fl; Osx-Cre+	Males	24	3 pairs	0.236±0.03	0.799±0.20	0.603±0.07	3.798±2.5	4.21[a] ±2.85
Osx-Cre WT	BMP2 fl/fl; Osx-Cre−	Males	12	5 pairs	0.251±0.02	0.987±0.15	0.686±0.09	6.308±2.6	10.73±4.63
Osx-Cre cKO	BMP2 fl/fl; Osx-Cre+	Males	12	4 pairs	0.226±0.03	0.714[a] ±0.06	0.575[a] ±0.02	2.760[a] ±0.62	3.88[a] ±0.63
Osx-Cre 1/2 cKO	BMP2 fl/+; Osx-Cre+	Males	12	8 pairs	0.232±0.03	0.835[b] ±0.06	0.631±0.03	4.711±1.3	7.95±3.28

[a] $p < 0.05$ WT v. cKO, [b] $p < 0.05$ WT v. 1/2 cKO (same ages).
*$p < 0.05$ 12wk v 24 wk (same genotype).

960 Δcm^{-1} bandwidth varied, indicating a small difference in atomic order, but was not statistically different by genotype ($p = 0.25$). The mineral-to-matrix ratio, as represented by the ratio of hydroxylapatite (area of the 960Δ cm^{-1} band) to collagen (area of the 1003 Δcm^{-1} band), was lower in the cKO mice than in WT for our pilot studies with 24-week-old humeri ($p = 0.04$), however the ratio did not differ by genotype for the 12-week-old femora ($p = 0.37$). No significant differences in features within the collagen spectral region were observed between the WT and cKO mice. To assess the degree of carbonate substitution, the area of the 1070 Δ cm^{-1} band (for Type-B carbonate substitution) was divided by the area of the 960 Δcm^{-1} band. The proportion of carbonate in the mineral varied slightly within and between specimens, as is normal in bone, but did not differ by genotype ($p = 0.84$). In summary, Raman spectroscopy revealed no obvious defects in the collagen or mineral aspect of Osx-Cre cKO bones that would account for the differences in mechanical and material properties.

Discussion

Our work shows that osteoblast-derived BMP2 is important to post-natal skeletal growth, structure and strength whereas vascular endothelial-derived BMP2 is not. Knockout of BMP2 using Osx-Cre affected both the structure and strength of long bones. Contrary to our hypothesis, the knockout of BMP2 from vascular endothelial cells did not affect any whole-body and few long-bone outcome measures for either sex, nor was the strength of the whole forelimb altered.

Structurally, Osx-Cre cKO resulted in a smaller mouse with slightly shorter limbs. This is a similar, but less severe, phenotype than when BMP2 is knocked out of all osteo- and chondro-progenitor cells using Prx1-Cre ($Bmp2^{fl/fl}$;Prx1-Cre, a.k.a, Prx1-Cre cKO) [9,10]. The shortness of the limbs we observed may be due to the off-target knockout in non-bone cells such as hypertrophic chondrocytes [31,34]. The Osx-Cre mouse is reported to target several non-bone cell types [31]. However, preliminary examination of growth plate morphology and cell proliferation did not identify any obvious dissimilarities that could account for the modest (10%) effect on tibial length. More importantly, the smaller bone width and reduced cortical bone volume, which would not be affected by hypertrophic chondro-cytes, supports the hypothesis that BMP2 is a key factor in periosteal osteoblasts. Furthermore, the similarity of the Osx-Cre cKO phenotype to the reported phenotype in a Col 1-Cre cKO [15] suggests that the effects are from bone cell deletion of BMP2.

Periosteal cells are responsible for radial bone expansion throughout life [35] and are the main cellular contributors to fracture repair [36]. The smaller total volume of Osx-Cre cKO cortical bones indicate that if the osteoblasts and osteocytes are unable to produce BMP2, the bone forming cells in the periosteal layer fail to create enough bone to circumferentially expand similar to controls. Recent work has suggested this maybe due to indirect effects of periosteal cell BMP2 knockout. Progenitor cell behavior and vasculature architecture is altered by BMP2 knockout in early stage osteoblasts [15]. More studies are necessary to determine the relative importance of direct effects on osteoblast function versus indirect effects from other sources such as defective signals from the osteocytes or bone matrix that does not contain BMP2.

An unexpected finding is that osteoblast-derived BMP2 is involved in bone quality. The mechanical properties of Osx-Cre cKO femora reflect a combination of their reduced size coupled with size-independent properties derived from three-point bending tests on the femora which revealed that bone material from Osx-

Cre cKO is stiffer (higher Young's modulus), marginally stronger (higher ultimate stress at 24 weeks) and less ductile (decreased post-yield displacement). This means that as a material the Osx-Cre cKO bones behave just as well or better than their controls under small deformations (i.e. normal loading conditions). However, because they are less ductile, once plastic deformation occurs (i.e. trauma) the bone material fails with less energy absorbed. While not directly measured, the spontaneous fractures sustained by the Prx1-Cre cKO mice suggest a similar but more severe material defect [9,10]. In both the Osx- and Prx1-Cre cKO lines the size discrepancy and material differences combine to create a weaker limb. Our findings are consistent with a recent report in which deletion of BMP2 using the 3.6Col1a1-Cre had a similar effect on postyield bone toughness [15].

In an initial effort to identify the source of the material property differences, we analyzed the femora with Raman spectroscopy, a technique that can characterize the structure-composition and degree of crystallinity of a material. Remarkably, there were no obvious spectroscopic differences in the mineral or collagen aspects of bone from cKO versus WT mice. Interestingly, the finding of normal bone mineral from Raman analysis of intact bones is in contradiction to the impaired in vitro mineralization in differentiated mesenchymal stem cell cultures from 3.6Col1a1-Cre; BMP2 cKO mice [15]. Nonetheless, given the strong link between bone toughness and the organic phase of bone material [37], further studies into the collagen alignment, cross linking, and structure are warranted.

A caveat to this research was off-target effects in Osx-Cre cKO teeth. All osteoblast knockout mice developed malocclusions that worsened as they aged (Figure S1). An obvious concern is that these mice could be malnourished, and the phenotype is due to diet not genetics. However, several observations argue against this possibility. First, there were no differences in percent fat in 12 week old Osx-Cre cKO mice and only modest differences at 24 weeks (Figure 2B). In mouse models of malnourishment percent fat is significantly lower ($\sim$10%) by 12 weeks of age [38]. Furthermore, none of the heterozygous knockout mice ($Bmp2^{fl/+}$;Osx-Cre+) presented malocclusions yet many of their structure and strength outcome measures fell between the knockouts and controls (see Figure S2). This shows a possible dose effect of the BMP2 knockout. Finally, a previous study by Feng et al. documented that this knockout not only causes malocclusions, but the mineralized tissue itself is altered; knockout teeth had extensive pitting which suggests that the teeth are brittle [39], similar to findings in our OSX-Cre cKO long bones. An additional limitation as a result of the malocclusions was that we had few Osx-Cre cKO mice at the later time point (24 weeks). Once the severity of the malocclusions was documented the experimental groups for Osx cKO were switched to a 12 week timepoint.

Knockout of BMP2 from vascular endothelial cells changed few aspects of skeletal growth up to 24 weeks of age. This was unexpected given the many links between vasculature and bone growth as well as between BMP2 and heart development, bone healing, and arterial calcification. It is possible that BMP2 from other cell types is capable of compensating for loss from vascular cells during development and maturation. Alternatively, other BMPs with overlapping functions (i.e. BMP4/7 [9]) may compensate for loss of BMP2. Further discrimination between these possibilities would require examination of BMP signaling at the cell level, which we did not evaluate here. The effects of BMP2 loss from vascular endothelial cells may only be evident in stressed situations such as a high fat diet or bone healing. It is known that BMP2 is highly elevated in vascular endothelial cells at early timepoints in healing via intramembranous bone formation (i.e. stress fracture healing and distraction osteogenesis) [13,28]. Further studies are needed to test the requirement for vascular BMP2 in these settings.

In conclusion, the knockout of osteoblast-derived BMP2 affects the structure and strength of long bones while knockout of vascular-endothelial cell BMP2 does not. The $Bmp2^{fl/fl}$;Osx-Cre+ cKO mouse could serve as model to investigate the relationship between bone mass density and fracture risk associated with $Bmp2$ polymorphisms in humans. The studies linking $Bmp2$ polymorphisms and osteoporosis are controversial and contradictory [40–43]. This is due in part to the rarity of the genetic mutation, the contribution of many different factors and genes to BMD, and the relatively mild effects. Using this mouse we can investigate mechanisms that may account for increased fracture risk and then potentially translate these findings to the clinic.

Supporting Information

Figure S1 The teeth of Osx-Cre cKO mice were abnormal. Example images demonstrate malocclusion in cKO mice. The teeth of ½ cKO mice were normal as were the teeth of Osx-Cre WT mice and Cre control mice (no $Bmp2$ floxing).

Figure S2 Results for various structural and strength measures from the Osx-Cre ½ cKO bones were between those of the Osx-Cre WT and Osx-Cre cKO.

Tables S1 Tables with DEXA (Table SA), micoCT (Tables SB and SC), and Raman Spectroscopy (Table SD) data for all experimental groups.

Author Contributions

Conceived and designed the experiments: SM JM BB JP VR MS. Performed the experiments: SM JM BB PK JP. Analyzed the data: SM JM BB PK JP. Contributed reagents/materials/analysis tools: SM JM JP VR MS. Wrote the paper: SM JM BB JP VR MS.

References

1. Brochmann EJ, Behnam K, Murray SS (2009), Bone morphogenetic protein-2 activity is regulated by secreted phosphoprotein-24 kd, an extracellular pseudoreceptor, the gene for which maps to a region of the human genome important for bone quality. Metabolism 58: 644–50.

2. Doss MX, Gaspar JA, Winkler J, Hescheler J, Schulz H, et al. (2012) Specific gene signatures and pathways in mesodermal cells and their derivatives derived from embryonic stem cells.Stem Cell Rev 8: 43–54.

3. Rosen V (2009) BMP2 signaling in bone development and repair. Cytokine Growth Factor Rev 20: 475–80.

4. Lian J B, Stein GS, Javed A, van Wijnen AJ, Stein JL, et al. (2006) Networks and hubs for the transcriptional control of osteoblastogenesis. Rev Endocr Metab Disord 7: 1–16.

5. Yamaguchi A, Katagiri T, Ikeda T, Wozney JM, Rosen V, et al. (1991) Recombinant human bone morphogenetic protein-2 stimulates osteoblastic maturation and inhibits myogenic differentiation in vitro. J Cell Biol 113: 681–7.

6. Chandler RL, Chandler KJ, McFarland KA, Mortlock DP (2007) Bmp2 transcription in osteoblast progenitors is regulated by a distant 3' enhancer located 156.3 kilobases from the promoter. Mol Cell Biol 27: 2934–51.

7. Fritz DT, Jiang S, Xu J, Rogers MB (2006) A polymorphism in a conserved posttranscriptional regulatory motif alters bone morphogenetic protein 2 (BMP2) RNA:protein interactions. Mol Endocrinol 20: 1574–86.

8. Wohl GR, Towler DA, Silva MJ (2009) Stress fracture healing: fatigue loading of the rat ulna induces upregulation in expression of osteogenic and angiogenic

genes that mimic the intramembranous portion of fracture repair. Bone 44: 320–30.

9. Bandyopadhyay A, Tsuji K, Cox K, Harfe BD, Rosen V, et al. (2006) Genetic analysis of the roles of BMP2, BMP4, and BMP7 in limb patterning and skeletogenesis PLoS Genet 2: e216.

10. Tsuji K, Bandyopadhyay A, Harfe BD, Cox K, Kakar S, et al. (2006) BMP2 activity, although dispensable for bone formation, is required for the initiation of fracture healing. Nat Genet 38: 1424–9.

11. Wu L, Feng J, Wang L, Mu Y, Baker A, et al. (2011) Development and characterization of a mouse floxed Bmp2 osteoblast cell line that retains osteoblast genotype and phenotype. Cell Tissue Res 343: 545–58.

12. McKenzie JA, Silva MJ (2011) Comparing histological, vascular and molecular responses associated with woven and lamellar bone formation induced by mechanical loading in the rat ulna. Bone 48: 250–8.

13. Matsubara H, Hogan DE, Morgan EF, Mortlock DP, Einhorn TA, et al. (2012) Vascular tissues are a primary source of BMP2 expression during bone formation induced by distraction osteogenesis. Bone 51: 168–80.

14. Zhang H, Bradley A (1996) Mice deficient for BMP2 are nonviable and have defects in amnion/chorion and cardiac development. Development 122: 2977–86.

15. Yang W, Guo D, Harris MA, Cui Y, Gluhak-Heinrich J, et al. (2013) Bmp2 gene in osteoblasts of periosteum and trabecular bone links bone formation to vascularization and mesenchymal stem cells. J Cell Sci 126: 4085–98.

16. Kronenberg HM (2003) Developmental regulation of the growth plate. Nature, 423: 332–6.

17. Simpson AH (1985) The blood supply of the periosteum. J Anat 140: 697–704.

18. Tomlinson RE, McKenzie JA, Schmieder AH, Wohl GR, Lanza GM, et al. (2013) Angiogenesis is required for stress fracture healing in rats. Bone 52: 212–9.

19. Tomlinson RE, McKenzie JA, Schmieder AH, Wohl GR, Lanza GM, et al. (2013) Nitric Oxide Mediated Vasodilation Increases Blood Flow During the Early Stages of Stress Fracture Healing. J App Physio. EPub December 19, 2013.

20. Jacobsen KA, Al-Aql ZS, Wan C, Fitch JL, Stapleton SN, et al. (2008) Bone formation during distraction osteogenesis is dependent on both VEGFR1 and VEGFR2 signaling. J Bone Miner Res 23: 596–609.

21. Hausman MR, Schaffler MB, Majeska RJ (2001) Prevention of fracture healing in rats by an inhibitor of angiogenesis. Bone 29: 560–4.

22. Hruska KA, Mathew S, Saab G (2005) Bone morphogenetic proteins in vascular calcification. Circ Res 97: 105–14.

23. Li X, Yang HY, Giachelli CM (2008) BMP-2 promotes phosphate uptake, phenotypic modulation, and calcification of human vascular smooth muscle cells. Atherosclerosis 199: 271–7.

24. Rodda SJ, McMahon AP (2006) Distinct roles for Hedgehog and canonical Wnt signaling in specification, differentiation and maintenance of osteoblast progenitors. Development 133: 3231–44.

25. Alva JA, Zovein AC, Monvoisin A, Murphy T, Salazar A, et al. (2006) VE-Cadherin-Cre-recombinase transgenic mouse: a tool for lineage analysis and gene deletion in endothelial cells. Dev Dyn 235: 759–67.

26. Muzumdar MD, Tasic B, Miyamichi K, Li L, Luo L (2007) A global double-fluorescent Cre reporter mouse. Genesis 45: 593–605.

27. Bouxsein ML, Boyd SK, Christiansen BA, Guldberg RE, Jepsen KJ, et al. (2010) Guidelines for assessment of bone microstructure in rodents using micro-computed tomography. J Bone Miner Res 25: 1468–86.

28. Martinez MD, Schmid GJ, McKenzie JA, Ornitz DM, Silva MJ (2010) Healing of non-displaced fractures produced by fatigue loading of the mouse ulna. Bone 46: 1604–12.

29. Wopenka B, Kent A, Pasteris JD, Yoon Y, Thomopoulos S (2008) The tendon-to-bone transition of the rotator cuff: a preliminary Raman spectroscopic study documenting the gradual mineralization across the insertion in rat tissue samples. Appl Spectrosc 62: 1285–94.

30. Penel G, Leroy G, Rey C, Bres E (1998) MicroRaman spectral study of the PO4 and CO3 vibrational modes in synthetic and biological apatites. Calcif Tissue Int 63: 475–81.

31. Chen J, Shi Y, Regan J, Karuppaiah K, Ornitz DM, et al. (2014) Osx-Cre targets multiple cell types besides osteoblast lineage in postnatal mice. PLoS One 9: e85161.

32. Skinner HCW (2005) Biominerals. Mineral Mag 69: 621–641.

33. Li Z, Pasteris JD (2014) Chemistry of bone mineral, based on teh hypermineralized rostrum of the beaked whale Mesoplodon densirostris. Am Mineral : In Press.

34. Oh JH, Park S, de Crombrugghe B, Kim JE (2012) Chondrocyte-specific ablation of Osterix leads to impaired endochondral ossification. Biochem Biophys Res Commun 418: 634–40.

35. Seeman E (2007) The periosteum–a surface for all seasons. Osteoporos Int 18: 123–8.

36. Colnot C, Zhang X, Knothe Tate ML (2012) Current insights on the regenerative potential of the periosteum: molecular, cellular, and endogenous engineering approaches. J. Orthop. Res. 30(12): 1869–78.

37. Nyman JS, Makowski AJ (2012) The contribution of the extracellular matrix to the fracture resistance of bone. Curr Osteoporos Rep 10: 169–77.

38. Devlin MJ, Cloutier AM, Thomas NA, Panus DA, Lotinun S, et al. (2010) Caloric restriction leads to high marrow adiposity and low bone mass in growing mice. J Bone Miner Res 25: 2078–88.

39. Feng J, Yang G, Yuan G, Gluhak-Heinrich J, Yang W, et al. (2011) Abnormalities in the enamel in bmp2-deficient mice. Cells Tissues Organs 194: 216–21.

40. Medici M, van Meurs JB, Rivadeneira F, Zhao H, Arp PP, et al. (2006) BMP-2 gene polymorphisms and osteoporosis: the Rotterdam Study. J Bone Miner Res 21: 845–54.

41. McGuigan FE, Larzenius E, Callreus M, Gerdhem P, Luthman H, et al. (2007) Variation in the BMP2 gene: bone mineral density and ultrasound in young adult and elderly women. Calcif Tissue Int 81: 254–62.

42. Styrkarsdottir U, Cazier JB, Kong A, Rolfsson O, Larsen H, et al. (2003) Linkage of osteoporosis to chromosome 20p12 and association to BMP2. PLoS Biol 1: E69.

43. Varanasi SS, Tuck SP, Mastana SS, Dennison E, Cooper C, et al. (2011) Lack of association of bone morphogenetic protein 2 gene haplotypes with bone mineral density, bone loss, or risk of fractures in men. J Osteoporos 2011: 243465.

26

Probiotics Protect Mice from Ovariectomy-Induced Cortical Bone Loss

Claes Ohlsson[1], Cecilia Engdahl[1,2], Frida Fåk[3], Annica Andersson[1,2], Sara H. Windahl[1], Helen H. Farman[1], Sofia Movérare-Skrtic[1], Ulrika Islander[1,2], Klara Sjögren[1]*

1 Centre for Bone and Arthritis Research, Institute of Medicine, Sahlgrenska Academy at University of Gothenburg, Gothenburg, Sweden, 2 Department of Rheumatology and Inflammation Research, Institute of Medicine, Sahlgrenska Academy at University of Gothenburg, Gothenburg, Sweden, 3 Applied Nutrition and Food Chemistry, Department of Food Technology, Engineering and Nutrition, Lund University, Lund, Sweden

Abstract

The gut microbiota (GM) modulates the hosts metabolism and immune system. Probiotic bacteria are defined as live microorganisms which when administered in adequate amounts confer a health benefit on the host and can alter the composition of the GM. Germ-free mice have increased bone mass associated with reduced bone resorption indicating that the GM also regulates bone mass. Ovariectomy (ovx) results in bone loss associated with altered immune status. The purpose of this study was to determine if probiotic treatment protects mice from ovx-induced bone loss. Mice were treated with either a single *Lactobacillus* (L) strain, *L. paracasei* DSM13434 (L. para) or a mixture of three strains, *L. paracasei* DSM13434, *L. plantarum* DSM 15312 and DSM 15313 (L. mix) given in the drinking water during 6 weeks, starting two weeks before ovx. Both the L. para and the L. mix treatment protected mice from ovx-induced cortical bone loss and bone resorption. Cortical bone mineral content was higher in both L. para and L. mix treated ovx mice compared to vehicle (veh) treated ovx mice. Serum levels of the resorption marker C-terminal telopeptides and the urinary fractional excretion of calcium were increased by ovx in the veh treated but not in the L. para or the L. mix treated mice. Probiotic treatment reduced the expression of the two inflammatory cytokines, TNFα and IL-1β, and increased the expression of OPG, a potent inhibitor of osteoclastogenesis, in cortical bone of ovx mice. In addition, ovx decreased the frequency of regulatory T cells in bone marrow of veh treated but not probiotic treated mice. In conclusion, treatment with L. para or the L. mix prevents ovx-induced cortical bone loss. Our findings indicate that these probiotic treatments alter the immune status in bone resulting in attenuated bone resorption in ovx mice.

Editor: Bernhard Ryffel, French National Centre for Scientific Research, France

Funding: This work was supported by the Swedish Research Council, Swedish Foundation for Strategic Research, COMBINE, Avtal om Läkarutbildning och Forskning/Läkarutbildningsavtalet research grant in Gothenburg, Lundberg Foundation, Torsten and Ragnar Söderberg Foundation, Novo Nordisk Foundation, Magnus Bergvall Foundation and Åke Wiberg Foundation. The BD FACS Canto II was bought thanks to generous support from the Inga-Britt and Arne Lundberg Foundation. The funders had no role in study design, data collection and analysis, decision to publish, or preparation of the manuscript.

Competing Interests: A pending patent application SE 1351571-3, where the main applicant is Probi AB, who provided the study product, but have not otherwise been involved in the conduction of the experiments and the analyses of data. Name of patent application: SE 1351571-3. Name of study products: Lactobacillus (L.) paracasei DSM13434 (8700:2), L. plantarum DSM 15312 (HEAL 9) and L. plantarum DSM 15313 (HEAL 19). The authors Klara Sjögren and Claes Ohlsson are included in the patent application as inventors but are not further involved in the activities of Probi AB.

* E-mail: Klara.Sjogren@medic.gu.se

Introduction

Fractures caused by osteoporosis constitute a major health concern and result in a huge economic burden on health care systems. In Sweden, the lifetime risk of any osteoporotic fracture is 47% and 24% in women and men, respectively [1]. In USA, the risk has been reported to be 40% and 13% in white women and men, respectively and fractures are associated with significant mortality and morbidity [2]. Cortical bone is the major contributor to non-vertebral fracture risk and comprises more than 80% of the skeleton.

The skeleton is remodeled by bone forming osteoblasts (OBs) and bone resorbing osteoclasts (OCLs). Macrophage colony stimulating factor (M-CSF) increases proliferation and survival of OCLs precursor cells as well as up-regulates expression of receptor activator of nuclear factor-κB (RANK) in OCL. This allows RANK ligand (RANKL) to bind and start the signaling cascade

that leads to OCL formation. The effect of RANKL can be inhibited by Osteoprotegerin (OPG), which is a decoy receptor for RANKL [3].

The association between inflammation and bone loss is well established. In autoimmune diseases, osteoclastic bone resorption is driven by inflammatory cytokines produced by immune cells e.g. activated T cells [4]. In addition, low-grade systemic inflammation, indicated by moderately elevated serum levels of high sensitivity C-reactive protein (hsCRP), associates with low bone mineral density (BMD), elevated bone resorption and increased fracture risk [5–8]. The estrogen deficiency that occurs after menopause results in increased formation and prolonged survival of OCLs. This is suggested to be due to a number of factors including loss of the immunosuppressive effects of estrogen, resulting in increased production of cytokines promoting osteoclastogenesis, and direct effects of estrogen on OCLs [9,10]. In line with these data, blockade of the inflammatory cytokines TNFα and IL-1 leads to a decrease in bone resorption markers in early postmenopausal women [11].

In recent years, the importance of the gut microbiota (GM) for both health and disease has been intensively studied. The GM constitutes of trillions of bacteria which collectively contain 150-fold more genes than our human genome. It is acquired at birth and, although a distinct entity, it has clearly coevolved with the human genome and can be considered a multicellular organ that communicates with and affects its host in numerous ways [12]. The composition of the GM is modulated by a number of environmental factors such as diet and antibiotic treatments. Molecules produced by the gut bacteria can be both beneficial and harmful and are known to affect the host's immune system [13]. Perturbed microbial composition has been postulated to be involved in a range of inflammatory conditions, within and outside the gut including Crohn's disease, ulcerative colitis, rheumatoid arthritis, multiple sclerosis, diabetes, food allergies, eczema and asthma as well as obesity and the metabolic syndrome [13,14]. We recently showed that absence of GM in germ-free (GF) mice leads to increased bone mass associated with reduced bone resorption and altered immune status in bone. Colonisation of GF mice with a normal gut microbiota led to a normalisation of bone mass and immune status in bone marrow [15]. A role of the GM for bone mass is supported by a recent study demonstrating that subtherapeutic antibiotic treatment in early life increases bone mass in young mice [16]. Although the low dose of antibiotics in this study did not cause a significant alteration in bacterial count it caused shifts in the composition of the GM. Furthermore, tetracycline treatment has been shown to prevent bone loss and improve mechanical properties of bone after ovariectomy (ovx) [17,18]. These studies, demonstrate that antibiotic treatment has the capacity to influence both the GM composition and bone mass, supporting the notion that the GM is a regulator of bone homeostasis.

Probiotic bacteria are defined as live microorganisms which when administered in adequate amounts confer a health benefit on the host. Probiotics act by altering the composition or the metabolic activity of the GM [19]. The suggested underlying mechanisms for how probiotics contribute to health are manifold including increased solubility and absorption of minerals, enhanced barrier function and modulation of the immune system [20,21]. Ovx in mice results in bone loss associated with altered immune status, resembling post-menopausal osteoporosis. The purpose of the present study was to determine if probiotic treatment protects mice from ovx-induced bone loss.

Materials and Methods

Ovx Mouse-model and Probiotic Treatment

Six-week-old C57BL/6N female mice were purchased from Charles River (Germany). The mice were housed in a standard animal facility under controlled temperature (22°C) and photoperiod (12-h light, 12-h dark) and had free access to fresh water and soy-free food pellets R70 (Lactamin AB, Stockholm, Sweden). The ovx model for osteoporosis is included in the FDA guidelines for preclinical and clinical evaluation for agents used for the treatment of postmenopausal osteoporosis [22]. Probiotic treatment started two weeks before ovx to study the preventive effect of probiotic treatment on ovx induced bone-loss (Fig. 1A). Mice were treated with either a single *Lactobacillus* (L) strain, *L. paracasei* DSM13434 (L. para) or a mixture of three strains, *L. paracasei* DSM13434, *L. plantarum* DSM 15312 and DSM 15313 referred to as L. mix during 6 weeks. The probiotic strains were selected based on their anti-inflammatory properties in an earlier study [23]. Mice were

randomized into six treatment groups with 10 mice in each as follows: 1. Veh-Ovx, 2. Veh-Sham, 3. L. Para-Ovx, 4. L. Para-Sham, 5. L. Mix-Ovx, 6. L. Mix-Sham (See also Figure 1). The L. strains were given in the drinking water at a concentration of 10^9 colony-forming units (cfu)/ml while control mice received tap water with vehicle (glycerol). Water bottles were changed every afternoon. The survival of the L. strains in the water bottles was checked regularly and after 24 h the concentration dropped one log unit to approximately 10^8 cfu/ml. Each mouse drank on average 4.5 ml water/day. After two weeks of probiotic treatment, the mice were either sham-operated or ovx under inhalation anesthesia with isoflurane (Forene; Abbot Scandinavia, Solna, Sweden). Four weeks after surgery, blood was collected from the axillary vein under anesthesia with Ketalar/Domitor vet, and the mice were subsequently killed by cervical dislocation. Tissues for RNA preparation were immediately removed and snap-frozen in liquid nitrogen for later analysis. Bones were excised and fixed in 4% paraformaldehyde.

A. Study Design

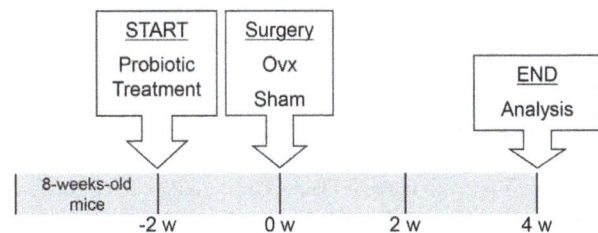

B. Body Weight

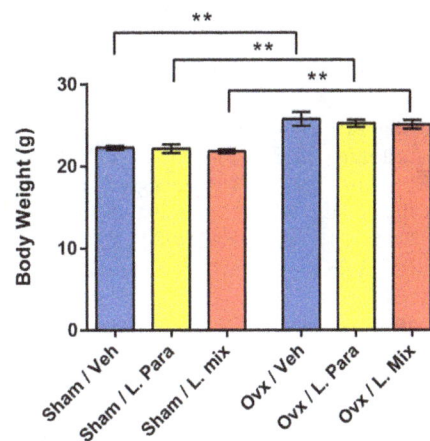

Figure 1. Study Design and Body Weight. Outline of study design (A). Eight-week-old mice were treated with either vehicle (veh), a single *Lactobacillus* (L) strain (L. para) or a mixture of three strains (L. mix) during 6 weeks, starting two weeks before ovx or sham surgery. The L. strains were given in the drinking water at a concentration of 10^9 colony-forming units (cfu)/ml while control mice received tap water with vehicle. Mice were 14-week-old at the end of the study, when tissues were collected for later analysis. Ovx resulted in an expected increased body weight compared to sham mice that was not different after probiotic treatment (B). Results are given as mean±SEM (n = 9–10), ** p≤0.01. Students *t* test ovx vs. sham.

Ethics Statement

All animal experiments had been approved by the local Ethical Committees for Animal Research at the University of Gothenburg.

Peripheral Quantitative Computed Tomography (pQCT)

Computed tomographic scans were performed with the pQCT XCT RESEARCH M (version 4.5B, Norland, Fort Atkinson, WI, USA) operating at a resolution of 70 μm, as described previously [24]. Cortical bone parameters were analyzed *ex vivo* in the mid-diaphyseal region of the femur.

High-resolution μCT

High-resolution μCT analyses were performed on the distal femur by using a 1172 model μCT (Bruker micro-CT, Aartselaar, Belgium). The femurs were imaged with an X-ray tube voltage of 50 kV and current of 201 μA, with a 0.5-mm aluminium filter. The scanning angular rotation was 180° and the angular increment 0.70°. The voxel size was 4.48 μm isotropically. The NRecon (version 1.6.9) was employed to perform the reconstruction following the scans. In the femur, the trabecular bone proximal to the distal growth plate was selected for analyses within a conforming volume of interest (cortical bone excluded) commencing at a distance of 538.5 μm from the growth plate, and extending a further longitudinal distance of 134.5 μm in the proximal direction. To illustrate the effect of probiotics on cortical bone in ovx mice, cortical μCT images of the diaphyseal region of one representative femur from each group were produced and are shown in Figure 2A. These CT images were derived from scans in the diaphyseal region of femur starting at a distance of 3.59 mm from the distal growth plate and extending a further longitudinal distance of 134.5 μm in the proximal direction. For BMD analysis, the equipment was calibrated with ceramic standard samples.

RNA Isolation and Real Time PCR

Total RNA was prepared from cortical bone (femur with the ends removed and bone marrow flushed out with PBS before freezing) and bone marrow using TriZol Reagent (Invitrogen, Lidingö, Sweden). The RNA was reverse transcribed into cDNA using High-Capacity cDNA Reverse Transcription Kit (#4368814, Applied Biosystems, Stockholm, Sweden). RT-PCR analyses were performed using the StepOnePlus Real-Time PCR system (Applied Biosystems). We used predesigned RT-PCR assays from Applied Biosystems (Sweden) for the analysis of IL-6 (Mm00446190_m1), IL-1β (Mm00434228_m1), TNFα (Mm00443258_m1), RANKL (Mm00441908_m1), OPG (Mm00435452_m1), Osterix (Mm04209856_m1), Col1α1 (Mm00801666_g1), osteocalcin (Mm01741771_g1) and TGFβ1 (Mm03024053_m1) mRNA levels. The mRNA abundance of each gene was calculated using the "standard curve method" (User Bulletin 2; PE Applied Biosystems) and adjusted for the expression of 18S (4308329) ribosomal RNA.

Serum and Urine Analysis

Analyses were performed according to the manufacturer's instructions for serum and urine calcium (Ca) (QuantiChrom™-Calcium Assay Kit (DICA-500), Bioassays systems, Hayward, CA, USA), serum and urine creatinine (Mouse Creatinine Kit, Crystal Chem, Downers Grove, IL, USA), serum 25-Hydroxy Vitamin D (EIA, Immunodiagnostic Systems, Herlev, Denmark). As a marker of bone resorption, serum levels of C-terminal telopeptides were assessed using an ELISA kit (Nordic Bioscience Diagnostics, Herlev, Denmark). Serum levels of osteocalcin, a marker of bone formation, were determined with a mouse osteocalcin immunoradiometric assay kit (Immutopics, San Clemente, CA).

Flow Cytometry

Bone marrow cells were harvested by flushing 5 ml PBS through the bone cavity of one femur using a syringe. After centrifugation at 473 g for 5 min, cells were resuspended in Tris-buffered 0.83% NH_4Cl solution (pH 7.29) for 5 min to lyse erythrocytes and then washed in PBS. For flow cytometry analyses, cells were extracellularly stained with BD Horizon v450-conjugated anti-CD4 (Becton Dickinson (BD), Franklin Lakes, NJ, USA) and allophycocyanin (APC) anti-CD25 (BD). By using anti-Mouse Foxp3 Staining Set (eBioscience, Vienna, Austria), Foxp3 was intracellularly stained with Phycoerythrin (PE)-conjugated anti-Foxp3, according to the manufacturer's instructions. Regulatory T cells were defined as $CD4^+CD25^+Foxp3^+$ and results are expressed as frequency of lymphocyte parent gate. Samples were run on a BD FACS Canto II and data was further processed using Flow Jo 8.8.6 software (Three Star Inc, Ashland, USA).

Statistical Analyses

We used GraphPad Prism for all statistical analysis. Results are presented as the means ± SEM. Between-group differences were calculated using unpaired t tests, ovx vs. veh. Comparisons between multiple groups were calculated using a one-way analysis of variance (ANOVA) followed by Dunnett's test to correct for multiple comparisons, within the sham and ovx groups respectively. A two-tailed $p \leq 0.05$ was considered significant.

Results

Probiotic Treatment Protects Mice from Ovx-induced Cortical Bone Loss and Increased Bone Resorption

To determine the preventive effect of probiotic treatment on ovx-induced bone-loss, eight-week-old mice were treated with vehicle (veh), a single *Lactobacillus* (L) strain (L. para) or a mixture of three strains (L. mix) during 6 weeks, starting two weeks before ovx or sham surgery (Figure 1A). Uterus weight can be used as an indicator of estrogen status and ovx resulted in an expected decrease in uterus weight that was similar for all treatments (Table 1). In addition, ovx increased body weight, fat mass and thymus weight in all treatment groups (Figure 1B, Table 1).

In the vehicle treated mice, ovx decreased the cortical bone mineral content (BMC) and cortical cross sectional bone area in the mid-diaphyseal region of femur ($p \leq 0.01$, Figure 2A, C, D). Importantly, ovx did not reduce cortical BMC or cortical cross sectional bone area in the L. para or the L. mix treated mice (Figure 2A, C, D). Cortical BMC was higher in both L. para and L. mix treated ovx mice compared to veh treated ovx mice ($p \leq 0.05$, Figure 2C). We analyzed C-terminal telopeptides to determine if the preventive effect of probiotics on cortical bone was mediated by changes in bone resorption. Ovx increased serum levels of C-terminal telopeptides in veh treated mice (+45±11%, $p \leq 0.05$ over sham) but not in L. para treated (20±9%, non-significant) or L. mix treated (23±9%, non-significant) mice (Table 2). Bone formation, as indicated by serum osteocalcin, was not significantly affected by probiotic treatment (Table 2). Trabecular bone parameters (BV/TV and trabecular BMD) in the distal metaphyseal region of femur were significantly reduced by ovx in all treatment groups ($p \leq 0.05$, Table 2, Figure 2B). These findings demonstrate that probiotic treatment protects mice from ovx-induced cortical bone loss and increased bone resorption.

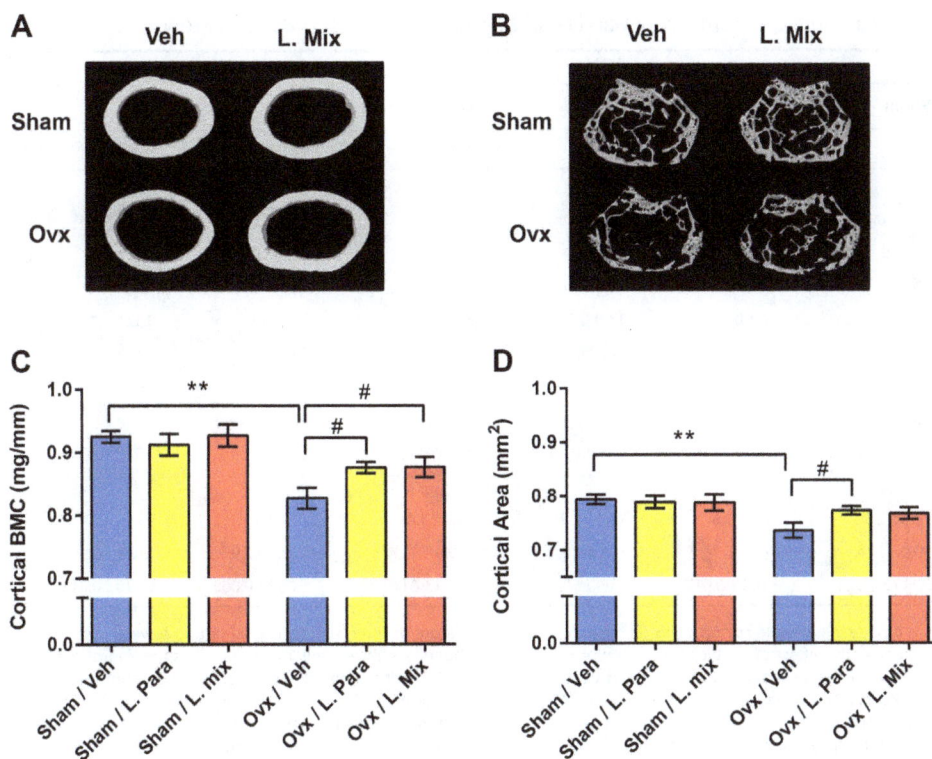

Figure 2. Probiotics Protect Mice from Ovx Induced Cortical Bone-loss. Eight-week-old mice were treated with either vehicle (veh), a single *Lactobacillus* (L) strain (L. para) or a mixture of three strains (L. mix) during 6 weeks, starting two weeks before ovx or sham surgery to study the preventive effect of probiotic treatment on ovx induced bone-loss. At the end of the experiment, dissected femurs were analysed with high-resolution μCT and peripheral quantitative computed tomography (pQCT). Representative μCT images of one cortical section from the veh and L. mix treated sham and ovx groups (A). Representative images of the trabecular bone volume (cortical bone excluded) from the distal metaphyseal region of femur (B). Cortical bone mineral content (BMC) (C) and cortical area (D) were measured by pQCT in the mid-diaphyseal region of femur. Values are given as mean±SEM, (n = 9–10). ** p≤0.01, * p≤0.05. Students *t* test ovx vs. sham. # p≤0.05, ANOVA followed by Dunnett's *post hoc* test within the groups, ovx L. Para and L. mix vs. ovx veh.

Probiotic treatment reduces expression of inflammatory cytokines and the RANKL/OPG ratio in cortical bone

To investigate the mechanism for the effect of probiotic treatment on ovx-induced cortical bone loss, we measured bone related mRNA transcripts in cortical bone (Figure 3). The mRNA levels of TNFα, an inflammatory cytokine produced by immune cells that promotes osteoclastogenesis, and IL-1β, a downstream regulator of the effects of TNFα on bone, were significantly decreased by probiotic treatment compared to vehicle treatment in ovx mice (TNFα −46%, p≤0.05; IL-1β −61%, p≤0.05, Figure 3A, B). The expression of IL-6 did not differ between

treatments although there was a tendency to decreased expression in the probiotic treatment group (−20%, p = 0.12, Figure 3C).

The RANKL/osteoprotegerin (OPG) ratio is a major determinant of osteoclastogenesis and bone resorption. Importantly, probiotic treatment decreased the RANKL/OPG ratio (−45%, p≤0.05 compared with veh) and this was mainly caused by an increased OPG expression (Figure 3 D–F). In contrast, the mRNA levels of three osteoblast-associated genes, Osterix, Col1α1 and osteocalcin, were not significantly affected by probiotic treatment (Figure 3G–H).

Table 1. Organ Weights.

	Sham			Ovx		
	Veh	L. Para	L. Mix	Veh	L. Para	L. Mix
Uterus weight (mg)	45.9±4.8	65.9±12.5	65.2±10.4	8.95±0.7**	11.0±3.2**	6.9±0.3**
Gonadal Fat (mg)	371±41	296±40	326±40	597±68*	630±28**	577±58**
Thymus weight (mg)	55.5±3.2	53.6±5.1	47.7±2.6	93.9±4.2**	90.0±5.1**	73.7±5.2**#

Eight-week-old mice were treated with either vehicle (veh), a single *Lactobacillus* (L) strain (L. para) or a mixture of three strains (L. mix) during 6 weeks, starting two weeks before ovx or sham surgery to study the preventive effect of probiotic treatment on ovx induced bone-loss. Mice were 14-weeks-old at the end of the study, when tissues were dissected and weighed. Results are given as mean±SEM, (n = 6–10). ** p≤0.01, * p≤0.05, Students *t* test ovx vs. sham. # p≤0.05, ANOVA followed by Dunnett's *post hoc* test within the groups, ovx L. Para and L. mix vs. ovx veh.

Table 2. Trabecular and Cortical Bone Parameters, Serum Bone Markers and Regulatory T cells in Bone Marrow.

	Sham			Ovx		
	Veh	**L. Para**	**L. Mix**	**Veh**	**L. Para**	**L. Mix**
Trabecular Bone						
BV/TV (%)	16.2±0.7	16.8±0.8	17.4±0.8	13.2±0.7**	14.4±0.6*	13.8±0.5**
BMD (mg/cm^3)	322±9	331±12	344±8	285±9*	302±7*	298±7**
Tb Th (µm)	45.3±0.7	46.0±0.7	47.9±1.0	43.2±0.8	42.7±0.8**	44.6±1.0*
Tb N (mm^{-1})	3.6±0.1	3.6±0.2	3.6±0.1	3.1±0.1*	3.4±0.1	3.1±0.1*
Tb Sp (µm)	124±1	124±1	124±1	126±1	124±1	127±1
Cortical Bone						
Crt Thk (µm)	181±2	180±3	186±3	168±2**	173±2	176±2#*
Tt Ar (mm^2)	1.96±0.02	1.96±0.04	1.86±0.04	1.92±0.07	2.00±0.03	1.92±0.03
Serum Bone Markers						
C-terminal telopeptides (ng/ml)	12.6±2.2	17.6±1.6	18.4±1.7	18.2±1.4*	21.1±1.6	22.6±1.7
Osteocalcin (ng/ml)	90.9±10.4	97.1±6.7	105.6±6.1	159.9±11.8**	142.1±7.9**	136.9±6.5**
Treg (%CD4+Foxp3+CD25+)	0.117±0.023	0.109±0.017	0.090±0.017	0.054±0.004*	0.069±0.008	0.070±0.014

Eight-week-old mice were treated with either vehicle (veh), a single *Lactobacillus* (L) strain (L. para) or a mixture of three strains (L. mix) during 6 weeks, starting two weeks before ovx or sham surgery to study the preventive effect of probiotic treatment on ovx induced bone-loss. Mice were 14-weeks-old at the end of the study, when tissues were dissected and weighed. Trabecular bone parameters were analysed by high resolution µCT in the distal metaphyseal region of femur; Trabecular bone volume as a percentage of tissue volume (BV/TV); Trabecular bone mineral density (BMD); Trabecular thickness (Tb Th); Trabecular number (Tb N); Trabecular separation (Tb Sp). Cortical bone was measured by pQCT in the mid-diaphyseal region of femur; Cortical thickness (Crt Thk); Total cross-sectional area inside the periosteal envelope (Tt Ar). The resorption marker, C-terminal telopeptides and the formation marker, osteocalcin were measured in serum. Femur bone marrow cells were stained with antibodies recognizing CD4, Foxp3 and CD25. Values represent the percentage of Treg (CD4+ Foxp3+ CD25+) of gated lymphocytes. Results are given as mean±SEM, (n = 6–10). ** p≤0.01, * p≤0.05, Students *t* test ovx vs. sham. # p≤0.05, ANOVA followed by Dunnett's *post hoc* test within the groups, ovx L. Para and L. mix vs. ovx veh.

Regulatory T cells in Bone Marrow

Some of the anti-inflammatory effects exerted by probiotic bacteria are thought to be mediated via the induction of regulatory T (Treg) cells [25]. FACS analysis of bone marrow showed that the frequency of Treg (CD4$^+$CD25$^+$Foxp3$^+$) cells was decreased by ovx in veh treated but not in probiotic treated mice (Table 1). Treg cells are dependent on TGFβ for their induction and maintenance and the expression of TGFβ1 in bone marrow was increased in bone marrow in probiotic compared to veh treated ovx mice (+77±19%, p≤0.01, Figure 3J).

Mineral Metabolism

The urinary fractional excretion of Ca (FECa = (urine Ca × serum creatinine)/(serumserum Ca × urine creatinine)) was increased by ovx in veh treated mice (+86%, p≤0.05, Figure 4). Interestingly, the ovx-induced increase in FECa was completely prevented by probiotic treatment (Figure 4). Serum levels of Ca were increased after ovx in veh but not probiotic treated mice (+13%, p≤0.05, Table 3). The urine Ca/creatinine ratio was not affected by ovx in any of the treatment groups (Table 3). 25-Hydroxy Vitamin D (25(OH)D$_3$) in serum was not affected by ovx or probiotic treatment (Table 3).

Discussion

The GM regulates bone mass and probiotic treatment can affect the GM composition or the metabolic activity of the GM. In the present study we show that probiotic treatment protects mice from ovx-induced cortical bone loss. Both the L. para and the L. mix treatments protected mice from ovx-induced cortical bone loss and increased bone resorption. The urinary fractional excretion of Ca and the bone resorption marker C-terminal telopeptides in serum

were increased by ovx in veh treated but not in probiotic treated mice, suggesting that the probiotic treatments reduced bone resorption in ovx mice. Probiotic treatment reduced the expression of the two inflammatory cytokines, TNFα and IL-1β, and increased the expression of OPG in cortical bone of ovx mice. These findings indicate that probiotic treatment alters the immune status in bone, resulting in attenuated bone resorption in ovx mice.

We have earlier shown that absence of GM leads to increased bone mass in GF mice and colonisation with a normal GM rapidly normalises bone mass [15]. The increased bone mass in GF mice was associated with an altered immune status reflected by decreased expression of inflammatory cytokines in bone. Estrogen deficiency increases inflammatory cytokines and reduces OPG in bone, resulting in bone loss [26]. Ovx mice have altered immune status and bone loss, resembling post-menopausal osteoporosis. Since probiotic treatment has the capacity to modulate the immune system, we hypothesized that probiotic treatment may attenuate ovx-induced increase in inflammatory cytokines and may, thereby, preserve the bone mass in ovx mice. The probiotic strains used, *L. paracasei* DSM13434 (L. para) or a mixture of three strains, *L. paracasei* DSM13434, *L. plantarum* DSM 15312 and DSM 15313 referred to as L. mix, in the present study were selected based on their anti-inflammatory properties in an earlier study [23]. In the study by Lavasani *et al* the selected lactobacilli strains had a suppressive effect on experimental autoimmune encephalomyelitis in an animal model of multiple sclerosis. L. para and L. mix prevented ovx-induced cortical bone loss to a similar extent. We can, therefore, conclude that treatment with L. para prevents ovx-induced cortical bone loss in mice while the possible independent roles of the two used *L. plantarum* strains for cortical bone remain to be determined. We believe that the main property of the L. para that explains the reversal effect of ovx on cortical

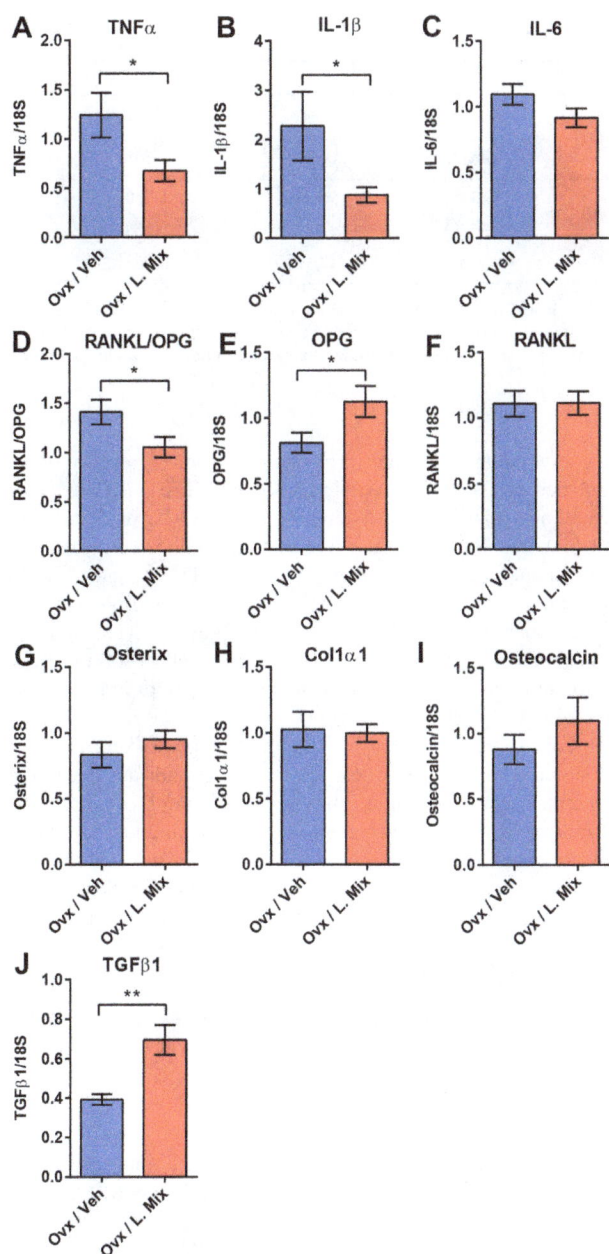

Figure 3. Probiotics Reduces Expression of Inflammatory Cytokines and the RANKL/OPG ratio in Cortical Bone and Increases Expression of TGFβ in Bone Marrow. QRT-PCR analysis of the expression of genes known to promote bone resorption; (A) Tumor Necrosis Factor alpha (TNFα), (B) Interleukin-1β (IL-1β), (C) Interleukin-6 (IL-6), (D) Ratio of Receptor activator of nuclear factor kappa-B ligand (RANKL) and Osteoprotegerin (OPG), and individual graphs for (E) OPG, (F) RANKL and genes known to promote bone formation; (G) Osterix, (H) Collagen, type I, α1 (Col1α1) and (I) osteocalcin in cortical bone and (J) transforming growth factor (TGF)β in bone marrow from 14-week-old ovariectomized (ovx) mice treated with either vehicle (veh) or a mixture of three probiotic Lactobacillus strains (L. mix) during 6 weeks, starting two weeks before ovx or sham surgery to study the preventive effect of probiotic treatment on ovx-induced bone-loss. Values are given as mean±SEM, n = 9–10. ** p≤0.01, * p≤0.05 versus veh treatment, Student's t-test.

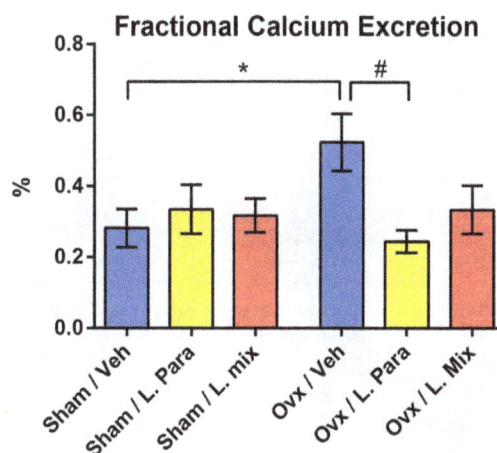

Figure 4. The Fractional Excretion of Ca was Increased by Ovx in the Veh Treated but not in the L. para or the L. mix Treated Mice. Ca and creatinine were measured in serum and urine from 14-week-old mice that had been treated with vehicle (veh), a single Lactobacillus (L) strain (L. para) or a mixture of three strains (L. mix) during 6 weeks, starting two weeks before ovx or sham surgery. Urinary fractional Ca excretion was calculated with the formula FECa = (urine Ca × serum creatinine)/(serum Ca × urine creatinine). Values are given as mean±SEM, n = 5–10 in each group. * p≤0.05. Students t test ovx vs. sham. # p≤0.05, ANOVA followed by Dunnett's post hoc test within the groups, ovx L. Para and L. mix vs. ovx veh.

bone is its anti-inflammatory capacity. However, further studies are required to in detail characterize its protective effect on ovx-induced cortical bone loss.

Cortical bone constitutes approximately 80% of the bone in the body and several studies demonstrate that cortical bone is the major determinant of bone strength and, thereby, fracture susceptibility [27–29]. Thus, the substantial cortical bone sparing effect of probiotic treatment in ovx mice in the present study indicates that this treatment might have the capacity to reduce non-vertebral fracture risk in postmenopausal women.

As expected, ovx increased bone resorption, as indicated by elevated serum levels of C-terminal telopeptides, in veh treated mice. In contrast, serum levels of C-terminal telopeptides were not significantly affected by ovx in probiotic treated mice. Bone formation, as indicated by serum osteocalcin was not influenced by probiotic treatment. Collectively, these findings indicate that the bone sparing effect of probiotics in ovx mice might be the result of attenuated bone resorption. A possible inhibitory effect on bone resorption is supported by the finding that the urinary fractional excretion of Ca was increased by ovx in the veh treated but not the probiotic treated mice. Estrogen therapy to post-menopausal women increases BMD associated with a reduced urinary fractional excretion of Ca [30,31]. We propose that treatment with probiotics supresses bone resorption and as a consequence the urinary fractional excretion of Ca is decreased. However, we cannot exclude other effects of probiotics on urinary fractional excretion of Ca. In addition, it has been proposed that biochemical bone markers might be more influenced by trabecular than cortical bone. Thus, it is possible that effects on the release of biochemical bone markers from cortical bone to serum might be confounded by abundant release from trabecular bone. Therefore, further analyses of other more specific cortical bone parameters, such as osteoclast number in cortical bone, are required to confirm that the protective effect of probiotics on ovx-induced cortical bone loss is mediated via altered cortical bone resorption.

Table 3. Mineral Metabolism.

	Sham			Ovx		
	Veh	L. Para	L. Mix	Veh	L. Para	L. Mix
Serum Ca (mg/dl)	9.1±0.4	9.2±0.4	8.5±0.3	10.3±0.4*	9.3±0.4	8.7±0.3#
Urine Ca/Creatinine Ratio	6.7±0.7	6.3±0.4	5.4±0.6	8.5±1.3	5.9±0.5	5.6±0.7
25(OH)D$_3$ (ng/ml)	16.5±1.3	17.5±1.7	16.5±1.8	16.7±1.1	17.6±1.0	16.8±1.2

Calcium (Ca) and Creatinine were measured in serum and urine and 25-Hydroxy Vitamin D (25(OH)D$_3$) was measured in serum from 14-week old mice that had been treated with vehicle (veh), a single *Lactobacillus* (L) strain (L. para) or a mixture of three strains (L. mix) during 6 weeks, starting two weeks before ovx or sham surgery. Results are given as mean±SEM, (n = 5–10). ** p≤0.01, * p≤0.05, Students *t* test ovx vs. sham, # p≤0.05, ANOVA followed by Dunnett's *post hoc* test within the groups, ovx L. Para and L. mix vs. ovx veh.

Mechanistic studies of the bone sparing effect of probiotic treatment in ovx mice revealed that the expression of several osteolytic cytokines such as TNFα and IL-1β as well as the RANKL/OPG ratio in cortical bone were suppressed by probiotic treatment. TNFα promotes osteoclastogenesis indirectly by stimulating RANKL expression by marrow stromal cells and osteoblasts and by direct stimulation of OCL precursors exposed to permissive levels of RANKL [32–34]. IL-1 is a downstream regulator of the effects of TNFα on osteoclastogenesis [35,36]. The inhibitory effect of probiotics on the RANKL/OPG ratio in the present study was mainly due to an increased expression of OPG in cortical bone. OPG directly inhibits OCL differentiation at a late stage in a dose dependant manner [37]. Together, these findings indicate that probiotic treatment suppress osteoclastogenesis, resulting in reduced OCL-mediated bone resorption.

Treg cells are critical for maintaining self-tolerance and negatively regulate immune responses. In an earlier study, Lavasani et al demonstrated that the probiotic strains used in the present study induce Treg cells [23]. Several probiotic L. strains have been described to have a therapeutic effect in experimental mouse models of inflammatory bowel disease, atopic dermatitis, and rheumatoid arthritis associated with enrichment of Treg cells in the inflamed regions [25]. This inhibitory effect of probiotic L. strains was recently shown to depend on suppressive motifs in the DNA enriched in these strains that potently prevented dendritic cell activation and maintained Treg cell conversion during inflammation [38]. TGFβ is crucial for the induction and activity of Treg cells [39]. Interestingly, ovx decreased Treg cells in bone marrow in veh but not probiotic treated mice in the present study. Furthermore, the expression of TGFβ1 was increased by probiotic compared to veh treatment

after ovx, suggesting that probiotic treatment prevents down regulation of Treg cells via an induction of TGFβ1. *In vitro* studies have shown that Treg cells directly inhibit OCL differentiation and function and that this effect of Treg cells is stimulated by estrogen and dependent on expression of TGFβ1 [40–42]. In addition, adoptive transfer of Treg cells decreases the number of OCLs and limits bone loss in ovx mice [43]. Collectively these findings may suggest that the suppressive effect of probiotic treatment on inflammatory cytokines and bone resorption involves effects by Treg cells.

In conclusion, treatment with L. para or the L. mix prevents ovx-induced cortical bone loss. Our findings indicate that these probiotic treatments alter the immune status in bone as demonstrated by reduced expression of inflammatory cytokines and increased expression of OPG, resulting in attenuated bone resorption in ovx mice. These data suggest a therapeutic potential for probiotics in the treatment of postmenopausal osteoporosis.

Acknowledgments

We would like to thank Irini Lazou Ahrén and Niklas Larsson at Probi AB, Lund, Sweden for providing the probiotic strains and Lotta Uggla and Biljana Aleksic for excellent technical assistance.

Author Contributions

Conceived and designed the experiments: CO CE FF AA UI KS. Performed the experiments: CO CE FF AA SW HF SMS KS. Analyzed the data: CO CE FF AA SW HF SMS UI KS. Contributed reagents/materials/analysis tools: CO CE FF AA SW HF SMS UI KS. Wrote the paper: CO CE FF AA SW HF SMS UI KS.

References

1. Kanis JA, Johnell O, Oden A, Sembo I, Redlund-Johnell I, et al. (2000) Long-term risk of osteoporotic fracture in Malmo. Osteoporos Int 11: 669–674.
2. Melton LJ, 3rd, Chrischilles EA, Cooper C, Lane AW, Riggs BL (1992) Perspective. How many women have osteoporosis? J Bone Miner Res 7: 1005–1010.
3. Boyle WJ, Simonet WS, Lacey DL (2003) Osteoclast differentiation and activation. Nature 423: 337–342.
4. Kong YY, Feige U, Sarosi I, Bolon B, Tafuri A, et al. (1999) Activated T cells regulate bone loss and joint destruction in adjuvant arthritis through osteoprotegerin ligand. Nature 402: 304–309.
5. Pasco JA, Kotowicz MA, Henry MJ, Nicholson GC, Spilsbury HJ, et al. (2006) High-sensitivity C-reactive protein and fracture risk in elderly women. JAMA 296: 1353–1355.
6. Ding C, Parameswaran V, Udayan R, Burgess J, Jones G (2008) Circulating levels of inflammatory markers predict change in bone mineral density and resorption in older adults: a longitudinal study. J Clin Endocrinol Metab 93: 1952–1958.

7. Schett G, Kiechl S, Weger S, Pederiva A, Mayr A, et al. (2006) High-sensitivity C-reactive protein and risk of nontraumatic fractures in the Bruneck study. Arch Intern Med 166: 2495–2501.
8. Eriksson AL, Moverare-Skrtic S, Ljunggren O, Karlsson M, Mellstrom D, et al. (2013) High sensitive CRP is an independent risk factor for all fractures and vertebral fractures in elderly men: The MrOS Sweden study. J Bone Miner Res.
9. Martin-Millan M, Almeida M, Ambrogini E, Han L, Zhao H, et al. (2010) The estrogen receptor-alpha in osteoclasts mediates the protective effects of estrogens on cancellous but not cortical bone. Mol Endocrinol 24: 323–334.
10. Nakamura T, Imai Y, Matsumoto T, Sato S, Takeuchi K, et al. (2007) Estrogen prevents bone loss via estrogen receptor alpha and induction of Fas ligand in osteoclasts. Cell 130: 811–823.
11. Charatcharoenwitthaya N, Khosla S, Atkinson EJ, McCready LK, Riggs BL (2007) Effect of blockade of TNF-alpha and interleukin-1 action on bone resorption in early postmenopausal women. J Bone Miner Res 22: 724–729.
12. Qin J, Li R, Raes J, Arumugam M, Burgdorf KS, et al. (2010) A human gut microbial gene catalogue established by metagenomic sequencing. Nature 464: 59–65.

13. Maynard CL, Elson CO, Hatton RD, Weaver CT (2012) Reciprocal interactions of the intestinal microbiota and immune system. Nature 489: 231–241.
14. Tremaroli V, Backhed F (2012) Functional interactions between the gut microbiota and host metabolism. Nature 489: 242–249.
15. Sjogren K, Engdahl C, Henning P, Lerner UH, Tremaroli V, et al. (2012) The gut microbiota regulates bone mass in mice. J Bone Miner Res 27: 1357–1367.
16. Cho I, Yamanishi S, Cox L, Methe BA, Zavadil J, et al. (2012) Antibiotics in early life alter the murine colonic microbiome and adiposity. Nature 488: 621–626.
17. Williams S, Wakisaka A, Zeng QQ, Barnes J, Martin G, et al. (1996) Minocycline prevents the decrease in bone mineral density and trabecular bone in ovariectomized aged rats. Bone 19: 637–644.
18. Pytlik M, Folwarczna J, Janiec W (2004) Effects of doxycycline on mechanical properties of bones in rats with ovariectomy-induced osteopenia. Calcif Tissue Int 75: 225–230.
19. Bron PA, van Baarlen P, Kleerebezem M (2012) Emerging molecular insights into the interaction between probiotics and the host intestinal mucosa. Nat Rev Microbiol 10: 66–78.
20. Yan F, Polk DB (2011) Probiotics and immune health. Curr Opin Gastroenterol 27: 496–501.
21. Scholz-Ahrens KE, Ade P, Marten B, Weber P, Timm W, et al. (2007) Prebiotics, probiotics, and synbiotics affect mineral absorption, bone mineral content, and bone structure. J Nutr 137: 838S–846S.
22. Thompson DD, Simmons HA, Pirie CM, Ke HZ (1995) FDA Guidelines and animal models for osteoporosis. Bone 17: 125S–133S.
23. Lavasani S, Dzhambazov B, Nouri M, Fak F, Buske S, et al. (2010) A novel probiotic mixture exerts a therapeutic effect on experimental autoimmune encephalomyelitis mediated by IL-10 producing regulatory T cells. PLoS One 5: e9009.
24. Windahl SH, Vidal O, Andersson G, Gustafsson JA, Ohlsson C (1999) Increased cortical bone mineral content but unchanged trabecular bone mineral density in female ERbeta(−/−) mice. J Clin Invest 104: 895–901.
25. Kwon HK, Lee CG, So JS, Chae CS, Hwang JS, et al. (2010) Generation of regulatory dendritic cells and CD4+Foxp3+ T cells by probiotics administration suppresses immune disorders. Proc Natl Acad Sci U S A 107: 2159–2164.
26. Clowes JA, Riggs BL, Khosla S (2005) The role of the immune system in the pathophysiology of osteoporosis. Immunol Rev 208: 207–227.
27. Zebaze RM, Ghasem-Zadeh A, Bohte A, Iuliano-Burns S, Mirams M, et al. (2010) Intracortical remodelling and porosity in the distal radius and post-mortem femurs of women: a cross-sectional study. Lancet 375: 1729–1736.
28. Holzer G, von Skrbensky G, Holzer LA, Pichl W (2009) Hip fractures and the contribution of cortical versus trabecular bone to femoral neck strength. J Bone Miner Res 24: 468–474.
29. Zheng HF, Tobias JH, Duncan E, Evans DM, Eriksson J, et al. (2012) WNT16 influences bone mineral density, cortical bone thickness, bone strength, and osteoporotic fracture risk. PLoS Genet 8: e1002745.
30. Bansal N, Katz R, de Boer IH, Kestenbaum B, Siscovick DS, et al. (2013) Influence of Estrogen Therapy on Calcium, Phosphorus, and Other Regulatory Hormones in Postmenopausal Women: The MESA Study. J Clin Endocrinol Metab.
31. McKane WR, Khosla S, Burritt MF, Kao PC, Wilson DM, et al. (1995) Mechanism of renal calcium conservation with estrogen replacement therapy in women in early postmenopause – a clinical research center study. J Clin Endocrinol Metab 80: 3458–3464.
32. Hofbauer LC, Lacey DL, Dunstan CR, Spelsberg TC, Riggs BL, et al. (1999) Interleukin-1beta and tumor necrosis factor-alpha, but not interleukin-6, stimulate osteoprotegerin ligand gene expression in human osteoblastic cells. Bone 25: 255–259.
33. Ochi S, Shinohara M, Sato K, Gober HJ, Koga T, et al. (2007) Pathological role of osteoclast costimulation in arthritis-induced bone loss. Proc Natl Acad Sci U S A 104: 11394–11399.
34. Lam J, Takeshita S, Barker JE, Kanagawa O, Ross FP, et al. (2000) TNF-alpha induces osteoclastogenesis by direct stimulation of macrophages exposed to permissive levels of RANK ligand. J Clin Invest 106: 1481–1488.
35. Zwerina J, Redlich K, Polzer K, Joosten L, Kronke G, et al. (2007) TNF-induced structural joint damage is mediated by IL-1. Proc Natl Acad Sci U S A 104: 11742–11747.
36. Wei S, Kitaura H, Zhou P, Ross FP, Teitelbaum SL (2005) IL-1 mediates TNF-induced osteoclastogenesis. J Clin Invest 115: 282–290.
37. Simonet WS, Lacey DL, Dunstan CR, Kelley M, Chang MS, et al. (1997) Osteoprotegerin: a novel secreted protein involved in the regulation of bone density. Cell 89: 309–319.
38. Bouladoux N, Hall JA, Grainger JR, dos Santos LM, Kann MG, et al. (2012) Regulatory role of suppressive motifs from commensal DNA. Mucosal Immunol 5: 623–634.
39. Marie JC, Letterio JJ, Gavin M, Rudensky AY (2005) TGF-beta1 maintains suppressor function and Foxp3 expression in CD4+CD25+ regulatory T cells. J Exp Med 201: 1061–1067.
40. Kim YG, Lee CK, Nah SS, Mun SH, Yoo B, et al. (2007) Human CD4+CD25+ regulatory T cells inhibit the differentiation of osteoclasts from peripheral blood mononuclear cells. Biochem Biophys Res Commun 357: 1046–1052.
41. Zaiss MM, Axmann R, Zwerina J, Polzer K, Guckel E, et al. (2007) Treg cells suppress osteoclast formation: a new link between the immune system and bone. Arthritis Rheum 56: 4104–4112.
42. Luo CY, Wang L, Sun C, Li DJ (2011) Estrogen enhances the functions of CD4(+)CD25(+)Foxp3(+) regulatory T cells that suppress osteoclast differentiation and bone resorption in vitro. Cell Mol Immunol 8: 50–58.
43. Buchwald ZS, Kiesel JR, Yang C, DiPaolo R, Novack DV, et al. (2013) Osteoclast-induced Foxp3+ CD8 T-cells limit bone loss in mice. Bone 56: 163–173.

Permissions

All chapters in this book were first published in PLOS ONE, by The Public Library of Science; hereby published with permission under the Creative Commons Attribution License or equivalent. Every chapter published in this book has been scrutinized by our experts. Their significance has been extensively debated. The topics covered herein carry significant findings which will fuel the growth of the discipline. They may even be implemented as practical applications or may be referred to as a beginning point for another development.

The contributors of this book come from diverse backgrounds, making this book a truly international effort. This book will bring forth new frontiers with its revolutionizing research information and detailed analysis of the nascent developments around the world.

We would like to thank all the contributing authors for lending their expertise to make the book truly unique. They have played a crucial role in the development of this book. Without their invaluable contributions this book wouldn't have been possible. They have made vital efforts to compile up to date information on the varied aspects of this subject to make this book a valuable addition to the collection of many professionals and students.

This book was conceptualized with the vision of imparting up-to-date information and advanced data in this field. To ensure the same, a matchless editorial board was set up. Every individual on the board went through rigorous rounds of assessment to prove their worth. After which they invested a large part of their time researching and compiling the most relevant data for our readers.

The editorial board has been involved in producing this book since its inception. They have spent rigorous hours researching and exploring the diverse topics which have resulted in the successful publishing of this book. They have passed on their knowledge of decades through this book. To expedite this challenging task, the publisher supported the team at every step. A small team of assistant editors was also appointed to further simplify the editing procedure and attain best results for the readers.

Apart from the editorial board, the designing team has also invested a significant amount of their time in understanding the subject and creating the most relevant covers. They scrutinized every image to scout for the most suitable representation of the subject and create an appropriate cover for the book.

The publishing team has been an ardent support to the editorial, designing and production team. Their endless efforts to recruit the best for this project, has resulted in the accomplishment of this book. They are a veteran in the field of academics and their pool of knowledge is as vast as their experience in printing. Their expertise and guidance has proved useful at every step. Their uncompromising quality standards have made this book an exceptional effort. Their encouragement from time to time has been an inspiration for everyone.

The publisher and the editorial board hope that this book will prove to be a valuable piece of knowledge for researchers, students, practitioners and scholars across the globe.

List of Contributors

Fan Fan, Wen-Qiong Xue, Bao-Hua Wu, Ming-Guang He, Hai-Li Xie, Wei-Fu Ouyang, Sulan Tu and Yu-Ming Chen
Guangdong Provincial Key Laboratory of Food, Nutrition and Health, School of Public Health, Sun Yat-sen University, Guangzhou, People's Republic of China

Bao-Hua Wu
Guangzhou Orthopaedics Trauma Hospital, Guangzhou, People's Republic of China

Ming-Guang He
Zhongshan Ophthalmic Center, Sun Yat-sen University, Guangzhou, People's Republic of China

Wei-Fu Ouyang
Guangdong General Hospital, Guangzhou, Guangdong, People's Republic of China

Sulan Tu
Orthopaedics Hospital of Baishi District, Jiangmen, Guangdong, People's Republic of China

Wen-Qiong Xue
Sun Yat-sen University Cancer Center, Guangzhou, People's Republic of China

Pei Feng and Cijun Shuai
State Key Laboratory of High Performance Complex Manufacturing, Central South University, Changsha, Hunan Province, P. R. China

Cijun Shuai
Department of Regenerative Medicine and Cell Biology, Medical University of South Carolina, Charleston, South Carolina, United States of America

Pingpin Wei and Shuping Peng
Cancer Research Institute, Central South University, Changsha, Hunan Province, P. R. China

Shuping Peng
Department of Obstetrics, Gynecology and Reproductive Sciences, Yale University School of Medicine, New Haven, Connecticut, United States of America

Guoyong Yin, Prashanthi Menon, Jinjiang Pang, Elaine Smolock, Chen Yan and Bradford C. Berk
Aab Cardiovascular Research Institute and the Department of Medicine, University of Rochester Medical Center, Rochester, New York, United States of America

Tzong-Jen Sheu, Hsin-Chiu Ho, Shanshan Shi, Chao Xie and Michael J. Zuscik
Center for Musculoskeletal Research and the Department of Orthopaedics and Rehabilitation, University of Rochester Medical Center, Rochester, New York, United States of America

Guoyong Yin
Orthopaedic Department, The First Affiliated Hospital of Nanjing Medical University, Jiangsu, China

Helena Hallström, Karl Michaëlsson and Liisa Byberg
Department of Surgical Sciences, Section of Orthopaedics, Uppsala University, Uppsala, Sweden

Alicja Wolk
Institute of Environmental Medicine, Division of Nutritional Epidemiology, Karolinska Institutet, Stockholm, Sweden

Anders Glynn
Risk and Benefit Assessment Department, National Food Agency, Uppsala, Sweden

Hila Haskelberg, Janaki Amin and Sean Emery
The Kirby Institute, University of New South Wales, Sydney, Australia

Nicholas Pocock
St. Vincent's Hospital, Sydney, Australia, 3 North West Academic Centre, University of Melbourne, Melbourne, Australia

Gaurav Garg, Fiona E. McGuigan and Kristina Åkesson
Clinical and Molecular Osteoporosis Research Unit, Department of Clinical Sciences, Lund University and Department of Orthopaedics, Skåne University Hospital, Malmö, Sweden

Jitender Kumar
Department of Medical Sciences, Molecular Epidemiology and Science for Life Laboratory, Uppsala University, Uppsala, Sweden

Martin Ridderstråle
Clinical Obesity Research, Department of Endocrinology, Skåne University Hospital, Malmö, Sweden

Paul Gerdhem
Department of Clinical Science, Intervention and Technology, Karolinska Institutet,Department of Orthopaedics, Karolinska University Hospital, Stockholm, Sweden

Holger Luthman
Medical Genetics Unit, Department of Clinical Sciences, Lund University, Malmö,Sweden

Stephanie Rossnagl, Anja von Au, Matthaeus Vasel and Inaam A. Nakchbandi
Max-Planck Institute of Biochemistry, Martinsried, Germany
Institute of Immunology, University of Heidelberg, Heidelberg, Germany

arco G. Cecchini
Department of Urology,University of Bern, Bern, Switzerland

Yong-Jun Liu, Qing Tian, Hui Shen, Inderpal S. Thethi and Hong-Wen Deng
School of Public Health and Tropical Medicine, Tulane University, New Orleans, Louisiana, United States of America

Shu Ran, Yu-Fang Pei, Lei Zhang, Ying-Ying Han, Yong Lin and Hong-Wen Deng
Center of System Biomedical Sciences, School of Medical Instrument and Food Engineering, University of Shanghai for Science and Technology, Shanghai, P. R. China

Rong Hai
Inner Mongolia People's Hospital, Hohhot, P. R.China

Tie-Lin Yang
School of Life Science and Technology, Xi'an Jiaotong University, Xi'an, Shanxi, P. R. China

Yan-Fang Guo
School of Basic Medical Science, Institute of Bioinformatics, Southern Medical University, Guangzhou, Guangdong, P. R. China

Jen-Hau Chen and Keh-Sung Tsai
Department of Geriatrics and Gerontology, National Taiwan University Hospital, No. 1, Taipei, Taiwan

Jen-Hau Chen and Keh-Sung Tsai
Department of Internal Medicine, National Taiwan University Hospital, No. 7, Taipei, Taiwan

Jen-Hau Chen, Yen-Ching Chen and Chien-Lin Mao
Institute of Epidemiology and Preventive Medicine, College of Public Health, National Taiwan University, Taipei, Taiwan

Jeng-Min Chiou
Institute of Statistical Science, Academia Sinica, Nankang, Taipei, Taiwan

Chwen Keng Tsao
MJ Health Management Institution, 12F., No. 413, Section 4, Taipei, Taiwan

Keh-Sung Tsai
Department of Laboratory Medicine, National Taiwan University Hospital, No. 7, Taipei, Taiwan

Hélène Coqueugniot, Olivier Dutour, Henri Duday,Bernard Vandermeersch and Anne-marie Tillier
Unitè Mixte de Recherche 5199 – De la Préhistoire àl'Actuel: Culture, Environnement et Anthropologie (PACEA), Centre National de la Recherche Scientifique (CNRS) – Université de Bordeaux, Pessac, France

Hélène Coqueugniot
Department of Human Evolution, Max Planck Institute for Evolutionary Anthropology, Leipzig, Germany

Olivier Dutour and Henri Duday
Laboratoire d'Anthropologie biologique Paul Broca, Ecole Pratique des Hautes Etudes (EPHE), Paris, France

Olivier Dutour
Department of Anthropology, University of Western Ontario, London,Ontario, Canada

Baruch Arensburg
Department of Anatomy and Anthropology, Sackler School of Medicine, Tel Aviv University, Ramat Aviv, Israel

Anne-marie Tillier
Museum of Archaeology and Anthropology, University of Pennsylvania, Philadelphia, Pennsylvania, United States of America

Rodrigo Guzmán,Ander Abarrategi and José Luis López-Lacomba
Instituto de Estudios Biofuncionales, Universidad Complutense de Madrid, Madrid, Spain

Stefania Nardecchia, María C. Gutiérrez, María Luisa Ferrer and Francisco del Monte
Instituto de Ciencia de Materiales de Madrid-ICMM, Consejo Superior de Investigaciones Científicas-CSIC, Campus de Cantoblanco, Madrid, Spain

Viviana Ramos
Noricum Inc, Departamento de I+D, Parque Científico de Madrid, Tres Cantos, Madrid, Spain

Chunlan Huang, Ming Xue, Hongli Chen, Regis J. O'Keefe and Xinping Zhang
Center for Musculoskeletal Research, University of Rochester, School of Medicine and Dentistry, Rochester, New York, United States of America

Jing Jiao and Harvey R. Herschman
Department of Molecular and Medical Pharmacology, David Geffen School of Medicine, University of California Los Angeles, Los Angeles, California, United States of America

Laufey Steingrimsdottir and Thorhallur I. Halldorsson
Unit for Nutrition Research, University of Iceland and Landspitali University Hospital, Reykjavik, Iceland

Kristin Siggeirsdottir, Berglind O. Einarsdottir, Gudny Eiriksdottir, Sigurdur Sigurdsson and Vilmundur Gudnason and Gunnar Sigurdsson
Icelandic Heart Association Research Institute, Kopavogur,Iceland

Lenore J. Launer and Tamara B. Harris
Intramural Research Program, Laboratory of Epidemiology, Demography and Biometry, National Institute of Aging, Bethesda, Maryland, United States of America

Mary Frances Cotch
Division of Epidemiology and Clinical Applications, National Eye Institute, Bethesda, Maryland, United States of America

Vilmundur Gudnason and Gunnar Sigurdsson
University of Iceland, Reykjavik,Iceland

Malte Steiner, Lutz Claes, Anita Ignatius, Ulrich Simon and Tim Wehner
Institute of Orthopaedic Research and Biomechanics, Center of Musculoskeletal Research Ulm, University Hospital Ulm, Ulm, Germany

Ulrich Simon
Scientific Computing Centre Ulm, University of Ulm, Ulm, Germany

Vedavathi Madhu, Ching-Ju Li, Abhijit S. Dighe, Gary Balian and Quanjun Cui
Orthopaedic Research Laboratories, Department of Orthopaedic Surgery, University of Virginia, Charlottesville, Virginia, United States of America

Zijie Wang, Zhijian Han, Jun Tao, Pei Lu, Xuzhong Liu, Jun Wang, Bian Wu, Zhengkai Huang, Changjun Yin, Ruoyun Tan and Min Gu
Department of urology, the first affiliated hospital of Nanjing Medical University, Nanjing, China

Takanobu Nishizuka, Toshikazu Kurahashi, Tatsuya Hara and Hitoshi Hirata
Department of Hand Surgery, Nagoya University Graduate School of Medicine, Nagoya, Japan

Toshihiro Kasuga
Department of Frontier Materials, Nagoya Institute of Technology,Nagoya, Japan

Andrea Ode, Georg N. Duda, Sven Geissler, Stephan Pauly, Jan-Erik Ode, Carsten Perka and Patrick Strube
Julius Wolff Institute, Charité - Universitätsmedizin, Berlin, Germany

Andrea Ode, Georg N. Duda, Sven Geissler and Carsten Perka
Berlin-Brandenburg Center for Regenerative Therapies, Berlin, Germany

Georg N. Duda, Stephan Pauly, Carsten Perka and Patrick Strube
Klinik für Orthopädie,Centrum für Muskuloskeletale Chirurgie, Charité – Universitäts medizin, Berlin, Germany

Peiran Zhou, Yi Liu, Fang Lv, Min Nie, Yan Jiang, Ou Wang, Weibo Xia and Xiaoping Xing, Mei Li
Department of Endocrinology, Key Laboratory of Endocrinology of Ministry of Health, Peking Union Medical College Hospital, Peking Union Medical College, Chinese Academy of Medical Sciences, Beijing, China

Astrid Liedert and Viktoria Röntgen and Anita Ignatius
Institute of Orthopaedic Research and Biomechanics, Center of Musculoskeletal Research, University of Ulm, Ulm, Germany

Thorsten Schinke and Michael Amling
Department of Osteology and Biomechanics, University Medical Center Hamburg-Eppendorf, Hamburg, Germany

Peggy Benisch, Regina Ebert and Franz Jakob
Orthopaedic Center for Musculoskeletal Research, University of Würzburg, Würzburg, Germany

Ludger Klein-Hitpass
Institute of Cell Biology, University of Duisburg-Essen, Duisburg, Germany

Jochen K. Lennerz
Institute of Pathology, University of Ulm, Ulm, Germany

Kathleen M. Hill Gallant, Maxime A. Gallant, Drew M. Brown, Amy Y. Sato, Justin N. Williams and David B. Burr
Department of Anatomy and Cell Biology, Indiana University School of Medicine, Indianapolis, Indiana, United States of America

Kathleen M. Hill Gallant
Department of Nutrition Science,Purdue University, West Lafayette, Indiana, United States of America

Fang-Yuan Wei, Kwok-Sui Leung, Gang Li, Jianghui Qin, Simon Kwoon-Ho Chow, Shuo Huang,Ming-Hui Sun, Ling Qin and Wing-Hoi Cheung
Department of Orthopaedics and Traumatology, Clinical Sciences Building, The Chinese University of Hong Kong, Shatin, New Territories, Hong Kong SAR, China

Kwok-Sui Leung, Ling Qin and Wing-Hoi Cheung
Translational Medicine Research and Development Center, Institute of Biomedical and Health Engineering, Shenzhen Institutes of Advanced Technology, Chinese Academy of Sciences, Shenzhen, China

Alison M. Greig
Department of Physical Therapy, University of British Columbia, Vancouver, Canada

Andrew M. Briggs
School of Physiotherapy and Exercise Science, Curtin University, Perth, Australia
Arthritis and Osteoporosis Victoria, Melbourne, Australia

Kim L. Bennell
Centre for Health, Exercise and Sports Medicine, The University of Melbourne, Melbourne, Australia

Paul W. Hodges
The University of Queensland, Centre for Clinical Research Excellence in Spinal Pain, Injury and Health, School of Health and Rehabilitation Sciences, Brisbane, Australia

Masahiro Ishikawa, Hiromu Ito, Toshiyuki Kitaori, Koichi Murata, Hideyuki Shibuya, Moritoshi Furu, Takayuki Fujii and Shuichi Matsuda
Department of Orthopaedic Surgery, Kyoto University Graduate School of Medicine, Kyoto, Japan

Masahiro Ishikawa and Moritoshi Furu
Department of the Control for Rheumatic Disease, Kyoto University Graduate School of Medicine, Kyoto, Japan

Hiroyuki Yoshitomi
The Center for Innovation in Immunoregulative Technology and Therapeutics, Kyoto University Graduate School of Medicine, Kyoto, Japan

Koji Yamamoto
Center for the Promotion of Interdisciplinary Education and Research, Kyoto University, Kyoto, Japan

Brian S. Bradke and Deepak Vashishth
Department of Biomedical Engineering, Rensselaer Polytechnic Institute, Troy, New York, United States of America

Yoshiaki Kitaura, Hironori Hojo, Yuske Komiyama and Tsuyoshi Takato
Department of Sensory and Motor System Medicine, The University of Tokyo Graduate School of Medicine, Bunkyo-ku, Tokyo, Japan

Yoshiaki Kitaura, Hironori Hojo, Yuske Komiyama, Ung-il Chung and Shinsuke Ohba
Division of Clinical Biotechnology,The University of Tokyo Graduate School of Medicine, Bunkyo-ku, Tokyo, Japan

Ung-il Chung and Shinsuke Ohba
Department of Bioengineering, The University of Tokyo Graduate School of Engineering, Bunkyo-ku, Tokyo, Japan

Sarah H. McBride, Jennifer A. McKenzie, Paige Kuhlmann and Matthew J. Silva
Department of Orthopaedic Surgery, Musculoskeletal Research Center, Washington University in St. Louis, St. Louis, Missouri, United States of America

Bronwyn S. Bedrick and Jill D. Pasteris
Department of Earth and Planetary Sciences, Washington University in St. Louis, St. Louis, Missouri, United States of America

Vicki Rosen
Department of Developmental Biology, Harvard School of Dental Medicine, Boston, Massachusetts, United States of America

Claes Ohlsson, Cecilia Engdahl, Annica Andersson, Sara H. Windahl, Helen H. Farman, Sofia Movérare-Skrtic, Ulrika Islander and Klara Sjögren
Centre for Bone and Arthritis Research, Institute of Medicine, Sahlgrenska Academy at University of Gothenburg, Gothenburg, Sweden

Cecilia Engdahl, Annica Andersson and Ulrika Islander
Department of Rheumatology and Inflammation Research, Institute of Medicine, Sahlgrenska Academy at University of Gothenburg, Gothenburg, Sweden

Frida Fåk
Applied Nutrition and Food Chemistry,Department of Food Technology, Engineering and Nutrition, Lund University, Lund, Sweden

Index

www.ingramcontent.com/pod-product-compliance
Lightning Source LLC
Chambersburg PA
CBHW080500200326
41458CB00012B/4040